4 31

METHODS IN CHEMICAL NEUROANATOMY

HANDBOOK OF CHEMICAL NEUROANATOMY

Edited by A. Björklund and T. Hökfelt

Volume 1:

METHODS IN CHEMICAL NEUROANATOMY

Editors:

A. BJÖRKLUND
Department of Histology
University of Lund, Lund, Sweden

T. HÖKFELT
Department of Histology
Karolinska Institute, Stockholm, Sweden

1983

ELSEVIER

Amsterdam – New York – Oxford

ISBN 0 444 90281 3
ISBN SERIES 0 444 90340 2

Published by:
Elsevier Science Publishers B.V.
P.O. Box 1126
1000 BC Amsterdam
The Netherlands

Sole Distributors for the USA and Canada:
Elsevier Science Publishing Co. Inc.
52 Vanderbilt Avenue
New York, NY 10017

Printed in The Netherlands by Casparie – Amsterdam

To the memory of Paula

List of contributors

A. BEAUDET
Montreal Neurological Institute and
    Department of Anatomy
McGill University
3801 University Street
Montréal, Québec H3A 2B4
Canada

A. BJÖRKLUND
Department of Histology
University of Lund
Biskopsgatan 5
S-223 62 Lund
Sweden

L.L. BUTCHER
Department of Psychology and
    Brain Research Institute
University of California
405 Hilgard Avenue
Los Angeles, CA 90024
U.S.A.

J.T. COYLE
Division of Child Psychiatry and
Departments of Psychiatry,
    Neuroscience and Pharmacology
The Johns Hopkins University School of
    Medicine
Baltimore, MD 21205
U.S.A.

R. COUTURE
Department of Pharmacology (Human
    Anatomy)
University of Oxford
South Parks Road
Oxford OX1 3QX
U.K.

A.C. CUELLO
Department of Pharmacology
University of Oxford
South Parks Road
Oxford OX1 3QT
U.K.

M. CUÉNOD
Brain Research Institute
University of Zürich
August Forel-Strasse 1
8029 Zürich
Switzerland

L. DESCARRIES
Centre de Recherche en Sciences
    Neurologiques (Département de
    Physiologie)
Faculté de Médecine
Université de Montréal
Montréal, Québec
Canada H3C 3T8

T. HÖKFELT
Department of Histology
Karolinska Institutet
P.O. Box 60400
S-104 01 Stockholm
Sweden

G. JONSSON
Department of Histology
Karolinska Institutet
P.O. Box 60400
S-104 01 Stockholm
Sweden

C. KENNEDY
Laboratory of Cerebral Metabolism
National Institute of Mental Health
U.S. Public Health Service
Department of Health, Education and
    Welfare
Bethesda, MD 20205
U.S.A.

List of contributors

M.J. KUHAR
Departments of Neuroscience,
  Pharmacology and Experimental
  Therapeutics and Psychiatry and the
  Behavioral Sciences
The Johns Hopkins University School of
  Medicine
Baltimore, MD 21205
U.S.A.

L.-I. LARSSON
Unit of Histochemistry
University Institut of Pathology
Frederik den V's vej 11
DK-2100 Copenhagen Ø
Denmark

G. RICHARDS
Pharmaceutical Research Department
F. Hoffman-La Roche and Co.
Grenzacherstrasse 124
4000 Basel
Switzerland

M. SAR
Department of Anatomy
School of Medicine
University of North Carolina
Chapel Hill, NC 27514
U.S.A.

R. SCHWARCZ
Maryland Psychiatric Research Center
University of Maryland
P.O. Box 3235
Baltimore, MD 21228
U.S.A.

G. SKAGERBERG
Department of Histology
University of Lund
Biskopsgatan 5
S-223 62 Lund
Sweden

L. SKIRBOLL
Clinical Neuroscience Branch and
  Endocrine Unit
National Institut of Mental Health
Building 10, Room 3N-256
Bethesda, MD 20205
U.S.A.

C.B. SMITH
Laboratory of Cerebral Metabolism
National Institute of Mental Health
U.S. Public Health Service
Department of Health, Education and
  Welfare
Bethesda, MD 20205
U.S.A.

M.V. SOFRONIEW
Department of Human Anatomy
University of Oxford
South Parks Road
Oxford OX1 3QX
U.K.

L. SOKOLOFF
Laboratory of Cerebral Metabolism
National Institute of Mental Health
U.S. Public Health, Service
Department of Health, Education and
  Welfare
Bethesda, MD 20205
U.S.A.

P. STREIT
Brain Research Institute
University of Zürich
August Forel-Strasse 1
8029 Zürich
Switzerland

W.E. STUMPF
Department of Anatomy
  School of Medicine
University of North Carolina
Chapel Hill, NC 27514
U.S.A.

Foreword

The appearance of this volume in what promises to be a continuing archive of Neurohistochemistry is like a milestone, for it marks the coming-of-age of a young form of Neuroscience that can be viewed as the chemical counterpart of traditional Neuroanatomy.

As one who first glimpsed the scene during the last few years before World War II, and has subsequently witnessed four decades of the development of Brain Sciences — most of it, of course, only as an interested bystander — I hope I may be permitted to indulge in some reminiscence. I remember that in the late nineteen-forties it was possible for an investigator to be familiar with the names, if not indeed with the main publications, of virtually all of the neuroanatomists publishing in internationally read journals. Activity in Neuroanatomy was at a low ebb, and I believe that it would have remained there much longer than it did if it had not been for the rapid progress in the neighboring fields of Neurophysiology and Neuroendocrinology. For quite a number of years, unexpected anatomical questions had been arising from studies with the then recent methods employing strychnine-neuronography, electroencephalography, and the recording of potentials evoked by focal electrical stimulation. Moreover, the development of the microelectrode-recording technique, which made it possible to register the activity of single neurons, raised numerous questions demanding an even sharper anatomical focus. It was becoming increasingly obvious with each passing year that Neuroanatomy — contrary to what I had been led to believe as a student by some of my mentors — was not '..a field already harvested to death...', that renewed exploration was necessary, and that part of that exploration would call for new and more adequate research techniques.

Under the circumstances it was no coincidence that the years around 1950 marked the opening of a new chapter in neuroanatomical research. This period saw the beginning of a vigorously renewed application of the Golgi method as a tool for circuit tracing. In the same period the Marchi method, for 60 years the only technique permitting direct tracing of fiber systems undergoing Wallerian degeneration, was gradually replaced by silver-impregnation methods less dependent on the degree of fiber myelination. And, last but not least, during that period the forbidding technical problems encountered in earlier electron-microscopic studies of brain tissue were surmounted stepwise, with the result that a whole new discipline of ultrastructural Neurohistology came into being which, incidentally, would later add crucially important new refinements to the strategies for experimental circuit tracing.

While all these new developments were taking place in the realm of what could be called 'dry' Neuromorphology, histochemical technology was making its debut in brain research, in the form of a neurohistological method for acetylcholinesterase and another one that selectively stained the axons of the supraoptic and paraventricular nuclei innervating the neurohypophysis. The latter, Gomori's chromalum-hematoxylin-phloxin method, naturally raised hopes for a whole arsenal of organic dyestuffs, each having a selective affinity for one or the other functionally defined neuron system. These hopes never materialized. And this brings to mind the fact, so obvious that it is often overlooked, that all histological staining methods are dependent on some degree of chemical specificity of the tissue element to be demonstrated. With certain notable exceptions (for example, stains for fatty substances, glycogen, heavy metals and certain enzymes such as esterases and phosphatases), such specificities vis-à-vis particular staining methods could, until very recently, be discovered only pragmatically. I vividly remember a comment from David McKenzie Rioch, founder of the Neuropsychiatry Division at the Walter Reed Army Institute of Research, and my chief at the time, when I showed him some diagrams of subcortical amygdaloid and hippocampal circuitry: '...there must be further detail hidden in those fiber systems, and I would not be amazed if much of it will require chemical rather than degeneration methods to be demonstrated.' The year must have been 1957, and I do not think anyone at that time could have predicted the nature of the chemical techniques Rioch expected to become necessary. That immunological methods would ever become crucial tools in the study of the brain's chemical anatomy could not even be foreseen five years later when the monoamine-histofluorescence methods were introduced.

And now the present. The last ten years could be viewed as the first ten of yet another new era in Neuroanatomy, but it is becoming more difficult to delineate eras when so many new techniques and research strategies are developed in such rapid succession. It is however certain that histochemical techniques have now become available that make it possible to demonstrate and localize any intra- or extracellular compound against which a specific antibody can be raised. The experimental circuit-tracing methods based upon lesion-induced degeneration, both anterograde and retrograde, during the past ten years have been all but superseded by new and far more sensitive methods utilizing the normal biological phenomenon of intra-axonal transport. The Golgi method and electron-microscopy have remained as useful as ever, and together with the axonal- transport methods they continue to form the technological backbone of 'dry' Neuroanatomy. However, this traditional discipline no longer proceeds alone; alongside it now strides the younger form of Chemical Neuroanatomy. There is every reason to expect that the two will be congenital fellow-explorers with an almost infinite potential for complementing and educating each other, each from its own specific background. Together, as true explorers, they march into a future that is known to no one.

WALLE J.H. NAUTA

Preface

The techniques for chemical coding of neurons have fundamentally changed our way of looking at the nervous system. Over the last two decades, a new image regarding the organization of the nervous system has gradually emerged, making it possible to analyze neuronal circuitries in a new dimension and in functionally relevant terms. As Walle Nauta has phrased it: 'classical neuroanatomy provided us with the blue-print of the nervous system, while chemical anatomy has added the red-print to the construction plan'. This 'new' neuroanatomy has also brought about a dynamic interplay between the structural analysis of the nervous system and modern developments in cellular neurophysiology, neurochemistry and neuropharmacology.

The roots of chemical neuroanatomy as we know it today can be traced back to the early studies on neurosecretion. During the first part of this century a group of researchers, most prominently Speidel (1), Ernst and Berta Scharrer (2,3) and Hanström (4), identified certain elements in the nervous system of vertebrates and invertebrates as being peculiar because of their 'secretory' features. This led to the important discovery by Bargmann in 1949 (5) that some specific neurons in the mammalian hypothalamus could be selectively stained with Gomori's chromalum-hematoxylin which is otherwise used for demonstrating 'secretory material' in endocrine cells. The most important feature of this stain was that it became possible to selectively visualize compounds – the neurophysins – which are intimately associated with the secretory process of these neurons. Thus, although the Gomori-positivity rested on an essentially nonspecific mechanism, it provided a very useful chemical 'tagging' of a functionally defined group of neurons. The subsequent history of neurosecretion also demonstrates how the 'neurosecretory stains' presented essentially new possibilities for studies on neuronal function at the cellular level.

Another important step in the cytochemical analysis of neurotransmission is represented by Koelle and Friedenwald's thiocholine method for acetylcholinesterase (AChE), introduced in 1949 (6). Although it is now known that this enzyme is not a specific marker for cholinergic neurons, it is abundantly present in association with the cell bodies, axons and terminals of such neurons. The Koelle method soon revealed that known cholinergic neurons and synapses in the peripheral nervous system stain heavily for AChE (7–10). Shute and Lewis (11–14) were the first to make a systematic mapping of the AChE-positive neurons in the CNS. The AChE method can therefore be stated as being the first neuroanatomical technique for the visualization of a transmitter-related neuronal marker. Butcher's chapter on the AChE methodology is hence a very natural introduction to this volume on Methods in Chemical Neuroanatomy.

The next decisive step in the development of chemical neuroanatomy was the introduction of the formaldehyde method for the visualization of biogenic monoamines. As early as 1932, Erös (15) and Hamperl (16) had described fluorescence in enterochromaffin cells, carcinoid cells and mast cells in formalin-fixed tissue. During the fifties, Eränkö (17,18) and Barter and Pearse (19,20) investigated this phenomenon further and provided evidence that the formaldehyde-induced fluorescence in both the adrenal chromaffin and intestinal enterochromaffin cells was due to the presence of catecholamines and indolamines in high concentrations. Later, Eränkö and Räisänen improved this method to be able to demonstrate also noradrenaline in sympathetic nerves (21);

however, in its original form Eränkö's 'wet' formalin method was not sensitive enough for visualizing neuronal monoamines. The breakthrough in aldehyde fluorescence histochemistry came in the early sixties when Falck, Hillarp and co-workers developed a method which was sufficiently sensitive to visualize intraneuronal stores of monoamines in both peripheral and central nervous tissue (22–25). The key feature of this method is to perform the formaldehyde reaction under essentially dry conditions. This was achieved by using either dried whole-mounts of thin tissue sheets (iris or mesentery) or freeze-dried tissue pieces, which were caused to react by exposure to formaldehyde vapors generated from paraformaldehyde powder at elevated temperatures (+80°C). Furthermore, extensive work by Hillarp in collaboration with Corrodi and Jonsson clarified the chemical reactions underlying the method and provided a sound basis for evaluating the specificity and sensitivity of the technique (see Chapter II).

The Falck-Hillarp method triggered a virtually explosive development in the study of monoamine-containing neuron systems, which, in turn, has given much of the momentum for the rapid developments that have subsequently taken place in the study of transmitter-identified systems at large. The Falck-Hillarp technique was the first histochemical method which allowed the direct visualization of the neurotransmitter itself. This made possible the tracing and mapping of both the central monoamine neurons, as demonstrated in the pioneering work of Fuxe and Dahlström (26–28), and on peripheral noradrenaline neurons (29,30). In addition, this technique also gave information on the intracellular distribution of the transmitter levels under normal and experimental conditions as exemplified in several of the above mentioned studies.

In parallel with the introduction of the formaldehyde-induced fluorescence technique, successful attempts were also made in many laboratories to identify peripheral noradrenaline neurons under the electron-microscope. Using conventional fixation techniques it could be shown that noradrenaline nerve endings are characterized by their content of synaptic vesicles with an electron-dense core (31–33), making possible the mapping of transmitter-characterized neuron populations also at the ultrastructural level (see Chapter III).

Subsequently, a whole range of methods – based on other principles – for identifying transmitter-specific neuron systems were developed and introduced. Of these, the autoradiographic and immunohistochemical methodologies have probably had the most significant impact. Marks et al. (34) and Wolfe et al. (35) in 1962 were the first to use autoradiography for transmitter visualization, based on specific neuronal uptake of exogenously administered [³H]noradrenaline. Thereafter, this approach was employed by Aghajanian and Bloom (36,37) for the study of central noradrenergic and serotoninergic neurons at the ultrastructural level after intraventricular administration of [³H]noradrenaline or [³H]serotonin. In the early seventies, several groups described amino acid-accumulating neurons at the light- and electron-microscopic levels with this technique (38–40). More recently Storm-Mathiesen and Iversen (41) have visualized glutamate- or aspartate-accumulating neurons.

Although these autoradiographic techniques all rest on an indirect principle, i.e. the ability of the neurons to accumulate exogenously labeled transmitters, they have been of great importance in the characterization of neurons and their synapses at the ultrastructural level (see Chapter VII). A more recent development in this approach – selective retrograde labeling of neurons after application of tritiated amines or amino acids in terminal regions – is presented in Chapter VIII. Autoradiography has also provided a fresh insight into the interplay between the brain and the endocrine system. As outlined in Chapter XI, autoradiography has revealed that specific neuron populations have the ability of accumulating steroids of different types, giving a neuroanatomical cue to the site of action of these hormones in the brain. Another new field – based on autoradiography – in which specific transmitter receptors can be visualized with radiolabeled ligands has recently opened up. The basic methodology for this novel type of mapping is presented in Chapter IX.

The immunohistochemistry of transmitter-related compounds was introduced by Geffen, Livett and Rush in 1969 (42). In their pioneer study they purified dopamine-ß-hydroxylase (the noradrenaline synthesizing enzyme), and the adrenergic vesicle protein chromogranine, raised antibodies against these two compounds and then localized them in tissue sections with Coon's indirect immunofluorescence technique (43). Several other groups used the same approach for mapping monoamine neurons, and during the last decade we have seen extensive developments in the immunohistochemical field. In part, this has been due to significant improvements of the techniques, such as the introduction of horseradish peroxidase (HRP) as antibody marker, which have allowed both light- and electron-microscopic analysis, as well as the development by Sternberger et al. (46) of the highly sensitive unlabelled enzyme method (peroxidase-antiperoxidase, or PAP method). This methodology has been described in Chapters IV and V.

Another methodology of great importance to anatomical studies of transmitter-specific neuronal systems has been the use of certain compounds for producing chemical lesions of varying types of specificity. This field was opened up by the pioneer work of Thoenen and Tranzer who demonstrated that the dopamine analogue, 6-hydroxydopamine, can induce degeneration of peripheral sympathetic, noradrenergic neurons, while leaving the cholinergic system intact (47). The current status of the methodology in this field has been presented in Chapters XII and XIII.

Axonal tracing in the modern sense dates back to the Nauta-Gygax method in 1951 (48) and its subsequent modifications (49). The major advance in neuroanatomical tracing since then has been the introduction of methods based on axonal transport for anterograde and retrograde tracing of neuronal connections. The methods are founded on two general principles: (a) anterograde transport of radiolabeled amino acids incorporated into proteins at the cell body level combined with autoradiographic detection (50,51), and (b) retrograde transport of the enzyme HRP, visualized with a suitable substrate (52). These methodologies are now available to the neuroanatomist in a multitude of modifications and variations. The present volume does not deal with this particular aspect (for refs. see, e.g. Cowan and Cuenod (53), Heimer and RoBards (54) and Mesulam (55)), but it is now clear that several types of transmitter histochemistry can be suitably combined with retrograde tracing techniques. Some of these aspects are dealt with in Chapter VI.

Finally, and as a conclusion to this historical survey, a completely different type of neurochemical anatomy is represented by the 'metabolic mapping' technique introduced in the mid-seventies by Sokoloff and collaborators (55). Using radiolabeled 2-deoxy-D-glucose – a competitive, non-metabolized substrate to glucose – maps of cerebral activity can be obtained with autoradiographic detection. The basis and application of this technique are described in Chapter X.

The use of histochemical, autoradiographic and immunohistochemical methods for the analysis of neuronal circuitries has meant no less than a revolution in neuro-anatomy. The introduction of methods for the microscopic visualization of neurotransmitters, neuropeptides and associated enzymes has provided a new neuroanatomical nomenclature. The new tools for the study of chemically identified systems have added new dimensions to the analysis of neuronal connections and in contrast to the classical neuroanatomical techniques, they have offered possibilities for selective neuroanatomical tracing of chemically defined neurons. The rapid development of this field has on the other hand resulted in a virtual explosion of new information. The assembled knowledge of the cholinergic, monoaminergic, amino acid-producing and peptidergic systems has, as a result, become highly complex and difficult to survey. A major objective behind the present book series, the *Handbook of Chemical Neuroanatomy*, is to assemble present-day knowledge on the organization of the chemically identified systems and provide an authoritative and comprehensive reference source for a broad spectrum of neuroscientists.

This first volume of the series seeks to cover the various methods that form the groundwork for current chemical neuroanatomy. At the same time the contents of this 'Methods' volume provide a broad delineation of the field that we intend to cover under the label Chemical Neuroanatomy, thus defining the scope of the future volumes. The chemical analysis of neuronal circuitries is likely to become increasingly more refined. During the last few years we have witnessed how transmitter localization has been supplemented with techniques for the localization of transmitter and hormonal binding sites at the cellular level, and regional metabolic mapping has opened new possibilities for the functional analysis of neuronal circuitries under resting conditions and after experimental or pharmacological intervention. Future progress and developments along such lines are also intended to be covered by the Handbook. It is our hope that the Handbook of Chemical Neuroanatomy will reflect at least some of the dynamics of this exciting field of neuroscience.

Lund and Stockholm in January 1983

ANDERS BJÖRKLUND   TOMAS HÖKFELT

References

1. Speidel CG (1919): Gland-cells of internal secretion in the spinal cord of the skates. *Carnegie Inst. Washington Publ.*, 131–31.
2. Scharrer B (1928): Die Lichtempfindlichkeit blinder Elritzen (Untersuchungen über das Zwischenhirn der Fische). *Z. Vgl. Physiol.*, 7, 1–38.
3. Scharrer E (1937): Über sekretorisch tätige Nervenzellen bei wirbellosen Tieren. *Naturwissenschaften*, 25, 131–138.
4. Hanström B (1937): Die Sinusdrüse und der hormonal bedingte Farbwechsel der Crustaceen. *K. Sven. Vetenskaps akad. Handl.*, 16, 1–99.
5. Bargmann W (1949): Über die neurosekretorische Verknüpfung von Hypothalamus und Neurohypophyse. *Z. Zellforsch. Mikrosk. Anat.*, 34, 610–634.
6. Koelle GB, Friedenwald JS (1949): A histochemical method for localizing cholinesterase activity. *Proc. Soc. Exp. Biol. Med.*, 70, 617–622.
7. Koelle GB (1950): The histochemical differentiation of types of cholinesterases and their localizations in tissues of the cat. *J. Pharmacol. Exp. Ther.*, 100, 158–179.
8. Koelle GB (1954): The histochemical localization of cholinesterases in the nervous system of the rat. *J. Comp. Neurol.*, 100, 211–235.
9. Koelle GB (1963): Cytological distributions and physiological functions of cholinesterases. *Handb. Exp. Pharmak.*, 15, 187–298.
10. Couteaux R (1958): Morphological and cytochemical observations on the postsynaptic membrane at motor endplates and ganglionic synapses. *Exp. Cell. Res. Suppl.*, 5, 294–322.

11. Shute CCD, Lewis PR (1963): Cholinesterase-containing system of the brain of the rat. *Nature (London) 199*, 1160–1164.

12. Shute CCD, Lewis PR (1965): Cholinesterase-containing pathways of the hindbrain: Afferent cerebellar and centrifugal cochlear fibres. *Nature (London) 205*, 242–246.

13. Shute CCD, Lewis PR (1967): The ascending cholinergic reticular system: Neocortical, olfactory and subcortical projections. *Brain, 90*, 497–520.

14. Lewis PR, Shute CCD (1967): The cholinergic limbic system projection to hippocampal formation, medial cortex, nuclei of the ascending cholinergic reticular system, and the subfornical organ and supraoptic crest. *Brain, 90*, 521–540.

15. Erös G (1932): Eine neue Darstellungsmethode der sogenannten 'gelben' argentaffinen Zellen des Magendarmtraktes. *Zentralbl. Allg. Pathol. Pathol. Anat., 54*, 385–391.

16. Hamperl H (1932): Was sind argentaffine Zellen? *Virchows Arch. A, 286*, 811–833.

17. Eränkö O (1952): On the histochemistry of the adrenal medulla of the rat, with special reference to acid phosphatase. *Acta Anat., 16, Suppl. 17*, 1–60.

18. Eränkö O (1955): Histochemistry of noradrenaline in the adrenal medulla of rats and mice. *Endocrinology, 57*, 363–368.

19. Barter R, Pearse AGE (1955): Detection of 5-hydroxytryptamine in mammalian enterochromaffin cells. *Nature (London) 172*, 810.

20. Barter R, Pearse AGE (1955): Mammalian enterochromaffin cells as the source of serotonin (5-hydroxytryptamine). *J. Pathol. Bacteriol., 69*, 25–31.

21. Eränkö O, Räisänen L (1966): Demonstration of catecholamines in adrenergic nerve fibers by fixation in aqueous formaldehyde solution and fluorescence microscope. *J. Histochem. Cytochem., 14*, 690–691.

22. Falck B, Torp A (1962): New evidence for the localization of noradrenaline in the adrenergic nerve terminals. *Med. Exp., 6*, 169–172.

23. Falck B (1962): Observations on the possibilities of the cellular localization of monoamines by a fluorescence method. *Acta Physiol. Scand., 56, Suppl. 197*, 1–25.

24. Falck B, Hillarp N-Å, Thieme G, Torp A (1962): Fluorescence of catecholamines and related compounds condensed with formaldehyde. *J. Histochem. Cytochem., 10*, 348–354.

25. Carlsson A, Falck B, Hillarp N-Å (1962): Cellular localization of brain monoamines. *Acta Physiol. Scand., 56, Suppl. 196*, 1–27.

26. Dahlström A, Fuxe K (1964): Evidence for the existence of monoamine neurons in the central nervous system. I. Demonstration of monoamines in the cell bodies of brain stem neurons. *Acta Physiol. Scand., 62, Suppl. 232*, 1–55.

27. Dahlström A, Fuxe K (1965): Evidence for the existence of monoamine neurons in the central nervous system. II. Experimentally induced changes in the intraneuronal amine levels of bulbospinal neuron systems. *Acta Physiol. Scand., 64, Suppl. 247*, 5–36.

28. Fuxe K (1965): Evidence for the existence of monoamine neurons in the central nervous system. IV. The distribution of monoamine nerve terminals in the central nervous system. *Acta Physiol. Scand., 64, Suppl. 247*, 39–85.

29. Norberg K-A, Hamberger B (1964): The sympathetic adrenergic neuron. Some characteristics revealed by histochemical studies on the intraneuronal distribution of the transmitter. *Acta Physiol. Scand., 63, Suppl. 238*, 1–48.

30. Malmfors T (1965): Studies on adrenergic nerves. The use of rat and mouse iris for direct observations on their physiology and pharmacology at cellular and subcellular levels. *Acta Physiol. Scand., 64, Suppl. 248*, 1–93.

31. De Robertis E, Pellegrino de Iraldi A (1961): Plurivesicular secretory processes and nerve endings in the pineal gland. *J. Biophys. Biochem. Cytol., 10*, 361–372.

32. Lever JD, Esterhuizen AC (1961): Fine structure of arteriolar nerves in the guinea-pig pancreas. *Nature (London) 192*, 566–567.

33. Richardson KC (1962): The fine structure of autonomic nerve endings in smooth muscle of the rat vas deferens. *J. Anat., 96*, 427–442.

34. Marks BH, Samorajski T, Webster EJ (1962): Radioautographic localization of norepinephrine-H^3 in the tissues of mice. *J. Pharmac. Exp. Ther., 138*, 376–381.

35. Wolfe DE, Axelrod J, Potter LT, Richardson KC (1962): Localization of tritiated norepinephrine in sympathetic axons by electron-microscope autoradiography. *Science, 138*, 440–442.

36. Aghajanian GK, Bloom FE (1966): Electron-microscopic autoradiography of rat hypothalamus after intraventricular ^{3}H-norepinephrine. *Science, 153*, 308–310.

37. Aghajanian GK, Bloom FE (1966): Localization of tritiated serotonin in rat brain by electron-microscopic autoradiography. *J. Pharmacol. Exp. Ther., 156*, 23–30.

38. Ehinger B (1970): Autoradiographic identification of rabbit retinal neurons that take up GABA. *Experientia, 26,* 1063.
39. Hökfelt T, Ljungdahl Å (1970): Cellular localization of labelled gamma-aminobutyric acid (^{3}H-GABA) in rat cerebellar cortex: An autoradiographic study. *Brain Res., 22,* 391–396.
40. Bloom F, Iversen LL (1971): Localizing ^{3}H-GABA in nerve terminals of rat cerebral cortex by electron-microscopic autoradiography. *Nature (London) 229,* 628–630.
41. Storm-Mathiesen J, Iversen LL (1979): Uptake of (^{3}H)glutamic acid in excitatory nerve endings: Light- and electron-microscopic observations in the hippocampal formation of the rat. *Neuroscience 4,* 1237–1253.
42. Geffen LB, Livett DG, Rush RA (1969): Immunohistochemical localization of protein components of catecholamine storage vesicles. *J. Physiol. (London), 204,* 593–605.
43. Coons AH (1958): Fluorescent antibody methods. In: Danielli JF (Ed), *General Cytochemical Methods,* pp. 394–422. Academic Press, New York.
44. Nakane PN Pierce GB (1967): Enzyme-labelled antibodies for the light- and electron-microscopic localization of tissue antigens and antibodies. *J. Cell Biol., 33,* 307–311.
45. Avrameas S (1969): Coupling of enzymes to proteins with glutaraldehyde. Use of the conjugates for the detection of antigens and antibodies. *Immunochemistry 6,* 43–47.
46. Sternberger LA, Hardy PH, Cuculis JJ, Meyer HG (1970): The unlabelled antibody-enzyme method of immunohistochemistry. Preparation and properties of soluble antigen-antibody complex (horseradish peroxidase-antihorseradish peroxidase) and its use in identification of spirochetes. *J. Histochem. Cytochem., 18,* 315–333.
47. Thoenen H, Tranzer JP (1968): Chemical sympathectomy by selective destruction of adrenergic nerve endings with 6-hydroxydopamine. *Naunyn-Schmiedebergs Arch. Exp. Pathol. Pharmakol., 261,* 271–288.
48. Nauta WJH, Gygax PA (1951): Silver impregnation of degenerating axon terminals in the central nervous system (1) technique (2) chemical notes. *Stain Technol., 26,* 5–11.
49. Fink RP, Heimer L (1967): Two methods for selective silver impregnation of degenerating axons and their synaptic endings in the central nervous system. *Brain Res., 4,* 369–374.
50. Lasek R, Joseph BS, Whitlock DG (1968): Evaluation of a radioautographic neuroanatomical tracing method. *Brain Res., 8,* 319–336.
51. Cowan WM, Gottlieb DI, Hendrickson AE, Price JL, Woolsey TA (1972): The autoradiographic demonstration of axonal connections in the central nervous system. *Brain Res., 37,* 21–51.
52. Kristensson K, Olsson Y, Sjöstrand J (1971): Axonal uptake and retrograde transport of exogenous proteins in the hypoglossal nerve. *Brain Res., 32,* 399–406.
53. Cowan M, Cuenod M (Eds) (1975): *The Use of Axonal Transport for Studies of Neuronal Connectivity.* Elsevier, Amsterdam.
54. Heimer L, Robards MJ (Eds) (1981): *Neuroanatomical Tract-tracing Methods.* Plenum Press, New York.
55. Mesulam MM (Ed) (1982): *Tracing Neural Connections with Horseradish Peroxidase.* John Wiley, Chichester.
56. Kennedy C, Des Roisers MH, Reivich M, Sharp F, Jehle JW, Sokoloff L (1975): Mapping of functional neural pathways by autoradiographic survey of local metabolic rate with (^{14}C)deoxyglucose. *Science, 187,* 850–853.

Contents

Contents

Contents

VIII. NEURONAL TRACING USING RETROGRADE MIGRATION OF LABELED TRANSMITTER-RELATED COMPOUNDS – M. CUÉNOD AND P. STREIT

Contents

Contents

CHAPTER I

Acetylcholinesterase histochemistry

LARRY L. BUTCHER

1. INTRODUCTION

A number of hydrolases exist that catalyze the hydrolysis of short-chain carboxylic esters such as acetylcholine. On the basis of their reaction with organophosphorous compounds like bis(1-methylethyl)phosphorofluoridate (DFP*), these enzymes have been organized into three groups by Eto (1974): A, B and C (see also Oosterbaan and Jansz 1965). Although this terminology, as well as an extensive array of related alphabetic nomenclature and other appellative schemata (see Pearse 1972; Florkin and Stotz 1973; Silver 1974; and Kiernan 1981), is no longer preferred, it has historical significance and permits some useful comparisons to be made among the relevant enzymes.

Categories A and C are comprised of one enzyme each (Eto 1974). The esterase in Group A, now named arylesterase (aryl-ester hydrolase, EC 3.1.1.2), hydrolyzes organophosphorous compounds but is not inhibited by them, whereas the esterase in Category C, now called acetylesterase (acetic-ester hydrolase, EC 3.1.1.6), neither hydrolyzes nor is inhibited by those substances. Esterases of the B-type, according to Eto (1974), include cholinesterases (EC 3.1.1.7 and 3.1.1.8) and carboxylesterase (carboxylic-ester hydrolase, EC 3.1.1.1) and are readily inhibited by organophosphorous compounds.

Cholinesterases differ from carboxylesterase in that, under the proper experimental conditions, they hydrolyze choline esters at faster rates than other esters and can be inhibited by physostigmine, also known as eserine, at low concentrations, 10^{-5} M in most organisms (Silver 1974). Although species differences exist (see, e.g. Bayliss and Todrick 1956), two basic types of cholinesterases have been recognized in mammals: (1) the type (EC 3.1.1.7) demonstrating a substrate preference for acetic esters such as acetylcholine, and (2) the type (EC 3.1.1.8) exhibiting a substrate preference for other kinds of esters such as butyrylcholine and propionylcholine. Of the two cholinesterases, the first has attracted most attention because of its known or presumed role in intercellular communication processes involving acetylcholine.

The existence of cholinesterases as naturally occurring substances was suggested orginally by investigators studying the pharmacologic and physiologic actions of choline and choline derivatives. In a paper published in 1899 and in publications appearing shortly thereafter, Hunt and his associates demonstrated that the decreases in

---

*The abbreviation DFP derives from an earlier, but no longer preferred, name for the organophosphorous compound, diisopropylfluorophosphate.

Handbook of Chemical Neuroanatomy. Vol. 1: Methods in Chemical Neuroanatomy.
A. Björklund and T. Hökfelt, editors.
© Elsevier Science Publishers B.V., 1983.

blood pressure observed after injection of extracts of suprarenal glands, the brain, or sympathetic ganglia were due, in part, to choline (Hunt 1899; Hunt and Taveau 1906, 1909). Because choline was pharmacologically less potent than certain choline esters, however, Hunt and Taveau (1906) reasoned that:

> '...it [is] very probable that at least some of these results were to be attributed to a precursor of cholin or some compound of cholin.... Acetyl-cholin, the first of this series, is a substance of extraordinary physiological activity. In fact, I think it safe to state that, as regards its effect upon the circulation, it is the most powerful substance known....' (p. 1789).

Taking into account the observations of Hunt and co-workers, Dale noted in 1914 that:

> '...The question of a possible physiological significance, in the resemblance between the action of choline esters and the effects of certain divisions of the involuntary nervous system, is one of great interest.... Acetyl-choline is, of all the substances examined, the one whose action is most suggestive in this direction. The fact that its action surpasses even that of adrenine, both in intensity and evanescence... gives plenty of scope for speculation. On the other hand, there is no known depôt of choline derivatives, corresponding to the adrenine depôt in the adrenal medulla, nor, indeed, any evidence that a substance resembling acetyl-choline exists in the body at all. Reid Hunt found evidence of the existence of a substance in the supra-renal gland, which was not choline itself, but easily yielded that base in the process of extraction. If acetyl-choline, however, or any substance of comparable activity, existed in the suprarenal gland in quantities sufficient for chemical detection, its action would inevitably overpower that of the adrenine in a gland extract. The possibility may, indeed, be admitted, of acetyl-choline, or some similarly active and unstable ester, arising in the body and being so rapidly hydrolyzed by the tissues that its detection is impossible by known methods....' (pp. 188-189).

Experimental support for the conjecture of Dale (1914) that acetylcholine might be catabolized in vivo was provided 12 years later by Loewi and Navratil (1926). These investigators observed that the 'depressor' action of acetylcholine on frog heart was prolonged by physostigmine, an effect they attributed to inhibition by the drug of a naturally occurring enzyme responsible for inactivating acetylcholine. In 1932, Stedman et al. purified and characterized an enzyme preparation from horse serum, for which they proposed the name choline-esterase, that hydrolyzed both acetylcholine and butyrylcholine, with the latter being the preferred substrate. Stedman and Stedman (1935) later reported that erythrocytes possessed a high degree of acetylcholine-hydrolyzing activity and that cholinesterase activity in the cat basal ganglia was twice as high as that in the cerebral cortex, a result roughly paralleling the finding of Dikshit (1934) that acetylcholine-like activity was greater in the basal ganglia than in the cerebral cortex. It is interesting that Dikshit (1934) not only proposed that '...humoral transmission may occur in the central nervous system....' (p. 409), but also referred to the crude enzyme preparation of Stedman et al. (1932) as acetylcholine esterase. In 1938, Marnay and Nachmansohn presented evidence that the enzyme they called choline esterase was more concentrated in nerves innervating frog sartorius muscle than in the muscle itself and concluded that the hydrolysis of released acetylcholine could '...occur with the rapidity necessary for the assumption of a chemical transmission of nerve impulses in such quickly reacting cells as fibres of voluntary muscle...' (p. 46). Two years later, Alles and Hawes (1940) characterized cholinesterase activity in human blood and observed that the serum and cell enzymes differed qualitatively in their ability to hydrolyze acetylcholine and varied significantly with respect to activity changes as a function of pH and salt concentration. They further noted that the blood-cell cholinesterase was most efficacious in hydrolyzing acetylcholine at low substrate concentrations but could suggest no function for the association of the enzyme with

2

erythrocytes except to prevent the '...circulating blood from transmitting a local activity of cholinergic nerve endings to remote sites...' (p. 389).

In related experiments, Mendel and his associates (Mendel et al. 1943; Mendel and Rudney 1943) reported that the serum enzyme hydrolyzed butyrylcholine or propionylcholine at a faster rate than acetylcholine (cf. Stedman et al. 1932) but that acetylcholine was the preferred substrate for the erythrocyte enzyme (cf. Alles and Hawes 1940). On the basis of these data, Mendel and Rudney (1943) suggested that two categories of cholinesterases existed: one that was associated with blood cells, for which they proposed the term cholinesterase or true cholinesterase, and one found in the serum, which they called nonspecific cholinesterase or pseudocholinesterase. In 1949, Augustinsson and Nachmansohn proposed that the appellation acetylcholinesterase be reserved for the 'true' or 'specific' cholinesterase and the sobriquet cholinesterase for the 'nonspecific' or 'pseudo'-cholinesterase, a terminology subsequently adopted by the Enzyme Commission (1964) for the trivial names of the two enzymes. These and other nomenclature schemata, as well as some of the properties of the two cholinesterases, are summarized in Table 1.

The terminology to be used in this chapter for the two types of cholinesterases

TABLE 1. *Nomenclature and properties of cholinesterases*

Characteristic	Enzyme EC 3.1.1.7	Enzyme EC 3.1.1.8
A. Systematic name	Acetylcholine acetylhydrolase	Acylcholine acylhydrolase
B. Trivial name	Acetylcholinesterase (AChE)	Cholinesterase (ChE)
C. Other names	ChE I; true cholinesterase; specific cholinesterase; erythrocyte cholinesterase; E-type cholinesterase	ChE II; pseudocholinesterase; nonspecific cholinesterase; serum cholinesterase; S-type cholinesterase; butyrylcholinesterase; Ψ-type cholinesterase
D. Main sources	Erythrocytes; neural tissue; thymus	Serum; pancreas; heart; liver
E. Substrate specificity		
1. Preferred substrate	Acetylcholine (ACh $>>$ PrCh $>$ BuCh)[a]	Butyrylcholine or propionylcholine (BuCh, PrCh $>$ ACh)[a]
2 Other substrates	Acetyl-β-methylcholine; various acetylesters[b]	Benzoylcholine; various butyrylesters and propionylesters[b]
F. Optimum pH	8.0–8.5	8.2–8.5
G. Isoelectric point	4.65–4.70[c]	4.36[c]
H. Optimum temperature	37–40°C	37–40°C
I. Molecular forms	Many collagen-tailed and tailless or globular entities[d]	Many collagen-tailed and tailless or globular entities[d]
J. Inhibitors[e]		
1. Eserine	Inhibition by 10^{-5}M	Inhibition by 10^{-5}M
2. DFP	Inhibition in range 10^{-6} to 10^{-5}M	Inhibition in range 10^{-8} to 10^{-7}M
3. BW284c51	Inhibition in range 10^{-6} to 10^{-5}M	No inhibition in range 10^{-6} to 10^{-5}M; approximately 75% inhibition at 10^{-3}M
4. Iso-OMPA	Relatively resistant in range 10^{-5} to 10^{-4}M (rat brain homogenate)[f]	Over 90% inhibition in range 10^{-5} to 10^{-4}M (rat intestinal mucosa)[f]
5. Ethopropazine	Resistant	Susceptible (10^{-4}M)

[a]Abbreviations: ACh = acetylcholine; BuCh = butyrylcholine; PrCh = propionylcholine.
[b]See Hawkins and Mendel (1946) and Adams (1949).
[c]Bergmeyer (1963).
[d]Massoulié and Bon (1982).
[e]Abbreviations: BW284c51 = 1:5-*bis*(4-allyl-dimethylammoniumphenyl)pentan-3-one dibromide [Burroughs-Wellcome Co., Research Triangle, NC, USA]; iso-OMPA = N,N'-*bis*(1-methylethyl)pyrophosphorodiamide anhydride [K and K Laboratories, Plainview, NY, USA]; for meaning of other symbols, see text.
[f]Bayliss and Todrick (1956).

reflects a histochemical bias, but, consistent with the classification schemata of enzymologists, takes into account both substrate preference and susceptibility to inhibitors. The name acetylcholinesterase (AChE) will be reserved for the enzyme that hydrolyzes acetylcholine or a related structural analogue in the presence of an inhibitor of acylcholine acylhydrolase (EC 3.1.1.8), and the appellation butyrylcholinesterase (BuChE) will be used for the enzyme that hydrolyzes butyrylcholine, or an analogue of it, in the presence of an inhibitor of acetylcholine acetylhydrolase (EC 3.1.1.7). As the name logically implies, but at variance with Enzyme Commission nomenclature, the sobriquet cholinesterase will refer to either AChE (EC 3.1.1.7) or BuChE (EC 3.1.1.8) or to both enzymes.

2. ENZYME HISTOCHEMISTRY: THEORETIC AND GENERAL METHODOLOGIC CONSIDERATIONS

2.1. STRATEGY AND RULES OF THE GAME

Histochemistry is an interdisciplinary endeavor whose *raison d'être* is to demonstrate biologically significant chemical compounds and processes in relation to the anatomic matrix in which they occur. Its conceptual framework and methodology derive significantly from biochemistry and allied disciplines on one hand and from histology on the other. Because the methods and goals of these two broad areas of scientific inquiry are not infrequently incompatible, however, it does not necessarily follow that the best biochemical procedure for assaying a particular substance or the best histologic protocol for demonstrating cellular morphology will be the most satisfactory for use in a histochemical technique. Considerably more often than not, if not always, compromises must be made, and the optimal histochemical method is one that enables the maximum amount of information to be obtained about the chemical compounds and processes being assayed while simultaneously minimizing loss of information concerning the precise structural entities with which those compounds and processes are associated. The application to histochemistry of this minimax strategy, as it might be referred to by mathematical game theorists (Davis 1973), will be illustrated repeatedly in the following discourse.

Ideally, all enzyme histochemical methods should satisfy the following three criteria. First, the method should demonstrate the enzyme selectively. Second, there should be no translocation of the enzyme or of final end-products during tissue processing. In other words, the distribution of an enzyme revealed by a particular histochemical method should correspond exactly to the distribution of the enzyme in vivo. And third, the property of an enzyme essential for its histochemical detection (e.g. active or antigenic site) should not be affected by the manipulations to which the tissue is subjected. (For further discussion of these issues, see Holt 1958; Holt and O'Sullivan 1958; Pearse 1961; Silver 1974; Kiernan 1981.)

The value or usefulness of a given histochemical method can be evaluated on the basis of how seriously the above three criteria are violated and the extent to which possible infractions can be controlled. Although the necessity of satisfying Criterion 1 is obvious, more needs to be discussed concerning Criteria 2 and 3 and the consequences of their inobservance.

Violations of Criterion 2 are relatively serious, because such infractions could result in the simultaneous generation of false-positive and false-negative errors. That is, enzyme activity could be indicated at sites where it is not normally found and absent at loci where it is present in vivo. For this reason, high priority must be assigned to protocols in a particular histochemical method that are aimed at minimizing enzyme and end-product diffusion.

Criterion 3 is possibly the condition that can be compromised most in the opinion of many histochemists, primarily because quantitative methods are not well-developed in histochemistry. It becomes more important, therefore, to demonstrate where an enzyme is located rather than how much of the enzyme or how much activity is present at those loci. Consider methods based on enzyme activity, for example. In such procedures, there must be detectable activity in tissue in order to avoid false-negative errors in enzyme identification. Experimental conditions that demonstrate enzyme activity maximally, however, may result in enzyme and end-product diffusion (see, e.g. Pearse 1961; Silver 1974), the consequence being poor localization. Preservation of localization, particularly of soluble enzymes, can be facilitated by fixation, but fixation usually decreases enzyme activity (Pearse 1961). We are now confronted with a situation that requires compromise, and the application of the minimax strategy becomes essential. That is, within the context of the goals of a particular experiment, how much loss of enzyme activity can be tolerated in order to achieve most accurate localization? Once this question has been answered, then length of fixation can be determined. In tissues in which enzyme activity is normally low, for example, fixation times may have to be relatively short in order to avoid false-negative errors, but a necessary cost will be a decrease in accuracy of localization. In tissues in which activity is high, however, much longer fixation times may be used, the increased benefit in accuracy of localization offsetting the cost of augmented loss of activity.

2.2. OVERVIEW OF TECHNIQUES

Enzyme histochemical methods fall into 2 general categories (Kiernan 1981): those procedures that do not necessarily require that the enzyme be active and those that do. The first category of methods includes immunohistochemical and affinity labeling techniques, and the second category is comprised of substrate-film and dissolved-substrate procedures. Most enzyme histochemical procedures are currently of the dissolved-substrate type, but immunohistochemical methods are becoming increasingly used, primarily as anatomic tools for the mapping of enzymes thought to be important for interneuronal communication processes (see Chapters IV and V).

Techniques not necessarily based on an enzyme's ability to catalyze a particular chemical reaction

Enzymes can be defined as proteins that catalyze biologic chemical reactions with a high degree of specificity and catalytic power in normal metabolic processes. Not all structural components of a particular enzyme appear to be involved in a given catalysis however, and the formation of an enzyme-substrate complex apparently occurs at a specific locus or loci on the protein, referred to as the active site or sites (e.g. the glutamic acid-serine-alanine amino acid sequence at the esterasic site of AChE). Other portions of the macromolecule may not be directly involved in or important for the catalytic process. The viability of affinity labeling and immunohistochemical methods does not necessarily depend on the active sites of enzymes, however. All that is required is that some structural component of the protein be antigenic or available for binding with drugs. This component may include the active sites, the nonactive sites, or both.

(a) The immunohistochemical technique

Immunohistochemical methods, including those for enzymes, have been reviewed extensively by Cuello (1978), Sternberger (1979), Vandesande (1979) and Larsson (This Volume, Chapter IV), and will not be considered extensively in the present chapter. Suffice it to say that, for accurate localization in tissue, it is necessary that the enzyme retain its antigenic properties following fixation and other prestaining procedures and that the enzyme does not diffuse from its normal site before or after being complexed by the antibodies directed against it. Immunohistochemical procedures have been developed for a variety of enzymes, including tyrosine hydroxylase (e.g. Joh et al. 1973), dopamine-β-hydroxylase (e.g. Hartman et al. 1972), AChE (e.g. Benda et al. 1970), choline-0-acetyltransferase (EC 2.1.1.6; see, e.g. Eckenstein and Thoenen 1982), and tryptophan hydroxylase (e.g. Pickel et al. 1976).

(b) The affinity labeling technique

Current affinity labeling methods are based essentially on the preferential or selective binding of inhibitors with enzymes. In many procedures, a radiolabeled inhibitor is incubated with the tissue being studied, and enzyme loci are detected with standard autoradiographic procedures (see, e.g. Edwards and Hendrickson 1981). Tritiated DFP, for example, has been used to identify AChE loci in motor end-plates of mouse diaphragm (Ostrowski and Barnard 1961). An advantage of this procedure is that it can be used at the electron-microscopic level. At the optical light-microscopic level, however, it possesses all of the disadvantages of any autoradiographic method: morphologic detail is poor compared to other techniques, and the autoradiographic method itself is usually time- consuming.

Other enzymes have been demonstrated with peroxidase-coupled or fluorescent inhibitors. Loci of sodium, potassium-adenosine triphosphatase activity, for example, have been demonstrated with peroxidase-coupled ouabain (Mazurkiewicz et al. 1978), and the fluorescent compound dimethylaminonaphthaline-5-sulfonamide has been used to demonstrate carbonic anhydrase (Pochhammer et al. 1979).

Techniques based on an enzyme's ability to catalyze a particular chemical reaction

As indicated previously in this chapter, individual reactions of normal metabolism are catalyzed, with few exceptions, by different enzymes possessing a high degree of specificity. Nonetheless, most of these enzymes are not absolutely specific for their particular physiologic substrates and can also catalyze reactions involving structural analogues of those substrates, both naturally occurring and synthetic. The drug methacholine, for example, can be catabolized by AChE but at a slower rate than acetylcholine. These characteristics of enzymes, relative substrate specificity in normal metabolic processes and the ability to catabolize non-naturally occurring but structurally related substrate analogues, have been exploited in the substrate-film and dissolved-substrate procedures considered in this section (see also Kiernan 1981).

(a) The substrate-film technique

In substrate-film procedures, the substrate itself is prepared in the form of a thin film or is suspended in a suitable carrier that can be placed in close contact with the surface of sectioned tissue (for review, see Lillie 1965). The following example for proteinases illustrates how such methods have been used (Cunningham 1967; Kiernan 1981): glass slides are coated with gelatin. The gelatin is then stained with some dye such as Fast Blue (Cunningham 1967) or Procion Brilliant Red (Kiernan 1981). Cryostat sections of various tissues are placed on the stained gelatin. Different proteinases, depending on pH and the tissue examined, will digest the gelatin, leaving a hole in the film which can be visualized against the stained surround and correlated with a corresponding region of the tissue placed on it. Substrate-film methods also have been used to localize sites of ribonuclease, deoxyribonuclease, and amylase activity (Daoust 1965; see also Lillie 1965).

For various reasons, the substrate-film procedures have not been widely used. First, and most importantly, because the enzyme must diffuse from the tissue section to the substrate film to catalyze a reaction, resolution is low (Cunningham 1967; Kiernan 1981). And second, the substrate must be applied as a thin film, a time-consuming and technically difficult, if not impossible, procedure for the substrates of most enzymes. Indeed, no method for AChE currently exists based on the substrate-film technique.

(b) The dissolved-substrate technique

In dissolved-substrate methods, the substrate, which may or may not be the natural substrate of the enzyme, and all other reagents necessary to effect a particular enzyme-catalyzed reaction and detection of tissue loci where the reaction occurs are in solution. Tissue sections, either free-floating or slide-mounted, are placed within this incubation medium. Under the proper conditions of prior tissue preparation, substrate and reagent concentration, temperature, pH, and duration of incubation, the enzyme in the tissue catalyzes the reaction, resulting in the formation of products. At least one of these, called the primary reaction product in histochemical parlance (Pearse 1961), must then be rendered insoluble, if it is not already insoluble, as close as possible to the locus where it was generated. Because the products of most enzyme-catalyzed reactions are soluble, however, it is necessary to include in the incubation medium a trapping or capture agent, typically a low-molecular weight chemical compound that penetrates tissue efficiently and reacts rapidly with the primary reaction product to form, under optimal conditions, a nondiffusible precipitate called the secondary reaction product. This latter compound can be colored or colorless. If it is colorless, then the secondary reaction product, in order to facilitate visualization of the locus where it was deposited, is usually converted to a colored compound, the tertiary reaction product, by means of another chemical reaction.

Similar to other histochemical methods, artifacts in dissolved-substrate methods can occur by diffusion of the enzyme and diffusion of the primary, secondary, or tertiary reaction products during tissue processing. In addition, detectable reaction deposits may be formed that do not derive from the action of the enzyme being studied. Such false-positive reactions may result from (1) other enzymes acting upon the components of the incubation medium, and (2) non-enzymatic reactions among the constituents of the incubation medium or among those constituents and tissue entities not involved in normal catalytic processes. Errors of the first type can be minimized or eliminated by exposing tissue to specific inhibitors of the interfering enzymes, if the identity of those enzymes is known. Relevant controls for errors of the second type include performing the histochemical reaction on tissue exposed to all incubation reagents except the substrate and assessing the extent to which a positive reaction occurs in the absence of tissue.

3. HISTOCHEMICAL METHODS FOR CHOLINESTERASES

3.1. HISTORY, PRINCIPLES, AND PRACTICALITIES

The fatty-acid ester procedure of Gomori

Gomori, extending his procedure for lipases, published the first histochemical method for cholinesterases in 1948. The substrates he used were long-chain, fatty-acid esters of choline, specifically lauroyl-, myristoyl-, palmitoyl-, and stearoylcholine. Of these, the first two were deemed satisfactory for use in histochemical studies, but palmitoyl-choline and stearoylcholine were not. The latter two cholinesters were precipitated by salts unless propylene glycol was added to the incubation medium. Furthermore, stearoylcholine was hydrolyzed at a very slow rate.

Tissue was fixed in cold acetone and double-embedded in celloidin and paraffin, and sections were covered with celloidin prior to incubation. Unfortunately, these procedures resulted in considerable loss of enzyme activity, and incubation times were correspondingly long to obtain a positive histochemical reaction (Table 2).

Tissue sections were incubated in the following medium, which was filtered before use (Gomori 1952):

0.0125 M cobalt acetate in 0.025 M Tris-maleate buffer (pH = 7.6)	50.0 ml
0.02 M lauroyl- or myristoylcholine	1.0 ml
0.2 M MnCl$_2$	0.5 ml
0.2 M MgCl$_2$	0.5 ml
0.2 M CaCl$_2$	0.5 ml

The Mn^{2+}, Mg^{2+}, and Ca^{2+} ions were added to activate the cholinesterases (see Nachmansohn 1940), and the free fatty-acid released by the hydrolytic action of esterases was postulated to combine with cobalt ions to form a white granular deposit. This precipitate was then converted to black cobalt sulfide by immersion of sections in a dilute solution of ammonium sulfide in 70% ethanol.

For various reasons, the fatty-acid ester procedure of Gomori (1948, 1952) has never achieved widespread acceptance. First, the method does not appear to demonstrate AChE efficaciously in peripheral tissues, although it does appear to demonstrate BuChE successfully (Koelle and Friedenwald 1949; Pearse 1972). Second, application of Gomori's regimen to the study of cholinesterases in the central nervous system has not yielded acceptable results, and Gomori (1948) himself showed that the hydrolysis of higher fatty-acid esters of choline was poor in rat brain homogenates. Third, the method apparently is capricious when used with fixed tissue (Pearse 1972), although Denz (1953) has reported that it gives satisfactory and reliable results with fresh material.

The thiocholine methods

(a) The procedures of Koelle and his associates

A new and perhaps the most important chapter in cholinesterase histochemistry was written in 1949 when Koelle and Friedenwald introduced the use of acetylthiocholine as a substrate. This compound is hydrolyzed by AChE and BuChE at a rate more rapid than acetylcholine itself, presumably because the sulfur linkage of the thiocholine molecule is weaker than the oxygen bond of cholinesters.

TABLE 2. *Selected dissolved substrate methods for cholinesterases*[a]

Variable	Gomori (1948)	Koelle and Friedenwald (1949)	Koelle (1951)	Crevier and Bélanger (1955)	Lewis (1961)	Karnovsky and Roots (1964)	Koelle and Gromadzki[b] (1966)	Eränkö et al. (1967)	Tsuji[c] (1974)
A. Tissue preparation	Cold acetone fixed; double embedded in cellodin and paraffin	Fresh or fresh frozen	Fresh frozen	Fresh frozen or fixed in 4% formaldehyde at 4°C overnight (12 h?)	Fixed in 10% formal-saline	Fixed overnight (12 h?) in cold 10% formalin, 1% CaCl2	Fixed at 4°C in 4% formaldehyde, sucrose, and maleate (pH = 7.4)	Fixed at 0°C in 4% formaldehyde-Krebs-Ringer-Ca solution, 2-4 h	Fresh frozen or fixed in 3% paraformaldehyde-0.1 M phosphate buffer (pH = 7.4)
B. Incubation medium									
1. Substrate	Higher fatty acid esters of choline, 0.4 mM	AcThCh iodide, 4.0 mM; iodide precipitated with CuSO4	AcThCh iodide or BuThCh iodide, 4.0 mM; iodide precipitated with CuSO4	Thioacetic acid, 0.12 M	AcThCh sulfate, 4.0 mM	AcThCh iodide or BuThCh iodide, 1.7 mM; iodide not precipitated	AcThCh iodide or BuThCh iodide; 4.0 mM iodide precipitated with AgNO3	AcThCh iodide, 1.7 mM; iodide precipitated with lead acetate	AcThCh iodide or BuThCh iodide
2. Buffer	0.1 M Tris	None	Maleate	Phosphate-citrate	Acetate	Maleate	Phosphate	0.17 M Tris-acetate	0.1 M Acetate
3. pH	7.5-7.8	8.06	6.0	6.2	≈ 4.9	6.0	5.6	6.0	5.0-6.0
4. Chelating agent	—	Glycine with KOH	Glycine	—	Glycine	Sodium citrate	—	Tris-acetate	Glycine
5. Capture agent	Cobalt (acetate)	Copper (sulfate)	Copper (sulfate)	Lead (nitrate)	Copper (sulfate)	Copper (sulfate)	$AuNa_3(S_2O_3)_2$	Lead (acetate)	Copper
6. Other reagents	Trace amounts of CaCl2, MgCl2, MnCl2	Trace amounts of copper thiocholine	MgCl2, Na2SO4, trace amounts of copper thiocholine	—	—	Potassium ferricyanide	AuThCH phosphate	Potassium ferricyanide and ferrocyanide	—
7. Inhibitors	—	DFP in 0.85% saline, 30 min	DFP	—	Ethopropazine or BW62c47	Eserine (?)	Eserine, BW284c51, DFP, Nu-683	Physostigmine, $1-3 \times 10^{-5}$ M	—
C. Incubation conditions									
1. Time	2-16 h	10-60 min	5-60 min	30-60 min	Variable depending on pH and temp.; author unclear	15 min-2 h	1.5-180 min	1-60 min	5 min-2 h
2. Temperature	37°C	37°C (?)	38°C	Room (22°C?)	23°C recommended	?	Room (22°C?)	0°C	Room (22°C?)
D. Developer	Yellow ammonium sulfide	Yellow ammonium sulfide	Yellow ammonium sulfide	—	Na2S in HCl	Not necessary	Acid-alcoholic (NH4)2S	Lead ferrocyanide observed directly but can be reacted with (NH4)2S	(NH4)2S

[a]Abbreviations: AcThCh = acetylthiocholine; BuThCh = butyrylthiocholine; BW62c47 = 1:5-*bis*(4-trimethylammoniumphenyl)pentan-3-one diiodide [Burroughs-Wellcome Co.; Research Triangle, NC; USA]; Nu-683 = dimethylcarbamate of 2-hydroxyphenyl-benzyl-trimethylammonium bromide [Roche, Inc., Nutley, NJ, USA]; for meaning of other symbols, see text and Table 1.

[b]These authors also presented data on a gold thioacetic acid procedure for the localization of cholinesterases.

[c]The author's modification of the Koelle method is depicted, but he also presented data on the Karnovsky-Roots procedure.

The original thiocholine histochemical procedure involved incubating fresh tissue in a medium essentially containing acetylthiocholine as substrate, glycine as the chelating agent, Cu^{2+} as the capture agent, and trace amounts of copper thiocholine (Koelle and Friedenwald 1949; for summary, see Table 2). The chelating agent was necessary to minimize the inhibitory effects of the heavy metal ion on cholinesterase, and copper thiocholine was added to attenuate diffusion of the reaction product. All reagents were dissolved in an unbuffered aqueous solution at pH = 8.06. Tissue was incubated at 37°C for 10 min (teased preparation of intercostal muscle) to 40 min (30-μm sections of myelencephalon), although the authors mention but do not elaborate on incubation times of 60 min. Following incubation, the tissue was placed in an ammonium sulfide solution to form a dark brown to black reaction product of copper sulfide. Controls consisted of tissue immersed in a saline solution of 10^{-3} M DFP for 30 min prior to incubation in the thiocholine medium.

In two subsequent papers Koelle (1950, 1951) introduced modifications into the original thiocholine procedure in order to distinguish AChE from BuChE and to minimize diffusion artifacts. The first goal was approached by use of acetylthiocholine and butyrylthiocholine as substrates in combination with DFP or more selective inhibitors of AChE and BuChE, Nu-1250 (N-p-chlorophenyl-N-methylcarbamate of m-hydroxyphenyltrimethylammonium iodide: Roche, Inc., Nutley, NJ, USA) and Nu-683 (dimethylcarbamate of 2-hydroxy-5-phenylbenzyl-trimethylammonium bromide: Roche, Inc., Nutley, NJ, USA), respectively. Attenuation of diffusion artifacts was attempted by (1) incubating tissue in a reaction mixture containing all reagents except the substrate prior to full reagent incubation, (2) adding sodium sulfate to the medium to precipitate AChE and BuChE, (3) saturating tissue with copper thiocholine prior to formation of the tertiary reaction product in order to minimize diffusion of the copper thiocholine complex, and (4) adding buffer to the incubation medium and reducing the pH from 8.06 (Koelle and Friedenwald 1949) to 6.4 (Koelle 1950) and 6.0 (Koelle 1951; Table 2). The lowering of pH from 8 to 6.4 resulted in 33 and 60.4% decreases in the rates of hydrolysis by AChE of acetylcholine and acetylthiocholine, respectively, but the improved localization was judged more important than loss of enzyme activity. Koelle (1950, 1951) attempted to partially offset such decrements in enzyme efficacy however, by adding $MgCl_2$ to the incubation medium in order to activate cholinesterases (see Nachmansohn 1940). Subsequent authors reported that decreasing the pH of the incubation medium to 5.0 or lower and making use of fixed tissue could further diminish end-product diffusion (Coutreaux 1951; Coutreaux and Taxi 1952; Cöers 1953).

The following thiocholine procedure represents a composite of the various modifications introduced and implemented by Koelle in the early 1950's (Koelle 1951, 1953, 1954, 1955):

Frozen sections are prepared and placed into one of 3 storage solutions:

A. 9 ml 40% Na_2SO_4; 6 ml H_2O
B. 10.5 ml 40% Na_2SO_4; 4.5 ml H_2O
C. 9 ml 40% Na_2SO_4; 4.5 ml H_2O; 1.5 ml DFP (10^{-6} M)

For the demonstration of AChE, the sections in storage Solution A are placed into the incubation medium detailed below:

3.75% glycine and 2.5% $CuSO_4 \cdot 5H_2O$	0.6 ml
H_2O	2.1 ml

maleate buffer, pH = 6	1.5 ml
aqueous solution containing 23 mg acetylthiocholine iodide	1.2 ml
40% Na_2SO_4 adjusted to pH = 6	9.0 ml
9.5% $MgCl_2$	0.6 ml
copper thiocholine	trace (?)
0.1 M $CuSO_4 \cdot 5H_2O$	0.4 ml

Sections are incubated at 37^0C for 5–60 min before being transferred sequentially to solutions of 20% Na_2SO_4 saturated with copper thiocholine, 10% Na_2SO_4 saturated with copper thiocholine, and water saturated with copper thiocholine. Following treatment with ammonium sulfide, the tissue is then rinsed, fixed in formalin, and mounted.

Tissue sections from storage Solution B are incubated in the same medium as those from Solution A except that butyrylthiocholine iodide is substituted for acetylthiocholine iodide in order to demonstrate sites of BuChE activity preferentially. Sections placed into Solution C, because they are exposed to DFP, serve as controls.

A persistent criticism of the Koelle procedures outlined in the preceding discourse is that they are too cumbersome and include a number of steps that are unnecessary (see, e.g. Tsuji 1974). The removal of copper thiocholine from all media, for example, has been shown to have little or no effect on the histochemical reaction (Gomori 1952; Coutreaux and Taxi 1952).

Although the chemical reactions that ensue in tissue placed in the original Koelle-Friedenwald incubation medium, or in subsequent modifications of it, are not completely understood, it has been suggested that the thiocholine liberated by the action of AChE reacts with glycine-chelated cupric ions to form a copper thiocholine complex, which has been proposed to have one of three structures (Table 3). Based on currently available experimental evidence, the compound in Table 3 proposed by Tsuji (1974) appears most plausible for at least 2 reasons: (1) substitution of $CuCl_2$, $Cu(NO_3)_2$, $Cu(HCOO)_2$, and $Cu(CH_3COO)_2$ for $CuSO_4$ in the histochemical medium results in a positive reaction, suggesting that SO_4^{2-} ions are not necessary to form a precipitate; and (2) when acetylthiocholine iodide is replaced by acetylthiocholine chloride, bromide, or perchlorate, a copper thiocholine complex is formed, but it is soluble. Addition of iodide results in precipitation of that complex. On the basis of these and other observations, Tsuji (1974) suggested that '...iodide seems absolutely necessary for the precipitation of the complex....' (p. 101) and that the practice of precipitating iodide in earlier histochemical protocols for the enzyme was actually detrimental to the success of the method. Fortunately, according to Tsuji (1974), only half of the iodide in solution was precipitated by those earlier procedures.

Regardless of structure, the copper thiocholine complexes postulated to be formed in

TABLE 3. *Copper thiocholine complexes postulated to exist following the secondary histochemical reaction in the original Koelle-Friedenwald or derived methods*

Name of complex	Structure	Color	Reference
A. Copper (cupric) thiocholine hydroxyde	$[(CH_3)_3N^+(OH^-)CH_2CH_2S^-]_2Cu^{2+}$	White	Bergner and Bayliss (1952)
B. Copper (cupric) thiocholine sulfate	$(CH_3)N^+(SO_4^{2-})CH_2CH_2S^-Cu^{2+}$	White	Malgren and Sylvén (1955)
C. Copper (cuprous) thiocholine iodide	$(CH_3)N^+(I^-)CH_2CH_2S^-Cu^+$	White	Tsuji (1974)

cholinesterase histochemical reactions are white (Table 3). Although these compounds can be visualized by phase-contrast microscopy, loci of precipitation are more conveniently visualized, as suggested by procedures in the methods outlined previously in this chapter, by reacting the copper thiocholine deposited in tissue with ammonium sulfide to form copper sulfide, which is dark brown or black (Table 4). Imprecisions can be introduced at any stage in dissolved substrate methods however, and Malmgren and Sylvén (1955) have found that, under certain conditions, copper sulfide may not completely replace copper thiocholine but, rather, may only coat the crystals of the secondary reaction product. A less intensely colored tertiary product could result that might lead to false-negative errors in enzyme identification in tissues possessing weak cholinesterase activity.

(b) The direct coloring method of Karnovsky and Roots

An entirely different principle was introduced into cholinesterase histochemistry with the publication in 1964 of the direct coloring method of Karnovsky and Roots (for summary, see Table 2). The incubation medium in this procedure consists essentially of acetylthiocholine and butyrylthiocholine as substrates, potassium ferricyanide, copper sulfate, and citrate to complex the cupric ions, thereby attenuating inhibition of cholinesterase and reducing the formation of copper ferricyanide. The following major reaction sequence is postulated (Silver 1974): enzymatically released thiocholine reduces the ferricyanide to ferrocyanide in situ. Cupric ions then react with the ferrocyanide to form at sites of enzyme activity copper ferrocyanide, an insoluble russet-colored precipitate also known as Hatchett's Brown (Table 4). In addition to this reaction, Tsuji (1974) has suggested that a secondary reaction takes place identical to that occurring in non-direct coloring thiocholinester procedures. That is, a cuprous thiocholine iodide complex is formed by the reduction of Cu^{2+} to Cu^+ by enzymatically released thiocholine and the reaction of Cu^+ with iodide-complexed thiocholine. A brownish red deposit of cuprous ferricyanide is then postulated to be formed by the reaction of cuprous thiocholine with potassium ferricyanide.

The advantages of the Karnovsky-Roots procedures are: (1) the final reaction product is very fine, allowing for precise localization of enzyme activity and comparatively good morphologic detail; (2) Hatchett's Brown is electron-opaque, and, therefore, the Karnovsky-Roots procedure can be used in electron-microscopic studies, as well as in optical light-microscopic investigations; and (3) the histochemical reaction can be visualized as it develops, thereby permitting the intensity of staining to be monitored precisely. Because of these features, particularly the first and the last, the Karnovsky-Roots procedure, with minor modifications, has been used almost exclusively in my laboratory. Details of this method will be given later in this chapter, and examples of its application to the study of the central nervous system are depicted in Figures 1 and 2.

(c) Concluding commentary

Since the publication of the original Koelle-Friedenwald procedure for cholinesterases and the appearance of the modifications and extensions of the thiocholine method introduced by Koelle and others in the early 1950's and by Karnovsky and Roots in 1964, most of the subsequent alterations in the method have been relatively minor (Table 2). These have included increased use of (1) fixed tissue incubated at lower temperatures

TABLE 4. *Physical characteristics of some final precipitated products in different cholinesterase histochemical methods[a]*

Name	Formula	Molecular weight	Color and crystalline form	Solubility (g/100 ml)[b]		Other solvents
				Cold water	Hot water	
A. Copper sulfide	Cu_2S	159.14	Black, rhombic	$\times 10^{-14}$	—	s HNO_3, NH_4OH; i acetone
	CuS	95.60	Black, monoclinic or hexagonal	0.000033[18]	—	s HNO_3, KCN, hot HCl, H_2SO_4; i alc, alk
B. Copper ferrocyanide	$Cu_2Fe(CN)_6 \cdot H_2O$ (Hatchett's Brown)	—	Red-brown	i	i	i acid, NH_3; s NH_4OH
C. Copper ferricyanide	$Cu_3Fe(CN)_6$	402.57	Brownish red	i	—	i HCl; s NH_4OH
D. Gold sulfide	Au_2S	426.00	Brown black powder	i	—	s aqua regia, KCN; i acid
E. Lead ferrocyanide	$Pb_2Fe(CN)_6 \cdot 3H_2O$	680.38	Yellow-white powder	i	—	Slightly s in H_2SO_4
F. Lead sulfide	PbS	239.25	Black, cubic	0.01244[20]	—	s acid; i alk, KOH

[a]Data pertaining to physical properties taken from *Handbook of Chemistry and Physics* (Weast 1970).
[b]Abbreviations: s = soluble; i = insoluble; alc = alcohol; alk = alkalai.

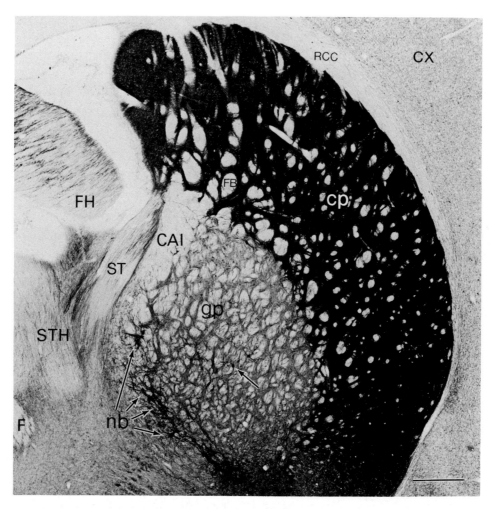

Fig. 1. Low-power portrayal of the distribution of AChE at one level of the rat forebrain. Slightly modified Karnovsky-Roots procedure without prior DFP treatment (Butcher et al. 1974). Compare with Figure 5. Unlabelled arrow points to a nucleus basalis neuron within globus pallidus proper (see Bigl et al. 1982). Scale, 500 μm. (Abbreviations used in this and subsequent figures: ad = nucleus anterior dorsalis thalami; av = nucleus anterior ventralis thalami; bla = basolateral amygdala; CAI = capsula interna; cp = caudate-putamen complex; cx = cortex cerebri; F = columna fornicis; FB = fiber bundle penetrating caudate-putamen complex; FH = fimbria hippocampi; gp = globus pallidus; nb = nucleus basalis; OT = tractus opticus; pc = substantia nigra, pars compacta; pr = substantia nigra, pars reticulata; RCC = radiatio corporis callosi; SM = stria medullaris thalami; ST = stria terminalis; STH = stria terminalis, pars hypothalamica.)

and pH to produce less diffusion and more precise localization of reaction products, and (2) the employment of different capture agents (e.g. lead acetate, aurous sodium thiosulfate) to produce finer intermediate and terminal precipitates more applicable to electron-microscopic investigations. Some physical properties of these and other end-products formed in dissolved substrate methods for cholinesterases are indicated in Table 4.

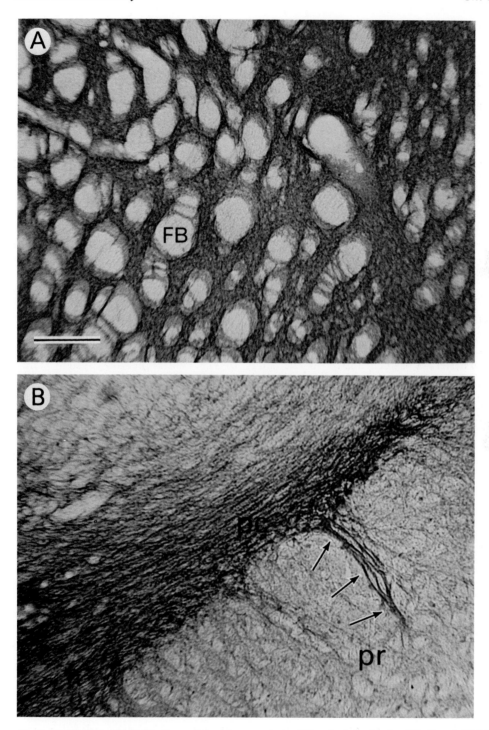

Fig. 2. Distribution of AChE in the caudate-putamen complex (A) and substantia nigra (B) of a rat. Slightly modified Karnovsky-Roots procedure (Butcher et al. 1974) without prior DFP treatment. Compare with Figure 6. Arrows point to AChE-containing processes projecting into pars reticulata. Scale in A, 200 μm (applies also to B). Rephotographed from a plate originally in color.

Methods not based on thiocholine or fatty-acid ester substrates

Procedures for cholinesterases based on the use of thioacetic acid (e.g. Crevier and Bélanger 1955; for summary, see Table 2), indoxyl compounds (e.g. Holt and Withers 1952), and β-naphthyl esters (e.g. Ravin et al. 1953) as substrates have been developed, but all of these compounds appear to demonstrate less substrate specificity than acetyl- or butyrylthiocholine (Silver 1974) and, therefore, are not preferred for use in most cholinesterase histochemical investigations. Similarly, those histochemical methods based on affinity labeling with ^{3}H-DFP or antibodies directed against AChE (see description earlier in this chapter) have proven to be more expensive and time-consuming and less specific, both morphologically and chemically, than dissolved-substrate procedures. Accordingly, they have not been used extensively.

3.2. THE OPTIMAL PROCEDURE FOR USE IN STUDIES OF THE CENTRAL NERVOUS SYSTEM

The choice of a histochemical method for cholinesterases depends on many factors, some of which are constant across different experimental situations and others which are dependent upon the goals of a particular experimenter. In the following discourse, some of these factors will be examined, especially as they relate to the application of cholinesterase histochemistry to the study of the central nervous system. Only dissolved-substrate methods will be considered because they are currently the most reliable, valid, and inexpensive procedures known. In addition, I will focus on methods suitable for use at the optical light-microscopic level. Electron-microscopic procedures have been discussed by Silver (1974), and the interested reader is referred to that excellent treatise.

Despite varying preferences among different histochemists, it is generally agreed that the optimal method for cholinesterases should currently incorporate the use of (1) fixed tissue, (2) specific inhibitors to distinguish AChE from BuChE, and (3) a thiocholine as substrate in an incubation medium having a pH between 5 and 6 and a temperature of approximately 22°C* (Pearse 1972; Silver 1974; see also Table 2). More needs to be said, however, about fixation parameters, the choice of inhibitors, and additional features of the use of acetylthiocholine and butyrylthiocholine.

Fixation parameters

Fixation is recommended in cholinesterase histochemistry for at least 6 reasons. First, cholinesterases are relatively resistant to the inactivating effects of fixation (e.g. Robinson 1971; Silver 1974). Second, fixation attenuates diffusion of AChE molecules, thereby permitting more accurate localization of enzyme activity (Eränkö et al. 1964; Koelle et al. 1970; see also Silver 1974). Third, the size of the crystals of the final reaction product is apparently reduced by prolonged fixation (formaldehyde), thereby increasing the accuracy of localization of AChE activity (Eränkö et al. 1967). Fourth,

---

*Although less but not appreciably different end-product diffusion can be observed at lower temperatures, incubation times are correspondingly increased. The choice of 22°C, therefore, represents yet another compromise.

penetration of incubation reagents into tissue is enhanced by fixation, thereby permitting reduced incubation times (Bell 1966; Brzin et al. 1966; Eränkö et al. 1967; Kokko et al. 1969; Silver 1974). Fifth, fixation may reveal sites of enzyme activity not seen in fresh tissue by removing lipoprotein structures surrounding the AChE molecule (Brzin et al. 1966). And sixth, although not peculiar to cholinesterase histochemistry, cellular morphology is preserved to a greater extent in fixed than in unfixed tissue. Indeed, Gatenby and Beams (1950), perhaps overstating their case, have contended that 'Without good fixation it is impossible to get good stains or good sections, or preparations good in any way' (p. 1).

Although formaldehyde and glutaraldehyde have been used most frequently as tissue fixatives in cholinesterase histochemical procedures (see, e.g. Koelle et al. 1974), formaldehyde is preferred primarily because it appears to produce less inhibition of enzyme activity than glutaraldehyde (Shimizu and Ishii 1966; Anderson 1967; Kokko et al. 1969; for a mitigating view see Koelle et al. 1974). In fact, Kiernan (1981), reviewing the advantages and disadvantages of several different fixatives, concluded that a '...neutral, buffered aqueous solution (pH = 7.2–7.4) containing 2–5% formaldehyde* and isotonic with tissue fluids, is probably the most generally useful of all fixatives for most histological and histochemical purposes' (p. 17). Nonetheless, loss of cholinesterase activity by fixation is not a trivial concern. One hour of immersion in a 2–4% glutaraldehyde solution, for example, reduces enzyme activity in different tissues of the frog and rat by 20–75% (Brzin et al. 1966; Anderson 1967; Tennyson et al. 1968). Similarly, cholinesterase activity is reduced by approximately 30–45% following 24-h exposure of various mammalian and non-mammalian tissues to 4% formaldehyde (Coutreaux and Taxi 1952; Taxi 1952; Ravin et al. 1953; Fukuda and Koelle 1959; Hardwick and Palmer 1961; Robinson 1971).

At least 3 factors appear to influence the degree to which fixation inhibits cholinesterase activity: the concentration of the fixative solution, its temperature, and the length of time the tissue is exposed to it. In the following discourse we will consider these factors but will restrict our discussion to formaldehyde because of the almost universal use of this chemical compound as a fixative in most cholinesterase histochemical procedures (Table 2).

(a) Concentration

In general, the more concentrated the fixative, the greater the inhibition of cholinesterase activity at a given temperature and for a particular length of exposure. Robinson (1971) showed, for example, that following 1 h immersion in 0.5, 1, 2, or 4% formaldehyde solutions, the cholinesterase activity of rabbit brain slices was 78, 70, 56, or 47% of normal, respectively.

(b) Temperature

Not unexpectedly, fixation taking place at higher temperatures results in greater inhibition of cholinesterase. Taxi (1952) demonstrated that exposure of bovine red blood

---

*Formaldehyde is a gas at room temperature ($\simeq 22°C$). Aqueous solutions of this gas can be expressed in terms of a percentage (g/100 ml). Confusion arises, however, with respect to formalin, which is a 38–40% formaldehyde solution in water. Histologists and histochemists often consider such a preparation to be a '100%' formalin solution. A 10% formalin solution in this nomenclature, therefore, is equivalent to a 3.8–4.0% formaldehyde solution.

cells to 4% formaldehyde for 1 h resulted in virtually complete loss of cholinesterase activity at 37°C, but approximately 31% of normal activity remained if fixation was carried out at 18°C. Similarly, exposure of erythrocytes to the same formaldehyde solution for 3 h produced a 72% decrease of enzyme activity at 18°C compared to a 65% reduction at 4°C (Taxi 1952). He further observed that cholinesterase activity in the dog pancreas was reduced by roughly 37% following 24 h of formaldehyde fixation at 4°C, but the loss (79%) was more than twice that amount when fixation procedures were conducted at 18°C. In neural tissue, Taxi (1952) reported a 74% decrease of cholinesterase activity following 1-h immersion in 4% formaldehyde at 18°C, whereas Robinson (1971) found, under similar conditions of tissue preparation and fixation, only a 53% loss at 0–4°C.

(c) Length of exposure

Just as increasing concentrations and temperatures of fixation solutions are correlated with increasing inhibition of cholinesterase activity, so is the same relationship observed with increasing times of tissue exposure to the fixative. Taxi (1952), for example, reported that fixation of dog pancreas in 4% formaldehyde at 18°C for 1, 3, 5, or 24 h produced reductions of cholinesterase activity by 26, 34, 44, or 79% of normal, respectively. As suggested by previous commentary in the present chapter, however, the rate of decrease of enzyme activity can be attenuated by lowering the temperature of fixatives. Sheep brain, for example, retains 46–54% of its normal cholinesterase activity following immersion of this tissue in 4% formaldehyde at 4°C for 16–17 h; even after 65 h of exposure, enzyme activity is 13% of normal (Hardwick and Palmer 1961). Using similar parameters, Austin and Phillis (1965) reported that, following fixation in 5% formaldehyde for 3, 10, 26, 34, or 46 h at room temperature (22°C?) for the first 3 h and at 4°C thereafter, cholinesterase activity in cat cerebellar folia was 90, 55, 28, 28, or 20% of normal, respectively.

Although duration of fixation is an important variable influencing loss of cholinesterase activity during pre-staining procedures, the interaction of that parameter with temperature appears to be highly significant. Temperature considerations, for example, may account for the observations that 24 h of fixation of cat ciliary ganglia in 10% neutral formalin produced virtually complete loss of histochemically detectable cholinesterase in the studies of Fukuda and Koelle (1959) but resulted in little or no decrements in enzyme activity under similar fixation conditions in the experiments of Martinez-Rodriquez et al. (1964) and Butcher et al. (1975). Although the temperature of fixation was not given by Fukuda and Koelle (1957), it was probably room temperature because in a subsequent paper, Koelle et al. (1974) reported that immersion of cat stellate ganglia in a 4% formaldehyde solution at 2–4°C resulted in a 17% retention of AChE activity and an approximately 40% preservation of BuChE after 21-h exposure. Both Martinez-Rodriguez et al. (1964) and Butcher et al. (1975) specified fixation of neural tissue in cold neutral buffered formaldehyde solutions. Indeed, in experiments performed in this laboratory during the past 12 yr, it has been found that 3–4 mm thick slabs of perfused rat brain can be maintained at 4°C in 4% formaldehyde solutions for up to 72 h with little or no histochemically detectable loss of cholinesterase activity. Nonetheless, control procedures should always be performed on fresh tissue to insure that the AChE or BuChE visualized after fixation is found in the same loci and in approximately the same ratios of intensity as that observed in unfixed material. Particularly important in this regard is the response to fixation of cholinesterases in places where enzyme activity is normally quite low (see discussion in Section 2.1 of this chapter).

Choice of inhibitors for use in combination with acetylthiocholine or butyrylthiocholine

A considerable number and wide variety of substances exist that inhibit cholinesterases, either reversibly or irreversibly. According to Pearse (1972), these compounds can be categorized into 3 major groups: (1) eserine and the urethanes; (2) quaternary ammonium compounds; and (3) organophosphorous compounds. Extensive treatments of inhibitors in the second and third groups can be found in Augustinsson (1948) and Eto (1974), respectively. Pearse (1972) and Silver (1974) have provided excellent discussions of substances in all 3 categories.

Many of the original histochemical procedures for cholinesterases specified prior or simultaneous incubation of tissue sections with DFP to distinguish AChE from BuChE (Table 2). It is known that this organophosphorous compound irreversibly inhibits BuChE to a greater extent than AChE (Pearse 1972; Table 1). In subsequent protocols, however, eserine (physostigmine), because of its lower toxicity, has been increasingly used to inhibit cholinesterases (Table 2), and more selective inhibitors of AChE and BuChE have been sought (Table 5). Among the most promising of the selective AChE and BuChE inhibitors for histochemical purposes have been BW284c51 and iso-OMPA (Pearse 1972). According to Bayliss and Todrick (1956), whose data are portrayed in Table 5, BW284c51 at a concentration of 3×10^{-5} M produces 100% inhibition of AChE with minimal effects on BuChE. Similarly, 10^{-5} m iso-OMPA results in a 90% inhibition of BuChE with negligible decreases in AChE activity. In my laboratory,

TABLE 5. *Inhibition of acetylcholinesterase (AChE, rat brain) and butyrylcholinesterase (BuChE, rat intestinal mucosa) by selective inhibitors*[a]

Inhibitor	Concentration	Percent inhibition	
	(M)	AChE	BuChE
Nu-1250[b]	5×10^{-7}	81	1
	2×10^{-6}	98	8
BW62c47[c]	5×10^{-6}	94	1
	2×10^{-5}	101	3
BW284c51[d]	3×10^{-5}	100	2
	1×10^{-4}	102	5
Ethopropazine	3×10^{-5}	−1	90
methosulfate	8×10^{-5}	9	95
Iso-OMPA[e]	1×10^{-5}	0.5[f]	90
	3×10^{-5}	8.5[f]	92
	1×10^{-4}	24	—

[a]Bayliss and Todrick (1956).
[b]N-*p*-chlorophenyl-N-methylcarbamate of *m*-hydroxyphenyl-trimethylammonium bromide [Roche, Inc., Nutley, NJ, USA].
[c]1:5-*bis*(4-trimethylammoniumphenyl)pentan-3-one diiodide [Burroughs-Wellcome Co., Research Triangle, NC, USA].
[d]1:5-*bis*(4-allyl-dimethylammoniumphenyl)pentan-3-one dibromide [Burroughs-Wellcome Co., Research Triangle, NC, USA].
[e]tetramonoisopropylpyrophosphortetramide [K and K Laboratories, Plainview, NY, USA]. For another chemical name see Table 1.
[f]Average of two values.

BW284c51 and iso-OMPA, in combination with acetylthiocholine and butyrylthiocholine as substrates, have been the inhibitors of choice to demonstrate AChE and BuChE selectively.

Although acetylthiocholine is the preferred substrate for AChE and butyrylthiocholine for BuChE, it is also true that butyrylthiocholine can be hydrolyzed by AChE and acetylthiocholine by BuChE (Figs 3 and 4). The BuChE associated primarily with blood vessels in the brain (Fig. 3B; for exception, see anteroventral and anterodorsal thalamus, Figs 4A and 4B) can also be visualized in sections incubated with acetylthiocholine (Fig. 3A) but not after incubation of that substrate with iso-OMPA, a selective inhibitor of BuChE (Fig. 3D, compare with Fig. 3A). Indeed, incubation of brain sections with acetylthiocholine in the presence of BW284c51 reveals sites of BuChE activity virtually identical to that observed after incubation with butyrylthiocholine alone (Fig. 3C, compare with Fig. 3B). Similarly, the slight background staining observed in the caudate–putamen complex and basolateral amygdala after incubation of brain sections with butyrylthiocholine is probably due to AChE hydrolysis of butyrylthiocholine because such staining is eliminated after incubation of that thiocholine with BW284c51, an inhibitor of AChE (Fig. 4B, compare with Fig. 4A). In addition, the staining seen in the substantia nigra after incubation of sections with butyrylthiocholine and iso-OMPA can be attributable to AChE hydrolysis of butyrylthiocholine because addition of BW284c51 abolishes that staining (Fig. 4F, compare with Fig. 4E). Incubation of brain sections with acetylthiocholine or butyrylthiocholine in the presence of eserine, an inhibitor of both AChE and BuChE, results in staining similar to that seen after incubation of sections with no substrate (Fig. 3F, compare with Fig. 3E) or in a medium containing both iso-OMPA and BW284c51 (Fig. 4F, compare with Fig. 4C).

What emerges from the above discourse is that use of acetylthiocholine or butyrylthiocholine alone is not sufficient to identify AChE and BuChE selectively and that specific inhibitors must also be employed.

Conspectus and recommended procedure

Regardless of the exact protocol used to demonstrate AChE and BuChE in neural tissue, most histochemists agree (see, e.g. Pearse 1972; Silver 1974) that the optimal procedure for most purposes should incorporate the following features. First, the animal should be perfused with a cold, neutral buffered solution of 2–5% formaldehyde isotonic with tissue fluids. Postfixation in the same fixative should be conducted in the cold and should probably not exceed 48 h. Controls for loss of enzyme activity due to fixation should be prepared from fresh tissue. Second, incubation of tissue sections should be carried out at room temperature at a pH of 5–6 with acetylthiocholine or butyrylthiocholine as substrates. And third, the specificity of the

---

Fig. 3. Cholinesterase histochemical reaction observed at one level of the rat forebrain following incubation of brain sections with different thiocholine substrates and enzyme inhibitors. Slightly modified Karnovsky-Roots procedure (Butcher et al. 1974) without prior DFP treatment. The substrate and inhibitor used are as follows. Frame A: acetylthiocholine, no inhibitor. Frame B: butyrylthiocholine, no inhibitor. Frame C: acetylthiocholine, 50 μM BW284c51. Frame D: acetylthiocholine, 30 μM iso-OMPA. Frame E: acetylthiocholine, 30 μM physostigmine. Frame F: no substrate, no inhibitor. Arrows in frames A-C point to blood vessels demonstrating cholinesterase activity, probably BuChE, within the corpus callosum. Observe the absence of such staining in Frames D-F. Scale, 2 mm (applies to all frames).

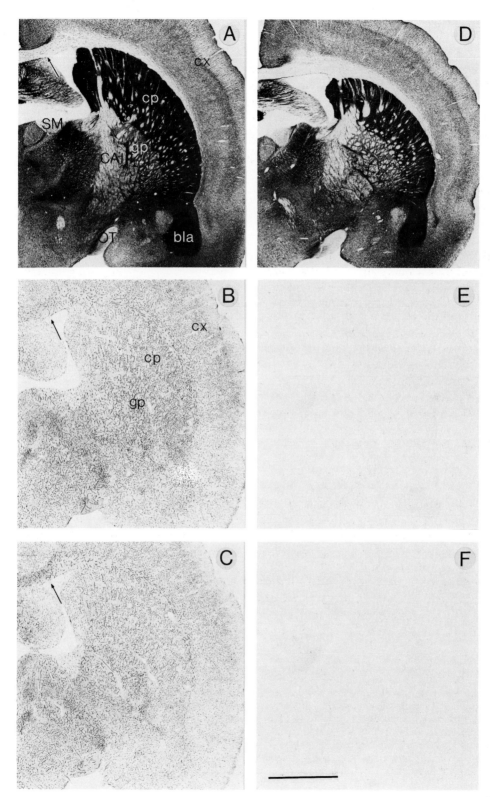

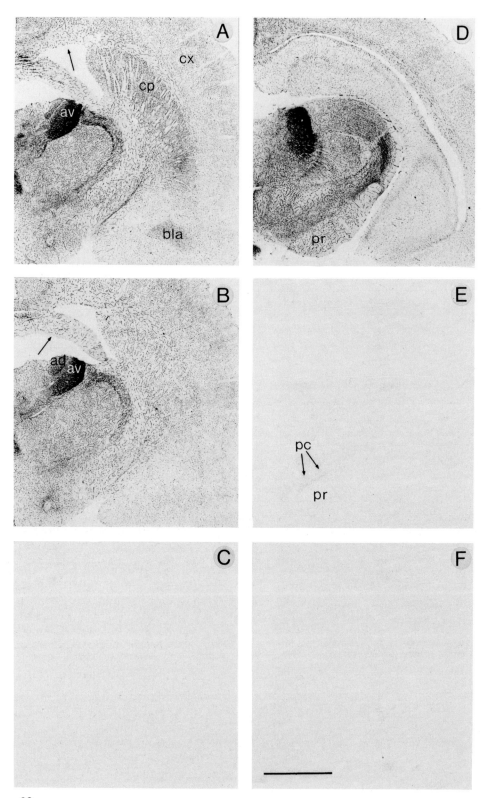

histochemical reaction for one or the other cholinesterase should be tested by assessing sites of non-enzymatic reaction (see Section 2.2, under 'Dissolved-substrate technique') and by determining possible confounds of AChE with BuChE activity.

One histochemical protocol that incorporates these tenets is detailed for AChE in the following discourse. Although this regimen employs a slightly modified Karnovsky-Roots procedure (Butcher and Bilezikjian 1975; Butcher et al. 1975), any of the thiocholine methods listed in Table 2 (or any one of numerous other variations published since 1949) that are comparable in terms of fixation, temperature, and pH parameters could be used in its stead.

Animals are anesthetized with an appropriate anesthetic (e.g. for the rat, 50 mg/kg sodium methohexital injected intraperitoneally) and, subsequently, are sacrificed by cardiac perfusion with 120 ml cold (4°C) 0.9% saline followed by 120 ml of a cold, neutral buffered 4% formaldehyde solution (pH = 7.4). The brain is then carefully extracted from the cranial cavity, cut into 4–6 mm slabs in the appropriate plane, and postfixed in cold, neutral buffered 4% formaldehyde for 16–48 h before being placed into a 30% sucrose solution for an additional 48 h or until the brain pieces sink. The time of formaldehyde fixation that we have employed was adopted after extensive parametric experimentation. Little or no histochemically detectable difference in the intensity of AChE staining is detected among sections fixed for 16–48 h, brain sections fixed only by perfusion with 20 ml of a cold 4% neutral buffered formaldehyde solution, and cryostat sections of unfixed brain tissue. Absence of fixation or minimal fixation results both in friable tissue and indistinct cellular morphology. In our studies of AChE in the nervous system, therefore, we have found brain fixed for 16–48 h preferable to fresh or minimally fixed material.

Following fixation and sucrose immersion, the brain slabs are rinsed in cold 0.9% saline for approximately 2 min and are then frozen on a microtome specimen holder by use of solid CO_2. Sections are cut at the appropriate interval, usually 16–50 μm, and collected into beakers containing chilled (0–4°C) 0.9% saline before being transferred to incubation vials. The reagents in a 10 ml volume of incubation medium are 5 mg acetylthiocholine iodide, 6.5 ml of 0.2 M Tris maleate buffer (pH = 5.7), 0.5 ml of 0.1 M sodium citrate, 1.0 ml of 0.03 M cupric sulfate, 1.0 ml of 0.005 M potassium ferricyanide, and 1.0 ml of distilled deionized water (cf. original Karnovsky-Roots protocol in Table 2). Brain sections are incubated with agitation at room temperature for 2 h or whatever time is necessary to demonstrate AChE optimally under the conditions of the experiment.

Following completion of incubation, sections are removed from the medium and placed in 0.9% saline before being mounted on glass slides coated with pig gelatin or chrome alum. Mounted sections are allowed to air-dry at 22°C for 12–14 h. They are then immersed in distilled, deionized water to remove NaCl crystals and are air-dried again or placed through a series of graded alcohols before being put into xylene and coverslipped under an appropriate medium such as Permount® (Fisher Scientific Co., Fairlawn, NJ, USA).

The specificity of the reaction for AChE is tested in several ways: (1) acetylthiocholine iodide is omitted from the Karnovsky-Roots incubation medium. (2) To give an indication of sites of butyrylcholinesterase activity, butyrylthiocholine iodide is substituted for acetylthiocholine iodide in the reaction mixture. (3) To inhibit butyrylcholinesterase, brain sections are preincubated in 30 μM iso-OMPA for 45 min followed by their incubation in the

---

Fig. 4. Cholinesterase histochemical reaction seen in the rat diencephalon (A-C) and mesencephalon (D-F) following incubation of brain sections with butyrylthiocholine and various enzyme inhibitors. Slightly modified Karnovsky-Roots procedure (Butcher et al. 1974) without prior DFP treatment. The inhibitors used in combination with butyrylthiocholine are as follows. Frame A: no inhibitor. Frame B: 50 μM BW284c51. Frame C: 30 μM physostigmine. Frame D: no inhibitor. Frame E: 30 μM iso-OMPA. Frame F: 30 μM iso-OMPA and 50 μM BW284c51. Arrows in frames A-B point to blood vessels demonstrating cholinesterase activity, probably BuChE, within myelinated fiber bundles. Scale, 2 mm (applies to all frames).

previously described Karnovsky-Roots medium having either butyrylthiocholine iodide or acetylthiocholine iodide as substrate and containing 30 μM iso-OMPA. (4) AChE is inhibited by placing brain sections in 50 μM BW 284c51 for 45 min prior to their incubation in a Karnovsky-Roots reaction mixture having either butyrylthiocholine iodide or acetylthiocholine iodide as substrate and containing 50 μM BW284c51. (5) To inhibit both butyrylcholinesterase and AChE, brain sections are preincubated in a 30 μM eserine sulfate solution; the sections are then incubated in a Karnovsky-Roots medium containing 30 μM eserine sulfate and either butyrylthiocholine iodide or acetylthiocholine iodide as substrate (see Figs 3 and 4).

4. THE PHARMACOHISTOCHEMICAL REGIMEN FOR AChE

4.1. BRIEF HISTORY, RATIONALE, AND GENERAL METHODOLOGIC CONSIDERATIONS

Both the Koelle-Friedenwald and Karnovsky-Roots procedures, or modifications of them (see, e.g. Table 2), have been applied to the study of cholinesterase systems in the brain and spinal cord, quite often in an attempt to map the distribution of cholinergic neurons (e.g. Shute and Lewis 1967; for caveats, see Butcher 1978; Butcher and Woolf 1982b). Indeed, the vast majority of AChE in the nervous system appears associated with neurons (e.g. Friede 1966). From a morphologic point of view, however, the cellular detail observed in some of these earlier studies was relatively indistinct in many neural regions, particularly those areas containing intensely staining neuropil (see, e.g. Figs 1 and 2; for further discussion, see Butcher and Bilezikjian 1975; Butcher et al. 1975; Butcher and Woolf 1982a,b). Recent developments in histochemical protocols for AChE, however, have largely overcome this problem (Figs 5 and 6, compare with Figs 1 and 2). The pharmacohistochemical regimen of Butcher et al. (1975), for example, based essentially on the observations of Fukuda and Koelle (1959) and Nichols and Koelle (1967, 1968) that AChE reappears first in neuronal somata following irreversible enzyme inhibition by DFP, has been used by many different laboratories to 'rewrite' the AChE neuroanatomy of the brain and spinal cord (e.g. Butcher et al. 1975; Parent and Butcher 1976; Poirier et al. 1977; Emson and Lindvall 1979; Woolf and Butcher 1981, 1982; Butcher and Woolf 1982a,b; Bigl et al. 1982).

As the name perhaps intimates, the pharmacohistochemical protocol for AChE involves administering a sublethal dose of a drug, in this case DFP, by a systemic route prior to animal euthanasia and subsequent histochemical processing. The rationale for the procedure derives from the following considerations: (1) DFP irreversibly phosphorylates serine residues of AChE and other serine enzymes (see Goldstein et al. 1974); (2) the reappearance of AChE after DFP administration is due primarily, if not exclusively, to de novo synthesis of the enzyme (Blaber and Creasey 1960); and (3) most AChE regeneration after DFP treatment is detectable first in neuronal somata and only later in cellular processes (Fig. 7; see also Butcher et al. 1975). It has been possible, therefore, to demonstrate morphologic features of AChE-containing neurons impossible to ascertain in pharmacologically unmanipulated material (Figs 5 and 6, compare with Figs 1 and 2; see also Butcher and Bilezikjian 1975; Butcher et al. 1975; Butcher and Woolf 1982a,b). In many areas of the central nervous system, particularly those containing fine-caliber neuronal processes, morphology can be improved further by dark-field illumination (Fig. 8; see also Butcher 1978; Butcher and Woolf 1982a,b).

Even in brain regions where individual AChE-containing cell bodies can be discerned without prior DFP injection (e.g. red nucleus; see Friede 1966), morphologic detail

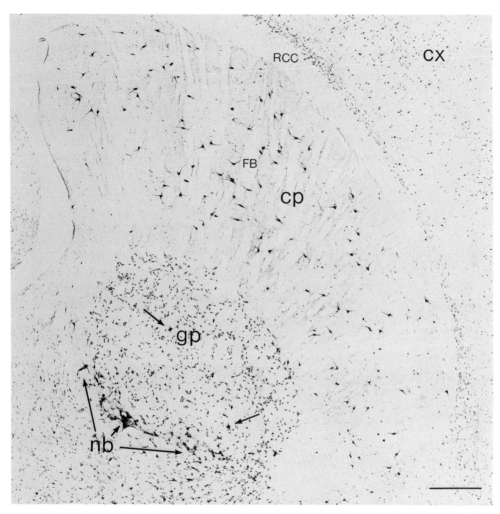

Fig. 5. Low-power portrayal of the distribution of AChE at one level of the rat forebrain. Pharmacohistochemical regimen (Butcher and Bilezikjian 1975; Butcher et al. 1975) in which the DFP (1.8 mg/kg)-euthanasia interval was 5 h. Compare with Figure 1. Unlabelled arrows point to nucleus basalis neurons within globus pallidus proper (see Bigl et al. 1982). Scale, 500 μm.

following systemic administration of the organophoshorous compound is improved considerably compared to that seen in pharmacologically unmanipulated organisms. A possible reason for this is that enzyme staining in AChE-containing neuronal somata and proximal processes may actually be intensified after systemic DFP treatment, perhaps to permit augmented supply of the enzyme to more distal portions of the cell by transport mechanisms. Such a conjecture is compatible with data presented by Nichols and Koelle (1968) on AChE regeneration in retinal amacrine cells following intravenous DFP administration:

> '...the acetylcholinesterase reappeared first in the somata of the amacrine cells.... It is then probably transported to the processes of the neurons.... The staining of these cells for acetylcholinesterase following diisopropyl phosphorofluoridate may represent a rebound, in this case from an initially sub-detectable to a demonstrable level of activity of the enzyme...' (p 5).

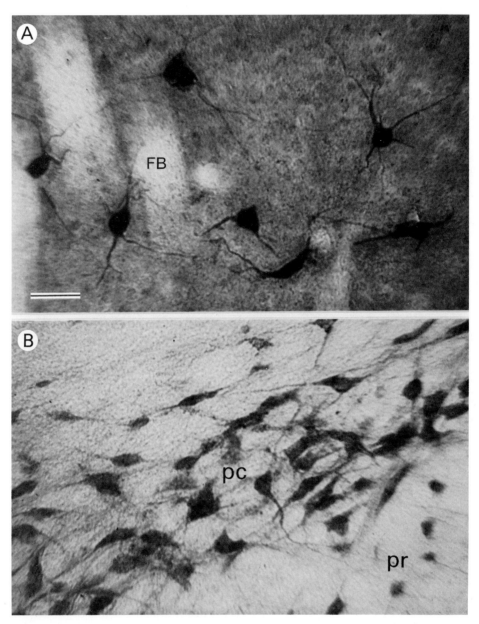

Fig. 6. Distribution of AChE in the caudate-putamen complex (A) and substantia nigra (B) of a rat. Pharmacohistochemical regimen (Butcher and Bilezikjian 1975; Butcher et al. 1975) in which the DFP (1.8 mg/kg)-euthanasia interval was 5 h. Compare with Figure 2. Observe the more intense staining of the neurons in the caudate-putamen complex than in the substantia nigra. Scale in A, 50 μm (applies also to B). Rephotographed from a plate originally in color.

In addition, in cholinergic neurons at least (i.e. those that synthesize and use acetylcholine to communicate with other tissue entities), it is possible that the increased acetylcholine resulting after DFP treatment might actually stimulate synthesis of AChE (Walker and Wilson 1976; Cisson and Wilson 1977; Gisiger and Vigny 1977; Brzin et al. 1980). Indeed, a critical feature of the pharmacohistochemical regimen for AChE is

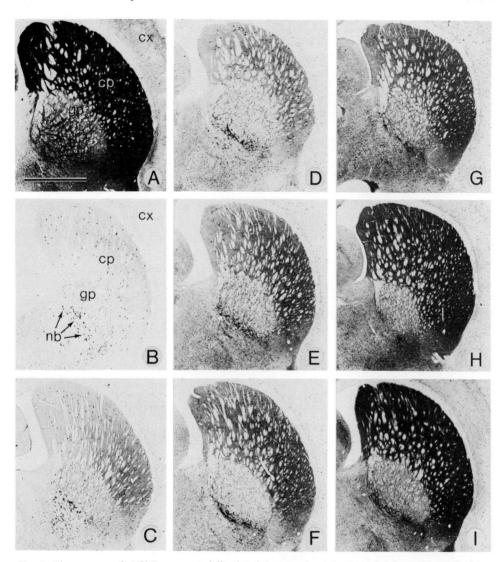

Fig. 7. Time-course of AChE recovery following intramuscular injection of 1.8 mg/kg DFP. Pharmacohistochemical regimen (Butcher and Bilezikjian 1975; Butcher et al. 1975). The DFP-euthanasia intervals were: A (no DFP treatment), B (2 h), C (4 h), D (8 h), E (12 h), F (16 h), G (24 h), H (48 h), and I (72 h). Scale, 2 mm (applies to all frames).

not enzyme inhibition per se but rather that the enzyme is inhibited irreversibly, thereby requiring AChE-containing neurons to synthesize new stores of the enzyme before cholinesterase activity recovers. It must be emphasized, however, that systemic DFP treatment, insofar as can be ascertained histochemically, does not induce AChE in neural regions and tissue constituents where the enzyme does not exist normally (Butcher and Bilezikjian 1975; Butcher et al. 1975).

Although DFP phosphorylates serine residues of enzymes such as AChE having an active serine site (Goldstein et al. 1974), it cannot be argued that the organophosphorous compound affects tissue constituents and processes nonselectively. In cor-

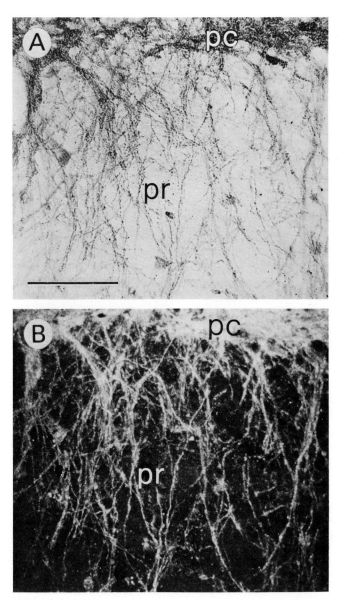

Fig. 8. Acetylcholinesterase-containing dendrites in the rat substantia nigra extending from pars compacta into pars reticulata. The same transverse brain section is shown with bright-field (A) and dark-field (B) illumination. Pharmacohistochemical regimen (Butcher and Bilezikjian 1975; Butcher et al. 1975) in which the DFP (1.5 mg/kg)-euthanasia interval was 48 h. Scale in A, 100 μm (applies also to B).

relative histochemical experiments on brain, it has been found that DFP has no effect on (1) Nissl staining (Woolf and Butcher 1981); (2) NADH-diaphorase activity (Butcher and Bilezikjian 1975; Butcher et al. 1975); (3) myelin staining (unpublished observations from this laboratory); (4) immunoreactivity for somatostatin, neurotensin, cholecystokinin, bombesin, enkephalins, or substance P (unpublished observations from this laboratory); (5) catecholamine fluorescence (Butcher and Marchand 1978;

Albanese and Butcher 1979, 1980); or (6) the retrograde or anterograde transport of horseradish peroxidase (unpublished observations from this laboratory) or various fluorescent markers useful for tracing neuronal pathways (see Section 5.3 of this chapter and Woolf and Butcher 1981, 1982; Bigl et al. 1982; Butcher and Woolf 1982a).

Despite the advantages of the pharmacohistochemical regimen detailed previously in this chapter for the demonstration of AChE-containing neuronal somata and proximal processes, the procedure should not be used if one wishes to visualize normal levels of the cholinesterase or the distribution of the terminal fields of neurons synthesizing the enzyme (e.g. AChE-containing terminals in the cerebral cortex; see Bigl et al. 1982). In addition, although the procedure could be used in conjunction with BuChE histochemistry, it has not yet been so used to any great extent, possibly because little interest currently exists in that cholinesterase.

4.2. PRACTICAL CONSIDERATIONS

Vehicle for DFP

At room temperature (22°C), the organophosphorous compound DFP is a clear, colorless, virtually odorless liquid of extreme toxicity. It has a density of 1.06 g/ml and is readily soluble in ethanol, benzene, chloroform, ether, and vegetable oils. Although it is soluble in water, such solutions are unstable, and DFP is hydrolyzed with a half-life of 16 h. Stable solutions can be prepared with vegetable oils, however, and arachis (peanut) oil has been employed most often as a vehicle for injections. In our hands, DFP-arachis oil solutions have been observed to be stable at 22°C for 1–2 yr. Although potency declines thereafter, this preparation is still usable at later times, but the dose must be increased to achieve the same pharmacologic effect.

Use of atropine methyl sulfate

As an irreversible inhibitor of cholinesterases (Volle 1971), sublethal doses of DFP can reduce brain levels of AChE and BuChE to 30–70% of normal for 1–10 days following injection (Koelle and Gilman 1946; Glow et al. 1966). The concomitant increase in acetylcholine levels will augment the functions subserved by cholinergic systems, and the effects of the organophosphorous compound are most noticeably manifested in the parasympathetic nervous system and at the neuromuscular junction. Readily observable signs of the action of DFP include fasciculation of skeletal muscles, head oscillations and extremity tremors, hyperactivity to touch, secretions of lacrimal glands, profuse salivation, and diarrhea. Although many of these symptoms are not life-threatening, the increased glandular secretions can produce respiratory difficulty, and it is advisable to attenuate these symptoms by pretreating the animal with the peripheral muscarinic blocker atropine methyl sulfate (dose for rat: 1–10 mg/kg administered intraperitoneally) prior to DFP administration.

Optimal dose of DFP

The optimal dose of DFP in the pharmacohistochemical regimen for AChE is defined as the dose that produces the greatest inactivation of the enzyme without being fatal. It follows from this stipulation that the optimal dose of DFP will be very close to the

LD$_{50}$ of the organophosphorous compound.

Factors determining the exact dose of DFP to be administered are the same as those governing the posology of any drug (see Levine 1978). Prominent among these are the route of administration and the health and species of the experimental animal. In this regard, the intramuscular route has been found to be highly satisfactory for most purposes (Butcher et al. 1975; Poirier et al. 1977; Butcher 1978; Woolf and Butcher 1981; Bigl et al. 1982), but we have also used subcutaneous infusions (unpublished procedure from this laboratory) and direct intracerebral injection of DFP (Butcher and Bilezikjian 1975).

Species differences are important, and Table 6 summarizes some of the doses of DFP that have been employed by various authors using the pharmacohistochemical regimen for AChE. For freshly prepared DFP-arachnis oil solutions, we have found 2.0 mg/kg DFP to be satisfactory for healthy adult rats. Rats experiencing respiratory difficulties should be given a lower dose of DFP, 1.5–1.8 mg/kg, preceded by an intraperitoneal injection of atropine methyl sulfate. Very young rats, 1 hour to 14 days postnatal, should be injected subcutaneously in the range 0.5-0.8 mg/kg (unpublished observations from this laboratory).

Choice of an optimal DFP-euthanasia interval

Shorter DFP-euthanasia times are best for visualizing AChE-containing somata and proximal portions of their processes (Fig. 7 and Butcher et al. 1975). With increasing intervals, increasingly more distal portions of processes are observed with a concomitant increase in neuropil activity (Fig. 7 and Butcher et al. 1975). The optimal DFP-euthanasia interval varies somewhat with the region of the nervous system examined but as a general rule cell bodies and their proximal processes are observed best from 4–8 h after DFP whereas distal processes are visualized better at later intervals, usually within the range 8–48 h (Table 7).

5. COMBINED PROCEDURES

5.1. PRELIMINARY COMMENTS AND GENERAL PRINCIPLES

Cholinesterase histochemistry has been and continues to be an extremely valuable tool in neuroanatomic studies alone. Several investigators have used the thiocholinester technique of Koelle and Friedenwald (1949), or variations of it (Table 2), to delineate and characterize, for example, (1) the non-homogeneous organization of the striatum (Butcher and Hodge 1976; Graybiel and Ragsdale 1978); (2) the various subdivisions of

TABLE 6. *Optimal dose of DFP for use in the pharmacohistochemical regimen for AChE*

Species	Adult dose (mg/kg)	Selected references
Rat	1.5–2.2	Butcher et al. (1975)
		Butcher and Talbot (1978)
		Woolf and Butcher (1981)
		Butcher and Woolf (1982a,b)
Cat	0.8–2.0	Parent and O'Reilly-Fromentin (1982)
		Parent et al. (1979)
Monkey	0.2–0.8	Poirier et al. (1977)
		Parent and De Bellefeuille (1982)

TABLE 7. *Optimal DFP-euthanasia intervals for various regions of the rat central nervous system*

Region	DFP-euthanasia interval[a] (h)
Cerebral cortex	12–24
Hippocampal complex	12–24
Basal forebrain (medial septal nucleus, nuclei of the diagonal band, ventral pallidum-substantia innominata region, nucleus basalis)	4–8
Caudate-putamen complex, Nucleus accumbens, and Olfactory tubercle	
Somata and proximal processes	4–8
Distal processes	12–72
Thalamus and Hypothalamus	5–10
Substantia nigra	
Somata and proximal processes	4–8
Distal processes	12–48
Pons and Medulla	6–8
Cerebellum	6–12
Spinal cord	
Somata and proximal processes	4–6
Distal processes	8–12

[a]The survival periods indicated are time-ranges reflecting not only variability in rates of distribution and metabolism of DFP in different neural regions, but also what constitutes optimal demonstration of AChE, defined as that providing the maximum figure-ground contrast necessary to attain the goals of a particular experiment. Counterstaining of AChE-processed material for Nissl substance, for example, requires that background be as light as possible, and, accordingly, the shortest indicated time-interval is most appropriate for such experiments. The time-ranges delimited, therefore, bracket DFP-euthanasia intervals found to be most satisfactory for Nissl counterstaining (lowest time-interval), optimal visualization of somata and proximal processes (interval intermediate between range extremes), and detection of more distal processes (upper time-interval). In some neural regions even more distal portions of AChE-containing processes, not necessarily continuous with neuronal somata, are revealed with even longer survival-times; these are specifically indicated.

the lateral thalamic complex (Graybiel and Berson 1980) and different nuclei in the amygdaloid area (Woolf and Butcher 1982); and (3) similar classes of neurons within the nervous system of given organisms (see, e.g. Das and Kreutzberg 1968; Heimer 1978) or across different species (Parent et al. 1979). As noted previously in this chapter, systemic administration of DFP prior to animal euthanasia permits AChE to be localized with a precision impossible to attain in pharmacologically unmanipulated material and, furthermore, reveals the morphologies of cholinesterase-containing neurons to an extent exceeded only by a few neuroanatomic techniques such as the Golgi methods and intracellular infusion of horseradish peroxidase (Butcher and Woolf 1982a,b). Although these features of cholinesterase histochemistry guarantee its continued use in neuroanatomic investigations alone, the power of the method can be increased by using it in combination with various lesion protocols and other histologic and histochemical procedures.

At the present time, AChE (and BuChE) can be simultaneously or sequentially demonstrated, either in pharmacologically unmanipulated or in DFP-treated animals, on the same tissue section with the following substances: (1) Nissl material and myelin; (2) horseradish peroxidase and a variety of neuronally transported fluorescent labels; (3) chemical compounds that can be processed autoradiographically; and (4) peptides (e.g. somatostatin, neurotensin), and other molecular entities that can be visualized by direct or indirect immunohistochemical methods. In addition, it is possible to sequentially visualize on the same tissue section neuronally transported labels, some immunohistochemically demonstrated compounds, cholinesterases, and Nissl material and myelin, as well as any combination of a lesser number of these substances (Woolf and Butcher 1981, 1982; Butcher and Woolf 1982a,b; Bigl et al. 1982).

In combined procedures, the general rule is that the perfusion, fixation, and other tissue processing protocols to be used are those that permit optimal demonstration of the most labile substance. Assume, for example, that the most labile substance in a particular experiment is one that is to be demonstrated immunohistochemically, but that it is also desired to demonstrate neuronally transported fluorescent labels, AChE and Nissl material on the same tissue section. The perfusion and fixation parameters to be employed in an experiment of this type will probably be those permitting optimal visualization of the immunohistochemically demonstrable compound. If immunohistochemistry is not to be performed in a combined method, however, perfusion and fixation parameters other than those appropriate for immunohistochemistry may be employed. The most important guideline in this regard is that the chemical compounds or cellular constituents being studied at a particular time, considered singly or in combination, are demonstrated optimally under the conditions of the experiment to answer the questions being asked.

In the following discourse, some of these combined procedures will be considered, with the focus being on methods developed primarily for use in conjunction with the pharmacohistochemical regimen for AChE. Combined methods based on other AChE protocols have been reviewed, although not extensively, by Silver (1974).

5.2. SIMULTANEOUS DEMONSTRATION OF AChE AND NISSL SUBSTANCE ON THE SAME TISSUE SECTION

Although a variety of Nissl stains can be used in conjunction with AChE histochemistry, thionine and cresyl violet have been employed most extensively. For most applications, the pharmacohistochemical protocol for AChE is the preferred combinative cholinesterase procedure because neuropil staining is attenuated with that regimen, thereby facilitating visualization of perikarya demonstrated by Nissl stains (Fig. 9B, compare with Fig. 2; see also Table 7).

The combined Nissl-AChE procedures used by us have been described in detail by Albanese and Butcher (1980) and Woolf and Butcher (1981). One such procedure is described briefly in the following discourse:

Sections of rat brain are processed for AChE as described previously. They are then mounted on glass slides coated with pig gelatin or chrome alum and allowed to dry at room temperature (22°C) for 12–24 h. The mounted sections are then placed in distilled, deionized water and transferred to absolute ethanol before being immersed for 5 min in a solution containing chloroform, absolute ethanol, and ether in the proportion 8:1:1. This procedure removes superficial lipids. Tissue sections are rehydrated in a graded series of alcohols (100, 95, 70, and 25% ethanol) and stained in a solution containing the following reagents: 2.0 g cresylecht violet, 185 ml 1 M acetic acid, 15 ml 1 M sodium acetate, 400 ml distilled deionized water and 200 ml absolute ethanol. The mounted sections are placed subsequently into successive alcohols of 50, 70, and 95% for 45 s each. The slides are then dipped into two solutions of absolute ethanol and chloroform in the proportion 3:1, rinsed twice in toluene, and coverslipped under Permount®. Microscopic evaluation and subsequent photography are then performed.

An example of the application of this procedure is shown in Figure 9.

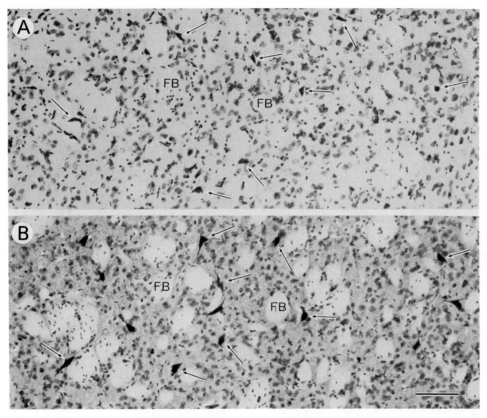

Fig. 9. Caudate-putamen complex of a rat stained with cresyl violet alone (A) or processed for both AChE and Nissl substance on the same brain section (B). Pharmacohistochemical regimen (Butcher and Bilezikjian 1975; Butcher et al. 1975) in B in which the DFP (1.8 mg/kg)-euthanasia interval was 4 h. Arrows point to possible correspondence between intensely chromophillic somata (A) and those large cells staining intensely for AChE (B). Observe that no intensely chromophillic neurons are apparent in B. Scale in B, 100 μm (applies also to A). Rephotographed from a plate originally in color.

5.3. USE OF PATHWAY TRACING PROCEDURES IN COMBINATION WITH AChE HISTOCHEMISTRY

Anterograde and retrograde neuronal degeneration

Among the oldest methods for tracing neuronal connections in the nervous system are those involving lesions and subsequent neuronal degeneration. A variety of lesion techniques (e.g. electrolytic and radio-frequency methods, intracerebral infusion of various cytotoxins such as 6-hydroxy-dopamine, kainic acid and cupric sulfate) can be used in conjunction with AChE histochemistry (Shute and Lewis 1967; Butcher et al. 1974; Butcher 1977, 1978; Butcher and Talbot 1978; Lehmann et al. 1979). After an appropriate survival time to allow for anterograde or retrograde degeneration, the animal is sacrificed, and its brain processed for AChE as described previously. If anterograde degeneration of terminal fields is to be assessed, DFP should not be given prior to euthanasia. If retrograde degeneration of cell bodies is to be assessed, however, then the pharmacohistochemical regimen should be employed because of the improved morphologic detail of somata and proximal processes that if affords. Usually the lesion–sacrifice interval is shorter in anterograde degeneration experiments than in retrograde experiments. An example of anterograde loss of AChE-containing nerve terminals is shown in Figure 10 and of retrograde degeneration in Figure 11.

The injury reaction in neuronal somata after axonal damage is more severe if the lesion is closer to the cell body. Retrograde loss of cell bodies in pars compacta of the substantia nigra, for example, is not complete until 3–4 weeks after a lesion in the

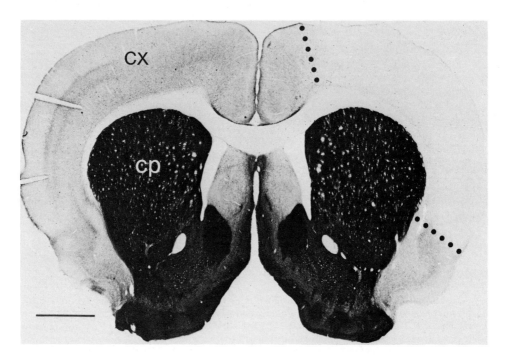

Fig. 10. Loss of AChE activity in the cerebral cortex (area on right between two lines of black dots; compare with left side) of a rat following an ipsilateral radio-frequency lesion of nucleus basalis. Slightly modified Karnovsky-Roots procedure (Butcher et al. 1974) without prior DFP treatment. Scale, 1.6 mm.

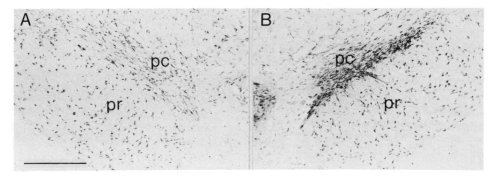

Fig. 11. Retrograde degeneration of AChE-containing neuronal somata in pars compacta of the rat substantia nigra (A, compare with B) following an ipsilateral radio-frequency lesion in the medial forebrain bundle at the level of the lateral hypothalamus. Pharmacohistochemical regimen (Butcher and Bilezikjian 1975); Butcher et al. 1975) in which the DFP (1.5 mg/kg)-euthanasia interval was 6 h. The lesion-sacrifice interval was 21 days. Scale in A, 500 μm (applies also to B).

globus pallidus, a region containing nigro-neostriatal axons relatively distant from their origin (Butcher and Talbot 1978). By comparison, retrograde degeneration of AChE-containing somata in pars compacta of the substantia nigra can be observed within 1 week after a lesion in the ventromedial mesencephalic tegmentum, an area through which axons of the nigro-neostriatal pathway initially course. At even shorter ablation–sacrifice intervals (<48 h), lesions in the ventromedial mesencephalic tegmentum produce accumulation of AChE within nigro-neostriatal axons (Butcher 1977; Butcher and Talbot 1978). A possible explanation for this last-mentioned finding is that the lesion, in addition to destroying neural tissue, disrupts transport mechanisms in nigro-neostriatal axons bordering on the region of cavitation. Since AChE synthesis and somato-axonal transport can continue for a limited time following axonal damage, build-up of the enzyme occurs within fibers between their somata of origin and near their point of severance.

Intracerebral infusion of colchicine

In addition to preventing mitosis by depolymerizing the microtubules of the mitotic spindle, colchicine disrupts the organization of neurotubules. Since neurotubules appear to be involved in axoplasmic transport, punctate intracerebral infusion of colchicine into regions through which AChE-containing axons project produces intracellular accumulation of the enzyme, thereby permitting enhanced visualization of those fibers (Butcher 1977; Butcher and Talbot 1978). In experiments on the trajectories of the nigrostriatal and septohippocampal pathways, it has been found that 0.05 or 0.10% solutions of colchicine (Sigma Chemical Co., St. Louis, MO, USA) are effective in blocking axonal transport of AChE (Butcher 1977; Butcher and Talbot 1978). The rate of infusion is 0.25 μl/min, and a total volume of 0.5 or 1.0 μl is administered (for other details of intracerebral infusion procedures, see Butcher et al. 1974 and elsewhere in this section). Rats are sacrificed 24, 32, or 72 h after colchicine injection, and the brains are subsequently processed for AChE according to the pharmacohistochemical regimen or in pharmacologically unmanipulated animals. When the pharmacohistochemical protocol is employed in combination with intracerebral colchicine infusion, DFP is infused intramuscularly 24 or 48 h prior to animal euthanasia. An example of the application of this combined procedure is shown in Figure 12.

Protein incorporation autoradiography

In this combined protocol, ^{3}H-proline or ^{3}H-leucine is infused into various brain regions according to procedures outlined by Cowan et al. (1972). At various times before or after intracerebral amino acid infusion the animals are given DFP intramuscularly. Choice of time of sacrifice is based on 2 considerations: (1) the interval between ^{3}H-proline or ^{3}H-leucine injection and euthanasia must be sufficient to allow the incorporation of the amino acid into protein and the transport of the protein along axons to terminals of the neuronal projection systems studied; and (2) the period between DFP administration and sacrifice must be appropriate to demonstrate those features of AChE-containing neurons being investigated. To reiterate, cell bodies are demonstrated best at short DFP-euthanasia intervals, but proximal and more distant portions of processes are visualized best at longer intervals (Butcher et al. 1975).

The animals are perfused and their brains are removed from the cranial cavity,

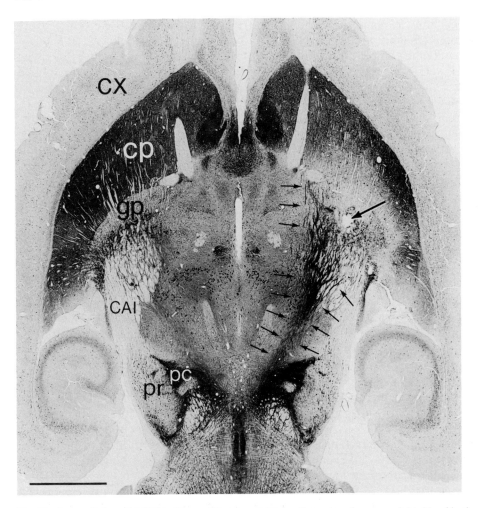

Fig. 12. Accumulation of AChE in fibers of the nigrostriatal pathway (small arrows, right side of brain section) following infusion of 0.05% colchicine into the globus pallidus (cannula tract indicated by large arrow). Rat sacrificed 72 h after intrapallidal colchicine injection. Pharmacohistochemical regimen (Butcher and Bilezikjian 1975; Butcher et al. 1975) in which the DFP (1.5 mg/kg)-euthanasia interval was 48 h. Scale, 2 mm.

postfixed, sectioned, stained for AChE as described previously in this chapter (see also Butcher et al. 1975; Butcher 1978), and mounted on glass slides. These slides are then coated with Kodak NTB-3 liquid emulsion and processed according to standard autoradiography procedures (Kopriwa and LeBlond 1962)*. An important consideration here is the choice of a developer. Although D-19 (Kodak Co., Rochester, NY, USA) is often used to develop autoradiograms and is thought by some investigators to

---

*This same basic procedure can be used to demonstrate on the same tissue section AChE and various radiolabeled compounds (e.g. ^{3}H-quinuclidinyl benzilate, ^{125}I-α-bungarotoxin, ^{3}H-propylbenzilylcholine mustard: New England Nuclear Co., Boston, MA, USA) binding muscarinic and nicotinic receptors (see, e.g. Butcher 1978 and Polz-Tejera et al. 1975; cf. Kuhar and Yamamura 1976).

give the best results in terms of background and contrast considerations (see, e.g. Edwards and Hendrickson 1981), the pH of this developer is 10.2. Hatchett's Brown, one of the final end-products in the Karnovsky-Roots procedure, is soluble in alkalai solutions (Table 4) and, therefore, considerable diffusion and loss of the copper ferrocyanide deposits will occur if D-19 is used to develop autoradiograms prepared in combination with AChE histochemistry based on the direct-coloring method (unpublished observations from this laboratory). A more appropriate developer in this case would be Microdol-X (Kodak Co., Rochester, NY, USA), which has a pH of 7.8 (see, e.g. Fig. 13). Alternatively, AChE could be demonstrated by a procedure that produces a final end-product that is insoluble in alkalai (e.g. lead sulfide in the procedure of Eränkö et al. 1967; see Tables 2 and 4).

Retrogradely and anterogradely transported labels

Horseradish peroxidase and a variety of fluorescent labels can be injected into the brain and spinal cord or applied to peripheral nerves and transported intraneuronally in anterograde and retrograde directions (see Kuypers 1981; Steward 1981; and Warr et al. 1981). Protocols have also been published in which these transported labels have been used in conjunction with AChE histochemistry, both in DFP-treated and in pharmacologically unmanipulated animals (Hardy et al. 1976; Mesulam 1976; Woolf and Butcher 1981, 1982; Bigl et al. 1982). Combined HRP-AChE protocols have been detailed elsewhere by other investigators (Hardy et al. 1976; Mesulam 1976) and will not be considered to any great extent here. Furthermore, as pointed out by us previously (Woolf and Butcher 1981; Bigl et al. 1982), fluorescent labels offer certain advantages compared to horseradish peroxidase when these markers are used in combination with AChE histochemistry. First, the chemical reactions necessary to demonstrate horseradish peroxidase frequently render AChE staining weak and indistinct (Lehmann et al. 1980), possibly increasing the probability of false-negatives in double-staining experiments (see Steward 1981). This problem is not as apparent with anterogradely or retrogradely transported fluorescent labels because they require no chemical processing for their visualization. Second, AChE loci are often difficult to detect in neurons also containing horseradish peroxidase because of the dark and intense color of the horseradish peroxidase reaction product. In combined procedures that we have developed and used *(vide infra),* fluorescent labels and AChE are demonstrated sequentially on the same tissue section under different illumination conditions. The presence of fluorescent compounds in the same neurons containing AChE, therefore, does not interfere significantly, if at all, with cholinesterase visualization. Third, fluorescent labels may be the most sensitive tools presently available for the demonstration of neuronal pathways. Sawchenko and Swanson (1981) found that considerably more cells were labelled in the paraventricular nucleus after spinal injections of True Blue or bisbenzimide than after spinal infusions of horseradish peroxidase. Finally, combined fluorescent tracer and AChE histochemical procedures are relatively simple and can be performed comparatively rapidly.

Among the fluorescent labels that have been used to trace neural pathways have been Evans Blue (Merck 3169), DAPI (4'-6-diamidino-2-phenylindol-dihydrochoride, Serva 18860), Primuline (Eastman 1039), bisbenzimide (Hoechst 33258), Nuclear Yellow (Hoechst S79121), propidium iodide (Sigma P-5264), True Blue [trans-1,2-bis(5-amido-2-benzofuramyl)ethylenedihydrochloride], granular blue {2-[4-(4-amidinophenoxy) phenyl]indol-6-carboxamidin-dihydrochloride}, and Fast Blue [trans-1-(5-amidino-2-

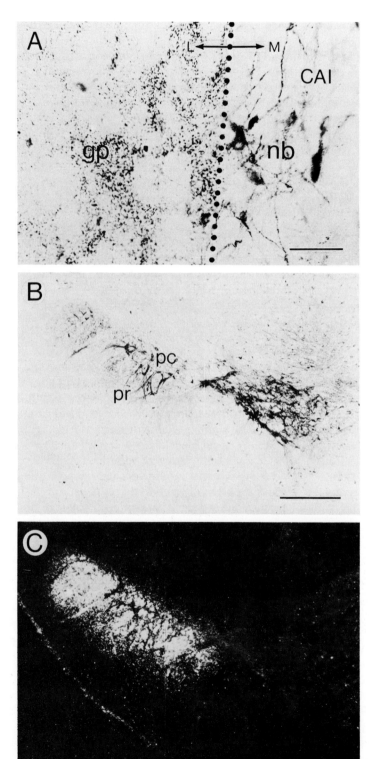

benzofumramyl)-2-(6-amidino-2-indolyl)ethylene-dihydrochloride)] (for further discussion, see Kuypers 1981).

Although many, if not all, of the above-delimited fluorescent labels could probably be used in conjunction with AChE histochemistry, Evans Blue and DAPI have been employed to the greatest extent in combined protocols at the present time (Woolf and Butcher 1981, 1982; Bigl et al. 1982). One such procedure is described below:

The solution of the fluorescent tracer is prepared immediately before infusion. Evans Blue, for example, is used as an aqueous solution or solution-suspension in concentrations of 10, 20, or 30% and DAPI is made up as a 2.5% aqueous solution. A 1-μl syringe with permanently attached cannula (outer diameter: 0.5 mm) or glass micropipettes (outer diameter: 50–100 μm) affixed to a microliter syringe are used to inject the fluorescent labels. Infusions are made slowly (0.005–0.02 μl/min) and the cannula is allowed to remain in place for 2–10 min following tracer delivery before being withdrawn slowly. Survival times vary and are determined experimentally to provide optimal labeling. Optimal labeling is defined as that giving most intense fluorescence, good morphologic detail, and absence of glial staining. For the nigrostriatal pathway, for example, we have found a survival time of 48 h to be optimal for labeling of nigral somata containing AChE following intrastriatal Evans Blue infusion (Woolf and Butcher 1981). Similar survival times were also found best for double-labeling of AChE-containing cell bodies in the basal forebrain following intracortical infusion of Evans Blue and a DAPI/primuline mixture (Bigl et al. 1982).

Following appropriate tracer infusion–euthanasia intervals, the animals are anesthetized with 350 mg/kg chloral hydrate or another appropriate agent. They are then perfused with saline and fixative as described previously for AChE histochemistry. After postfixation and sucrose immersion, sections of appropriate thickness (e.g. 40 μm) are prepared and collected into cold 0.9% saline before being mounted on glass slides precoated with pig gelatin or chrome alum. The sections are then dried at 22°C, rinsed in distilled deionized water, air-dried again, and coverslipped under mineral oil (Nujol®, Plough, Inc., Memphis, TN, USA). The slides thus prepared are examined within 48 h with a fluorescence microscope equipped with filters appropriate to visualize the tracers being used (see Kuypers 1981; Steward 1981).

Following photography and the recording of the location on the microscope stage of the regions photographed, the slides are taken from the stage and their coverslips removed manually. The slides are blotted on absorbent paper, immersed in xylene for 1 min to remove the mineral coverslipping medium, blotted again to remove excess xylene, and allowed to air-dry. The mounted brain sections are then rinsed in 0.9% saline for 2 min and subsequently processed for AChE. Three to six glass slides are first placed for 30 min into Coplin jars containing 30 μM iso-OMPA to inhibit BuChE. The iso-OMPA solution is then poured out and replaced with the AChE reaction mixture described previously in this chapter (see Section 3.2, under 'Conspectus and recommended procedure'). Incubation with mild agitation is carried out at 22°C for 4–12 h, depending on the length of time necessary to visualize the AChE reaction product most clearly in the neurons being studied. Appropriate control experiments for the specificity of the reaction are also performed (see Section 3.2, under 'Conspectus and recommended procedure').

After the histochemical reaction for AChE is complete, the slides are removed from the

---

Fig. 13. Simultaneous demonstration of ³H-proline and AChE on the same rat brain section. Frames B and C show the same region of the substantia nigra visualized with bright-field (B) and dark-field (C) illumination. For the data portrayed in all frames, ³H-proline was infused into the caudate-putamen complex 60 h prior to animal sacrifice. Pharmacohistochemical regimen for AChE (Butcher and Bilezikjian 1975; Butcher et al. 1975) in which the DFP (1.5 mg/kg)-euthanasia interval was 4 (A) or 16 (B, C) h. In Frame *A*, most of the exposed silver grains (dark puncta to the left of the line of black dots) representing the terminals of the striatopallidal pathway are found in association with globus pallidus and not nucleus basalis. In addition, most of the terminals of the striatonigral pathway are found in pars reticulata and not pars compacta of the substantia nigra (B, C). L = lateral; M = medial. Scale in A, 50 μm. Scale in B, 400 μm (applies also to C).

Coplin jars, rinsed in distilled water, air-dried, immersed in xylene, and coverslipped under Permount® . The same regions of the brain examined for neurons labeled with fluorescent tracer are then analyzed with bright- or dark-field illumination for the presence of AChE-containing cells. Some or all of these brain sections may be additionally counterstained with cresyl violet as described elsewhere in this chapter.

An example of brain tissue processed sequentially for a fluorescent tracer and AChE (pharmacohistochemical regimen) is shown in Figure 14.

5.4. SEQUENTIAL DEMONSTRATION OF CATECHOLAMINES AND AChE ON THE SAME TISSUE SECTION

In this procedure animals are prepared either with or without systemic DFP treatment. In some cases, nialamide, a monoamine oxidase inhibitor (Pfizer Inc., Brooklyn, NY, USA), may also be given prior to euthanasia in order to enhance catecholamine fluorescence. Nialamide pretreatment does not affect AChE staining. Similarly, DFP does not affect catecholamine fluorescence, at least as assessed histochemically (Albanese and Butcher 1979, 1980).

Animals are then killed by decapitation. Their brains are removed within 1.5 min from the cranial cavity, cut into 4–6 mm slabs, mounted on brass specimen holders, frozen in a cryostat maintained at −25°C, and cut at 6-, 8-, or 10-μm intervals. The brain sections are mounted on glass slides and reacted with glyoxylic acid according to the procedure of De La Torre and Surgeon (1976). The slides are then coverslipped under mineral oil and are subsequently examined in fluorescence microscope. (For further details on the aldehyde histofluorescence procedure for monoamines, the reader is referred to Chapter II).

Following the recording of the location of the slide on the microscope stage and subsequent photography of catecholamines, the coverslip is removed manually and the brain section processed for AChE as described in Section 5.3 under 'Retrogradely and anterogradely transported labels'. After AChE staining, the brain sections are coverslipped under mineral oil if further thionin or cresyl violet staining is to be done later or under Permount® if no further processing is deemed necessary or if Nissl substance is demonstrated immediately after AChE for simultaneous visualization. The same areas of the brain photographed after catecholamine histochemistry are then photographed for AChE. Examples of the application of this combined protocol are shown in Figure 15.

5.5. SEQUENTIAL VISUALIZATION OF IMMUNOHISTOCHEMICALLY DE-MONSTRABLE SUBSTANCES AND AChE ON THE SAME TISSUE SECTION

The immunohistochemical procedure currently most satisfactory for use in conjunction with AChE histochemistry is the indirect method described first by Weller and Coons (1954). One such combined protocol for rats is described in the following discourse (cf. also Chapter IV):

Animals are anesthetized with chloral hydrate (350 mg/kg) or ethyl carbamate (1.5 g/kg). They are then perfused transcardially with 50 ml cold (3–6°C) phosphate-buffered saline (PBS, pH = 7.2) during a 2-min period followed by perfusion with 300–500 ml of a fixative consisting of 4% paraformaldehyde in 0.1 M phosphate buffer for 30 min. The brain and spinal cord are then extracted and immersed in the above fixative for 90 min at 4°C. The fixative is removed and replaced with 5% sucrose in 0.1 M phosphate buffer (pH = 7.2). The tissue remains in this last solution for 12–14 h. The brain (or spinal cord) is then blocked, plac-

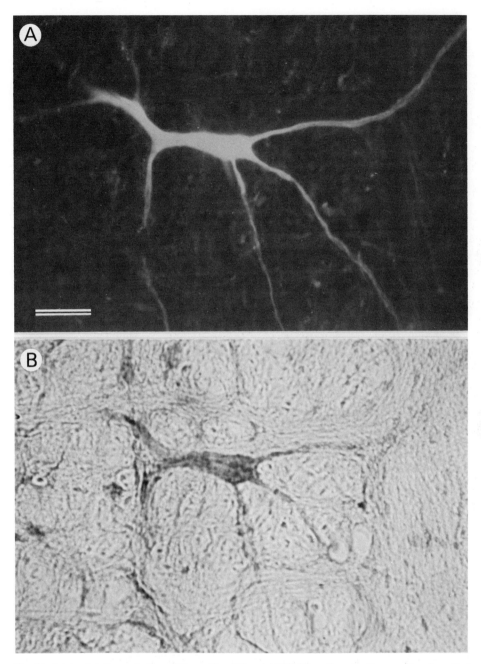

Fig. 14. Sequential demonstration of Evans Blue (A) and AChE (B) on the same tissue section from the brain stem raphe of the rat. The red fluorescent label (30% solution, 0.1 μl) was infused into the substantia nigra 48 h prior to animal sacrifice. Pharmacohistochemical regimen for AChE (Butcher and Bilezikjian 1975; Butcher et al. 1975) in which the DFP (1.8 mg/kg)-euthanasia interval was 4 h. Scale in A, 35 μm (applies also to B). Rephotographed from a plate originally in color.

ed on a brass specimen holder, and cut at 8–10 μm intervals in a cryostat maintained at -20 to $-30°$C. The resulting sections are mounted on glass slides precoated with 0.5% gelatin in

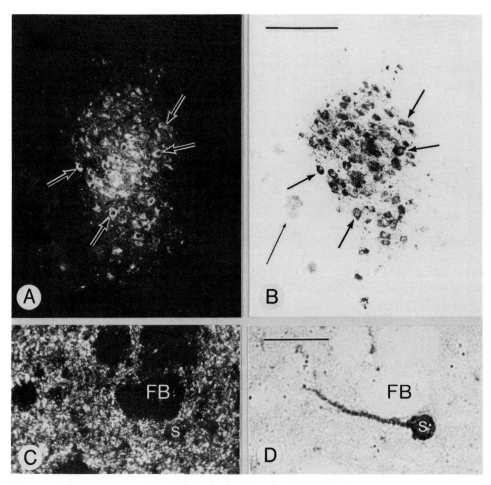

Fig. 15. Sequential demonstration of catecholamines (A, C) and AChE (B, D) on the same rat brain section. Frames A and B depict the locus ceruleus, and Frames C and D show the caudate-putamen complex. Pharmacohistochemical regimen for AChE (Butcher and Bilezikjian 1975; Butcher et al. 1975) in which the DFP (1.8 mg/kg)-euthanasia interval was 4 h. S = soma. Scale in B, 200 μm (applies also to A). Scale in D, 50 μm (applies also to C).

0.05% chromium potassium sulfate·12H$_2$0. Slides are maintained at 4°C until processed, usually within 24 h.

The tissue sections are brought to room temperature (22°C) and encircled with nail polish. A solution of 0.3% Triton X-100 in PBS is then added dropwise to cover each tissue section for 15–45 min. The Triton X-PBS is removed with a Pasteur pipette. The primary antibody, diluted appropriately in Triton X-PBS, is applied and the sections incubated for 12–14 h in a closed, high-humidity chamber. Excess antibody solution is removed from the tissue and the slides immersed in PBS for 15 min. Excess PBS is blotted from the slide and fluorescein-conjugated second antibody, diluted 1:10 or higher in Triton X-PBS, is applied to the tissue sections; incubation continues at 37°C for 30 min in a closed, high-humidity chamber. The slides are then rinsed with PBS as described previously and coverslipped under glycerine/PBS (3:1; v/v). Controls for specificity are performed on adjacent tissue sections subjected to above procedures except that the primary antibody is pretreated with an excess of antigen prior to tissue section incubation.

Following fluorescence microscopic examination of slides, the coverslips are removed and the brain sections processed for AChE and/or other histologic and histochemical entities as outlined elsewhere in this section.

An example of this combined protocol, in which choline-0-acetyltransferase and AChE (pharmacohistochemical regimen) are demonstrated on the same brain section, is shown in Figure 16.

6. FUTURE OF AChE HISTOCHEMISTRY

Some neuroscientists believe that the value of AChE histochemistry can be judged only to the extent that the enzyme co-exists in cholinergic neurons (i.e. those that synthesize and use acetylcholine to communicate with other tissue entities). As indicated in this chapter, however, the histochemical analysis of AChE in the nervous system has proven extremely worthwhile in anatomic investigations alone. Furthermore, when correlative experiments are done comparing the distribution of neurons demonstrating choline-0-acetyltransferase-like immunoreactivity with those demonstrating AChE, it is possible that all cholinergic neurons will have a characteristic pattern of cholinesterase activity, particularly following a DFP challenge (Butcher and Woolf 1982a,b). If so, then the study of AChE-containing neurons having that unique staining profile will, in fact, be a study of cholinergic neurons, and a whole host of proven combinative procedures can be brought to bear to investigate central cholinergic systems and their relationships with other histochemically identifiable cellular aggregates. The future of AChE histochemistry would appear, therefore, to be indeed bright.

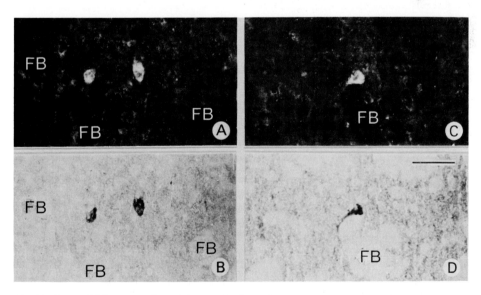

Fig. 16. Sequential demonstration on the same brain section of neuronal somata in the rat caudate-putamen complex demonstrating choline-O-acetyltransferase-like immunoreactivity (A, C) and AChE (B, D). Pharmacohistochemical regimen for AChE (Butcher and Bilezikjian 1975; Butcher et al. 1975) in which the DFP (1.8 mg/kg)-euthanasia interval was 4 h. All striatal neurons displaying intense AChE activity and having the reaction product mosaically organized in the somata and proximal processes also demonstrated choline-O-acetyltransferase-like immunoreactivity (see also Butcher and Woolf 1982a,b). Scale, 50 μm (applies to all frames).

7. ACKNOWLEDGEMENTS

I wish to thank all of those individuals who, at one time or another, were members of my laboratory and who contributed to the development and use of many of the procedures indicated in this chapter. Without them the writing of this chapter would have been impossible.

8. REFERENCES

Adams DH (1949): The specificity of the human erythrocyte cholinesterase. *Biochim. Biophys. Acta, 3,* 1–14.

Albanese A, Butcher LL (1979): Locus ceruleus somata contain both acetylcholinesterase and norepinephrine: Direct histochemical demonstration on the same tissue section. *Neurosci. Lett., 14,* 101–104.

Albanese A, Butcher LL (1980): Acetylcholinesterase and catecholamine distribution in the locus ceruleus of the rat. *Brain Res. Bull., 5,* 127–134.

Alles GA, Hawes RC (1940): Cholinesterases in the blood of man. *J. Biol. Chem., 133,* 375–390.

Anderson PJ (1967): Purification and quantitation of glutaraldehyde and its effect on several enzyme activities in skeletal muscle. *J. Histochem. Cytochem., 15,* 652–661.

Augustinsson K-B (1948): Cholinesterases. A study in comparative enzymology. *Acta Physiol. Scand., 15, Suppl. 52,* 1–182.

Augustinsson K-B, Nachmansohn D (1949): Distinction between acetylcholinesterase and other cholinester-splitting enzymes. *Science, 110,* 98-99.

Austin L, Phillis JW (1965): The distribution of cerebellar cholinesterases in several species. *J. Neurochem., 12,* 709–717.

Bayliss BJ, Todrick A (1956): The use of a selective acetylcholinesterase inhibitor in the estimation of pseudo-cholinesterase activity in rat brain. *Biochem. J., 62,* 62–67.

Bell C (1966): Use of the direct-coloring thiocholine technique for demonstration of intracellular neuronal cholinesterases. *J. Histochem. Cytochem., 14,* 567–570.

Benda P, Tsuji S, Daussant J, Changeux J-P (1970): Localization of acetylcholinesterase by immunofluorescence in eel electroplax. *Nature, 225,* 1149–1150.

Bergmeyer HU (1963): *Methods of Enzymatic Analysis.* Academic Press, New York.

Bergner AD, Bayliss MW (1952): Histochemical detection of fatal anticholinesterase poisoning. *US Armed Forces Med. J., 3,* 1637–1644.

Bigl V, Woolf NJ, Butcher LL (1982): Cholinergic projections form the basal forebrain to frontal, parietal, temporal, occipital, and cingulate cortices: A combined fluorescent tracer and acetylcholinesterase analysis. *Brain Res. Bull., 8,* 727–749.

Blaber LC, Creasey NH (1960): The mode of recovery of cholinesterase activity in vivo after organophosphorus poisoning. 2. Brain cholinesterase. *Biochem. J., 77,* 597–604.

Brzin M, Tennyson VM, Duffy PE (1966): Acetylcholinesterase in frog sympathetic and dorsal root ganglia. A study by electron-microscope cytochemistry and microgasometric analysis with the magnetic diver. *J. Cell Biol., 31,* 215–242.

Butcher LL (1977): Nature and mechanisms of cholinergicmonoaminergic interactions in the brain. *Life Sci., 21,* 1207–1226.

Butcher LL (1978): Recent advances in histochemical techniques for the study of central cholinergic mechanisms. In: Jenden DJ (Ed), *Cholinergic Mechanisms and Psychopharmacology,* pp. 93–124. Plenum Press, New York.

Butcher LL, Bilezikjian L (1975): Acetylcholinesterase-containing neurons in the neostriatum and substantia nigra revealed after punctate intracerebral injection of di-isopropylfluorophosphate. *Eur. J. Pharmacol., 34,* 115–125.

Butcher LL, Hodge GK (1976): Postnatal development of acetylcholinesterase in the caudate-putamen nucleus and substantia nigra of rats. *Brain Res., 106,* 223–240.

Butcher LL, Marchand R (1978): Dopamine neurons in pars compacta of the substantia nigra contain acetylcholinesterase: Histochemical correlations on the same brain section. *Eur. J. Pharmacol., 52,* 415–417.

Butcher LL, Talbot K (1978): Acetylcholinesterase in rat nigro-neostriatal neurons: Experimental verification and evidence for cholinergic-dopaminergic interactions in the substantia nigra and caudate-putamen complex. In: Butcher LL (Ed), *Cholinergic-Monoaminergic Interactions in the Brain,* pp. 25–95. Academic Press, New York.

Butcher LL, Woolf NJ (1982a): Monoaminergic-cholinergic relationships and the chemical communication matrix of the substantia nigra and neostriatum. *Brain Res. Bull., 9,* 10–280.

Butcher LL, Woolf NJ (1982b): Cholinergic and serotonergic systems in the brain and spinal cord: Anatomic organization, role in intercellular communication processes, and interactive mechanisms. In: Buijs RM, Pévet P, Swaab DF (Eds), *Chemical Transmission in the Brain, Progress in Brain Research, Vol. 55,* pp. 3–40. Elsevier Biomedical Press, Amsterdam.

Butcher LL, Eastgate SM, Hodge GK (1974): Evidence that punctate intracerebral administration of 6-hydroxydopamine fails to produce selective neuronal degeneration: Comparison with copper sulfate and factors governing the deportment of fluids injected into the brain. *Naunyn-Schmiedeberg's Arch. Pharmacol., 285,* 31–70.

Butcher LL, Talbot K, Bilezikjian L (1975): Acetylcholinesterase neurons in dopamine-containing regions of the brain. *J. Neural Transm., 37,* 127–153.

Cisson CM, Wilson BW (1977): Recovery of acetylcholinesterase in cultured chick embryo muscle treated with paraoxon. *Biochem. Pharmacol., 26,* 1955–1960.

Coërs C (1953): La détection histochimique de la cholinestérase au niveau de la jonction neuro-musculaire. *Rev. Belge Pathol. Med. Exp., 22,* 306–315.

Coutreaux R (1951): Remarques sur les méthodes actuelles de détection histochimique des activités cholinestérasiques. *Arch. Intern. Physiol., 59,* 526–537.

Coutreaux R, Taxi J (1952): Recherches histochimiques sur la distribution des activités cholinestérasiques au niveau de la synapse myoneurale. *Arch. Anat. Microsc. Morphol. Exp., 41,* 352–392.

Cowan WM, Gottlieb DI, Hendrickson AE, Price JL, Woolsey TA (1972): The autoradiographic demonstration of axonal connections in the central nervous system. *Brain Res., 37,* 21–51.

Crevier M, Bélanger LF (1955): Simple method for histochemical detection of esterase activity. *Science, 122,* 556.

Cuello AC (1978): Immunocytochemical studies of the distribution of neurotransmitters and related substances in CNS. In: Iversen LL, Iversen SD, Snyder SH (Eds), *Handbook of Psychopharmacology, Vol. 9,* pp. 69–137. Plenum Press, New York.

Cunningham L (1967): Histochemical observations of the enzymatic hydrolysis of gelatin films. *J. Histochem. Cytochem., 15,* 292–298.

Dale HH (1914): The action of certain esters and ethers of choline, and their relation to muscarine. *J. Pharmacol. Exp. Ther., 6,* 147–190.

Daoust R (1965): Histochemical localization of enzyme activities by substrate film methods: Ribonucleases, deoxyribonucleases, proteases, amylase and hyaluronidase. *Int. Rev. Cytol., 18,* 191–221.

Das GD, Kreutzberg GW (1968): Evaluation of interstitial nerve cells in the central nervous system: A correlative study using acetylcholinesterase and Golgi techniques. *Ergeb. Anat. Entwicklungsgesch., 41,* 1–58.

Davis MD (1973): *Game Theory.* Basic Books Inc., New York.

De La Torre JC, Surgeon JW (1976): A methodological approach to rapid and sensitive monoamine histofluorescence using a modified glyoxylic acid technique: The SPG method. *Histochemistry, 49,* 81–93.

Denz FA (1953): On the histochemistry of the myoneural junction. *Br. J. Exp. Pathol., 34,* 329–339.

Dikshit BB (1934): Action of acetylcholine on the brain and its occurrence therein. *J. Physiol., 80,* 409–421.

Eckenstein F, Thoenen H (1982): Production of specific antisera and monoclonal antibodies to choline acetyltransferase: Characterization and use of identification of cholinergic neurons, *EMBO J., 1,* 363–368.

Edwards SB, Hendrickson A (1981): The autoradiographic tracing of axonal connections in the central nervous system. In: Heimer L, RoBards MJ (Eds), *Neuroanatomical Tract-tracing Methods,* pp. 171–205. Plenum Press, New York.

Emson PC, Lindvall O (1979): Distribution of putative neurotransmitters in the neocortex. *Neuroscience, 4,* 1–30.

Enzyme Commission (1965): *Enzyme Nomenclature. Recommendations (1964) of the International Union of Biochemistry on the Nomenclature and Classification of Enzymes together with their Units and the Symbols of Enzyme Kinetics.* Elsevier, Amsterdam.

Eränkö O, Härkönen M, Kokko A, Räisänen L (1964): Histochemical and starch gel electrophoretic characterization of desmo- and lyo-esterases in the sympathetic and spinal ganglia of the rat. *J. Histochem. Cytochem., 12,* 570–581.

Eränkö O, Koelle GB, Räisänen L (1967): A thiocholine-lead ferrocyanide method for acetylcholinesterase. *J. Histochem. Cytochem., 15,* 674–679.

Eto M (1974): *Organophosphorus Pesticides: Organic and Biological Chemistry.* CRC Press, Cleveland, OH.

Florkin M, Stotz EH (Eds) (1973): *Comprehensive Biochemistry, Vol. 13, Enzyme Nomenclature, 3rd ed.* Elsevier, Amsterdam.

Friede RL (1966): *Topographic Brain Chemistry.* Academic Press, New York.

Fukuda T, Koelle GB (1959): The cytological localization of intracellular neuronal acetylcholinesterase. *J. Biophys. Biochem. Cytol., 5,* 433–440.

Gatenby JB, Beams HW (1950): *The Microtomist's Vademecum (Bolles Lee), 11th ed.* Churchill, London.

Gisiger V, Vigny M (1977): A specific form of acetylcholinesterase is secreted by rat sympathetic ganglia. *FEBS Lett., 84,* 253–256.

Glow PH, Rose S, Richardson A (1966): The effect of acute and chronic treatment with diisopropyl fluorophosphate on cholinesterase activities of some tissues of the rat. *Aust. J. Exp. Biol. Med. Sci., 44,* 73–86.

Goldstein A, Aronow L, Kalman SM (1974): *Principles of Drug Action: The Basis of Pharmacology, 2nd ed.,* pp. 7–9. Wiley, New York.

Gomori G (1948): Histochemical demonstration of sites of choline esterase activity. *Proc. Soc. Exp. Biol., 68,* 354–358.

Gomori G (1952): *Microscopic Histochemistry.* University of Chicago Press, Chicago.

Graybiel AM, Berson DM (1980): Histochemical identification and afferent connections of subdivisions in the lateralis posterior-pulvinar complex and related thalamic nuclei in the cat. *Neuroscience, 5,* 1175–1238.

Graybiel AM, Ragsdale Jr CW (1978): Histochemically distinct compartments in the striatum of human, monkey, and cat demonstrated by acetylthiocholinesterase staining. *Proc. Nat. Acad. Sci. USA, 75,* 5723–5726.

Grubić Z, Sketelj J, Klinar B, Brzin M (1981): Recovery of acetylcholinesterase in the diaphragm, brain, and plasma of the rat after irreversible inhibition by soman: A study of cytochemical localization and molecular forms of the enzyme in the motor end plate. *J. Neurochem., 37,* 909–916.

Hardwick DC, Palmer AC (1961): Effect of formalin fixation on cholinesterase activity in sheep brain. *Q. J. Exp. Physiol., 46,* 350–352.

Hardy H, Heimer L, Switzer R, Watkins D (1976): Simultaneous demonstration of horseradish peroxidase and acetylcholinesterase. *Neurosci. Lett., 3,* 1–5.

Hartman BK, Zide D, Udenfriend S (1972): The use of dopamine-β-hydroxylase as a marker for the central noradrenergic nervous system in rat brain. *Proc. Nat. Acad. Sci. USA, 69,* 2722–2726.

Hawkins RD, Mendel B (1946): True cholinesterases with pronounced resistance to eserine. *J. Cell. Comp. Physiol., 27,* 69–85.

Heimer L (1978): The olfactory cortex and the ventral striatum. In: Livingston KE, Hornykiewicz O (Eds), *Limbic Mechanisms: The Continuing Evolution of the Limbic System Concept,* pp. 95–187. Plenum Press, New York.

Holt SJ (1958): Indogogenic staining methods for esterases. In: Danelli JF (Ed), *General Cytochemical Methods,* pp. 375–398. Academic Press, New York.

Holt SJ, O'Sullivan DG (1958): Studies in enzyme cytochemistry. I. Principles of cytochemical staining methods. *Proc. R. Soc. London, Ser. B., 148,* 465–480.

Holt SJ, Withers RFJ (1952): Cytochemical localization of esterase using indoxyl derivatives. *Nature, 170,* 1012–1014.

Hunt R (1899): Direct and reflex acceleration of the mammalian heart with some observations on the relations of the inhibitory and accelerator nerves. *Am. J. Physiol., 2,* 395–470.

Hunt R, Taveau R de M (1906): On the physiological action of certain choline derivatives and new methods for detecting choline. *Brit. Med. J., 2,* 1788–1791.

Hunt R, Taveau R de M (1909): On the relation between the toxicity and chemical constitution of a number of derivatives of choline and analogous compounds. *J. Pharmacol. Exp. Ther., 1,* 303–339.

Joh TH, Geghman C, Reis D (1973): Immunochemical demonstration of increased accumulation of tyrosine hydroxylase protein in sympathetic ganglia and adrenal medulla elicited by reserpine. *Proc. Nat. Acad. Sci. USA, 70,* 2767–2771.

Karnovsky MJ, Roots L (1964): A 'direct-coloring' thiocholine method for cholinesterase. *J. Histochem. Cytochem., 12,* 219–221.

Kiernan JA (1981): *Histological and Histochemical Methods: Theory and Practice.* Pergamon Press. Oxford.

Koelle GB (1950): The histochemical differentiation of types of cholinesterases and their localizations in tissues of the cat. *J. Pharmacol. Exp. Ther., 100,* 158–179.

Koelle GB (1951): The elimination of enzyme diffusion artifacts in the histochemical localization of cholinesterases and a survey of their cellular distributions. *J. Pharmacol. Exp. Ther., 103,* 153–171.

Koelle GB (1953): Cholinesterase of the tissues and sera of rabbits. *Biochem. J., 53,* 217–226.

Koelle GB (1954): The histochemical localization of cholinesterases in the central nervous system of the rat, *J. Comp. Neurol., 100,* 211–235.

Koelle GB (1955): Cholinesterases of the central nervous system. *J. Neuropathol., 14,* 23–27.

Koelle GB, Friedenwald JS (1949): A histochemical method for localizing cholinesterase activity. *Proc. Soc. Exp. Biol., 70,* 617–622.

Koelle GB, Gilman A (1946): The relationship between cholinesterase inhibition and the pharmacological action of di-isopropyl fluorophosphate (DFP). *J. Pharmacol. Exp. Ther., 87,* 421–434.

Koelle GB, Gromadzki CG (1966): Comparison of the gold-thiocholine and gold-thiolacetic acid methods for the histochemical localization of acetylcholinesterase and cholinesterases. *J. Histochem. Cytochem., 14,* 443–454.

Koelle WA, Hossaini KS, Akbarzadeh P, Koelle GB (1970): Histochemical evidence and consequences of the occurrence of isoenzymes of acetylcholinesterase. *J. Histochem. Cytochem., 18,* 812–819.

Koelle GB, Davis R, Koelle WA (1974): Effects of aldehyde fixation and of preganglionic denervation on acetylcholinesterase and butyrocholinesterase of cat autonomic ganglia. *J. Histochem. Cytochem., 22,* 244–251.

Kokko A, Mautner HG, Barrnett RJ (1969): Fine structural localization of acetylcholinesterase using acetyl-β-methylthiocholine and acetylselenocholine as substrates. *J. Histochem. Cytochem., 17,* 625–640.

Kopriwa BM, LeBlond CP (1962): Improvements in the coating technique of radioautography. *J. Histochem. Cytochem., 10,* 269–284.

Kuhar MJ, Yamamura HI (1976): Localization of cholinergic muscarinic receptors in rat brain by light-microscopic radioautography. *Brain Res., 110,* 229–243.

Kuypers HGJM (1981): Procedure for retrograde double labeling with fluorescent substances. In: Heimer L, RoBards MJ (Eds), *Neuroanatomical Tract-tracing Methods,* pp. 299–303. Plenum Press, New York.

Lehmann J, Fibiger HC, Butcher LL (1979): The localization of acetylcholinesterase in the corpus striatum and substantia nigra of the rat following kainic acid lesion of the corpus striatum: A biochemical and histochemical study. *Neuroscience, 4,* 217–225.

Lehmann J, Nagy JI, Atmadja S, Fibiger HC (1980): The nucleus basalis magnocellularis: The origin of a cholinergic projection to the neocortex of the rat. *Neuroscience, 5,* 1161–1174.

Levine RR (1978): *Pharmacology: Drug Actions and Reactions, 2nd ed.* Little, Brown and Co, Boston.

Lewis PR (1961): The effect of varying the conditions in the Koelle technique. *Bibl. Anat., 2,* 11–20.

Lillie RD (1965): *Histopathologic Technic and Practical Histochemistry, 3rd ed.* McGraw-Hill, New York.

Loewi O, Navratil E (1926): Über humorale Übertragbarkeit der Herznervenwirkung. XI. Über den Mechanismus der Vaguswirkung von Physostigmin und Ergotamin. *Pflügers Arch., 214,* 689–696.

Malmgren H, Sylvén B (1955): On the chemistry of the thiocholine method of Koelle. *J. Histochem. Cytochem., 3,* 441–445.

Marnay A, Nachmansohn D (1938): Cholinesterase in voluntary muscle. *J. Physiol. (London), 92,* 37–47.

Martinez Rodriguez R, Riba Soto A, Moya Mangas J (1964): Demostración de la activad acetilcolinesterasica con un nuevo metado histoquimica. *Trab. Inst. Cajal Invest. Biol., 56,* 27–39.

Massoulié J, Bon S (1982): The molecular forms of cholinesterase and acetylcholinesterase in vertebrates. In: Cowan WM, Hall ZW, Kandel ER (Eds), *Annual Review of Neuroscience, Vol. 5,* pp. 57–106. Annual Reviews, Palo Alto, CA.

Mazurkiewicz JE, Hossler FE, Barrnett RJ (1978): Cytochemical demonstration of sodium, potassium-adenosine triphosphatase by a hemepeptide derivative of ouabain. *J. Histochem. Cytochem., 26,* 1042–1052.

McGeer PL, McGeer EG, Singh VK, Chase WH (1974): Choline acetyltransferase localization in the central nervous system by immunohistochemistry. *Brain Res., 81,* 373–379.

Mendel B, Rudney H (1943): Studies on cholinesterase. 1. Cholinesterase and pseudo-cholinesterase. *Biochem. J., 37,* 59–63.

Mendel B, Mundell DB, Rudney H (1943): Studies on cholinesterase. 3. Specific tests for true cholinesterase and pseudo-cholinesterase. *Biochem. J., 37,* 473–476.

Mesulam M-M (1976): A horseradish peroxidase method for the identification of the efferents of acetylcholinesterase-containing neurons. *J. Histochem. Cytochem., 24,* 1281–1286.

Nachmansohn D (1940): Cholinesterase in brain and spinal cord of sheep embryos. *J. Neurophysiol., 3,* 396–402.

Nichols CW, Koelle GB (1967): Acetylcholinesterase: Method for demonstration in amacrine cells of rabbit retina. *Science, 155,* 477–478.

Nichols CW, Koelle GB (1968): Comparison of the localization of acetylcholinesterase and nonspecific cholinesterase activities in mammalian and avian retinas. *J. Comp. Neurol., 133*, 1–16.

Oosterbaan RA, Jansz HS (1965): Cholinesterases, esterases and lipases. In: Florkin M, Stotz EH (Eds), *Comprehensive Biochemistry, Vol. 16*, pp. 1–73. Elsevier, Amsterdam.

Ostrowski K, Barnard EA (1961): Application of isotopically-labelled specific inhibitors as a method in enzyme cytochemistry. *Exp. Cell. Res., 25*, 465–468.

Parent A, Butcher LL (1976): Organization and morphologies of acetylcholinesterase-containing neurons in the thalamus and hypothalamus of the rat. *J. Comp. Neurol., 170*, 205–226.

Parent A, De Bellefeuille L (1982): Organization of efferent projections from the internal segment of globus pallidus in primate as revealed by fluorescence retrograde labeling method. *Brain Res., 245*, 201–213.

Parent A, O'Reilly-Fromentin J (1982): Distribution and morphological characteristics of acetylcholinesterase-containing neurons in the basal forebrain of the cat. *Brain Res. Bull., 8*, 183–196.

Parent A, Gravel S, Olivier A (1979): The extrapyramidal and limbic systems relationship at the globus pallidus level: A comparative histochemical study in the rat, cat and monkey. In: Poirier LJ, Sourkes TL, Bédard PJ (Eds), *Advances in Neurology, Vol. 24, The Extrapyramidal System and its Disorders*, pp. 1–11. Raven Press, New York.

Pearse AGE (1961): *Histochemistry: Theoretical and Applied, 2nd ed.* Little, Brown and Co, Boston.

Pearse AGE (1972): *Histochemistry: Theoretical and Applied, 3rd ed., Vol. 2.* Williams and Wilkins Co, Baltimore.

Pickel VM, Joh TH, Reis DJ (1976): Monoamine-synthesizing enzymes in central dopaminergic, noradrenergic and serotonergic neurons. Immunocytochemical localization by light- and electron-microscopy. *J. Histochem. Cytochem., 24*, 792–806.

Pochhammer C, Dietsch P, Siegmund PR (1979): Histochemical detection of carbonic anhydrase with dimethylaminonaphthalene-5-sulfonamide. *J. Histochem. Cytochem., 27*, 1103–1107.

Poirier LJ, Parent A, Marchand R, Butcher LL (1977) Morphological characteristics of the acetylcholinesterase-containing neurons in the CNS of DFP-treated monkeys. Part 1. Extrapyramidal and related structures. *J. Neurol. Sci., 31*, 181–198.

Polz-Tejera G, Schmidt J, Karten HJ (1975): Autoradiographic localization of α-bungarotoxin binding sites in the central nervous system. *Nature, 258*, 349–351.

Ravin HA, Zacks SI, Seligman AM (1953): The histochemical localization of acetylcholinesterase in nervous tissue. *J. Pharmacol. Exp. Ther., 107*, 37–53.

Robinson PM (1971): The demonstration of acetylcholinesterase in autonomic axons with the electron-microscope. *Prog. Brain Res., 34*, 357–370.

Rossier J (1981): Serum monospecificity: A prerequisite for reliable immunohistochemical localization of neuronal markers including choline acetyltransferase. *Neuroscience, 6*, 989–991.

Sawchenko PE, Swanson LW (1981): A method for tracing biochemically defined pathways in the central nervous system using combined fluorescence retrograde transport and immunohistochemical techniques. *Brain Res., 210*, 31–51.

Shimizu N, Ishii S (1966): Electron-microscopic histochemistry of acetylcholinesterase of rat brain by Karnovsky's method. *Histochemie, 6*, 24–33.

Shute CCD, Lewis PR (1967): The ascending cholinergic reticular system: Neocortical, olfactory and subcortical projections. *Brain, 90*, 497–520.

Silver A (1974): *The Biology of Cholinesterases.* American Elsevier, New York.

Stedman E, Stedman E (1935): The relative cholinesterase activities of serum and corpuscles from the blood of certain species. *Biochem. J., 29*, 2107–2111.

Stedman E, Stedman E, Easson LH (1932): Cholinesterase. An enzyme present in the blood-serum of the horse. *Biochem. J., 26*, 2056–2066.

Sternberger LA (1979): *Immunocytochemistry, 2nd ed.*, John Wiley and Sons, Inc, New York.

Steward O (1981): Horseradish peroxidase and fluorescent substances and their combination with other techniques. In: Heimer L, RoBards MJ (Eds), *Neuroanatomical Tract-tracing Methods*, pp. 279–310. Plenum Press, New York.

Taxi J (1952): Action du formol sur l'activité de diverses préparations de cholinestérases. *J. Physiol. (Paris), 44*, 595–599.

Tennyson VM, Brzin M, Duffy P (1968): Electron-microscopic cytochemistry and microgasometric analysis of cholinesterase in the nervous system. In: Lajtha A, Ford DH (Eds), *Progress in Brain Research, Vol. 29*, pp. 41–62. Elsevier, Amsterdam.

Tsuji S (1974): On the chemical basis of thiocholine methods for demonstration of acetylcholinesterase activities. *Histochemistry, 42*, 99–110.

Vandesande F (1979): A critical review of immunocytochemical methods for light-microscopy. *J. Neurosci. Meth., 1*, 3–23.

Volle RL (1971): Cholinomimetic drugs. In: DiPalma JR (Ed), *Drill's Pharmacology in Medicine,* pp. 584–607. McGraw-Hill, New York.

Walker CR, Wilson BW (1976): Regulation of acetylcholinesterase in chick muscle cultures after treatment with diisopropylphosphorofluoridate: Ribonucleic acid and protein synthesis. *Neuroscience, 1,* 509–513.

Warr WB, De Olmos JS, Heimer L (1981): Horseradish peroxidase: The basic procedure. In: Heimer L, RoBards MJ (Eds), *Neuroanatomical Tract-tracing Methods,* pp. 207–262. Plenum Press, New York.

Weast RC (Ed) (1970): *Handbook of Chemistry and Physics, 50th ed.* CRC Press, Cleveland, OH.

Weller TH, Coons AH (1954): Fluorescent antibody studies with agents of varicella and herpes zoster propagated in vitro. *Proc. Soc. Exp. Biol., 86,* 789–794.

Woolf NJ, Butcher LL (1981): Cholinergic neurons in the caudate-putamen complex proper are intrinsically organized: A combined Evans Blue and acetylcholinesterase analysis. *Brain Res. Bull., 7,* 487–507.

Woolf NJ, Butcher LL (1982): Cholinergic projections to the basolateral amygdala: A combined Evans Blue and acetylcholinesterase analysis. *Brain Res. Bull., 8,* 751–763.

CHAPTER II

Fluorescence histochemistry of biogenic monoamines

ANDERS BJÖRKLUND

1. INTRODUCTION

The origins of the fluorescence histochemical technique for monoamines date back to the observations of Erös (1932), Eränkö (1952) and Barter and Pearse (1953, 1955) about formalin-induced fluorescence in enterochromaffin and chromaffin cells in regular formalin-fixed tissue, as well as to the biochemical fluorimetric method of Hess and Udenfriend (1959) for the determination of tryptamine, based on formaldehyde condensation in solution. Since then, the histofluorescence methodology has undergone a continuous development, and today we have at our disposal a wide variety of alternative methods and procedures for the visualization and quantitation of cellular stores of, above all, catecholamines and indolamines by fluorescence microscopy. While this wide selection of available methods represents a powerful arsenal for the researcher, the multitude of alternative procedures currently in use is difficult to overview for anyone who is not well into the field. The present chapter is intended both as an introduction to the monoamine histofluorescence methodology for the newcomer, and as a guide and manual for the active lab worker. Emphasis will thus be placed on both the general features and the chemical background of the aldehyde-based histofluorescence methodology, and on the practical performance of currently available methods, their potentials, pitfalls and limitations.

2. THE MONOAMINE NEURON

The biogenic monoamines can be defined as a family of compounds formed — in one or more steps — from the aromatic amino acids tyrosine, phenylalanine and tryptophan. Tyrosine and phenylalanine give rise to one class of monoamines, the β-phenylethylamines. The catecholamines dopamine, noradrenaline and adrenaline, belong to this class, as do the 'minor' amines tyramine, octopamine and phenylethylamine. Tryptophan gives rise to the β-indolylethylamine class of monoamines, to which 5-hydroxytryptamine (serotonin), tryptamine, and melatonin belong. Histamine, though sharing many features with the monoamines, is a diamine (formed by decarboxylation from histidine) and falls therefore outside the scope of the present review.

Figures 1 and 2 show the generally accepted biosynthetic pathways and main degradation routes for the biogenic phenylethylamines and indolylethylamines. In addition, the principles used to number the carbon atoms in the phenylethylamine and indolylethylamine skeletons is shown in Figure 3. This numbering has been used to label

Handbook of Chemical Neuroanatomy. Vol. 1: Methods in Chemical Neuroanatomy.
A. Björklund and T. Hökfelt, editors.
© Elsevier Science Publishers B.V., 1983.

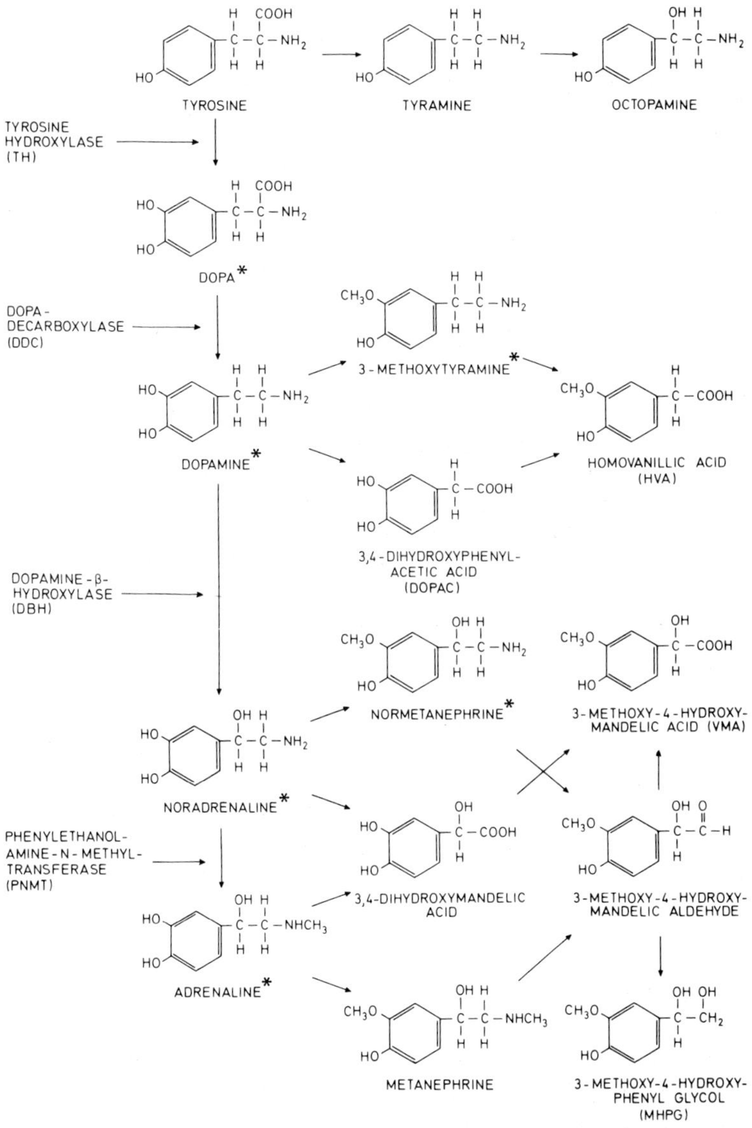

Fig. 1. In vivo synthesis and degradation of some biogenic phenylethylamines. Compounds that yield significant fluorescence in any of the FA or GA reactions are labeled with asterisks. (Modified from Axelrod 1971.)

substituents on the molecules in Figures 1 and 2. The asterisks in Figures 1 and 2 indicate those compounds which are *fluorogenic* in the aldehyde histofluorescence methods, i.e. those compounds which can be made fluorescent in any of the formaldehyde (FA)- or glyoxylic acid (GA)-based histochemical reactions, as described in further detail in Section 3.

The catecholamines (Fig. 1) are formed from tyrosine by two enzymes, tyrosine hydroxylase (TH) and aromatic amino acid decarboxylase (DOPA decarboxylase, DDC). All three catecholamines, dopamine (DA), noradrenaline (NA) and adrenaline (A), are fluorogenic in the FA reaction, while DA and NA, but not A, give intense fluorescence in the GA reaction. Among the catecholamine precursors and metabolites,

51

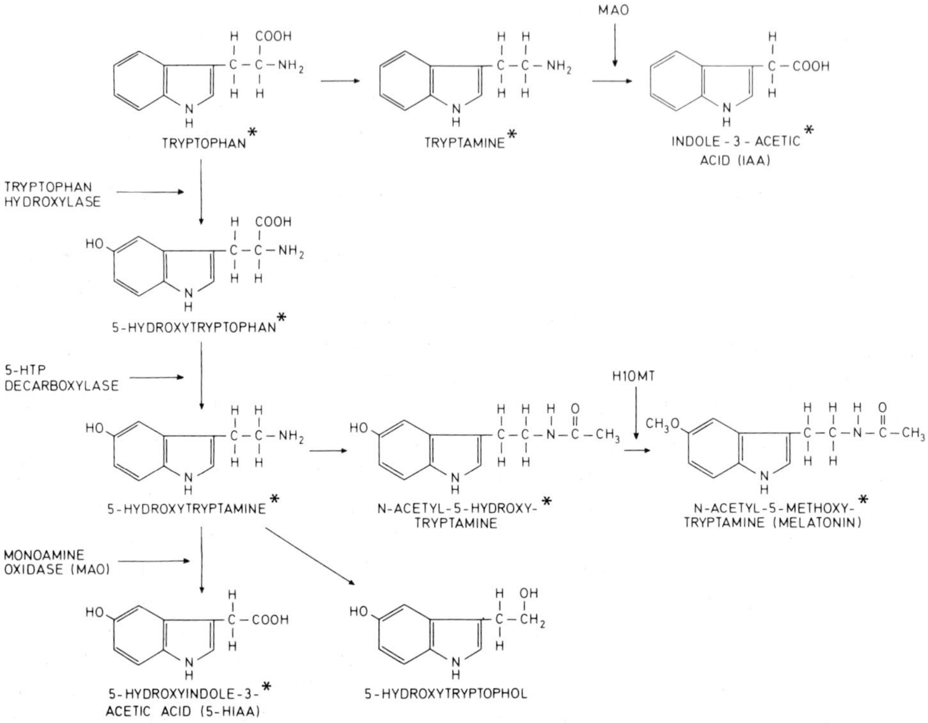

Fig. 2. In vivo synthesis and degradation of some biogenic indolylethylamines. Compounds that yield fluorescence in any of the FA or GA reactions are labeled with asteriscs. (Modified from Wurtman et al. 1968.)

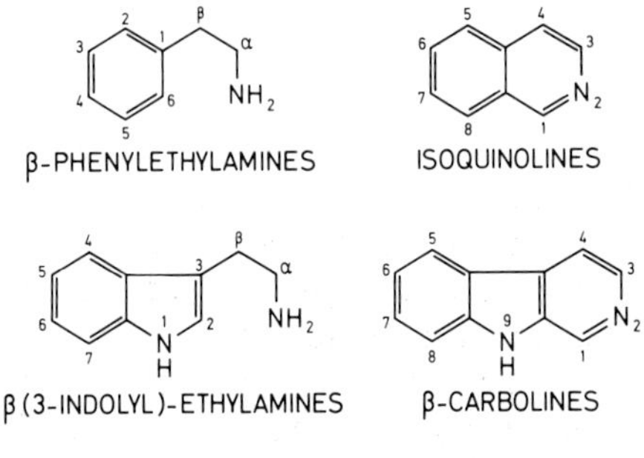

Fig. 3. Convention used for the numbering of substituent positions in phenylethylamines, indolylethylamines and their corresponding aldehyde-induced fluorophores, i.e. the isoquinolines and β-carbolines.

only three compounds are fluorogenic: 3,4-dihydroxyphenylalanine (DOPA), 3-methoxy-4-hydroxy-phenylethylamine (3-methoxytyramine), and 3-methoxy-4,β-dihydroxy-phenylethylamine (normetanephrine). DOPA, which is the immediate biological precursor of DA, yields as intense a fluorescence as DA in both the FA and GA reactions. DOPA occurs, however, normally in negligible concentrations in tissue. 3-Methoxy-tyramine and normetanephrine yield significant fluorescence only in the GA reaction. These metabolites are likely to occur primarily extracellularly, and have so far proved impossible to demonstrate with the fluorescence histochemical techniques.

Amines are known to be formed in tissue from tyrosine and phenylalanine also through direct decarboxylation. These 'minor' monoamines, tyramine and octopamine (formed from tyrosine: see Fig. 1) and β-phenylethylamine (formed from phenylalanine, not shown in Fig. 1) are known to occur in neural tissue, but usually at considerably lower concentrations than the catecholamines (Boulton 1976; Saavedra and Axelrod 1976). None of these non-catecholic amines are fluorogenic in the FA or GA reactions.

Indolamines are formed from tryptophan by one of two routes (Fig. 2): either by 5-hydroxylation (with the assistance of tryptophan hydroxylase) and further decarboxylation to 5-hydroxytryptamine (5-HT), or by direct decarboxylation to tryptamine. Both 5-HT and tryptamine, as well as the 5-HT precursor 5-hydroxytryptophan are fluorogenic in the FA and GA methods. In contrast to tyrosine and phenylalanine, tryptophan itself is also fluorogenic in the FA and GA reactions. This is the case for both free tryptophan and tryptophan in the N-terminal position in peptides and proteins (Håkanson and Sundler 1971; Björklund et al. 1973b; cf. below). So far, it has been impossible to demonstrate the break-down products of 5-HT and tryptamine (5-HIAA, IAA and 5-hydroxytryptophol) in tissue, despite the fact that under certain conditions they can yield fluorescence in the FA and GA reactions (see Section 3.3).

In pinealocytes, and probably also in certain neural tissues, 5-HT can serve as a precursor for N-acetylated amines (N-acetyl-5-HT and melatonin: see Fig. 2). These amines are fluorogenic both in the aluminum-catalyzed FA method and in the GA method (see Section 3.3). Other indolamines, not depicted in Figure 2, may also occur in tissue. Thus, bufotenine (N,N-dimethyl-5-hydroxytryptamine) has been demonstrated in toad brain in concentrations similar to those of 5-HT (Axelsson et al. 1972a; Seiler and Bruder 1975) and 5-methoxytryptamine has been claimed to occur besides 5-HT and tryptamine in the rat brain (Green et al. 1973). Such biogenic indolamines are also fluorogenic in the histochemical aldehyde reactions.

3. CHEMICAL BASIS OF FLUOROPHORE FORMATION

The underlying principle of the histofluorescence methods is the conversion of the essentially non-fluorescent catecholamines and indolamines to strongly fluorescent compounds. This is achieved through a ring-closure of the ethylamine side-chain, induced by reactive carbonyl compounds (in particular reactive aldehydes) to form isoquinoline and β-carboline derivatives of the type illustrated in Figure 3. This cyclization reaction has been known for a long time in organic chemistry as the Pictet-Spengler reaction (Pictet and Spengler 1911: see Whaley and Govindachari 1951; Abramovitch and Spencer 1964, for reviews). Hess and Udenfriend (1959) were the first to make use of this reaction for fluorescence analysis of biogenic monoamines, and Falck et al. (1962) and Corrodi and Hillarp (1963, 1964) adopted this principle for histochemical purposes in their formaldehyde vapor reaction.

The Pictet-Spengler cyclization reaction can, especially in the presence of strong mineral acids in solution, be carried out with a variety of carbonyl compounds, such as aldehydes, α-keto acids, and carboxylic acids (for further details, see Axelsson et al. 1972b). Under the mild reaction conditions present in tissue, however, only the most reactive reagents are useful. A reagent useful for histochemical purposes must, furthermore, combine high reactivity with a high degree of selectivity, so that the specific induction of fluorescence takes place under conditions when general tissue constituents (present in the 'background' of the sections) will remain essentially non-fluorescent. This criterion has so far only been fulfilled by two reagents, formaldehyde (CHO) and glyoxylic acid (HOOC-CHO) (Axelsson et al. 1972b, 1973). Alone or together these two highly reactive aldehydes serve as the fluorophore-forming reagents in the monoamine histofluorescence methods currently in use.

3.1. FLUOROPHORE FORMATION IN THE FORMALDEHYDE METHOD

The pioneering work on the chemical reactions underlying the development of fluorescence from catecholamines and indolamines under histochemical conditions was carried out during the mid-sixties by Hans Corrodi and Gösta Jonsson (see Corrodi and Jonsson 1967, for a review of this work). As a result we have today a good understanding of the chemical specificity of the histochemical aldehyde reactions.

The fluorophore forming reactions between the biogenic monoamines and FA are summarized in Figures 4A and B. The reactions occur in two steps (Corrodi and

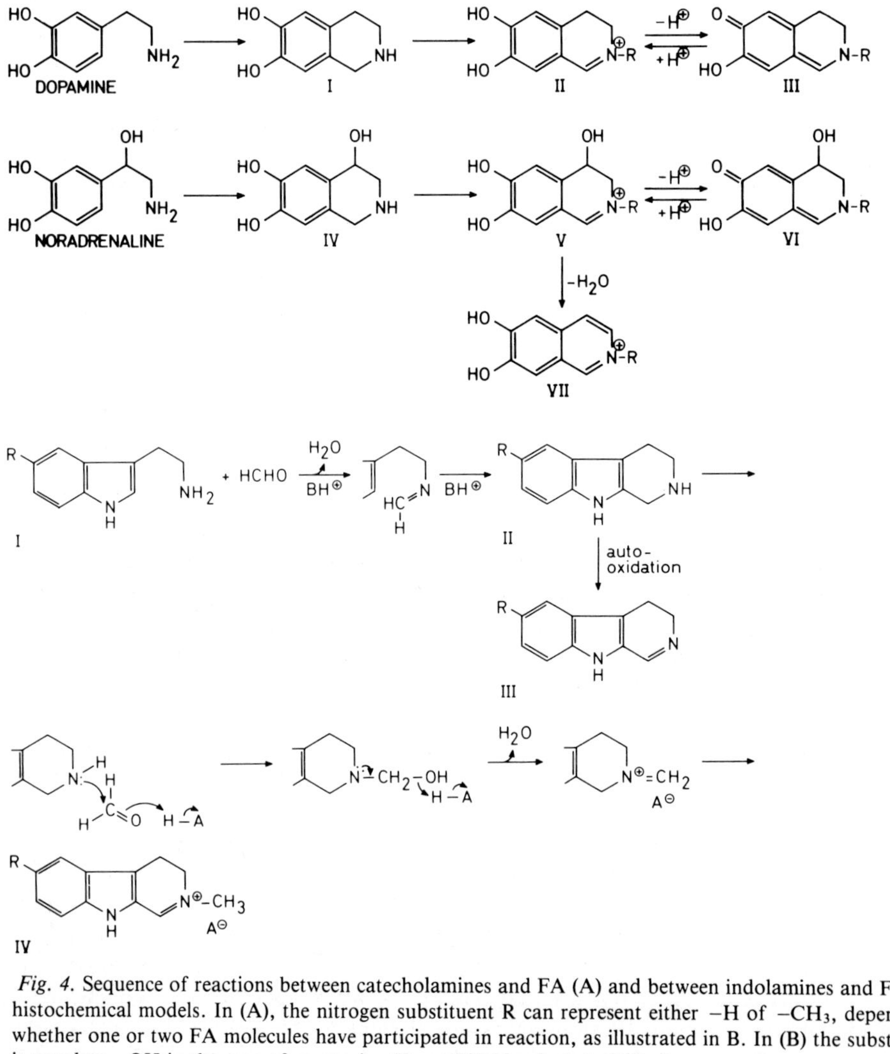

Fig. 4. Sequence of reactions between catecholamines and FA (A) and between indolamines and FA (B) in histochemical models. In (A), the nitrogen substituent R can represent either −H of −CH₃, depending on whether one or two FA molecules have participated in reaction, as illustrated in B. In (B) the substituent R is equal to −OH in the case of serotonin. (From Björklund et al. 1973a.)

Hillarp, 1963, 1964; Corrodi and Jonsson 1965b; Björklund et al. 1973a): In the first step, the catecholamine or indolamine reacts with FA in a Pictet-Spengler condensation, yielding the weakly fluorescent or non-fluorescent 1,2,3,4-tetrahydroisoquinoline (I and IV in Fig. 4A) or 1,2,3,4-tetrahydro-β-carboline (II in Fig. 4B), respectively, via a Schiff's base (for numbering of the positions in the molecules, see Fig. 3). When the amines are enclosed in a dried protein matrix, as in freeze-dried or air-dried tissue, these initially formed tetrahydro-derivatives are converted to strongly fluorescent molecules. This second step can proceed in two ways (Björklund et al. 1973a): either through autoxidation to the 3,4-dihydroisoquinoline (II and V in Fig. 4A: R = H) or 3,4-dihydro-β-carboline (III in Fig.4B), or through a second, acid-catalyzed reaction with FA yielding the 2-methyl-3,4-dihydroisoquinolinium compound (II and V in Fig. 4A: R = CH$_3$) or the 2-methyl-3,4-dihydro-β-carbolinium compound (IV in Fig. 4B). At least in the reaction with tryptamine the yield of highly fluorescent molecules in these two alternative fluorophore-forming pathways seems to be fairly equal (Björklund et al. 1973a).

Through the above reactions, 3-hydroxylated phenylethylamines (such as the catecholamines) will be converted to 6-hydroxylated 3,4-dihydroisoquinoline derivatives. At neutral pH, as occurs in tissue, these fluorophores are in their quinoidal forms (III and VI in Fig. 4A), whereas the non-quinoidal forms (II and V) are predominating at lower pH (Jonsson 1966; Björklund et al. 1968a, 1972a). This pH-dependent tautomerism between two states of the fluorophores is reflected in characteristic changes in their spectral properties (cf. Section 8.1). In addition, the fluorophores having a 4-hydroxy group (formed from phenylethylamines with a β-hydroxy group on the side-chain, such as occurs in NA and A) can be transformed into the fully aromatic compounds (VII) by splitting-off the hydroxy group with acid (Corrodi and Jonsson 1965a; Björklund et al. 1968a, 1972a). Since the conversion is followed by characteristic spectral changes, microspectrofluorometric differentiation between DA and NA is possible after acidification of the specimen (see Section 8.1; Björklund et al. 1968a, 1972a).

The formation of fluorophores from the initially formed tetrahydro-derivatives in the second step of the reaction is known to be promoted by FA and catalyzed by certain amino acids, peptides and proteins (Corrodi and Hillarp 1964). Thus, tissue amino acids can probably act as acid catalysts of the reaction of a second FA molecule with the initially formed tetrahydroisoquinolines or tetrahydro-β-carbolines to yield the strongly fluorescent 2-methyl-dihydro-derivatives (II-IV in Fig. 4B) (Björklund et al. 1973a). This probably explains why the second step of the fluorophore-forming reaction runs so much better under nearly dry conditions in tissue than in solutions (Corrodi and Hillarp 1963, 1964; Jonsson 1967).

The first step of the fluorophore formation, the Pictet-Spengler cyclization reaction, is facilitated by high electron-density at the point of ring closure of the amine (the 2-position of indolylethylamines and the 6-position of phenylethylamines: see Fig. 3; Whaley and Govindachari 1951). These requirements are fulfilled in 3-hydroxylated β-phenylethylamines (e.g. the catecholamines) and in β-(3-indolyl) ethylamines (e.g. 5-HT), whereas the phenylethylamines lacking electron-releasing substituents in the 3-position are much less reactive (Whaley and Govindachari 1951; Jonsson 1967; Björklund and Stenevi 1970). Furthermore, unsubstituted indolylethylamines are known to be less reactive in the Pictet-Spengler condensation than those having a hydroxy or methoxy group in the 5-position of the indole nucleus (Späth and Lederer 1930). Finally, the Pictet-Spengler condensation is limited to primary and secondary amines; tertiary amines and amides do not react.

The differences in reactivity of closely related phenylethylamine and indolylethylamine derivatives are important in determining the specificity of both the FA and the GA reactions. In the standard FA reaction, primary 3-hydroxylated phenylethylamines (including the catecholamines and the corresponding amino acids, including DOPA) give the highest fluorescence yields (Table 1; Falck et al. 1962; Jonsson 1967; Björklund et al. 1971). The fluorescence induced from 3-methoxylated phenylethylamines (such as the catecholamine metabolites, 3-methoxytyramine, normetanephrine and metanephrine) is much weaker, probably due to less activation exerted by the 3-methoxy- than by the 3-hydroxy-group at the point of ring closure in the Pictet-Spengler condensation. Phenylethylamines lacking activating substituents in the 3-position (such as tyramine and octopamine, and the amino acids phenylalanine and tyrosine) give no fluorescence in the reaction. In the case of indolylethylamines, the 5- or 6-hydroxylated derivatives give the strongest fluorescence in the standard FA reaction (Table 1).

Secondary amines generally give weaker fluorescence than the corresponding primary amines (Table 1; Corrodi and Hillarp 1963; Falck et al. 1963; Corrodi and Jonsson 1967) and they require more severe reaction conditions (i.e. higher temperature and/or longer reaction time) for maximum fluorescence. This difference between the primary and secondary amines, which is more pronounced for the phenylethylamines than for the indolylethylamines, can be explained by the fact that the second FA molecule (Fig. 4B) cannot react with the pyridine ring nitrogen of the 2-methyl-1,2,3,4-tetrahydroisoquinoline or the 2-methyl-1,2,3,4-tetrahydro-β-carboline derivatives formed from the secondary amines in the initial Pictet-Spengler reac-

TABLE 1. *Fluorescence yields of a number of biogenic phenylethylamine and indolylethylamine derivates (enclosed in dried protein films) in the FA, ALFA and GA reactions. The fluorescence intensities are expressed with the intensity obtained from noradrenaline and dopamine in the standard formaldehyde vapor reaction as 100.*

Substance	FA vapor[a]	ALFA + FA vapor[b]	GA + heating[c]	GA + GA vapor[c]
1. 3,4-Dihydroxyphenylalanine (DOPA)	120	70	130	570
2. 3,4-Dihydroxyphenylethylamine (dopamine)	100	175–200	670	810
3. 3,4-β-Trihydroxyphenylethylamine (noradrenaline)	100	85–195	460	445
4. N-Methyl-3,4-β-trihydroxyphenylethylamine (adrenaline)	40	10	10	45
5. 3-Methoxy-4-hydroxyphenylethylamine (3-methoxytyramine)	0	25	0	80
6. 3-Methoxy-4,β-dihydroxyphenylethylamine (normetanephrine)	0		0	35
7. 5-Hydroxytryptamine	30	50–255	10	125
8. 5-Hydroxytryptophan	10	30	0	130
9. Tryptamine (β(3-indolyl)ethylamine)	10	140–180	25	305
10. Tryptophan	10	25–115	0	375
11. 5-Methoxytryptamine	20	115–170	15	115
12. N-acetyl-5-hydroxytryptamine	0	160	0	60
13. N-acetyl-5-methoxytryptamine (melatonin)	0	105	0	80
14. N,N-dimethyl-5-hydroxytryptamine (bufotenin)	0	95	0	35
15. 5-Hydroxyindoleacetic acid	0	60	0	

[a]Formaldehyde vapor treatment at +80°C for 1 h. Data from Björklund et al. (1971b).
[b]Data compiled from Björklund et al. (1980) and Lindvall et al. (1981). The range given represents values recorded at different concentrations of aluminium sulphate (10–100 mM). FA vapor treatment as in a.
[c]Data from Lindvall and Björklund (1974). Reaction at +100°C for 3–6 min.

tion. Therefore, the secondary amines can be transformed into the strongly fluorescent dihydro-derivatives only via the less efficient autoxidative pathway (II-III in Fig. 4b) (Björklund et al. 1973a).

Acid catalysis In solution, the Pictet-Spengler reaction is catalyzed by hydrogen ions (Whaley and Govindachari 1951). Several attempts have been made to utilize such acid catalysis also in the histochemical FA reaction. As shown in Figure 4B, both the cyclization and the dehydrogenation steps in the fluorophore-forming reactions are catalyzed by acid. Consistent with this it has been shown that the fluorescence yields from tryptamine and 3-methoxylated catecholamines are dramatically increased when the FA reaction is performed in the presence of minute amounts of HCl (Björklund and Stenevi 1970; Björklund et al. 1971a). Acid catalysis of the fluorophore formation has subsequently found its application in the GA reaction (in which the carboxyl group of the GA molecule exerts an internal acid catalysis of the reaction: see below), as well as in the aluminum- and magnesium-catalyzed FA reactions (Lorén et al. 1976, 1980). Both these reactions represent a significant improvement in the sensitivity of monoamine visualization.

Magnesium ions (Lorén et al. 1976) and aluminum ions in particular (Lorén et al. 1980; Björklund et al. 1980) are efficient fluorescence-promoting agents in the histochemical FA reaction. This effect is, at least partly, probably due to the so-called Lewis' acid properties of these metal ions. As elaborated in further detail in the papers by Lorén et al. (1976), Björklund et al. (1980) and Lindvall et al. (1980), the positive effects of magnesium and aluminum in the FA method can probably be explained by a combination of four different mechanisms: (a) an acid catalysis of the fluorophore forming reaction; (b) a direct, fluorescence-enhancing action on the fluorophores formed; (c) a 'locking-in' effect of the ions on the monoamine-storing neurons in the tissue; and (d) in the case of N-acetylated and tertiary indolamines and indole acids, the promotion of an alternative route of fluorophore formation, via the so-called 2-methylene reaction (Lindvall et al. 1981) (see Section 3.3).

Ozone oxidation Ozone (produced in low amounts through electric discharge between two electrodes) can be used as a gaseous oxidant to promote fluorophore formation from tryptamine and peptides with tryptophan in the N-terminal position (Björklund et al. 1968b; Håkanson and Sundler 1971). Although the mechanism by which ozone promotes the fluorophore formation from tryptamine and tryptophanyl-peptides has not yet been clarified, it seems probable that the effect of ozone is, at least partly, to bring about an increased oxidative conversion of the initially formed 1,2,3,4-tetrahydro-β-carboline (II-III in Fig. 4B). The ozone concentration is important for optimum fluorescence yield in the reaction. The fact that too much ozone in the reaction vessel decreases the fluorescence induced from tryptamine and that the CAs and 5-HT give a strongly reduced fluorescence in the combined FA-ozone reaction is most likely due to oxidation of the fluorophores or of the amines themselves to products with low or no visible fluorescence. The FA-ozone technique has also been found useful for the histochemical visualization of peptides with NH$_2$-terminal tryptophan in endocrine tissues (Håkanson and Sundler 1971). It is likely that these peptides react as α-substituted tryptamine derivatives, and that the mechanism of fluorophore formation is similar to that of tryptamine itself.

3.2. FLUOROPHORE FORMATION IN THE GLYOXYLIC ACID METHOD

As in the FA method, the fluorophore formation from catecholamines and indolamines in the GA method has been shown to proceed in two steps (Figs 5A and B) (Björklund et al. 1972c; Lindvall et al. 1974c). In the first step, the monoamines react

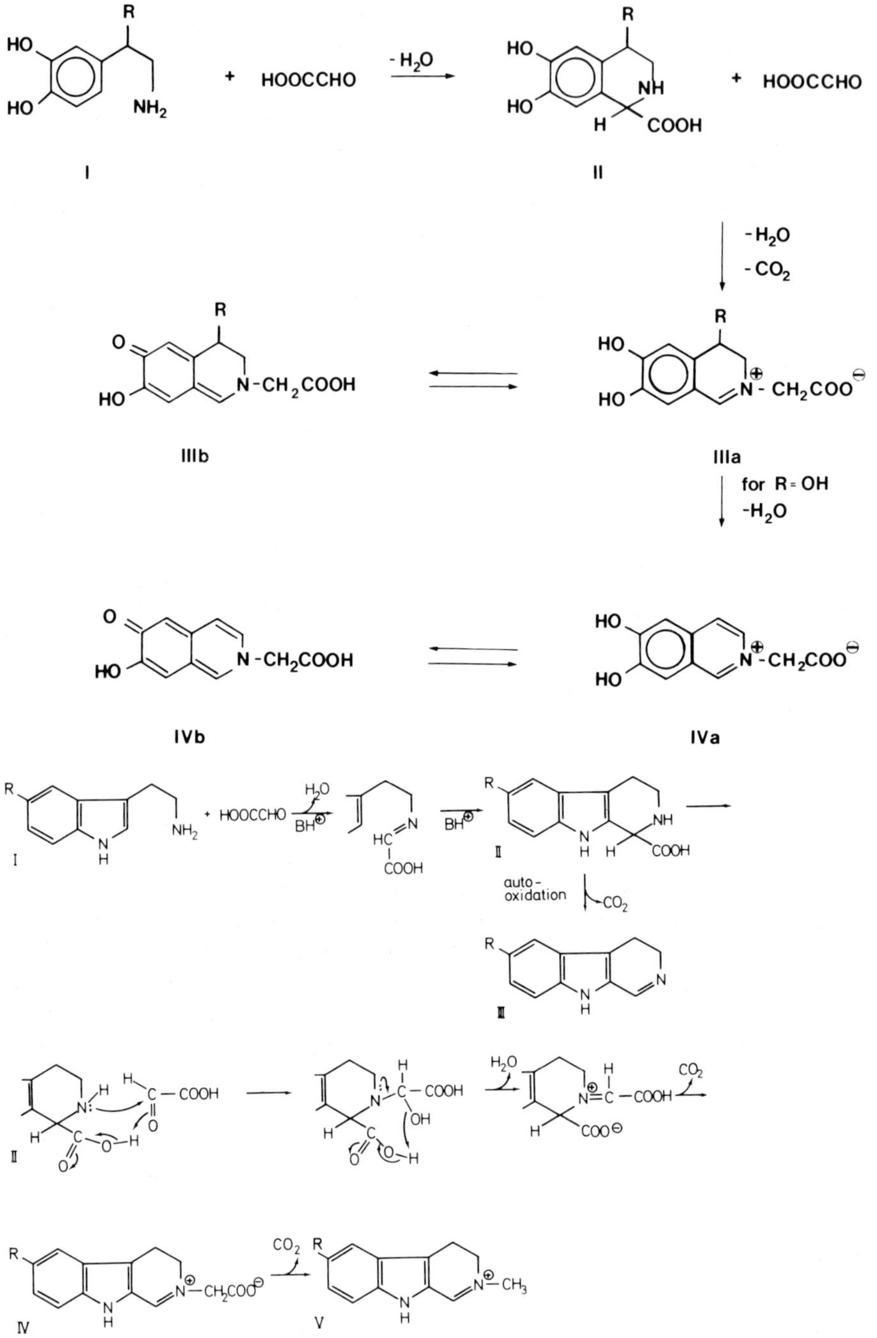

Fig. 5. Sequence of reactions between catecholamines and GA (A), and between indolamines and GA (B), in histochemical models. In (A), R = H for DA and R = OH for NA. In (B), R = OH for serotonin. (From Björklund et al. 1972c; and Lindvall et al. 1974c.)

with GA in an acid-catalyzed Pictet-Spengler condensation yielding the 1,2,3,4-tetra-hydroisoquinoline-1-carboxylic acid or 1,2,3,4-tetrahydro-β-carboline-1-carboxylic acid, respectively, via a Schiff's base (I-II in Fig. 5). These very weakly fluorescent compounds can be transformed into strongly fluorescent molecules in two alternative ways: via autoxidative decarboxylation to the 3,4-dihydroisoquinoline or 3,4-dihydro-β-carboline (II-III in Fig. 5), or through a second, intramolecularly acid-catalyzed, reaction with GA to the 2-carboxymethyl-3,4-dihydroisoquinolinium or 2-carboxy-methyl-3,4-dihydro-β-carbolinium compound (II-IV in Fig. 5B and II-III in Fig. 5A). A further decarboxylation to the 2-methylated compounds (V in Fig. 5B) is possible.

The dihydroisoquinoline fluorophores formed from catecholamines will exhibit a pH-dependent tautomerism similar to that described above for the corresponding FA-induced fluorophores (cf. Figs 4A and 5A). At neutral pH they will be in their quinoidal forms (IIIb in Fig. 5A) and in an acid environment the fluorophores will exist in the non-quinoidal forms (IIIa). By splitting-off the 4-hydroxy group with acid from the dihydroisoquinoline fluorophores formed from β-hydroxylated phenylethylamines, such as NA, they can be converted into the fully aromatic compounds (IV in Fig. 5A).

As demonstrated in model experiments, GA treatment induced stronger fluorescence than FA treatment from several phenylethylamines and indolylethylamines (Table 1; Axelsson et al. 1973; Lindvall and Björklund 1974a; Lindvall et al. 1974c). As in the FA reaction, the highest fluorescence yields in the GA reaction are obtained from 3-hydroxylated phenylethylamines and their corresponding amino acids. The strong fluorescence induced from 3-methoxylated phenylethylamines, which are less activated at the point of ring closure, indicates that GA is more efficient than FA in the initial cyclization step, and the reactions proceed considerably faster.

The high fluorescence yields in the GA reaction can be referred to several phenomena (see Björklund et al. 1972c; Lindvall et al. 1974c; Svensson et al. 1975): (a) The forma-tion of the strongly fluorescent 2-carboxymethyl-3,4-dihydroisoquinolinium and 2-car-boxymethyl-3,4-dihydro-β-carbolinium compounds through intramolecular acid cata-lysis, exerted by the carboxyl group on the 1-carbon of the tetrahydroisoquinoline or tetrahydro-β-carboline molecules (II-IV in Fig. 5B and II-III in Fig. 5A). (b) Because acid catalysis is of importance in both steps of the fluorophore formation, GA is also able to promote the initial cyclic step. Thus, the fact that GA induces fluorescence from 3-methoxylated phenylethylamines, which are less reactive in the Pictet-Spengler cyclization reaction, may well be explained by a catalysis of this step of the reaction. (c) Acidification is known to increase the fluorescence intensity of some amine fluorophores (Björklund et al. 1968a, 1972a). This should also contribute to the higher fluorescence yields induced from these amines in the GA reaction. (d) N-acetylated and tertiary indolamines, which are non-fluorescent in the standard FA reaction, yield fluorescence after more intense GA treatment (Table 1). This is probably due to a dif-ferent type of GA-induced fluorophore reaction, in which fluorescent 2-methylated derivatives of these indole compounds are formed. This reaction will be dealt with in some further detail in the following section.

3.3. THE 2-METHYLENE REACTION

It is known that GA, or FA in the presence of aluminum ions, can induce fluorescence from indolylethylamine compounds which cannot cyclize in a Pictet-Spengler type reaction (Lindvall et al. 1981). Such compounds are N-acetylated indolamines (e.g. melatonin), tertiary indolamines (e.g. bufotenin), and indole acids (5-HIAA and IAA).

Lindvall et al. (1981) proposed that the fluorophores responsible for the fluorescence induced from such compounds are formed through a reaction of GA or FA with the 2-carbon atom of the indole nucleus to form fluorescent, conjugated 2-methylene derivatives of the amine compounds.

The histofluorescence detection of N-acetylated or tertiary indolamines, or indole acids, by the 2-methylene reaction has so far not found any biological application. Judged by the model experiments, the sensitivity of detection of these compounds in the GA and ALFA methods should be well in the range of, say, 5-HT. Nevertheless the use of these methods for the detection of known or unknown stores of, for example, melatonin (N-acetyl-5-methoxytryptamine) or bufotenin (N,N-dimethyl-5-HT) meets with problems. In pinealocytes, where melatonin is known to occur, the high levels of 5-HT present will disguise any melatonin fluorescence formed. Another problem in the identification of any stores of N-acetylated and tertiary indolamines in nervous tissue is that the fluorescence color and spectral characteristics of the induced fluorophores are not easily distinguished from those of the catecholamine fluorophores. Bufotenin is, however, known to occur in relatively high concentrations in toad brain (Axelsson et al. 1972a; Seiler and Bruder 1975), and there are indications that melatonin may occur in the mammalian CNS (Green et al. 1973; Bubenik et al. 1974, 1976). Thus, the role of these little explored indolamines in neuronal function may very well deserve further exploration.

4. GENERAL PRINCIPLES FOR THE PREPARATION AND REACTION OF TISSUES

The original Falck-Hillarp method, as introduced in 1962, was based on exposure of air-dried or freeze-dried tissue to hot formaldehyde (FA) vapors. Earlier experimentation had shown that the water-soluble monoamines were very easily lost or dislocated through diffusion from their storage sites in unfixed tissue. The gas-phase reaction principle solved this problem, although it was found that a minimum amount of water had to be present during the FA reaction in order to facilitate the fluorophore reaction (Falck and Owman 1965; Hamberger et al. 1965; Hamberger 1967).

Subsequent work has shown, however, that, provided the monoamines are properly fixed (usually by formalin at low temperature), the histochemical reaction can, at least partly, be carried out also in solution. The first successful attempts along this line were made by Eränkö and Räisänen (1966), Laties et al. (1967), Sakharova and Sakharov (1971), and Hökfelt and Ljungdahl (1972). This has opened up the possibility to apply the FA or GA reagents via intravascular perfusion of the living animal, a principle that has been essential for the development of the highly sensitive aldehyde fluorescence methods currently in use.

4.1. THE ROLE OF WATER

Water plays an important role in the development and intensity of monoamine fluorescence in the histochemical preparation. As demonstrated, for example, in Hess' and Udenfriend's FA-based biochemical assay method from 1959, the first Pictet-Spengler cyclization step of the fluorophore-forming reaction proceeds very efficiently in solution. By contrast, the subsequent dehydrogenation of the initially formed tetrahydroisoquinolines or tetrahydro-β-carbolines (see Fig. 4) runs very slowly in water (Jonsson 1967). Corrodi and Hillarp (1963, 1964) and Jonsson (1967) have shown that this reaction is facilitated in a dry protein matrix. Under such simulated histochemical conditions proteins and amino acids seem to be necessary as catalysts of this reaction step in the FA method, while the COOH group of the GA molecule provides for a particularly efficient so-called internal catalysis of the fluorophore-forming reaction in the GA method (see Section 3.2).

This explains why removal of the water, often combined with or followed by heating, seems to be necessary for the full development of fluorescence in the tissue. Thus, while the initial cyclization between the amine and the FA or GA reagent can readily take place in wet tissue, the final transformation of the cyclized molecules into fluorophores is in most procedures obtained by air drying or freeze-drying.

The combined FA and glutaraldehyde reaction mixture, introduced by Furness et al. (1977a,b, 1978), is an interesting exception to this principle. Here, fluorescence develops from intraneuronal catecholamines while the tissue is still wet, although the intensity increases upon subsequent drying. Furness et al. (1977b) have suggested that glutaraldehyde may facilitate the dehydrogenation of the non-fluorescent tetrahydroisoquinoline intermediates through a reaction with the nitrogen in 2-position (Reaction II-IV in Fig. 4B).

In the FA method, Hamberger et al. (1965) have shown that a minimum amount of water has to be present during the histochemical FA reaction for optimum development of the monoamine fluorophores. In the FA vapor reaction this is regulated by controlling the water content of the paraformaldehyde powder used in the reaction of the tissue. This is less critical in the GA reaction however where the residual tissue water content seems to be sufficient for optimum fluorescence yields. This difference may well be explained by the stronger catalytic powers of the GA molecule.

4.2. TISSUE PERFUSION AND FIXATION

Tissue perfusion is made for several reasons. First, intravascular perfusion is an efficient way to introduce the FA and GA reagents into the tissue. Secondly, the perfusion solution can contain fixatives, such as FA or glutaraldehyde, in order to bind the monoamines firmer at their storage sites and to obtain better structural and ultrastructural preservation of the tissue. Finally, the perfusion step provides a means of cooling the still living tissue down to temperatures where enzymatic degradation processes cease.

It is a general rule that perfusion solutions of FA and GA, alone or in combination, should be ice-cold (0-5°C) for the amines to be retained in neuronal structures (Eränkö and Räisänen 1966; Hökfelt and Ljungdahl 1972; Lindvall et al. 1973; Watson and Ellison 1976). Formaldehyde solutions at room temperature, although compatible with visualization of rich amine stores in, e.g. adrenal medulla and mast cells, give very poor results in nervous tissue. Interestingly, perfusion with formaldehyde (4%) in combination with glutaraldehyde (0.5 - 1.0%) (the Faglu mixture of Furness et al. 1977, 1978) can succesfully be used also at room temperature (see Section 5.2). The probable reason for this is that glutaraldehyde, being a very good fixative, can bind the amines strongly enough to prevent their dislocation during processing. Glutaraldehyde in higher concentrations, alone or in mixture, is not useful as a fixative for monoamine histofluorescence because of the high background fluorescence induced.

The retention of the amines at their intraneuronal storage sites can be improved by manipulations of the salt content of the perfusion or immersion solutions. Hökfelt (see

Fuxe et al. 1968; Hökfelt and Ljungdahl 1972) reported that perfusion with hypertonic salt solution improved the visualization of fine NA terminals in the brain. Subsequently, Lorén et al. (1976, 1977, 1980) discovered that high concentrations of magnesium or aluminum salts (in combination with acid pH) have a striking fluorescence-promoting effect in the aldehyde histofluorescence procedures. This effect is not caused by the hypertonicity per se, and appears to be specific for metal ions having the property of Lewis' acids. The positive effect has been ascribed to both a 'locking in' effect on the amines within the neurons, a catalytic effect on the fluorophore-forming reactions, and a direct fluorescence-enhancing effect on the dihydroisoquinoline and dihydro-β-carboline fluorophores formed in the reaction (see Section 3.1). This principle forms the basis of the so-called ALFA method which is described in further detail below.

The actual technique used for the intravascular perfusion seems to be of less importance. In our own laboratory we have used manual perfusion with a 150 ml syringe (Lindvall and Björklund 1974a; Lorén et al. 1976), gravity perfusion (Hökfelt and Ljungdahl 1972; Lindvall et al. 1973) or perfusion with a pressurized system (Lorén et al. 1980, 1982). The manual perfusion, which is rapid and simple, has proven fully adequate for the different versions of the GA method where the purpose of the perfusion is to introduce the reagent into the tissue rather than to obtain any fixation. With FA and FA-glutaraldehyde solutions, most authors use gravity perfusion or pressurized systems, although the amount of fluid is kept rather small (usually 200-250 ml for rats) and the time short (usually up to 10-15 min). A convenient pressurized perfusion system, which allows perfusion under adjustable and controlled pressure has been described by Furness et al. (1978). This apparatus is illustrated in Figure 6A. For perfusions of ALFA solution (4% FA with high content of aluminum sulfate) a pressurized system of the type shown in Figure 6B is necessary. This is because even tissue penetration of the strongly hypertonic ALFA solution requires high pressure (2 atmospheres for adult rats).

Immersion can serve the same purpose as perfusion in some cases. This approach has been employed with good results for whole mount specimens of thin tissue sheets (e.g. iris, mesentery or intestinal mucosa) (Eränkö and Räisänen 1966; Lindvall and Björklund 1974a; Furness and Costa 1975; Furness et al. 1977a; Lorén et al. 1977; Ajelis et al. 1979), and for Vibratome and cryostat sections of nonperfused tissue (Hökfelt and Ljungdahl 1972; Lindvall and Björklund 1974a; De La Torre and Surgeon 1976; Watson and Barchas 1977). GA and Faglu solutions are clearly superior to FA in such procedures. GA immersion has also proved convenient and efficient for demonstration of catecholamines in tissue cultures (Schlumpf et al. 1977; Victorov et al. 1979; Dreyfus et al. 1979; Hendelman et al. 1982). In general, those procedures in which the reagent is applied through an immersion step provide the most rapid processing of specimens for monoamine visualization, and are easy to perform, which may have distinct advantages for certain purposes. These aspects will be dealt with further in Section 5.

4.3. TISSUE DRYING

As pointed out above, removal of the water from the tissue, at some stage of tissue processing, is necessary for optimal development of monoamine fluorescence. Generally stated, 3 alternative drying procedures are being used: freeze-drying, drying over phosphorous pentoxide (P_2O_5) in a vacuum dessicator, or air-drying with or without

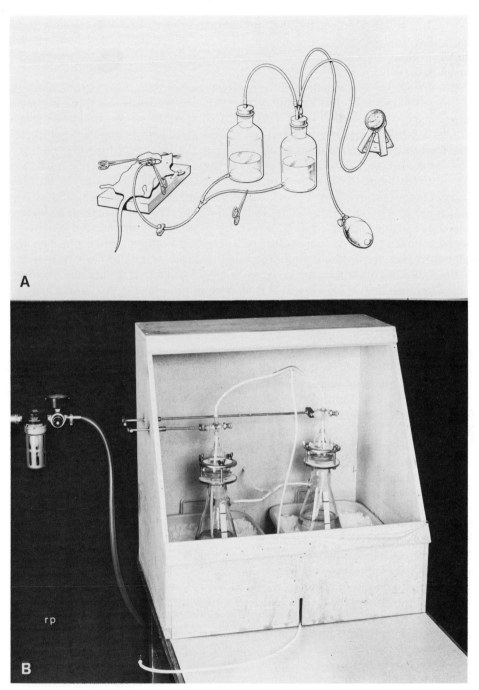

Fig. 6. Equipment suitable for intravascular perfusions for aldehyde fluorescence histochemistry. (A) shows the set-up used by Furness et al. (1978) in the Faglu method. The pressure used (120 Torr) is produced manually with the rubber ball. (B) shows the pressurized and cooled system used by Lorén et al. (1980) in the ALFA method. The pressure (up to 2 bar) is regulated by the manometer to the left, and led into the vessels via a tube entering through the back wall.

heating. The two latter procedures are applicable to cryostat and Vibratome sections and whole mounts (including the so-called 'smear' preparations and tissue culture specimens), while freeze-drying is the only reliable way to dry fresh or perfused blocks of tissue, prior to sectioning.

Freeze-drying, in combination with paraffin embedding, was introduced into monoamine fluorescence histochemistry in 1961 independently by three different groups (Eränkö 1961; Falck and Torp 1961; Lagunoff et al. 1961). Different laboratories have subsequently worked out standardized and reproducible protocols for the freeze-drying paraffin-embedding procedure (Falck and Owman 1965; Eränkö 1967; Fuxe et al. 1970; Björklund et al. 1972b). These involve rapid freezing of the wet (fresh or fixed) tissue to very low temperature (below $-80°C$) and drying in high vacuum at temperatures below $-20°C$. The dry tissue is subsequently embedded, e.g. in paraffin or plastic, before sectioning. During the sixties, freeze-drying was also widely applied to cryostat sections. This is however an unnecessary complication and drying of sections (made from wet nonembedded tissue) is nowadays carried out with the simpler air-drying or vacuum-drying procedures. Further aspects of the freeze-drying paraffin-embedding technique are given in Section 5.1, and air-drying and vacuum-drying of sections and whole mounts is dealt with in Sections 5.2, 5.3, and 5.4.

4.4. SPECIFICITY TESTS

The monoamines become fluorescent in the histochemical reaction, i.e. after treatment with FA or GA. The first criterion, therefore, of any monoamine fluorescence is that it is specific, i.e. induced by the FA or GA treatment. The literature contains many examples of misinterpretations in which a nonspecific autofluorescence is ascribed to the presence of monoamines. In particular, one should be aware of the fact that elastin (e.g. in blood vessels) displays a greenish autofluorescence similar to the color of the CA fluorophores, and that lipofuchsin pigment (e.g. in macrophages) has a yellow-orange color that can be mistaken for serotonin fluorescence. Such mistakes can be avoided by the application of some simple specificity tests.

(a) A test of basic importance is to establish that the observed fluorescence does not appear when the FA or GA step is omitted. It should be noted that even slight contamination with FA in the room air or the paraffin wax can induce significant monoamine fluorescence.

(b) The catecholamine and 5-hydroxytryptamine (5-HT) fluorophores exhibit a marked photodecomposition on irradiation with UV or blue-violet light. Such a photodecomposition is usually not observed with autofluorescent structures. The 5-HT fluorophore shows a much faster photodecomposition than the catecholamine fluorophores (Ritzén 1966a,b). This feature is often helpful in distinguishing 5-HT at low and moderate concentrations from catecholamines in the microscope.

(c) The catecholamine and 5-HT fluorophores display only very weak fluorescence in the presence of water (Ritzén 1966a,b), and hence the fluorescence is quenched when the section is mounted in water. Such fluorescence-quenching has not been reported for autofluorescent structures.

(d) Treatment with sodium borohydride ($NaBH_4$) in alcoholic solutions was introduced as a specificity test in the FA method (Corrodi et al. 1964). With this treatment, the fluorescent dihydroisoquinolines and dihydro-β-carbolines are reduced to their corresponding nonfluorescent tetrahydroderivatives (cf. Figs 4 and 5). The fluorescence can be regained by renewed FA treatment. It must be remembered that the

64

essential step of the test is this regeneration of the fluorescence and that proper controls, as devised by Corrodi et al. (1964), must be performed. Watson and Barchas (1977) have reported that the NaBH$_4$ test is also useful for GA-treated material.

(e) Since the autofluorescent structures usually have spectral characteristics and colors different from those of the amine fluorophores, they are revealed by spectral analysis. When working with previously uncharacterized systems, microspectrofluorometric analysis should always be performed.

(f) In conjunction with the histochemical tests, the use of pharmacological tests can be recommended. Such tests involve, for example, disappearance of the fluorescence after depletion of the amine with reserpine or α-methyl-m-tyrosine treatment, or after amine-synthesis inhibition, e.g. with α-methyl-p-tyrosine or p-chlorophenylalanine (for further details, see Corrodi and Jonsson 1967).

5. METHODS

The aldehyde histofluorescence methods currently in use fall into 4 general categories: (1) methods based on freeze-drying followed by paraffin or plastic embedding; (2) methods based on Vibratome sectioning of wet unfrozen tissue, followed by air- or vacuum-drying of the sections; (3) methods based on cryostat sectioning of frozen wet tissue, followed by air- or vacuum-drying of the sections; and (4) methods based on whole mounts of specimens that are thin enough to be viewed directly under the microscope, without sectioning. This section will survey the different methods outlining their principal design and the equipment necessary for their performance. Detailed protocols for some selected procedures are given in the Appendix at the end of the chapter.

5.1. FREEZE-DRY METHODS

The principal steps of the freeze-dry paraffin-embedding procedures are summarized in the block diagram in Figure 7. The original Falck-Hillarp procedure (Falck 1962; Dahlström and Fuxe 1964; Falck and Owman 1965) is based on direct processing of nonperfused tissue. Minor variations of this technique have been worked out in several other laboratories (Eränkö 1967; L'Hermite 1969; Fuxe et al. 1970; Hoffman and Sladek 1973). The sensitivity and precision of this procedure has subsequently been greatly enhanced through perfusion of the tissue with ice-cold FA and/or GA solutions containing high concentrations of aluminum or magnesium salts (Lorén et al. 1976, 1980, 1982; Ajelis et al. 1979). The original procedure and its improved versions are summarized in Protocols I and II A-C in the Appendix.

Preparation of tissues

Perfusion

The effect of various types of perfusion solutions has been reported in some detail by Lorén et al. (1976). Perfusion with ice-cold buffered FA, in 1-10% concentration, provides good fixation of the tissue but gives only minor improvements in the fluorescence microscopic picture, as compared to nonperfused tissue processed in parallel. Addition

FREEZE DRY METHODS

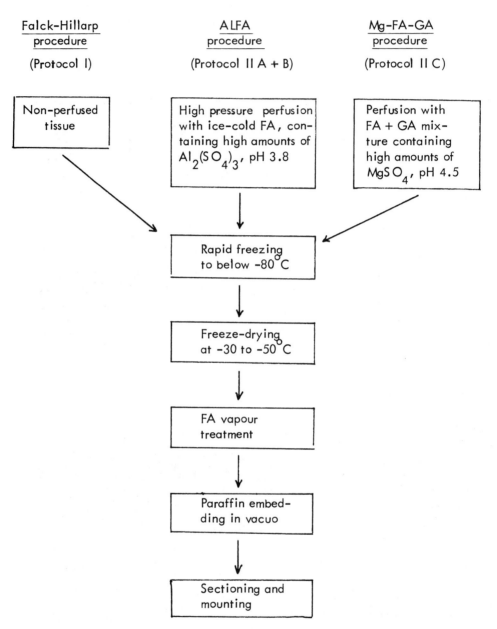

Falck–Hillarp procedure	ALFA procedure	Mg-FA-GA procedure
(Protocol I)	(Protocol II A + B)	(Protocol II C)

Non-perfused tissue

High pressure perfusion with ice-cold FA, containing high amounts of $Al_2(SO_4)_3$, pH 3.8

Perfusion with FA + GA mixture containing high amounts of $MgSO_4$, pH 4.5

Rapid freezing to below $-80\,°C$

Freeze-drying at -30 to $-50\,°C$

FA vapour treatment

Paraffin embedding in vacuo

Sectioning and mounting

Fig. 7. Principal steps of the freeze-dry, paraffin-embedding methods described in the text.

of $MgSO_4$, and $Al_2(SO_4)_3$ in particular, in high concentrations to the perfusion buffer has a strikingly positive effect. This is reflected, first, in an increased fluorescence intensity of intraneuronal catecholamines, and to a lesser degree also of indolamines. In animals perfused with the aluminum-formaldehyde (ALFA) solution this increase has been estimated to be about 4-5 fold (as registered microfluorimetrically from the DA-containing nerve terminal network in the neostriatum) (Björklund et al. 1980). Secondly, the metal salt perfusions give considerably sharper definition of fluorescent fibres and cell bodies due to less diffusion of the amines or their fluorophores during processing (Fig. 8).

The positive effects of magnesium and aluminum salts are observed to some extent also with solutions free of aldehydes. Optimum results are obtained however with solu-

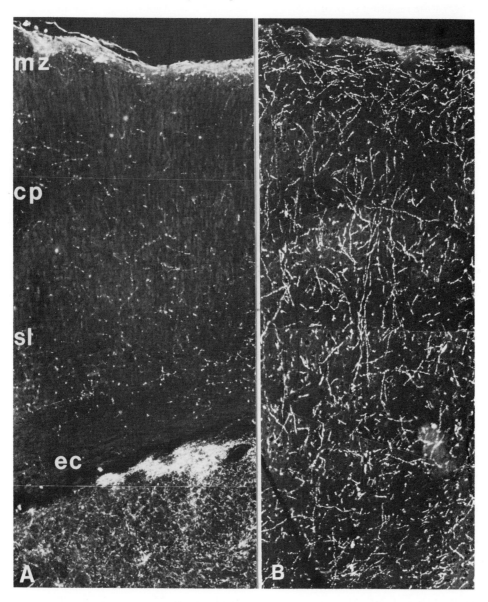

Fig. 8. Examples of results obtained with the ALFA method in freeze-dried, paraffin-embedded tissue, showing the NA-containing locus ceruleus innervation in the parietal cortex in the newborn (A) and in the adult rat (B). (A) also shows the developing DA innervation of the caudate-putamen (bottom). ec = external capsule; sl = subplate layer; cp = cortical plate; mz = marginal zone. (From Lorén et al. 1980, 1982.)

tions containing both aldehydes and the metal salts together, at acid pH. The recommended mixtures are 10% $Al_2(SO_4)_3 \cdot 18H_2O$ and 2% FA at pH 3.8 in the ALFA procedure (see Protocol IIA), and 27% $MgSO_4 \cdot 7H_2O$, 2% GA monohydrate and 0.5% FA at pH 4.5, in the Mg-FA-GA procedure (see Protocol IIC).

As pointed out above (Section 3), the action of aluminum and magnesium is specific and probably related to the property of these metal ions to act as Lewis' acids with the capacity to catalyze the fluorophore-forming reaction and enhancing the fluorescence intensity of the resulting fluorophores (see Björklund et al. 1980). Thus, aluminum has stronger Lewis' acid properties than magnesium and is also more efficient as fluorescence promoting agent in the perfusate. The effect is not seen with other salts, e.g. sodium or potassium sulfate, and not with solutions made hypertonic with sucrose (Lorén et al. 1976). Thr metal salt action is, however, pH-dependent, the optimum being at acid pH (about 3.5-5).

Equipment

The Mg-FA-GA solution can be perfused without preceding preperfusion with buffer, and can be made with any simple device. We have obtained good results with a hand-held 150 ml syringe connected to a perfusion cannula (Lorén et al., 1976), but gravity perfusion and perfusion apparatuses of the type shown in Figure 6 may provide more reliable results. It is preferable, however, that the perfusion is rather quick (150 ml in about 1 min).

The ALFA solution is more problematic. As indicated in the Protocol (IIA) the ALFA solution causes immediate precipitation of blood, and a thorough preperfusion with buffer to wash all blood out of the vessels is therefore needed. A second problem is that perfusion of the brain with high concentrations of $Al_2(SO_4)_3$ will be uneven and patchy unless a high perfusion pressure is used. Since it is desirable to reach about 2 atmospheres (bar) pressure, a system driven by pressurized air or nitrogen has to be used. Such an equipment, with two interchangeable fluid reservoirs, is illustrated in Figure 6B. It should be remembered that glass vials, used at such high pressure, must be housed in a protecting box (a wooden box with a movable thick clear plastic front is used in our laboratory). A modification of this setup, suitable for preperfusions of neonatal and embryonic rats, has been described by Lorén et al. (1982).

Freezing

The performance of the freezing and subsequent freeze-drying (see below) steps is critical for the final outcome of the processed specimens. Work has therefore to go into monitoring and optimizing these steps before good results can be expected. Once established in a laboratory, however, the freezing and freeze-drying procedures are reasonably reliable and very well suited for routine processing of large numbers of specimens. The reproducibility of results within each batch of specimens is also very good.

The single most important factor for the freezing of fresh or perfused tissue ('quenching') is the speed of freezing (for a more detailed discussion of the theoretical and practical aspects of tissue freezing the reader is referred to Meryman 1956, 1960; and Pearse 1968). During freezing the tissue water inevitably forms crystals. Too slow a freezing will allow these crystals to grow large, which destroys the tissue and gives a 'honeycomb-like' appearance to the sections. An essentially noncrystalline or microcrystalline structure of the ice is obtained if the tissue is rapidly brought down to temperatures below $-40°C$. At this temperature, the rate of formation of new crystals (so-called crystal nuclei) is very high and this keeps the size of the individual crystals down. To achieve this, low temperatures must be reached throughout the tissue piece within a few seconds.

Three main factors are of importance in determining the speed of freezing: the size of the tissue block; the temperature of the cooling medium; and the thermal conductivity of the cooling medium. Trump et al. (1964) monitored freezing rates in tissue blocks of approximately $5 \times 3 \times 1$ mm size. They found that with dry ice as cooling medium it took close to 2 min for the center to reach $-79°C$, with isopentane cooled by liquid air or liquid nitrogen $-150°C$ was reached within 10 sec, and with liquid propane cooled by liquid nitrogen $-175°C$ was reached within 6 sec.

Dry ice is thus unsuitable for freezing unless the tissue is infiltrated with some cryoprotective agent, such as 5-30% sucrose, which is widely used in the freezing for cryostat sectioning (see Section 5.3). Liquid air or liquid nitrogen, which have a temperature of about $-195°C$, are by themselves poor freezing media, since the formation of a layer of evaporized air or nitrogen around the specimens will isolate the specimen and thus reduce the heat conductance. This is overcome by using a liquid intermedium with a higher boiling point. The best intermedia are liquid propane and Freon 22 (monochloro-difluoro-methane), which can be used at temperatures close to $-195°C$ (propane solidifies below $-185°C$, but this can be reduced further by adding propylene to the propane; see Protocol I in the Appendix). Isopentane can be used at cooling temperatures down to about $-165°C$ (for further details on intermedia, see Pearse 1968).

Ideal results with respect to crystal artifacts will be obtained with very small specimens (up to $1 \times 1 \times 1$ mm) and with liquid propane or Freon (cooled by liquid nitrogen or liquid air) as cooling medium. In practice, however, one will often have to compromise with this principle. For CNS work larger specimens are desirable in order to provide reasonable overview. Freezing of larger specimens introduces, on the other hand, another problem, i.e. cracking of the tissue during freezing. Cracking is explained by the fact that the tissue is reduced about 2% in volume upon freezing (Pearse 1968). In larger tissue blocks the center will freeze much slower than the periphery, which will cause tensions in the shrinking, frozen parts of the block. Cracking is quite extensive when 3-5 mm thick slices of rat brain are frozen *at $-195°C$*. Such large pieces will be free of, or almost free of, cracks when frozen in isopentane *at $-50°C$*, but at this temperature crystal artifacts are abundant. Moreover, pieces frozen at this temperature have poor or no intraneuronal monoamine fluorescence. This is probably due to diffusion of the amines during slow freezing. As Meryman (1956) has pointed out, slowly growing ice crystals will extract the non-frozen water out of their environment, very much like a desiccation process. This process, which obviously can occur also during the freeze-drying step (see below), may partly explain why temperatures close to the freezing point (0 to $-15°C$) are deleterious to the retention of amines in the specimens.

Good retention of monoamines in CNS specimens is seen with cooling temperatures of *-80 to $-90°C$*, but at these temperatures crystal artifacts are still present, although the crystal holes in the section are now of subcellular size. Pieces as large as the lower brain stem of the rat (medulla pons + cerebellum) can be frozen at -80 to $-90°C$ without disturbing cracks. Whole transverse slices of the rat brain can be frozen without disturbing crystal artifacts *at $-100°C$*, or lower. Freezing at $-100°C$ causes less extensive cracking than freezing at $-195°C$ and may thus represent a good compromise for the freezing of larger specimens (cf. Hoffman and Sladek, 1973).

Equipment

Freezing should be made at temperatures below −80°C, which is most conveniently obtained with liquid nitrogen, or liquid air. The intermedium (best propane or Freon, but isopentane can also be used for smaller specimens) is held in a metal container immersed in the liquid nitrogen within a Dewar vessel. Propane and Freon, which are gases at room temperature, are liquidized by passage through a thin copper tube (attached to the gas tube outlet). The copper tube is bent so that it first passes through the liquid nitrogen (here the gas is cooled and turned into liquid) and ends above the metal container. Alternatively, the gas can be blown into a round-bottom flask immersed in liquid nitrogen. The liquid collected there is then transferred to the metal container.

For those who want to circumvent the use of liquid nitrogen or liquid air, Zlotnik (1960) has described a freezing procedure using a mixture of dry ice and propane cooled by vacuum. After 1 h under vacuum the temperature of the propane phase of this mixture is reported to fall to about −125°C, which should be sufficient for cooling of specimens of moderate size. We cannot, however, refer to any personal experience of this procedure.

Freeze-drying

Considerations on the principles underlying the freeze-drying process can be found, e.g. in Meryman (1960) and Pearse (1968). The following summarizes the experience gathered in our own department in work with freeze-drying for monoamine fluorescence visualization. For a more complete treatment of the subject the reader is referred to the quoted reviews.

Freeze-drying is performed at a low temperature and in a high vacuum. The simple rule is: the lower the temperature and the higher the vacuum the better the results. For practical purposes, most laboratories keep the specimens at −30 to −50°C and the vacuum below 10^{-3} Torr. Ideally, the tissue should, during the drying, be kept below the temperature where any diffusion of ions or water-soluble molecules can occur, i.e. below what is called the eutectic point of the tissue. This point is probably well below −50°C (see Pearse 1968; and Roth 1969). In ALFA or Mg-FA-GA perfused tissue we have found that a cooling temperature of −35°C is sufficient to prevent any disturbing diffusion of monoamines, whereas in non-fixed tissue Eränkö (1972) has reported that further reduction (down to −50°C) is advantageous.

The control of the temperature of the specimens during freeze-drying is critical. Specimens kept below −30°C will remain completely frozen and contain very little liquid water. At higher temperatures (approx. in the interval −15 to −25°C) the ice will start to melt. This increases the risk of diffusion artifacts. It also makes possible recrystallization of the tissue water and growth of the ice crystals, thus creating greater risks for freezing artifacts. Since the removal of water from the frozen tissue is progressively slower when the temperature is reduced, it is from a practical point of view disadvantageous to run the freeze-dryer at too low a temperature. Pearse (1968) states that sublimation of water from ice is 10 times slower at −60°C than at −40°C. A drying temperature of −30 to −40°C seems therefore to be a good compromise. When running the freeze- dryer at this relatively high temperature it becomes important, however, to make sure that the inflow of heat from the surrounding (i.e. by irradiation from the room) is kept to a minimum. Although the supply of heat to the frozen specimens from the outside will speed-up the drying process it will raise the temperature of the specimen into the critical range in an uncontrolled way. The best way to speed-up the drying process is to use as high a vacuum as possible, and to use a freeze-dryer equipment with an efficient system for the removal of evaporated water from the vacuum chamber.

Equipment

The freeze-dryer is essentially a vacuum-chamber, cooled to the desired temperature, and equipped with a water vapor trap of some sort. The systems commonly in use are based either on the use of a dessicant (usually phosphorous pentoxide, P_2O_5) or a cold finger as water trap. The cold finger principle ensures more efficient drying and, in our experience, also more reproducible results. Freeze-dryers using P_2O_5 as water trap are easier to run, however, and give in most cases adequate results.

Several freeze-dryers, suitable for monoamine fluorescence histochemistry, have been described in the literature (Falck and Owman 1965; Eränkö 1967; Pearse 1968; Olson and Understedt 1970a; Björklund et al. 1972b; Baumgarten 1972; Tilders et al. 1974). Some of these are also commercially available[1]. Freeze-dryers can, however, be assembled fairly easily by any instrument workshop, as evident from the above quoted papers.

The construction of the freeze-dryers used in our laboratory has been described previously (Björklund et al. 1972b). Like the construction developed by Olson and Ungerstedt (1970a) these apparatuses have a high tissue capacity and are convenient for routine laboratory work.

FA Vapor treatment

The reaction of the freeze-dried specimens is performed in a paraformaldehyde-containing sealed glass vessel in an oven at $+80°C$ for 1-2 h, as described in the Appendix. As mentioned above (Section 4.1) the amount of water present during the reaction is the most critical aspect of this step. This is usually regulated by using paraformaldehyde powder with a controlled water content, as described by Hamberger et al. (1965) and Hamberger (1967). They recommend equilibration of the paraformaldehyde to a preset air humidity. This can be done by storing the paraformaldehyde over different concentrations of sulfuric acid in desiccators, prior to use. Once used, a paraformaldehyde batch is then discarded.

Optimal results are usually obtained with paraformaldehyde equilibrated at 50-90% relative humidity. The optimal value usually varies from laboratory to laboratory and should thus be tested out individually by each laboratory.

Equipment

We use simple 1-liter glass jars with a plastic or metal lid as reaction vessels, and the heating is performed in a regular laboratory oven set at $+80°C$.

---

[1]The equipment used in our laboratory (Björklund et al. 1972b) is available from Eltronic AB, Furulund, Sweden. The equipment developed by Olson and Ungerstedt (1970a) is available from Bergman and Beving AB, Karlavägen 74, S-10055 Stockholm, Sweden. The freeze-dryer used by Tilders et al. (1974) is available from the Virtis Co. Inc., Gardiner, NY 12525, USA.

Embedding and sectioning

Vacuum-embedding in regular or synthetic paraffin is the standard technique used for freeze-dried specimens. Good results are, however, obtained also with embedding in araldite epoxy resin (Hökfelt 1965) and in methacrylate plastic (Hess et al. 1976; Lyon et al. 1982). A recent modification using polyethylene glycol (Schöler and Armstrong 1982; Smithson et al. 1983) should also be useful. These embedding media allow cutting of thinner sections.

Paraffin-embedding should be done in degassed paraffin in vacuo to ensure rapid and complete penetration. The time of embedding varies depending on the size of the pieces. Since the monoamine fluorophores are in some cases extractable in hot paraffin, it is recommendable to keep the infiltration time short, usually not longer than a few minutes (Björklund and Falck 1968).

Mounting of sections can be done in several types of non-fluorescent media. Entellan (Merck, Darmstadt, FRG), mixed with xylene is routinely used in our laboratory. Fluoromount (E. Gurr, London, UK), paraffin oil, and immersion oil are suitable as well, while xylene alone should be avoided (see Björklund and Falck 1968). Of the latter media, paraffin oil and immersion oil do not solidify upon storage, which is usually a disadvantage; this may be useful, however, if one wants to remove the coverslip, e.g. for subsequent staining of the sections.

Blocked specimens and deparaffinized, unmounted or mounted sections deteriorate rather quickly at room temperature. Mounted sections are also sensitive to light. Thus, within days or weeks there is a gradual fading of the specific fluorescence and a general increase in the background fluorescence unless the specimens are stored dark and cool. Specimens stored in a freezer (−20°C) will, however, retain their quality for at least several months. Freezing of Entellan-mounted sections should, however, not be done until all xylene has evaporated (1-2 days at +4°C); disturbing bubbles will otherwise appear in the polymerized Entellan.

Equipment

Specially designed glass containers for vacuum embedding have been described by Björklund et al. (1972b) and Dahlström and Fuxe (1964). These are designed so that the container can be evacuated with the specimen on a shelf above the melted paraffin. The specimen is then tipped into the paraffin. However, desiccators or similar vials with melted paraffin at the bottom are also suitable.

Usefulness and field of application of the freeze-dry methods

The freeze-drying, paraffin-embedding methods have several important advantages over other procedures, such as cryostat and Vibratome sectioning, dealt with below. *First*, en bloc reaction is the only way to obtain consistent and reproducible fluorescence yields throughout large series of sections and throughout series of parallelly processed specimens. This is essential for microfluorometric quantitation of the monoamines and important also for the evaluation, e.g. of lesions or drug effects. *Second*, many specimens can be processed simultaneously, and several regions can be taken from each brain. This meets with greater difficulty in the cryostat techniques, and it is virtually impossible to obtain with the Vibratome methods. *Third*, the en bloc processing allows very convenient storage and transportation of the specimens.

72

Without any loss in quality, frozen specimens can be stored and shipped in liquid nitrogen, or (air-tight) in dry-ice, to be freeze-dried and processed at a later stage or in another laboratory. Once paraffin-embedded, the specimens can again be stored for prolonged periods in a deep-freeze. *Fourth*, paraffin sectioning allows complete, uninterrupted serial sectioning of large tissue blocks. The entire section series can be kept and sections picked out of the band for parallel processing with other techniques. We have thus used the ALFA-treated material with excellent results for immunohistochemistry, for cresyl violet-, silver-, and Klüver-Barrera staining, as well as for simultaneous visualization of monoamine fluorophores and fluorescent retrograde tracers (see Section 6).

The standard Falck-Hillarp procedure, employing nonperfused tissue, is still very useful for studies in peripheral tissue, as well as for visualization of indolamine-containing systems in the CNS. The demonstration of serotonin-containing neurons with aldehyde fluorescence methods is, however, clearly inferior to that obtained with serotonin immunohistochemistry (Steinbusch et al., 1968). For studies on central catecholamine systems, on the other hand, the use of nonperfused tissue has several disadvantages. This procedure gives suboptimal visualization of many systems (some systems cannot be visualized at all) and diffusion artifacts are usually difficult to avoid. The metal salt perfusion procedures, and the ALFA procedure in particular, are considerably more sensitive and precise and are thus recommended in all cases where intravascular perfusion is possible.

In comparison with the method applied to nonperfused tissue, the ALFA perfusion procedure has a considerably higher sensitivity in the detection of both central and periphal catecholamine-containing structures. In the CNS, the nonterminal portions of the catecholamine axons, which are poorly detectable in specimens processed according to the Falck-Hillarp procedure, become visualized throughout their full extent (Fig. 8). This allows the tracing, in the intact untreated animal, of catecholamine axon pathways such as the dorsal tegmental bundle, the central tegmental tract, and the nigrostriatal bundle. The ALFA technique also demonstrates catecholamine systems which are only partly detectable, or which cannot be visualized at all, with the Falck-Hillarp method. This is the case with those systems originally discovered with the GA-Vibratome method, e.g. the periventricular system (Lindvall et al. 1974a; Lindvall and Björklund 1974b), the incerto-hypothalamic DA system (Lindvall et al. 1974a; Björklund et al. 1975b), and the DA terminal systems in the lateral septal nucleus (Lindvall 1975) and neocortex (Lindvall et al. 1974b).

The ALFA procedure for freeze-dried, paraffin-embedded tissue has a sensitivity for NA- and DA-containing structures comparable to that of the GA-Vibratome method, and is thus a good alternative to the GA-Vibratome method. The ALFA method is particularly nice for studies on the noradrenergic neurons in the locus ceruleus. Both their axon pathways and terminal systems (in, e.g. thalamus, hippocampus, and cerebral and cerebellar cortices) are demonstrated with high intensity, precision, and reproducibility. Another attractive feature of the ALFA method is that the fluorescence is usually without any signs of diffusion. This makes the fluorescence picture of the catecholamine-containing structures very distinct and rich in detail. In addition, the general background fluorescence tends to be lower in the perfused specimens, thus improving the contrast between the specifically fluorescent structures and the background.

Studies on fetal and neonatal rats have shown that the metal salt perfusion procedures can be applied with excellent results also to such material (Fig. 8A) (Lorén et al. 1982). The ALFA perfusion technique is thus the method of choice for ontogenetic studies in the CNS, particularly since the brains of young animals are difficult to section on the Vibratome. When applied to immature brains in combination with systemic injections of α-methyl-noradrenaline, even catecholamine systems with very low transmitter content are visualized. This procedure greatly improves the possibilities for studies on the early development of the catecholamine neuron systems.

5.2. METHODS APPLIED TO VIBRATOME SECTIONS

Vibratome sectioning was first introduced for monoamine histofluorescence by Hökfelt and Ljungdahl in 1972. They made use of nonperfused or FA-perfused tissue. Subsequent variants of this technique have employed GA (Lindvall et al. 1973; Lindvall and Björklund 1974a), the FA-glutaraldehyde (Faglu) combination (Furness et al. 1977a, 1978) and the aluminum catalyzed formaldehyde reaction (Lorén et al. 1980). The block diagram in Figure 9 summarizes the principal steps of the three main Vibratome-based protocols currently in use. Further details are found in Protocols III-V in the Appendix.

Perfusion and fixation

Intravascular perfusion in the Vibratome procedures is recommendable in order to improve the consistency of the tissue prior to the Vibratome sectioning. Hökfelt and Ljungdahl (1972) have reported their experience with nonperfused brain tissue. Although good results can be achieved, it is often very difficult to obtain reasonably thin sections and the sections are often uneven and fragmented. It is obvious, however, that these problems vary from region to region, and from one tissue type to the other (see below). Sectioning of brain tissue is made easier, however, simply by perfusion with ice-cold buffer, which improves tissue consistency. This is recommended, therefore, when using Vibratome sections of nonperfused tissue, for example for monoamine uptake experiments (see below, Section 6.7).

The choice of fixative/reagent in the perfusion step will depend on the purpose of the study to be undertaken. The FA-glutaraldehyde (Faglu) mixture at room temperature gives clearly the best fixation, and this fixation is even sufficient for good EM studies (Furness et al. 1978) (see Section 6.6). Although visualization of catecholamine cell bodies is good with this fixative (Fig. 11), the intensity of fluorescence is lower than that in the FA or GA procedures and may, in our experience, not always provide a complete demonstration of fibers and terminals. According to Wreford et al. (1982) perfusion with the Faglu mixture at alkaline pH (pH 10) markedly enhances serotonin fluorescence in raphe cell bodies. The intensity of the catecholamine fluorescence is at the same time reduced.

The GA perfusion procedure offers the most sensitive technique, giving brilliant and sharp visualization of all parts of the catecholamine-containing neurons (Fig. 10). GA is a poor fixative, however, and the sectioning of GA-perfused brain tissue can therefore be tricky. The addition of 0.5% FA to the GA solution, as introduced by Berger et al. (1976), is helpful in this respect.

Perfusion with ice-cold FA represents somewhat of a compromise: the tissue will be better fixed than after GA perfusion — and hence easier to section — and the sensitivity of catecholamine visualization is good. In fact, in combination with immersion of the sections in ALFA solution (see Fig. 9), as introduced by Lorén et al. (1980), the FA

VIBRATOME METHODS

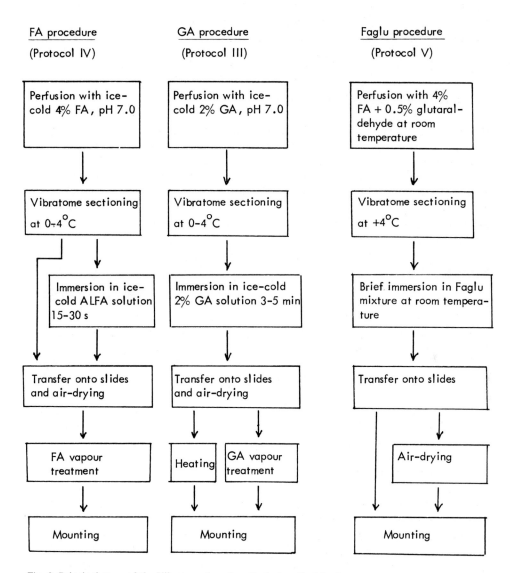

FA procedure
(Protocol IV)

Perfusion with ice-cold 4% FA, pH 7.0

Vibratome sectioning at 0–4°C

Immersion in ice-cold ALFA solution 15–30 s

Transfer onto slides and air-drying

FA vapour treatment

Mounting

GA procedure
(Protocol III)

Perfusion with ice-cold 2% GA, pH 7.0

Vibratome sectioning at 0–4°C

Immersion in ice-cold 2% GA solution 3–5 min

Transfer onto slides and air-drying

Heating | GA vapour treatment

Mounting

Faglu procedure
(Protocol V)

Perfusion with 4% FA + 0.5% glutaraldehyde at room temperature

Vibratome sectioning at +4°C

Brief immersion in Faglu mixture at room temperature

Transfer onto slides

Air-drying

Mounting

Fig. 9. Principal steps of the Vibratome based methods described in the text.

perfusion protocol will provide results on central catecholamine systems comparable to those obtained with GA perfusion. Additions of metal ions to the perfusion fluid, as used in the freeze-dry methods, offer little advantage. In fact, at higher concentrations magnesium and aluminum salts make the tissue 'sticky' and more difficult to section.

Sectioning

The procedure used in our laboratory (Lindvall and Björklund 1974a) essentially follows that described by Hökfelt and Ljungdahl (1972). After perfusion, the tissue is

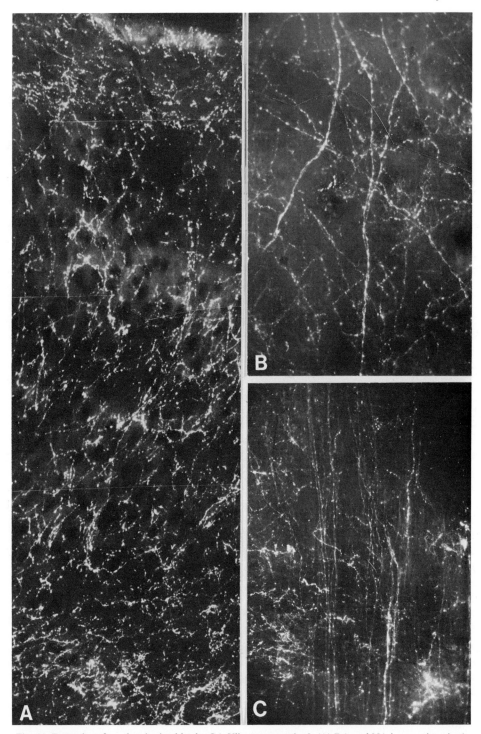

Fig. 10. Examples of results obtained in the GA-Vibratome method. (A) DA and NA innervations in the rat prefrontal cortex; (B) Locus ceruleus axons in the molecular layer of the cingulate cortex in a section parallel to the surface; (C) Bundles of locus ceruleus NA axons running in the dorsal tegmental bundle (From Lindvall et al. 1978; Lindvall and Björklund 1974a.)

rapidly taken out and cooled with ice-cold Tyrode's or Krebs-Ringer buffer and the desired piece is dissected out. The tissue is sectioned in the Vibratome intrument and, during this procedure, immersed in the ice-cold buffer. A low temperature (between 0 and +5°C) in the sectioning bath is essential in the FA and GA protocols; otherwise, the catecholamine fluorophores will diffuse away and in addition, the tissue piece softens, making the sectioning more difficult. In order to keep the sectioning bath at the necessary low temperature, we use noncorroding metal bars, cooled to a very low temperature in a solid carbon dioxide-ethanol mixture. These cold metal bars are placed in the buffer trough and are changed at suitable intervals. In the Faglu method (Furness et al. 1977a) the sectioning is done without any buffer in the bath. Instead, the sectioning is carried out in a cold room and the specimen is kept moist with the Faglu mixture.

The sectioning procedure and the quality of the sections are influenced by several factors: (1) Consistency of the tissue. As described above, this is to a large extent determined by the perfusion step. (2) Size of the tissue pieces. Brain tissue pieces as large as frontal sections trough the rat di- and telencephalon can be sectioned. The thickness of the dissected tissue piece can be up to 5-6 mm, but 3-4 mm is better. In case of tissues difficult to section on the Vibratome (see below), it is helpful to use even smaller pieces. (3) Type of tissue. The possibilities of obtaining sections of useful quality on the Vibratome depend very much on the type of tissue. Sections of good quality have been produced from, for example, GA-perfused ovary and uterus, tissues that are much more difficult to section than GA- or FA-perfused brain tissue. Certain areas of the brain are markedly easier to section than others. Homogeneous brain regions such as the cerebral cortex, caudate nucleus, and diencephalon (in the sagittal plane) are easiest, while regions with a heterogeneous build-up, e.g. heavily myelinated regions, such as the lower brain stem and spinal cord, and regions including large ventricle spaces, such as the hypothalamus in the frontal plane, are more difficult.

For brain tissue, it has been found that sections of 30-35 μm thickness are useful for the study of innervation density and denervation effects because they can be obtained from most brain areas and in all planes of section. However, in the most favorable areas, and in FA- or Faglu-perfused tissue in particular, sections can be obtained with a thickness down to about 20 μm. A thickness greater than about 40 μm is not useful for fluorescence microscopy, since the opacity of the thicker sections decreases the contrast and, finally, disguises the catecholamine structures.

GA- or FA-perfused tissue pieces will remain in an acceptable condition in the cold buffer for a maximum of 4-6 h. This means that several pieces from each animal can be sectioned, the pieces being stored in the ice-cold buffer until they are sectioned. From each piece, one can expect to obtain a maximum of 15-20 good sections. For GA-perfused tissue, at least, it is recommended that the buffer in the trough is oxygenated and that it is changed at regular intervals during the day. It is important for the sectioning that the tissue piece be firmly glued to the holder of the Vibratome. If the tissue piece loosens, partly or completely, the quality of the sections declines or no sections at all will be obtained. The tissue piece can in most cases be reglued to the holder.

Equipment

The Vibratome instrument is commercially available from Oxford Instruments, San Mateo, California, USA. The instrument and its general application to histochemical work has been dealt with in some further detail by Smith (1970) and Hökfelt et al.

(1974). An instrument of equivalent design ('Vibroslice') is offered by Campden Instruments Ltd., 186 Campden Hill Road, London, UK.

Immersion and drying

The immersion step can be omitted in the processing of FA-perfused specimens, but is essential in the GA and Faglu procedures. However, also in the FA procedure immersion is advantageous. Thus, the inclusion of the ALFA immersion step, as indicated in Figure 9, gives a clear-cut improvement in the visualization of catecholamine-containing structures (see Lorén et al. 1980). The immersion is carried out on free-floating sections, and the sections are then transferred onto glass slides, as described in Protocol III in the Appendix.

Drying of the sections is most reliably done in a 2-step procedure: First under the warm air-stream of a hair dryer for about 15 min, and then in a vacuum desiccator over fresh granular P_2O_5 for at least 1 h (preferably overnight). Complete drying is essential for the development and retention of catecholamines in the FA and GA methods, while some fluorescence (especially in cell bodies and more intensely fluorescent fibers) is visible already in wet sections after Faglu perfusion. This is advantageous when using Faglu sections for combined fluorescence and electron-microscopy. Also in Faglu sections, however, optimum fluorescence develops only after thorough drying.

Reaction and mounting

In the GA and FA methods the final development of the monoamine fluorophores takes place during heating and FA vapor treatment, respectively. The FA vapor treatment is the same as that used in the freeze-dry FA methods (see Section 5.1, under 'FA vapor treatment'), with the precaution that the slides are preheated to $+80°C$ before they are put in the room-tempered paraformaldehyde reaction vessel. This is done in order to minimize the risk of water condensation onto the sections. GA vapor treatment (see Lindvall and Björklund 1974a), is an alternative to simple heating in the GA method; but since this offers little advantage it is seldom used.

Mounting is done in a non-fluorescent medium, such as paraffin oil, immersion oil, xylene or Fluoromount.

Usefulness and field of application of the Vibratome methods

The Vibratome-sectioning procedures have several advantages for the visualization of central CA neurons. Thus, the Vibratome procedure is easier to perform than freeze-drying and requires less elaborate equipment, and specimens are more rapidly available for fluorescence microscopy when processed according to the Vibratome technique. Also, in the Vibratome sections, cracks and other freezing artifacts are avoided. On the other hand, the sectioning in the Vibratome of fresh or perfused tissue is much more time-consuming than for paraffin-embedded tissue in an ordinary microtome, and considerably fewer sections are obtained from each specimen. In addition, it is not always easy to obtain acceptable sections, especially when sectioning unfixed tissue of regions with a heterogeneous architecture, e.g. those containing ventricle systems or consisting of a mixture of white and gray matter. Also under favorable circumstances the Vibratome sections are often uneven in thickness.

The high sensitivity of the GA-Vibratome method made possible a more complete tracing of catecholamine axon pathways in the rat brain (Lindvall and Björklund 1974b). Furthermore, several previously unknown fiber systems have been discovered with this technique. This is the case, for example, for the incertohypothalamic DA system (Lindvall et al. 1974a; Björklund et al. 1975b), the periventricular CA system (Lindvall et al. 1974a), the DA terminal systems in the cerebral cortex (Lindvall et al. 1974b) and in the septum (Lindvall 1975), and the DA-containing dendrites of the neurons in the substantia nigra (Björklund and Lindvall 1975).

A most advantageous feature of the Vibratome methods, and of the GA-Vibratome method in particular, is the very distinct and precise picture of the CA-containing structures that is obtained (Figs 10 and 11). This allows observations on details of the systems such as axonal morphology, branching patterns, and terminal arrangements. Of particular interest for neuroanatomical tracing is that in GA-treated Vibratome sections, axons of the same origin but localized in different brain regions in several cases have very similar fluorescence appearance, and in the relatively thick Vibratome sections they can be traced over long distances. This offers possibilities to distinguish both preterminal and terminal axons of the same origin in an area where they are mixed with axons of other origins. Knowing the characteristic morphological features, it is therefore possible to study, in the intact animal, the pathways and terminal arrangements of the different CA afferents to an area. The Vibratome methods thus have

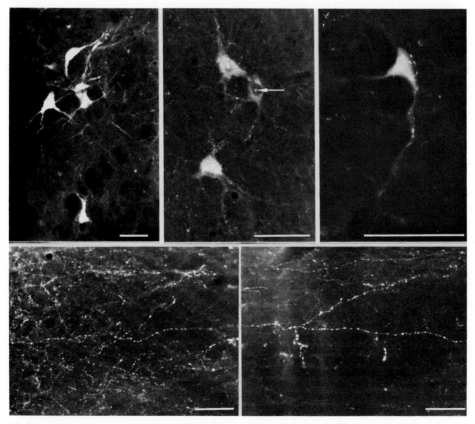

Fig. 11. Examples of results obtained with the Faglu-Vibratome method, showing brain stem NA cell bodies, and NA terminals in the hypothalamic periventricular nucleus (bottom left) and in the cerebal cortex (bottom right). (From Furness et al. 1978.)

their greatest potential in neuroanatomical studies of the central DA and NA neurons. Although the ALFA perfusion technique for freeze-dried, paraffin-embedded specimens (see Section 5.1) has a sensitivity for CA neurons that is similar to that of the GA-Vibratome method, the latter technique has several attractive features that make it particularly valuable in certain situations.

Vibratome sections are well suited for correlative studies with different histochemical techniques (see Section 6). They can be used for catecholamine fluorescence in combination with acetylcholinesterase staining, on the same or consecutive sections (Hökfelt et al. 1974; Lindvall 1977; Bieger and Harley 1982), in combination with HRP tracing (Blessing et al. 1978; Berger et al. 1978), and in combination with Fink-Heimer fiber degeneration staining (Hökfelt et al. 1974). Vibratome sections of unfixed (usually buffer-perfused) tissue are also useful for monoamine uptake experiments in vitro. As elaborated in further detail in Section 6.7, such uptake studies offer a possibility to differentiate between different types of axons (NA, DA or 5-HT-containing) in the microscope (Lindvall and Björklund 1974a; Berger and Glowinski 1978).

5.3. METHODS APPLIED TO CRYOSTAT SECTIONS

FA-induced fluorescence from catecholamines in cryostat sections was first described by Eränkö (1955 a-c). Eränkö demonstrated fluorescent NA-containing cells in the adrenal medulla after immersion of adrenal glands in a formalin solution, followed by cryostat sectioning. Similar results were subsequently obtained in cardiac tissue after intracranial perfusion with a 4% paraformaldehyde solution just prior to cryostat sectioning (Laties et al. 1967). The latter authors also reported that heating of the sections further improved the fluorescence picture, but that the best results were obtained after FA vapor treatment according to the original Falck-Hillarp method. During the sixties and early seventies attempts were made to apply the Falck-Hillarp FA vapor method to cryostat sections. Most of them were based upon rapid freezing of freshly dissected tissue specimens, sectioning in the cryostat, drying of the sections, and finally development of the fluorophores by FA vapor treatment (Hamberger and Norberg 1964; Spriggs et al. 1966; Csilik and Kàlmàn 1967; El-Badawi and Schenk 1967; Heene 1968; Nelson and Wakefield 1968; Placidi and Masuoka 1968; Masuoka et al. 1971; Winckler 1970). In most of these studies freeze-drying of freshly cut sections was used in order to enhance the fluorescence picture and to reduce the diffusion artifacts. Laties et al. (1967) and Watson and Ellison (1976) have shown that perfusion of the animals with a 4% paraformaldehyde solution improves the sensitivity and reduces the problems of diffusion artifacts in the FA-cryostat method. This was demonstrated in NA-containing nerves of cardiac tissue (Laties et al. 1967) and later in NA-, DA- and 5-HT-containing neurons of the central nervous system (Watson and Ellison 1976). The failure to visualize catecholamine neurons in the CNS by Laties et al. depended probably partly on the high sectioning temperature ($-10°C$) as compared to that used by Watson and Ellison ($-25°C$).

Despite the considerable efforts made, the FA-based cryostat procedures remain to be of limited value, above all because of their unsatisfactory reproducibility, the risk of diffusion artifacts, and their limited sensitivity, particulary in the visualization of central monoamine neurons. The application of the GA reagent to cryostat sections, therefore, came to represent a decisive improvement of the cryostat method (De La Torre and Surgeon 1976; De La Torre 1980; Bloom and Battenberg 1976; Nygren 1976; Watson and Barchas 1977). Due to their relative simplicity these GA-cryostat protocols are now the most popular procedures for catecholamine visualization.

The present account will focus on these more recently introduced versions of the cryostat procedure, based on GA or GA in combination with FA. The principles of these methods are summarized in the block diagram in Figure 12. Detailed protocols are found in the Appendix (Protocols VI-VIII).

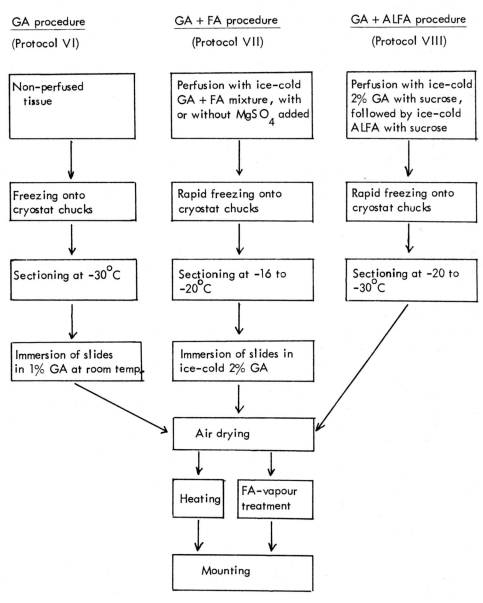

Fig. 12. Principal steps of the cryostat-based methods described in the text.

Perfusion

Although several authors have recommended the use of nonperfused tissue (De La Torre and Surgeon 1976; De La Torre 1980; Watson and Barchas 1977), perfusion with GA or combined GA and FA solutions will, according to our experience, provide a general improvement of the results in CNS tissue (Lorén et al. 1977,1980). As in the freeze-dry method addition of aluminum or magnesium salts in high concentrations to the perfusion fluid offers advantages also in the cryostat procedures. Lorén et al. (1977) have thus reported improved results with a modification of Bloom and Battenberg's (1976) and Nygren's (1976) protocols, in which $MgSO_4$(40 g/150 ml) is added to the FA-GA perfusion mixture. The best results were obtained with a combined GA-ALFA perfusion, according to Protocol VIII in the Appendix (Ajelis et al. 1979; Lorén et al. 1980). In this procedure the animal is first perfused with ice-cold 2% GA at moderate pressure, followed by ice-cold ALFA solution at high pressure.

A word of caution should however be inserted when trying to compare different perfusion techniques for cryostat sectioning, and that is that the further handling of the specimens (through the freezing, sectioning and drying steps) is much more critical for the final outcome of the procedure. The perfusion step plays a secondary role in this respect.

The technique and equipment used for perfusion in the cryostat methods are essentially the same as those dealt with in Section 5.1, in conjunction with the freeze-dry methods.

Freezing and sectioning

The considerations on tissue freezing and freezing artifacts, given in Section 5.1, are also valid for the handling of specimens for cryostat sectioning. Thus, freezing artifacts and diffusion of the water soluble monoamines from the cellular storage sites are the most obvious problems to be overcome. The freezing should be as rapid as possible. As in the freeze-dry technique the safest freezing medium is liquid propane or isopentane, cooled by liquid air or liquid nitrogen. This provides cooling temperatures of $-165°C$ or lower, and is the one generally recommended for histochemistry or autoradiography of diffusible substances (Pearse 1968; Stumpf and Roth 1969; Stumpf and Sar 1975; Lojda et al. 1976). Many labs compromise with this principle, however, in order to avoid the use of liquid nitrogen and in order to be able to work with larger pieces which will crack unless they are frozen more slowly. In most of the published catecholamine histofluorescence procedures, therefore, freezing on precooled chucks in powdered dry-ice has been used (Watson and Barchas 1977; Bloom and Battenberg 1976; Lorén et al. 1980). One should however be aware that the freezing temperature provided by dry-ice (approx. $-70°C$) is on the margin, both with respect to the formation of crystal artifacts and with respect to loss of catecholamine fluorescence through diffusion. It is important therefore to ensure that the freezing in dry-ice is as efficient as possible: the dry-ice should be finely powdered and the chuck plus the entire specimen should be immediately covered deeply in the ice.

Freezing with CO_2 or Freon expansion coolers (as used, e.g. by Watson and Ellison, 1976) is an excellent alternative to dry-ice powder. Slow freezing in the cryostat chamber, as recommended by De La Torre and Surgeon (1976), has given extremely variable results in our hands. Slower freezing is safer if a cryoprotective agent, like sucrose, can be infiltrated into the tissue. This is commonly employed, e.g. for immunohistochemistry of serotonin in cryostat sections (Steinbusch et al. 1968). In the immunohistochemical method the monoamine is, however, sufficiently well fixed to allow overnight immersion in cold 5% sucrose-buffer. In the ALFA procedure of Lorén et al. (1980), 2.5-5% sucrose is included in both the GA- and the ALFA-perfusion steps (see Protocol VIII in the Appendix). Although this certainly is an inefficient way to get sucrose into the tissue, Lorén et al. report some positive effect of the sucrose.

Good results in the cryostat sectioning step of the procedure is a matter of trial and error. Pearse (1968) and Lojda et al. (1976) have discussed some general principles of the technique and the cryo-microtome equipment, and the reader is referred to these books for a more detailed treatment of the subject. Sectioning of frozen tissue is usually done in the temperature range −10 to −30°C. This temperature is obviously partly in the range of incipient melting of the frozen tissue (see Section 5.1, under 'Freezing'). In this range, approx. −15 to −25°C, the risk of diffusion artifacts and recrystallization of the tissue water is increased. The principle is therefore to seek the lowest possible cutting temperature where sections of good quality can be obtained. This is usually possible at −25 to −30°C, as recommended by Lorén et al. (1976, 1980) and by De La Torre and Surgeon (1976). Interestingly, Bloom and Battenberg (1976) and Watson and Barchas (1977) report good results also with cryostat chamber temperatures set at −16 to −20°C. We feel, though, that when such high temperatures are employed (in order to obtain sections of higher quality) one should try to keep the specimens (and the sections) for as short a time as possible at this temperature.

Equipment

A large number of cryostats of varying designs are commercially available. Suitable machines should allow to keep a constant, low temperature (in the −25 to −30°C range) throughout sectioning. This should be checked by recording the temperature frequently *at the specimen and at the knife.* Cryostats with a closed chamber design have therefore been found to be the most satisfactory ones in our laboratory.

Immersion and drying

Immersion of the sections in a GA solution is generally advantageous in the GA methods, while this step can be omitted in the GA-ALFA procedure (see Fig. 12). The immersion is done immediately after the sections have been transferred onto microscope slides, and is directly followed by air drying, essentially as described above for Vibratome sections. Bloom and Battenberg (1976), Watson and Borchas (1977) and Lorén et al. (1977) recommend an ice-cold buffered 2% GA solution as immersion fluid, while the fluid used by De La Torre and Surgeon (1976) is a room-temperature 1% GA solution with sucrose.

Reaction and mounting

A reaction step, performed on the dried sections, is essential for full development of fluorescence in the sections. The reaction is performed either by heating at +95-100°C for 2.5-10 min (De La Torre 1980; Bloom and Battenberg 1976), by GA vapor treatment in a closed vessel at 100°C for 2-5 min (Watson and Barchas 1977), or by FA vapor treatment at +80°C for 1 h (Nygren 1976; Lorén et al. 1977, 1980). Consistent with Nygren's (1976) findings we have had the best experience with FA vapor treatment, performed in a closed vessel over paraformaldehyde of controlled humidity, as used in the freeze-dry methods (see Section 5.1, under 'FA vapor treatment').

Mounting is done in non-fluorescent media (Entellan, Fluoromont, paraffin oil or immersion oil) as in the previously described procedures.

Usefulness and field of application of the cryostat methods

The major advantages of the cryostat procedures are their short processing time and their relative simplicity which make them accessible to many laboratories. In fact, in De La Torre's (1980) procedure, based on nonperfused tissue, results can be obtained within 15-20 min after freezing of the tissue. The main disadvantages are their relatively low sensitivity and the risks of freezing and diffusion artifacts which make the results variable not only in between specimens but also within a section series.

All the cryostat techniques described above have a sensitivity in the detection of central catecholamine neurons that is markedly higher than that of the earlier FA-based methods. In our hands, the GA-ALFA technique has given the most reproducible and sensitive visualization of central catecholamine neurons. All known catecholamine systems can be demonstrated except those having a very low amine content, e.g. the DA-containing terminal systems in the anterior hypothalamus and the anterior cingulate cortex. The cryostat methods visualize the catecholamine cell bodies and the preterminal and terminal parts of the axons of the principal dopaminergic and noradrenergic projection systems well. These techniques are also useful for studies on peripheral catecholamine-containing structures. The fluorescence yield from central indolamine neurons is low. The cryostat sectioning procedure has several practical advantages for fluorescence histochemical work. As compared to Vibratome sectioning, the cryostat allows serial sections of large pieces. Furthermore, the cryostat sections can be larger than Vibratome sections; they are thinner and of an even thickness. Since the frozen tissue can be stored in sealed vials in a low temperature freezer (below $-50°C$) for at least several days, many specimens can be taken from each animal, and from groups of animals sacrificed at the same time.

The cryostat methods are most practical for routine work involving, e.g. evaluation of denervating lesions or localization of lesions, electrodes, or cannula tracks in relation to catecholamine pathways or cell groups. For neuroanatomical work or reliable and complete visualization of terminal systems in the CNS, the more sensitive and reproducible freeze-dry and Vibratome techniques, dealt with above, are to be preferred.

5.4. WHOLE-MOUNT AND SMEAR PREPARATIONS

Tissues which are thin enough to be spread directly on microscope slides can be used for direct visualization of cellular stores of catecholamines and 5-HT, without the need of any embedding, freezing or sectioning. Such procedures have been developed on the basis of the original FA-vapor method of Falck and Hillarp (Falck 1962; Malmfors 1965), and on the basis of the GA and Faglu techniques (Lindvall and Björklund 1974a; Furness and Costa 1975; Furness et al. 1977b). These so-called whole-mount procedures are summarized in the block diagram in Figure 13.

WHOLE-MOUNT PREPARATIONS

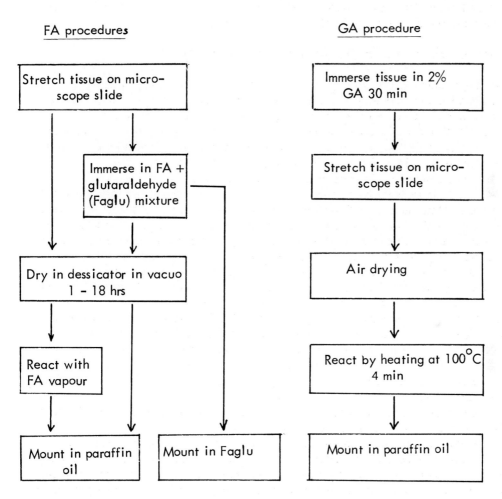

FA procedures   GA procedure

Stretch tissue on micro-   Immerse tissue in 2%
scope slide   GA 30 min

Immerse in FA +
glutaraldehyde
(Faglu) mixture   Stretch tissue on micro-
                                  scope slide

Dry in dessicator in vacuo   Air drying
1 – 18 hrs

React with   React by heating at 100°C
FA vapour   4 min

Mount in paraffin   Mount in Faglu   Mount in paraffin oil
oil

Fig. 13. Principal steps of the whole-mount procedure described in the text.

Procedures

The FA method has been applied to whole-mounts of iris and mesentery (Falck 1962; Malmfors 1965) (Fig. 14A), vascular walls and meninges (Nielsen and Owman 1967), heart atria (Sachs 1970), urinary bladder (McLean and Burnstock 1966), peripheral nerve (Olson 1969), and tissue sheets prepared from the digestive tract and the genital organs (Furness and Malmfors 1971). The technique is simple: the tissue membranes are spread on microscope slides and dried — preferably in a dessicator — over fresh granular phosphorous pentoxide for at least 1 h and then exposed to gaseous FA (see Section 5.1, under 'FA vapor treatment'). Mounting in, for example, Entellan (Merck) or liquid paraffin is recommended but not essential. The whole-mount technique is simple, rapid and versatile, and has therefore been extensively used (cf. Furness and

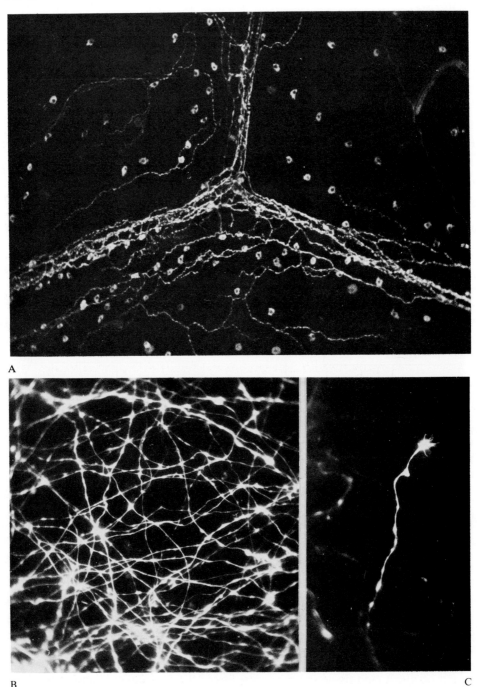

Fig. 14. A: FA-vapor treated whole-mount specimen of rat mesenterium, from one of the first successful series obtained with the Falck-Hillarp method. Adrenergic nerves around vessels and 5-HT-containing mast cells. (From Falck 1962). B and C: Whole-mounts of an explant culture of *Locus ceruleus*, processed according to a modified GA-immersion technique (Victorov et al. 1979). B shows a network of adrenergic neurites in the outgrowth zone by 10 days of culture (×620). C shows an outgrowing adrenergic fiber with a fluorescent growth cone (5 days, ×720). Courtesy of Dr. I. Victorov.

Malmfors 1971). FA-induced fluorescence has also been studied in smears of, for ex-
ample, peritoneal fluid containing mast cells (Ritzén 1966a), CNS tissue (Olson and
Ungerstedt 1970b), and subcellular fractions of homogenized tissues (Jonsson and
Sachs 1969).

Ajelis et al. (1979) have reported that immersion of the tissue in an aluminum-FA
(ALFA) solution, before stretching on slides, will improve the result in the standard FA
vapor procedure. Even better results were obtained if the animal was perfused with the
ALFA solution prior to sacrifice.

Fluorescence-histochemical demonstration of peripheral catecholamine stores in
whole-mount preparations by immersion in GA solution was first described by Lindvall
and Björklund (1974a). In this procedure, the thin tissue sheets (iris and mesentery) are
processed similar to the Vibratome sections (i.e. soaked in the ice-cold GA solution,
dried under a warm air stream, and then mounted in paraffin oil). This procedure has
been further developed by Furness and Costa (1975), who have applied the technique
to whole-mounts from several peripheral organs. Briefly, their procedure is as follows:
The freshly dissected tissue is immersed for 30 min at room temperature in a 2% GA
solution (0.1 M phoshate buffer, pH 7.0). The preparations are then freed of excess
moisture with the use of absorbent paper and stretched on clean glass slides, to which
they adhere as they dry. The slides are left on the laboratory bench for 3-5 min and are
then placed in an oven, set at $+100°C$, for 4 min. The specimens are mounted in paraffin oil. Furness and Costa (1975) found that the development of fluorescence is favored
by an initial excess of moisture in the tissue that is driven off during the fluorophore
formation. This is achieved by heating the tissue that has been partially dried (on the
laboratory bench) and then covering it with paraffin oil.

The whole-mount GA technique can also be used for demonstration of peripheral 5-
HT stores, e.g. in mast cells (Furness and Costa 1975). Furness and Costa (1975)
reported fairly selective visualization of peripheral 5-HT stores by immersing the
whole-mounts in acid 2% GA solution at pH 3.5, for 30 min at room temperature,
followed by air-drying and heating at $+100°C$ for 10 min. To induce fluorescence from
both 5-HT and NA, the tissue was first incubated in 2% GA at pH 7.0 for 30 min at
room temperature, followed by air-drying and exposure to FA vapor ($+80°C$ for 1 h).
A similar procedure has also been applied to catecholamine neurons in explant cultures
with excellent results (Figs 14B and C).

The Faglu technique is also excellent for visualization of catecholamine and 5-HT in
whole-mounts (Furness et al. 1977b). The preparations, adhering to glass slides, are
placed in a mixture of 4% FA and 0.5% glutaraldehyde in 0.1 M phosphate buffer (pH
7.0; Faglu mixture) at room temperature for 1-3 h. The specimens are then examined
in the fluorescence microscope with the Faglu as mounting medium. A further
enhancement of the fluorescence intensity is obtained if the preparations are dried over
phosphorous pentoxide for 1-2 h and then mounted in paraffin oil. With this technique, the fluorescence intensity in the noradrenergic axons seems to be similar to that
obtained with the GA method (Furness et al. 1977b). The major advantage with the
Faglu technique is that the specimens can be used for electron-microscopy, thus allowing direct correlations between the fluorescence- and electron-microscopic pictures (see
Section 6.6).

Usefulness and field of application

The whole mount and smear procedures for catecholamine and serotonin visualization are attractive because they are simple and quick and do not require any expensive or specialized equipment. The whole-mounts are, moreover, particularly useful in that they give a total overview, without any cumbersome reconstructions from series of sections, of the entire architecture of an innervated organ. Whole-mounts of, e.g. iris and heart atrium, have also been used very successfully as model systems for pharmacological and functional studies on sympathetic noradrenergic axons and terminal networks (see, e.g. Malmfors 1965; Sachs 1970; Olson and Malmfors 1970; Burnstock and Costa 1975).

The use of whole-mounts is limited to tissues that can be spread into sufficiently thin sheets. However, Furness and Malmfors (1971), in particular, have demonstrated that many thicker peripheral tissues (e.g. intestine and genital tract) can be divided into layers of thin sheets. The only part of the CNS that can be prepared as whole-mount is the filum terminale (i.e. the most caudal portion of the sacral spinal cord) (Olson and Nygren 1972). For other parts of the CNS, Olson and Ungerstedt (1970b) have described a quick smear-technique. Such preparations can visualize NA-, DA- and 5-HT-containing varicosities, but without any anatomical preservation of the region analyzed.

Finally, it should be pointed out that whole-mounts of iris, which has a rich noradrenergic innervation, has been widely used as a convenient preparation to help the investigator to standardize and optimize the immersion and reaction steps in the histofluorescence procedures, and also to help to assess that these steps are working properly once the method is set up. The irides are easy to prepare and can be obtained from the experimental rats when other tissues are being taken for analysis. Only albinos can be used, however, since pigmented irides are unsuitable for fluorescence microscopy. A detailed description on the preparation of iris whole-mounts is found in Malmfors (1965).

6. COMBINED TECHNIQUES

The monoamine histofluorescence techniques are nowadays widely combined with other microscopic, histochemical or neuroanatomical, methods in order to obtain more information from the specimens. The wide variety of alternative procedures for processing of tissue for monoamine visualization, summarized in the preceeding section, provides almost unlimited possibilities for such technical combinations. The following comments can thus only serve to exemplify some of the more commonly used combined procedures. For a more detailed account on combinations of monoamine histochemistry with retrograde axonal tracing and autoradiography, the reader is referred to Chapters VI and XI.

6.1. CONVENTIONAL HISTOLOGICAL STAINS

For identification purposes it is sometimes sufficient to perform the fluorescence microscopy in combination with a Zernicke-type phase-contrast condenser (and corresponding objectives) in a system allowing simultaneous mixing of the UV light with ordinary visible light. Better results are obtained in a microscope equipped with illuminating systems for both incident and transmitted light. Histological staining can be carried out successfully on sections processed with FA fixation or FA vapor reaction. The FA vapor treatment ensures a mild fixation of the tissues, and the dry conditions of this procedure facilitate good cytological preservation as well as excellent staining of the tissue components (cf. McNeill and Sladek 1980). For staining purposes, it is necessary to secure the paraffin sections on microscope slides coated with a thin layer of albumin-glycerine, or a similar substance. Xylene, liquid paraffin, or immersion oil is used for mounting. After photography in the fluorescence microscope, the coverslip can then be easily removed for subsequent staining. Additional fixation of the sections before staining is advantageous in certain cases (cf. Jennings 1965). The staining is followed by re-photography of the section and identification of the fluorescent structures.

6.2. ACETYLCHOLINESTERASE STAINING

Adrenergic and cholinergic neurons can be demonstrated in the peripheral nervous system by applying the FA and acetylcholinesterase (AChE) methods *consecutively* on one and the same section or whole-mount (Ehinger and Falck 1965, 1966; Eränkö and Räisänen 1965; Jacobowitz and Koelle 1965). Because of the enzyme inactivation produced by FA it is necessary to find an FA treatment sufficiently mild to give adequate fluorescence and still preserve enough AChE activity to enable its subsequent visualization. Treatment of the dried tissue for 0.5-1 h in FA gas generated at 37°C, or for 3-4 h at room temperature (Svengaard et al. 1975) has been found optimal. As a rule, the incubation time then required for the demonstration of AChE according to the Koelle technique has to be increased to 6-10 h to get pictures equivalent to those obtained without previous FA treatment (Ehinger and Falck 1966).

Since consecutive staining with re-photography is cumbersome, attempts have been made to apply catecholamine histofluorescence and AChE-staining *simultaneously* on the same section or whole-mount. Such procedures, useful on peripheral tissue, have been described by El-Badawi and Shenk (1967) and Ellison and Olander (1972) using the FA vapor method. More recently Waris et al. (1977) and Waris and Rechardt (1977) developed a similar technique in which GA is used instead of FA for the demonstration of catecholamine neurons. This modification seems superior to the combined FA-AChE procedures because of the stronger fluorescence and more limited diffusion seen with the GA-AChE technique. After immersion of the tissue pieces in a GA solution, they are processed for the demonstration of AChE. The pieces are then again immersed in the GA solution, dried and heated. In the fluorescence microscope, both NA fluorescent and AChE-positive fibers can be observed, the latter being distinguishable as dark profiles against the weakly fluorescent background.

Combined procedures applicable to CNS tissue have been described by Hökfelt et al. (1974), Lindvall (1977) and Bieger and Harley (1982) using Vibratome sections of FA-, GA- or Faglu-perfused tissue (see Section 5.2). Hökfelt et al. used consecutive sections for catecholamine and AChE visualization, whereas Lindvall's and Bieger and Harley's protocols have the advantage of using consecutive staining of the same section. In Lindvall's (1977) method, the brains are first processed according to the GA-Vibratome method (see Protocol III in the Appendix), i.e. it is perfused with an ice-cold GA solution, sectioned on a Vibratome instrument immersed in a GA solution, and dried under a stream of warm air. The unmounted sections are examined and photographed in the fluorescence microscope and then stained for AChE according to the Koelle technique (incubation 4-6 h). The sections are then examined in the light-microscope and re-photographed, and the two pictures are compared.

6.3. IMMUNOCYTOCHEMISTRY

Correlative microscopic studies of monoamine- and neuropeptide-containing systems have most often employed sequential staining with different antibodies on cryostat sections. The section is then first stained with an antibody directed, e.g. against tyrosine hydroxylase, DOPA decarboxylase, DBH, PNMT or serotonin, in order to visualize a monoaminergic marker. After photography and elusion of the first antibody, according to the technique of Tramu et al. (1978), the same section can be restained with a second antibody (directed, e.g. against a neuropeptide) and re-photographed (see, for example, Hökfelt et al. 1980a,b; and Chapter IV).

Aldehyde-induced fluorescence can, however, also be combined with immunocytochemistry in sequential procedures. This has been achieved both with FA-vapor fixed, freeze-dried and paraffin-embedded material (Alumets et al. 1978; Ibata et al. 1979; Johnson et al. 1979; McNeil and Sladek 1980; Schröder et al. 1982), with GA-treated cryostat sections (König 1979) and with Faglu-treated Vibratome sections (Howe et al. 1980). All these procedures involve photography of the monoamine fluorescence, restaining of the sections with antibodies, using the FITC, TRITC, MRITC or PAP techniques, and finally re-photography of the same area. Since the aldehyde-induced monoamine fluorescence can remain quite strong also after application of the antibody, several authors recommend the use of the red-fluorescent rhodamine-labeled antibodies, or the PAP technique, rather than FITC for this purpose.

When using freeze-dried, paraffin-embedded material for combination with immunocytochemistry, a special problem has been to secure the sections sufficiently well to the slides without causing diffusion of the monoamine fluorophores. McNeil and Sladek (1980) have recommended the use of paraffin sections finger-pressed onto gelatin-coated slides, and Larsson (Chapter IV) reports good results with sections floated out and stretched onto slides coated with a mixture of glycerin and gelatin. For floatation he recommends a mixture of 2% FA and 3% glutaraldehyde. For further details on this combined procedure see Chapter IV.

Recently, Smithson et al. (1983) and Schöler and Armstrong (1982) have introduced Faglu-perfused tissue embedded in polyethylene glycol (PEG) as an alternative to paraffin-embedded FA-vapor fixed material and Faglu-treated Vibratome sections. Since PEG-embedded specimens can be sectioned as thin as $1-2$ μm, this technique has the advantage that correlations can be done not only with the sequential procedure, but also by comparisons of adjacent sections. In case of cell bodies therefore, several 2 μm sections can be obtained from the same cell body, which thus can be compared in, e.g. a split image or superimposition microscope set-up (cf. McNeill and Sladek 1980).

6.4. RETROGRADE AXONAL TRACING METHODS

The combination of fluorescence histochemistry with retrograde tracing, using horseradish peroxidase (HRP) or fluorescent tracers, has provided a powerful 'transmitter-specific' neuroanatomical tracing technique which has greatly improved the possibilities for detailed analyses of monoaminergic projection systems, particularly in the CNS.

The first method of this kind was described by Ljungdahl et al. (1975). Their procedure involves sequential visualization of tyrosine hydroxylase and retrogradely transported horseradish peroxidase (HRP) in the same Vibratome section. Later, Satoh et al. (1977) introduced a combined, simultaneous staining of monoamine oxidase (MAO) and HRP in the same cryostat section, which enabled the observation of the purple formazane deposits from the MAO staining and the brown HRP granules from the diaminobenzidine reaction in the same cells. This procedure is, however, complicated by the fact that MAO is not an absolutely specific marker for monoaminergic neurons, and it is not a very sensitive stain for such neurons.

Procedures combining aldehyde histofluorescence and HRP staining have been published by Berger et al. (1978), Blessing et al. (1978), Smolen et al. (1979), and Hwang and Williams (1982). All these methods use a sequential procedure where catecholamine fluorescence is first visualized and photographed in the fluorescence microscope. The same section is then reacted for HRP staining and re-photographed in normal light. This combination has been carried out in Vibratome sections from brains perfused with either GA (Berger et al.), GA plus FA and glutaraldehyde (Smolen et al.) or FA plus glutaraldehyde (Blessing et al.); and on cryostat sections of tissue perfused with glyoxylic acid plus formaldehyde and glutaraldehyde (Berger et al.).

All these sequential procedures have the drawback of being very time-consuming. The re-photography and comparisons by means of photographs also make screening of large areas difficult. Blessing et al. (1982) have, however, recently modified their combined fluorescence-HRP procedure so that it is possible to view catecholamine fluorescence and HRP labeling concomitantly in the sections, an improvement which offers great advantage over the sequential procedures.

In our laboratory (Björklund and Skagerberg, 1979a,b) we have adopted an alternative approach, taking advantage of the different fluorescent retrograde tracers which have been introduced by Kuypers and collaborators (Kuypers et al. 1977, 1979; Bentivoglio et al. 1979). Such fluorescent tracers can be used concomitantly with aldehyde-induced monoamine fluorescence, provided that: (1) the tracer has a fluorescence color sufficiently different from the monoamine fluorophores; (2) the tracer has an excitation maximum different from the monoamine fluorescence; and/or (3) the tracer has a subcellular localization that is different from that of the monoamine fluorophores. 'True Blue' and Propidium Iodide fulfill at least two of these criteria. Subsequently, we have found that the compound called 'Nuclear Yellow' would also be useful for this purpose. True Blue, which fluoresces in an ice-blue color, and Propidium Iodide, which fluoresces brick-red, are ideally suited for combination with the greenish-yellow catecholamine fluorophore and the yellow serotonin fluorophore. The procedure currently used in our laboratory involves the following steps. After sufficient survival time following the tracer injection the rats are perfused according to the ALFA or Mg-FA-GA methods (see above), the brains are freeze-dried, reacted with formaldehyde vapor, paraffin-embedded, and finally sectioned for fluorescence microscopy. This processing gives excellent retention of the fluorescent tracers, which are now visible concomitantly with the formaldehyde-induced monoamine fluorophores in the same section.

For further details of the transmitter specific retrograde tracing procedures, and detailed protocols, the reader is referred to Chapter VI.

6.5. AUTORADIOGRAPHY

Studies on the binding and storage of exogenous amines and on compounds that interfere with their metabolism and function require techniques for concomitant demonstration of the amine structures and the compound administered. This can be obtained with microautoradiographic methods for water-soluble substances carried out under dry conditions (Masuoka and Placidi 1968; Masuoka et al. 1971; Stumpf and Roth 1969; Ullberg and Appelgren 1969; Hökfelt and Ljungdahl 1971). These procedures utilize whole-mounts, cryostat-sectioned material or sections from freeze-dried tissues, and they have all employed FA-vapor treatment for the visualization of CA and 5-HT. The reacted sections are photographed in the fluorescence microscope before application of the autoradiographic emulsion. After development, the sections are again examined for autoradiographic grains.

Combined autoradiographic and fluorescence-histochemical techniques have been used also to study the morphological relationships between CA neurons and estrogen target neurons. In the technique of Grant and Stumpf (1981), cryostat sections from animals injected with [³H]estradiol are freeze-dried and reacted with FA vapor. The sections are then dry-mounted onto emulsion coated slide for autoradiographic localization of [³H]estradiol-uptake sites. After exposure and development, the [³H]estradiol-uptake sites and CA neurons can be localized simultaneously in the same section by using a microscope with a combination of UV and regular tungsten light. For further details of this procedure, the reader is referred to Chapter XI.

6.6. ELECTRON-MICROSCOPY

Early attempts to combine monoamine fluorescence histochemistry and electron-microscopy on the same specimens were hampered by the inadequacies of the reagents, formaldehyde and glyoxylic acid, as fixatives for the preservation of good ultrastructure. Important progress in this field has, however, been made, first by Chiba et al. (1976) and later by Furness et al. (1977a,b, 1978) through the development of their Faglu method (see Section 5.2).

The critical feature of both these procedures is the introduction of glutaraldehyde into the perfusion fluid. In the method of Chiba et al. (1976), the animal is first perfused with ice-cold GA, followed by an ice-cold mixture of 4% FA and 0.5% glutaraldehyde. Sections are cut with either cryostat or Vibratome at 20-50 μm, incubated briefly in the GA solution, and mounted for fluorescence microscopy (omitting the otherwise-used drying and heating steps). The same sections are finally processed for electron-microscopy.

In the Faglu procedure (Protocol V in the Appendix), the brains are fixed through perfusion with a mixture of 4% formaldehyde and 0.5-1.0% glutaraldehyde at room temperature. Vibratome sections are immersed in this mixture for 15 min. An interesting feature of this method is that catecholamine fluorescence can be viewed (particularly in cell bodies and strongly fluorescent processes) in the wet sections mounted in the Faglu mixture. In this solution the fluorescence develops without drying of the tissue. Furness et al. (1978) have suggested that this is due to a stabilization and binding of the fluorophore by glutaraldehyde. However, also in the Faglu-processed sections the intensity of the catecholamine fluorescence is markedly increased by thorough drying.

Furness et al. (1978) have reported excellent ultrastructural preservation in the Faglu-processed Vibratome sections, particularly if the glutaraldehyde concentration is raised to 1% and cacodylate buffer is used. Figure 15 gives examples from a locus ceruleus cell body and from synapses in the paraventricular nucleus of the hypothalamus, taken from material processed in this way. This method should help greatly to bridge the gap between light and electron-microscopy of monoaminergic systems.

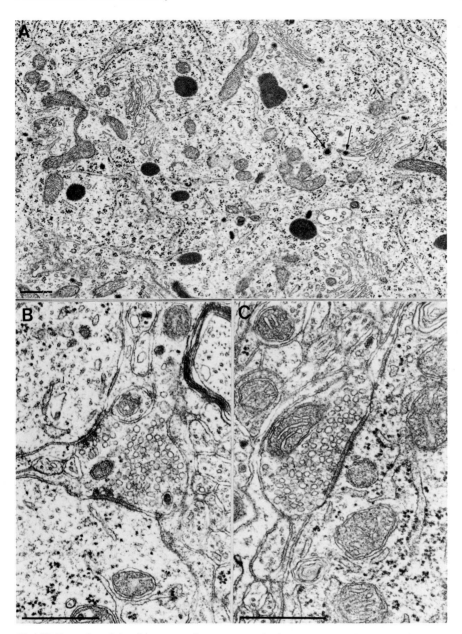

Fig. 15. Examples of the ultrastructural appearance of a locus ceruleus cell body (A) and synapses in the paraventricular hypothalamic nucleus (B and C) in Vibratome sections of Faglu-processed tissue. Calibration: 0.5 μm. Arrows in (A) denote granular vesicles. (From Furness et al. 1978.)

6.7. IN VITRO UPTAKE EXPERIMENTS

As described in Section 8.1, DA- and NA-containing structures can be differentiated in the FA method by microspectrofluorometric analysis (see Fig. 17). In the GA method applied to Vibratome sections, this is not possible. However, DA neurons can be nialamide (to inhibit monoamine oxidase). They are then perfused with ice-cold, neutral Krebs-Ringer bicarbonate buffer. Sections cut in the Vibratome instrument are then preincubated at $+37°C$ for 15 min either in buffer alone or in the presence of desipramine (10^{-5} M). Desipramine is an inhibitor of neuronal CA uptake that is about 1000 times more potent on the uptake into NA neurons than on the uptake into DA neurons (Horn et al. 1971). This selective blocking effect of desipramine has previously been utilized for both biochemical and histochemical differentiation between DA and NA terminals in the CNS (Hamberger 1967; Cuello et al. 1973). Following the preincubation, the sections are incubated in the presence of DA (10^{-6} M) for 20 min. They are then processed according to the GA-Vibratome method (see Section 5.2). In sections preincubated without desipramine (A and C in Fig. 16) *both* noradrenergic and dopaminergic axons are fluorescent, whereas in the adjacent sections preincubated with desipramine (B and D) only the dopaminergic axons are fluorescent.

Berger and Glowinski (1978) have developed this approach further in order to provide selective visualization of NA-, DA- and 5-HT-containing terminals in the CNS. In

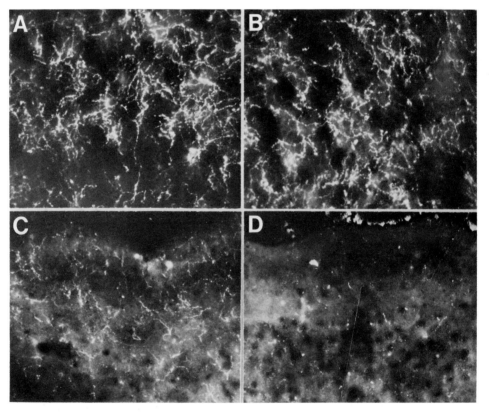

Fig. 16. Illustrations of the fluorescence-microscopic picture in Vibratome sections prepared for differentiation between dopaminergic and noradrenergic neurons. For details on the methodology, see the text. (A,B) From adjacent sections through the supragenual anteromedial cortex. (C,D) From adjacent sections through the sensorimotor cortex. (A,C) Incubated in DA alone; in this case, both dopaminergic (A) and noradrenergic (C) axons became visible after treatment with GA. (B,D) Incubated in DA in the presence of desipramine, which is a blocker of CA uptake into noradrenergic neurons; in this case, only dopaminergic axons are demonstrated (B), whereas the noradrenergic axons are not visible (D). (From Lindvall et al. 1978.)

their procedure the animals are pretreated with the tyrosine hydroxylase inhibitor, α-methyl-p-tyrosine, in order to deplete endogenous catecholamines. Vibratome sections are then incubated, as above, in the presence of exogenous amines and uptake inhibitors of the different catecholamine and serotonin uptake systems. Thus, NA terminals were visualized by incubation in NA (10^{-6} M) in the presence of 10^{-5} M benzatropine and DA terminals by incubation in DA (10^{-6} M) in the presence of 5×10^{-6} M DMI. Incubation in DA, with and without selective serotonin uptake blockers, gave a further possibility to identify presumed 5-HT terminals.

7. FLUORESCENCE-MICROSCOPY

In fluorescence-microscopy of biogenic monoamines the specimen is illuminated with light in the blue-violet to ultraviolet range. Fluorescence is a special form of luminescence in which a molecule absorbes light and re-emits the absorbed energy as light of lower energy, i.e. longer wavelenght. As will be dealt with in the following section, the FA- and GA-induced monoamine fluorophores are maximally excited by light in the blue-violet to ultraviolet range, and the emitted light is in the blue to yellow range.

The principal construction of a standard fluorescence-microscope using transmitted light (sub-stage illumination) is schematically illustrated in Figure 17A. The instrument is equipped with a UV light source for activation or exitation of the fluorophores in the microscopic specimen and with two sets of filters. The light source is usually a high-pressure mercury lamp giving a high intensity of UV and blue-violet light. The light is

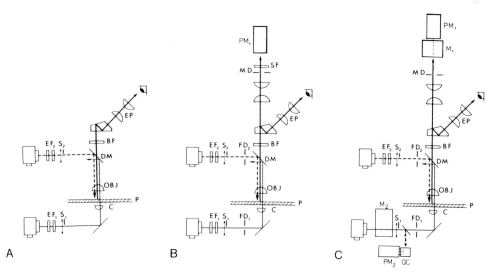

Fig. 17. Principal design of a fluorescence-microscope equipped for both incident and transmitted illumination (A), of a fluorescence-microscope equipped for intensity measurements (B), and a fluorescence-microscope equipped for recordings of excitation and emission spectra. For explanation, see text. Abbreviations: BF = barrier filter; C = condenser; DM = dichroic mirror; EF_1 and EF_2 = excitation filters; EP = eyepiece; FD_1 and FD_2 = field diaphragms; OBJ = objective; P = preparation; M_1 and M_2 = emission and excitation monochromators; PM_1 and PM_2 = photomultipliers connected to recording units; QC = quantum counter device; S_1 and S_2 = shutters; SF = band interference selection filter. (Modified after Schipper and Tilders 1982; and Wreford and Smith 1982.)

is equipped with a UV light source for activation or excitation of the fluorophores in the microscopic specimen and with two sets of filters. The light source is usually a high-pressure mercury lamp giving a high intensity of UV and blue-violet light. The light is passed through a heat-absorption filter (Schott KG l) and through suitable primary filters (EF_1 in Fig. 17A, thick enough to minimize unwanted excitation light and, thus, disturbing background fluorescence) to select optimum wavelength. The light is then focused by a metallized front-surface mirror into a dark-field condenser (c). Oil-immersion condensers usually give higher light intensity, and are thus preferable. The emitted light is passed through the so-called secondary filters (BF) placed after the objective (OBJ), in order to cut-off the stray light from the lamp. The lamp filter or filters are selected to filter-through light with a wavelength as close as possible to the excitation (absorption) maximum of the fluorophores. For the FA- and GA-induced fluorophores this maximum is at 390-410 nm. As evident from the spectral curves shown in Figure 18, the catecholamine and 5-HT fluorophores are, however, efficiently excited over a wider wavelength range, approx. between 360 and 450 nm. When selecting filters it is important to remember that the light of the mercury lamp is discontinuous and confined to a few bands (or lines), as illustrated by the lamp spectrum shown in Fig. 3 in Chapter VI of this volume. For the present purposes the 365, 405, and 435 nm lines are all useful for excitation of monoamine fluorescence. The most intense fluorescence is, in fact, obtained if two or all three of these lines are used to activate the fluorescence. When using transmitted light this is achieved with Schott's filters BG 12 or BG 3 as lamp filters. A 1 mm BG 12 filter transmits about 75% of the 365 nm line, about 85% of the 405 nm line and about 80% of the 435 nm line; and a 1 mm BG 3 filter transmits about 90% of the 365 nm line, about 90% of the 405 nm line, and about 70% of the 435 nm line. The thickness of the filters should be variable, so that more filters are used when the lamp is new, and less filters as the lamp gets older. To allow this, the microscope should be equipped with a holder for at least two lamp filters. In addition, a red-absorbing filter (e.g. Schott BG 38) may be used, particularly in combination with the BG 3 filter which has high transmission of light in the red part of the spectrum (over 90%). This reduces disturbing red stray-light.

The secondary (so-called cut-off or barrier) filter is selected so that it absorbs the lamp light that shines through the specimen, but lets the fluorescent light pass through. These cut-off barrier filters are designed so that they absorb all, or almost all, light below a certain cut-off wavelength, and transmit all, or almost all, light above the cut-off wavelength. With BG 12 or BG 3 lamp filters, secondary barrier filters with a cut-off wavelength of 470-500 nm are suitable. Such barrier filters will, however, cut-off some of the low-wavelength part of the catecholamine fluorescence. This will make the otherwise blue catecholamine fluorescence appear greenish or yellow-green.

Many fluorescence microscopes are equipped for incident illumination (epi-illumination) of the specimen, i.e. illumination where the objective is used both as condenser and objective. These microscopes are equipped with a filter-mirror package that is inserted into the light path, above the objective (see Ploem 1967). The light is first passed through a lamp filter (often a band-pass interference filter; EF_2 in Fig. 17A) and then reflected down, through the objective onto the specimen, with a dichroic mirror (DM). This dichroic mirror has the property of reflecting the lamp light but allowing the fluorescent light (which is of longer wavelength) to pass. The fluorescence coming back through the objective is thus passed through the mirror and a barrier filter to the observer's eyes. The manufacturers usually offer packages with selected lamp filter-mirror-barrier filter combinations; for monoamine histofluorescence work combinations designed for illumination in the violet and ultraviolet range (the 365 and 405 nm peaks of the mercury lamp) are normally recommended.

Although the microscopes employing incident illumination are more expensive than the standard type with sub-stage illumination, they offer little advantage for most types of monoamine fluorescence histochemical work. Sub-stage illumination is usually superior to incident illumination at lower magnifications (up to 25× objective), whereas incident illumination is superior at higher magnifications (25× objective or higher). Thus, microscopes which allow both sub-stage and epi-illumination, like the one illustrated in Figure 17A, will be the most optimal and flexible equipment. In either case, the use of objectives with high numerical apertures (neofluars or planapochromates) are essential to obtain a sensitive system suitable for studies also of delicate and weakly fluorescent fiber systems. With incident light, not only the transmittance of the emitted fluorescent light, but also the intensity of illumination is directly proportional to the numerical aperture of the objective used. Thus, the quality of the objectives is even more critical in microscopes with this type of illumination.

One final practical comment should be made about the high-pressure mercury lamp used in most fluorescence microscopes. One should be aware that these lamps do not 'burn out' in the conventional way; instead, they age and decline gradually in intensity over time. A new lamp will perform at maximum intensity for, usually, at least 100 burning hours, and sometimes for up to 250-300 burning hours. At this point they start to decline in intensity, although they will continue to burn at progressively lower intensity for several hundred hours more. For optimum performance of the microscope it is important, therefore, to keep records of the burning time of each new lamp. This is most easily done with a timer attached to the electric switch for the lamp. We usually change our lamps after a burning time of about 150-200 h. Some lamps will, however, decline in intensity earlier, and occasionally a new lamp may not reach acceptable intensity even when it is new.

8. MICROFLUOROMETRY

The microspectrofluorometer (Figs. 17B and C) is principally a fluorescence-microscope with attachments allowing qualitative and quantitative analysis of intracellular fluorophores. For fluorescence quantitation a comparatively simple equipment can be used. Thus, any fluorescence-microscope with epi-illumination, with a stabilized light source and a suitable photodetector can be sufficient (see, e.g. Lichtensteiger 1970; Van Orden 1970; Tilders et al. 1974; Geyer et al. 1978; Rundqvist 1981). Although the instrumentation for fluorescence quantitation can be rather uncomplicated, the theoretical and practical problems inherent in this technique, particularly when applied to quantitation of monoamines in tissue, are quite substantial. These methodological problems have been dealt with in reviews by Jonsson (1971), Ritzén (1973), Sernetz and Thaer (1973), Ploem (1977), Schipper and Tilders (1982) and Wreford and Smith (1982).

More advanced instruments are required for qualitative spectral analysis of fluorophores at high sensitivity. For complete fluorophore characterization the microspectrofluorometer must permit recordings of both emission and excitation spectra, which means that it must be equipped with monochromators for both the exciting and the emitted light, as illustrated in Figure 17C. Such instruments are commercially available, and for details on the construction and operation of such instruments the

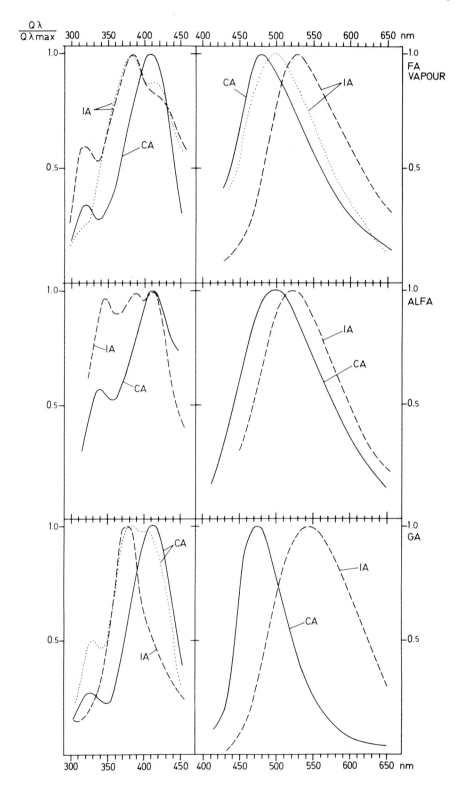

reader is referred to Casperson et al. (1965), Björklund et al. (1968a, 1972a), Rost and Pearse (1971), Ruch and Leeman (1973), Mayer and Novacek (1974), Cova et al. (1974), Ploem et al. (1974), Wreford and Schofield (1975), Jotz et al. (1976), Klig et al. (1976), Reinhold and Hartwig (1982), and Wreford and Smith (1982).

8.1. SPECTRAL ANALYSIS OF MONOAMINE FLUOROPHORES

Technical considerations

Qualitative microspectrofluorometric analysis is based on the recording of two types of spectral of the fluorophores: the emission and the excitation spectrum. These spectra are physical entities related to the molecular configuration of the fluorescent compounds, i.e. the fluorophores formed from the monoamines in the histochemical reactions. For this reason, the spectral analysis has high analytical value for structural identification of biogenic monoamines at their cellular storage sites.

The emission spectrum gives the spectral distribution of the emitted light and can be considered independent of the wavelength of the exciting (activating) light. It is recorded at a fixed wavelength of the exciting light (preferably close to the wavelength of maximal excitation), and the relative distribution of the emitted light in the visual part of the spectrum is registered. The excitation spectrum expresses the efficiency by which the exciting light of different wavelength induces fluorescence. This type of spectrum is obtained by varying the wavelength of the exciting light while the intensity of the emitted light is measured at a fixed wavelength. The excitation spectrum of a fluorescent substance is practically identical with its absorption spectrum and is for this reason especially helpful for identification purposes. While emission spectra can be recorded with a mercury lamp as the exciting light source, excitation spectra can only be made with a light source that has a more continuous light spectrum. Xenon arc lamps are those most commonly employed in microspectrofluorometry. Excellent reviews on the theory of fluorescence and fluorescence spectra have been published, e.g. by Hercules (1966), Parker (1968) and Pesce et al. (1971).

Both the excitation and emission spectra are distorted by a number of factors in the instrument, and the registered spectra (i.e. the uncorrected instrument values) usually deviate considerably from the true spectra (see Ritzén 1967; Parker 1968). The emission spectrum is influenced by the secondary filters used, the transmission of the optics, the transmission and band width of the analyzing monochromator, and the sensitivity of the photomultiplier. Similarly, the excitation spectrum is influenced by the varying transmission of the excitation monochromator and optics; it is also strongly influenced by the varying intensity of the light source at different wavelengths. Altogether, these factors will make the values distorted in a way that is characteristic for each individual instrument. For this reason, all published spectra should be corrected and expressed in

Fig. 18. Fluorescence excitation (left) and emission (right) spectra, recorded in tissue processed according to the FA vapor method (top), according to the ALFA method (middle), and according to the GA method (bottom). *Solid lines* give typical spectra recorded from catecholamine-containing neurons in the rat CNS. *Dashed lines* give typical spectra recorded from serotonin-containing cell bodies in the rat brain stem (top and middle) or serotonin-containing enterochromaffin cells in the rat stomach (bottom). *Dotted line in top panel* shows the deviating type of indolamine spectrum recorded in FA-treated specimens of the rat CNS (see Björklund et al. 1971c). *Dotted line in bottom panel* shows the excitation spectrum of the GA-induced catecholamine fluorophore in its acid form, sometimes recorded in GA-treated Vibratome sections.

standardized units, which will allow direct comparison between spectra obtained in different laboratories.

The correction of the emission spectrum requires the preparation of an instrument calibration curve, which can be obtained, for instance, from measurements with a calibrated tungsten lamp or by measuring the fluorescence of a fluorescent reference solution with known emission characteristics. For *the correction of the excitation spectrum,* some kind of device for the continuous measurement of the intensity of the exciting light is necessary as the characteristics of the exciting light will vary between the individual lamps and throughout the lifetime of a lamp. The correction procedures employed in our laboratory have been introduced and described by Ritzén (1967). The reader should also consult the papers by Van Orden (1970), Rost and Pearse (1971) and Ploem et al. (1974).

For excitation spectra below 360 nm, the optical pathway for the exciting light must be entirely made up of quartz (quartz optics and quartz condenser) and the excitation monochromator must have a high transmittance in this low wavelength range. For this reason, we have found grating monochromators superior to prism monochromators for the recording of excitation spectra of monoamine fluorophores. The specimens cannot be mounted on glass microscope slides which absorb too much light below 360 nm and are strongly fluorescent at these lower wavelengths. Instead we have used either quartz slides or non-fluorescent coverslips. When coverslips are used, the specimens are mounted upside-down, on the under surface of the slip, and liquid paraffin (which has less absorption in the low UV range than immersion oil) is used as condenser liquid. Ritzén (1967) has pointed out that the quartz slides commonly used for ultraviolet microscopy (Hereaus-Schott's Suprasil[R]) have a weak fluorescence at about 370-390 nm, which is excited near 310 nm.

Another potentially complicating factor in fluorescence analysis is *fluorescence fading*. The indolamine fluorophores, in particular, show marked photocomposition under irradiation with ultraviolet or blue-violet light. If this occurs during the registration of the spectra, it will naturally distort the shape of the spectrum. Consequently, the spectral recordings should be made at a speed that ensures that the fading during registration is negligible. If significant fading of the fluorescence occurs during the course of the spectral registration, the spectrum can be corrected afterwards, provided that the rate of photodecomposition of the fluorophores is known.

Spectral properties of catecholamine and indolamine fluorophores

The spectral properties of the FA- and GA-induced fluorophores from various phenylethylamine and indolylethylamine compounds, and the influence of changes in the physical environment and in molecular substituents, have been dealt with in detail in the reviews by Björklund and Falck (1973) and Björklund et al. (1975a). Here we will focus on some of the key features of the catecholamine and indolamine fluorophores produced in FA and GA-treated nervous tissues.

Table 2 and Figure 18 summarize the fluorescence intensities and spectral properties of the fluorogenic catecholamines and indolamines, and their amino acid precursors, in the FA, ALFA and GA reactions. As seen in Figure 18 the monoamine fluorophores are all maximally excited in the UV-blue violet range (excitation maxima at 370-415 nm), and the emission maxima are in the blue to yellow range of the spectrum (emission maxima at 475-535 nm).

In both the FA and GA reactions, the catecholamine and indolamine fluorophores

TABLE 2. *Fluorescence yields and excitation (ex. max.) and emission peak maxima (em. max.) of some fluorogenic catecholamines and indolamines in the FA, ALFA and GA methods, as registered in dried protein films. The variation in the peak values is at least ± 5 nm.*

	FA reaction[a]			ALFA reaction[a,b]			GA reaction[c]		
	Relative intensity	Exc. max.[d] (nm)	Em. max. (nm)	Relative intensity	Exc. max.[d] (nm)	Em. max. (nm)	Relative intensity	Exc. max.[d] (nm)	Em. max. (nm)
Dopamine	100	320 and 410	475	200	(330)(350), 410	490–530	670	(330)415	475
Noradrenaline	100	320 and 410	475	85	(320)350, 410	490–530	460	(330)415	475
Adrenaline	40	320 and 410	475	10	(330)350(410)	510	10	(335)370[e]	485[e]
DOPA	120	320 and 410	475	70	(330)355(405)	510	130	(330)415	480
Tryptamine	10	370	495	140	360	500	25		
5-Hydroxy-tryptamine	30	(315)385, 415	520–540	55	365(410)	525	10	375[e]	520–550[e]
5-Methoxy-tryptamine	20	(330) and 380	505	115	365	535	15		
Tryptophan	10	375	435 or 500	25	360	500	0		
5-Hydroxy-tryptophan	10	310, 385, 415	520–540	30	365(410)	525	0		

[a] FA vapor treatment at +80°C for 1 h. Data from Björklund et al. (1971).
[b] Recorded in protein models containing 10 mM $Al_2(SO_4)_3$. Data from Björklund et al. (1980).
[c] Recorded in protein models containing 2% GA (pH 7.0) and heated at +100°C for 6 min. Data from Lindvall and Björklund (1974a).
[d] Figures in brackets denote low peak or shoulder in the excitation spectrum.
[e] Values obtained from models reacted with GA vapor (100°C, 3 min). From Lindvall and Björklund (1974a).

can usually be distinguished by their fluorescence color: the catecholamine fluorescence being blue (em.max. at about 475 nm) and the 5-HT and 5-HTP fluorescence being yellow (em.max. at 520-540 nm) (Fig. 18, top and bottom). This difference is, however, abolished in the aluminum-catalyzed FA reaction (ALFA reaction) where both catecholamines and indolamines fluoresce in the yellow range (em.max. at 495-525 nm) (Fig. 18, middle). Also in the standard FA reaction, distinction between catecholamines and indolamines on the basis of fluorescence color has to be made with caution. In certain cases when dealing with high concentrations of catecholamines the emitted light from the FA-induced fluorophores appears yellowish in the fluorescence-microscope even though the microspectrofluorometric recording shows an emission maximum at about 480 nm (Norberg et al. 1966; Jonsson 1967). This is because the maximum sensitivity of the human eye is shifted toward longer wavelengths with increasing intensity of the light (the so-called Bezold-Brücke effect). To avoid misinterpretations of catecholamine fluorescence as being due to, for example, 5-HT, it is important in all doubtful cases to perform spectral analyses.

Whereas the Bezold-Brücke effect means that the color impression of the fluorescence is changed without a corresponding change in the emission spectrum, there are instances in which a true change of the emission spectrum does occur. Thus, the FA-induced fluorescence from catecholamines will exhibit a shift in the emission maximum from 480 nm to 500-550 nm when the amine concentration is very high, as in adrenal medullary cells (Caspersson et al. 1966; Jonsson 1967). This is most probably due to a concentration-dependent side-reaction, e.g. polymerization or oxidation, or both (Jonsson 1967), and can be prevented by using milder reaction conditions (less humid FA gas, lower temperature, and shorter reaction time). The shift in the emission spectrum has never been reported in central or peripheral catecholamine-containing neurons after the standard FA reaction, or in GA-treated specimens, but it occurs consistently in specimens processed according to the ALFA method (Fig. 18, middle). The emission maximum of the NA and DA fluorophores in ALFA treated specimens can thus vary from 490 nm up to about 530 nm in extreme cases. The spectral distinction between catecholamines and serotonin is thus less clear-cut in the ALFA method than in the standard Falck-Hillarp procedure (cf. top and middle panels in Fig. 18).

The catecholamines and DOPA show all indistinguishable spectra in both the FA, ALFA and GA reactions. The excitation spectrum of these fluorophores are, however, pH-dependent. Thus, at neutral pH the maximum is at 410-415 nm and at acid pH at 370-380 nm. This is due to the pH-dependent tautomerism and non-quinoidal forms of the dihydroisoquinole fluorophores, illustrated in Figure 4A, above (Corrodi and Hillarp 1964; Jonsson 1966; Björklund et al. 1968a). Figure 4A also illustrates that the fluorophores induced by FA treatment from the β-hydroxylated catecholamines, NA and adrenaline, have a labile 4-hydroxy group that can be split-off by acid (Corrodi and Jonsson 1965a; Björklund et al. 1968a). Those fluorophores which lose this group are converted to fully aromatic compounds. This is followed by a shift in the main excitation peak down to 320-330 nm. The DA fluorophore, lacking the 4-hydroxy group cannot be transformed into the fully aromatic compound in this way, and consequently its main excitation peak after acid treatment remains at 370 nm. This difference in the behavior of the DA and NA fluorophores on treatment with acid, can be utilized for differentiating intracellular DA from NA by microspectrofluorometric analysis (Björklund et al. 1968a, 1972a). In this method, the FA-treated tissue sections are exposed to hydrochloric acid vapor for various times at room temperature and the behavior of the peaks at 370 and 320 nm is carefully studied. For further details on the practical performance, the limitations, and the pitfalls of this differentiation technique, the reader should consult the papers by Björklund et al. (1972a) and Reinhold and Hartwig (1982). Reinhold and Hartwig (1982) have recently shown that the spectral differentiation between the various catecholamine fluorophores after acidification can be further improved if the excitation spectra are recorded further down into the low UV-range (down to 250 nm). This requires, however, a more advanced equipment. Although these pH-dependent changes occur also with the GA-induced catecholamine fluorophores, the accompanying spectral shifts are more sluggish and more difficult to obtain in tissue sections (Lindvall et al. 1974c). The spectral differentiation between DA and NA is therefore not useful in GA-treated material. In ALFA-treated material, the expected spectral changes are known to occur in DA- and NA-containing models, but it is so far not known whether the differentiation can be made in tissues.

5-HT and its immediate precursor 5-HTP give fluorophores that are spectrally very similar to each other. These 5-hydroxylated indolamines differ, however, from their non-hydroxylated or methoxylated congeners, such as tryptamine, tryptophan and 5-methoxytryptamine (Table 2). All indolamine fluorophores have a fluorescence color in the yellow range, but the fluorophores of the non-hydroxylated indolamines have 20-30 nm lower emission and excitation peak maxima than those of 5-HT and 5-HTP. Interestingly, in FA-vapor treated material fluorophores with spectral properties of both these kinds are found in the brain stem raphe nuclei (see dashed and dotted curves in Fig. 18, top panel) (Björklund et al. 1971b). Parallel biochemical observations suggest that this may be due to the presence of non-hydroxylated indolamines (such as tryptamine or 5-methoxytryptamine) (besides 5-HT) in some indolaminergic raphe neurons (Björklund et al. 1976).

8.2. MICROFLUOROMETRIC QUANTITATION

Fluorescence intensity can be used as a measure of amine concentration in cells provided that certain conditions are fulfilled: (i) the histochemical reaction must be standardized and consistent throughout a series of specimens and standards; (ii) variations in section thickness and intensity of the activating light must be controlled; (iii) the measuring technique must avoid errors due to fluorescence fading; and (iv) the measurements must be confined to the concentration range where fluorescence is linearly related to the fluorophore concentration.

The last point, i.e. the problem of concentration quenching, is potentially the most serious limitation to fluorometric quantitation in cells. In air-dried protein droplets the fluorescence-concentration curve is linear up to over 10^{-2} M concentration of catecholamines and 5-HT, both after FA (Ritzén 1966a,b, 1967; Geyer et al. 1978; Wreford and Smith 1982) and GA treatment (Lindvall et al. 1974c). In freeze-dried models concentration quenching appears to occur at lower concentration, about 10^{-3} M (Schipper and Tilders 1982). The first experiments in tissue (Jonssons 1969, 1971; Van Orden et al. 1970), performed on peripheral adrenergic nerve terminals, indicated that the normal concentrations of NA in such nerve terminals were well above the linear range. This is in contrast to the more recent findings of Schipper et al. (1980), using smaller measuring fields (100-700 μm^2) or scanning with a 0.5×0.5 μm measuring spot, demonstrating a linear relationship between NA concentration and nerve terminal fluorescence in FA-treated whole-mounts of rat iris. Such linear relationship has also been demonstrated in DA- and 5-HT-containing cell bodies in the CNS (Lichtensteiger

1970; Jonsson et al. 1975; Geyer et al. 1978), in 5-HT-containing pinealocytes (Tilders et al. 1974) and mastcells (Enerbäck et al. 1977), and in DA-containing terminals in the median eminence (Bacopoulus et al. 1975; Löfström et al. 1976a,b) and neostriatum (Einarsson et al. 1975; Agnati et al. 1978). In central NA-containing terminals, the situation seems to be more variable. Lidbrink and Jonsson (1971), using a semiquantitative technique, have reported that in cortical NA terminals, the relationship between fluorescence intensity and concentration is linear up to the normal endogenous NA level, whereas this linear relationship is broken at approximately 50% of the normal level in hypothalamic NA terminals.

Taken together, these data indicate that microfluorometry can be used for quantitation in a wide variety of monoaminergic cell systems. Nevertheless, since the problem of linearity may vary from system to system and depend on variations in the fluorescence yields, i.e. the amount of fluorophores formed in the histochemical reaction, each investigator will have to establish that the above quoted conditions are fulfilled for his or her own system. Such caution is even more warranted since the physical environment of the fluorophores, and interactions between the fluorophores and surrounding matrix, is known to influence the fluorescence yields of monoamine fluorophores in ways that are so far not fully understood (Lindvall et al. 1980).

Standardization of the histochemical processing is essiential for reliable quantitation. All published studies so far have employed either freeze-dried, paraffin-embedded material or whole-mount preparations, and it is evident that these preparative techniques are well suited to provide well standardized results throughout large series of specimens. Under such conditions relative quantitative data, comparable within a series of specimens processed in parallel, can be made without the use of internal fluorescence standards. In such cases 'normal' or untreated tissue often serves as a reference standard, allowing the results to be expressed as 'percent of normal'. However, since the fluorescence yield of the monoamines in the FA reaction is influenced by the reaction conditions and since this yield is difficult or impossible to reproduce exactly from one experiment to another, fluorescence reference standards must be used in all cases when different experiments are compared, or when attempts are made to express results in absolute units. When the measurements are performed on whole cells (e.g. isolated mast cells) or on structures in whole mounts (e.g. adrenergic terminals in stretch preparations of the iris), identically treated dried albumin droplets with known amine concentration have been used as reference standards (Ritzén 1967; Jonsson 1969). When the measurements are performed on tissue sections, the recordings are obtained from only part of a cell or from a nerve-terminal area. In this case, the amount of amine measured will depend not only on the measuring area but also on the section thickness. The fluorescence standard used must therefore correct for variations in the reaction conditions as well as in section thickness. For this purpose, Lichtensteiger (1970), Einarsson et al. (1975) and Tilders et al. (1974) used freeze-dried gelatin or protein cylinders and Löfström et al. (1976a,b) freeze-dried agar-protein cylinders with a known amine concentration. The cylinders are treated identically with the tissue specimens, and the cylinder and the specimens are embedded and sectioned in the same paraffin block. If each section has a reasonably even thickness, the fluorescence standard will thus correct for variation in thickness among different sections.

Although quantitation of fluorescence intensities is done most accurately with the aid of a microfluorometer, subjective semiquantitative estimations are often useful provided that a double-blind procedure with coded slides is used (see Jonsson 1971).

Agnati et al. (1978) have introduced an alternative photographic procedure based on fluorescent varicosity counts after photography using gratings of different transmittance.

Microfluorometric quantitation will have a great potential in all those systems in which concentration quenching does not occur or in which it can be eliminated by, for example, alterations in the histochemical reaction conditions. Lichtensteiger (1969, 1970), Tilders and Schipper (Tilders et al. 1974; Schipper et al. 1980), Jonsson and co-workers (Einarsson et al. 1975; Löfström et al. 1976a,b) and Fuxe, Agnati and co-workers (Fuxe et al. 1978; Agnati et al. 1979) have shown very elegantly how microfluorometric quantitation can be used for functional studies on single neurons and defined populations of nerve terminals. Using the tyrosine hydroxylase inhibition model for transmitter-turnover measurements, Einarsson et al. (1975), Löfström et al. (1976a,b) and Agnati et al. (1979) have shown that by measuring the rate of decline of CA fluorescence after inhibition of the synthesizing enzyme, microfluorometry can be used for estimation of DA and NA turnover in discrete terminal areas in the CNS. Similarly, Schipper et al. (1980) have shown that this method works well also in peripheral adrenergic nerve terminals. The great virtue of microfluorometric quantitation and turnover measurements over, for example, biochemical microdissection or punch techniques is that amine content and turnover changes can be analyzed in different and defined neuronal populations within the same area.

For further considerations in the use of the microfluorometric quantitation technique for monoamines and monoamine turnover measurements, the reader is referred to the papers by Ritzén (1967, 1973), Jonsson (1971, 1973), Einarsson et al. (1975), Löfström et al. (1976b), Agnati et al. (1978, 1979) and Schipper and Tilders (1982).

9. APPENDIX

PROTOCOL I: THE FALCK-HILLARP FA-VAPOR METHOD FOR FREEZE-DRIED TISSUE

Sources: Falck (1962), Falck and Owman (1965), Björklund et al. (1972b). See Section 5.1, for further comments.

1. *Dissection*. Nonperfused, unfixed tissue is used. The tissue should be frozen as soon as possible after the death of the animal. Good results, especially with peripheral tissues, are obtained from e.g. slaughterhouse material as long as 1 h after death of the animal (cf. El Badawi et al. 1970). The same is true for embryonic CNS tissue (Nobin and Björklund 1973).
2. *Freezing*. The tissues are cut into pieces as small as possible. Whole rat brain stem + cerebellum, and long strips of the spinal cord can be frozen as individual pieces. The rat brain should be frozen in 2-5 mm thick slices. Place the tissue piece on a piece of cardboard paper, carrying an identification number. With larger pieces it is advisable to wrap them up in cotton gauze to keep the tissues intact even if they crack. Holding the cardboard with a pair of precooled forceps, the tissue piece is immersed for at least 20 sec in liquid propane (preferably mixed with propylene), cooled by liquid nitrogen or liquid air. The tissue is then transferred to liquid nitrogen for storage.

   The liquid propane is prepared by passing domestic propane gas through liquid nitrogen or liquid air, as described in Section 5.1, under 'Preparation of tissues'. Carry out the entire process in a fume cupboard, and cover afterwards the Dewar container with a cloth to prevent water and oxygen condensation into the liquid propane, so avoiding explosion risks.
3. *Freeze-drying*. Transfer the specimens from the liquid nitrogen storage to the cold specimen

holder of the freeze-dryer. The temperature of the specimens should be kept at −35 to −40°C throughout the drying. Immediately before they are taken out of the freeze-dryer the specimens should be heated to above room temperature in order to avoid condensation of water onto the dried tissue pieces. The dried pieces are immidiately placed in a dessicator over fresh P_2O_5 and kept in darkness until they are embedded. Note that the freeze-dried specimens are fragile and should be handled with great care, e.g. with soft entomologist's forceps.

4. *FA-vapor treatment.* Place the specimens in a suitable receptacle, which is placed together with 5 g paraformaldehyde in a 1 liter closed glass vessel. We put the paraformaldehyde powder at the bottom of the vessel and the specimens on a tray (made of nylon net) placed 1-2 cm above the powder. The vessel is placed in a +80°C oven for 1-2 h.

   The water content of the paraformaldehyde is regulated prior to use. The commercial powder is first dried at about +100°C for 1 h in an open vial placed in an efficient fume-cupboard. Batches of the dried powder are then stored in dessicators over different sulfuric acid-water mixtures for at least 5-7 days, as described by Hamberger et al. (1965) and Hamberger (1967). These solutions produce a constant air humidity and, hence, a constant water content of the paraformaldehyde. Relative humidities of 50-90% usually give the best results. For optimum visualization of indolamines, a 2-step FA vapor treatment is recommended (Fuxe and Jonsson 1967). First treatment takes place at +80°C for 1 h with paraformaldehyde equilibrated in 50% relative humidity, followed by a second treatment (1 h, +80°C) with paraformaldehyde equilibrated in 90% relative humidity.

Composition of H_2SO_4-H_2O mixtures used to obtain different relative humidities. The paraformaldehyde is first dried in a +100°C oven for ½–1 hr, and then stored over the sulfuric acid for at least 1 week. (After Hamberger 1967 and Heym 1981.)

Relative humidity %	Density of H_2SO_4 solution	Weight % of H_2SO_4
20	1.49	59.24
30	1.44	59.49
40	1.39	49.48
50	1.34	44.17
60	1.29	38.53
70	1.25	33.28
80	1.20	27.72
90	1.14	20.08

Note that the mixing is done by adding the H_2SO_4 very slowly into the water, and not in the reverse order. Calculate weight of H_2SO_4 by using a specific density (g/ml) of 1.84 for pure sulfuric acid.

5. *Paraffin embedding.* The specimens are embedded in previously degassed paraffin in vacuo. The embedding is done in special vials or in a desiccator as described in Section 5.1, under 'Embedding and sectioning'. The embedding time should not exceed a few minutes. The paraffin-embedded specimens are stored dark and cold (preferably in a −20°C freezer) until sectioning.

6. *Sectioning.* Remove the cardboard identification tag and remove the cotton-gauze with the aid of warm forceps. The block-embedding should be made so that the paraffin in the core of the piece remains solid. This prevents cracked specimens from falling apart in the block embedding step. Sectioning is best done in a rotary microtome at 6-15 μm thickness. Mounting on slides is done in the following way: Use especially clean slides and check that the glass of the slides is non-fluorescent and that it is free of fluorescent stains or films on its surface. Place the paraffin sections on a dry slide, and flatten them out as much as possible with a fine brush or spatula. Transfer the slide to a hot plate for a short time, allowing the paraffin to melt and the sections to spread. Remove the slide from the hot plate and allow the paraffin to reharden. Scrape-off excess paraffin with a pointer or a spatula. Cover the sections with

a few drops of Entellan-xylene mixture (5-8 ml xylene in 30 ml Entellan[R], Merck, Darmstadt, FRG) to dissolve the paraffin of the sections, and add coverslip. Return the slide to the hot plate (about $+60°C$) for 1.5-2 h. The paraffin should be almost completely dissolved by the mounting medium.

7. *Indolamine visualization.* In the mammalian CNS the intraneuronal indolamine fluorescence is very weak unless the amine content is raised through pharmacological pretreatment. This can be done by administering a MAO-inhibitor in a high dose, 3-5 h before killing (nialamide, Pfizer, at a dose of 300 mg/kg, i.p., or pargyline hydrochloride, Sigma, at a dose of 150 mg/kg, i.p.). The increase in intraneuronal indolamines is further enhanced after combined MAO-inhibition and L-tryptophan treatment according to Aghajanian et al. (1973): Chloral hydrate (300 mg/kg, i.p.) followed 10 min later by nialamide (300 mg/kg, i.p.) and 15 min later by L-tryptophan (100 mg/kg, i.p.). The rats are killed 1-3 h after the last injection. Suitable procedure for cats is: Nialamide, 50-100 mg/kg, followed 1 h later by 25-50 mg/kg L-tryptophan. The cats are killed 1 h after the last injection. Chloral hydrate is omitted in this schedule.

PROTOCOL II: METAL SALT CATALYZED METHODS FOR FREEZE-DRIED TISSUE

IIA: The ALFA method for adult animals

Sources: Ajelis et al. (1979), Lorén et al. (1980). See Section 5.1.

1. *Perfusion procedure.* The animals are perfused via the ascending aorta in 2 steps using a pressurized perfusion apparatus of the type shown in Figure 6B, first with a *preperfusion* solution to rinse the blood out of the vessels and then with the *main perfusion* solution. General barbiturate or chloral hydrate anesthesia is used. The preperfusion is made with 150-300 ml of ice-cold Tyrode's buffer, pH 7.2 (8.0 g NaCl, 0.2 g KCl, 0.26 g $CaCl_2 \times 2H_2O$, 0.1 g $MgCl_2 \times 6H_2O$, 1.0 g Na HCO_3, 0.05 g $NaH_2PO_4 \times 1 H_2O$ and 1.0 g D-glucose per liter distilled water). This volume is usually adequate for rats when the descending aorta is clamped (perfusion of brain and upper spinal cord) but the volume may be increased further (300-450 ml) when the descending aorta is open (perfusion of the entire body). The perfusion pressure should be kept at 0.4-0.8 bar/cm^2. Check that the outflowing perfusion fluid is free of blood by the end of the perfusion.

The aluminum perfusion is performed with either of two alternative solutions. (a) *Aluminum alone:* Dissolve 10 g $Al_2(SO_4)_3 \cdot 18H_2O$ per 100 ml of Tyrode's buffer. The salt should be dissolved in the ice-cold buffer immediately before use. The dissolution of the $Al_2(SO_4)_3$ crystals occurs slowly but can be speeded-up by stirring and mechanical crushing of the crystals. The pH of the solution is adjusted to about 3.8 by adding 0.38 g $Na_2B_4O_7 \cdot 10H_2O$ per 100 ml. Check that the solution is completely clear, filter otherwise. (b) *Aluminum plus FA:* Dissolve 20 g of paraformaldehyde in 500 ml distilled water with 4-6 drops of 1 M NaOH added. The solution is allowed to stand in a boiling water bath until all paraformaldehyde is dissolved. This solution is cooled to room temperature and then mixed with 500 ml of ice-cold Tyrode's buffer of double strength. When ice-cold, 10 g of $Al_2(SO_4)_3 \cdot 18H_2O$ per 100 ml is added and the pH is adjusted with sodium borate, as in (a). Check that the solution is completely clear. Filter the solution free of undissolved crystals if necessary.

When switching from the preperfusion to the aluminum perfusion (which should be made without introducing air bubbles), the perfusion pressure is gradually raised to about 2.0 bar/cm^2. The perfusion volume is at least 300 ml with clamp over the descending aorta and at least 450 ml without clamp. The entire perfusion is completed within about 30 sec. Marked swelling of the neck and head region is a bad sign and signifies that intravascular precipitation has taken place. When starting a new animal, remember to wash the tubing free of ALFA solution before the next preperfusion is made.

2. *Further processing.* Freezing, freeze-drying, FA vapor treatment, paraffin embedding and sectioning are done as in Protocol I.

IIB: The ALFA method for young animals or fetuses
Source: Lorén et al. (1982).

1. *Perfusion.* Also for this method it is essential to have a pressure perfusion system similar to that shown in Figure 6B. For immature animals the two perfusion solution reservoirs are connected via teflon tubing to a 3-way needle valve which permits rapid shifting between them, as illustrated in Figure 1 in Lorén et al. (1980). Extending from the valve is a short piece of tubing leading to the perfusion cannula. The entire system is pressurized by a compressed air source which is adjustable between 0.3-2 bar. Perfusion is conducted, under deep methoxy barbital (Brietal, Lilly) anesthesia, in 2 stages because the aluminum-containing solution causes severe intravascular blood precipitation. When beginning a perfusion it is important to rinse the valve, tubing and cannula free of any remaining ALFA solution with the preperfusion solution. The perfusion is done via the left heart ventricle.

The *preperfusion* solution consists of a Tyrode's buffer, pH 7.2 (8.0 g NaCl, 0.2 g KCl, 0.26 g $CaCl_2 \times 2H_2O$, 0.1 g $MgCl_2 \times 6 H_2O$, 1.0 g $NaHCO_3$, 0.05 g $NaH_2PO_4 \times 1 H_2O$ and 1.0 g D-glucose per liter distilled water) supplemented with 2 g $MgSO_4 \times 7H_2O$ and 1 g procaine chloride per liter. This solution is used at room temperature, which, together with the added magnesium and procaine, counteracts vasoconstriction and helps to assure even, reproducible perfusions in young animals.

The second, or *main perfusion* solution is prepared as follows: 20 g of paraformaldehyde powder is depolymerized in 500 ml distilled water containing 4-6 drops 1 N NaOH in a boiling water bath. After cooling, 500 ml ice-cold, double-strength Tyrode's buffer is added and the solution kept on ice. Before use, 100 g $Al_2(SO_4)_3 \times 18 H_2O$ and 3.8 g $Na_2B_4O_7 \times 10 H_2O$ are added with continued mixing, and the final solution (pH about 3.8) is filtered free of any undissolved crystals.

The preperfusion solution is introduced with a pressure of 0.3-0.5 bar and continued for 45-60 sec in order to rinse out all blood and establish an even perfusion. After this has been completed the needle valve is rapidly shifted to introduce the ice-cold main perfusion solution. The perfusion is continued for 2-4 min during which the pressure is gradually increased to 1.0-2.0 bar (the higher pressures are used with older rats). The perfused volumes of the pre- and main perfusion solutions are at least 20 and 80 ml, respectively.

2. *Further processing.* Freezing, freeze-drying, FA reaction, paraffin embedding and sectioning are done as in Protocol I.

IIC: The Mg-FA-GA method
Sources: Lorén et al. (1976, 1982).

1. *Perfusion procedure.* The animals are perfused in 2 steps, either by a pressurized system, as above, or simply by means of a syringe driven by hand. A *preperfusion* step is not necessary, since the perfusate does not cause intravascular precipitation. A wash-out with cold buffer gives, however, minor improvements of the fluorescence picture and tissue morphology, and can thus be recommended. The perfusion pressure should be kept high. Too low a pressure gives inferior results.

The *preperfusion solution* consists of 150 ml of an ice-cold Tyrode's or Krebs-Ringer bicarbonate buffer (pH 7.4) and the *main perfusion* (the magnesium perfusion) consists of 150-450 ml of an ice-cold phosphate buffer with 40 g/150 ml of $MgSO_4 \times 7H_2O$, 2% GA and 0.5% FA added (pH 4.5). The larger volumes are used when the descending aorta is open. Either sodium glyoxylate or glyoxylic acid monohydrate can be used. Sodium glyoxylate: A 0.5% FA solution (0.75 g paraformaldehyde/150 ml) in 0.1 M phosphate buffer is made as in IIA and IIB above. When the FA solution has reached room temperature sodium glyoxylate is added to a final concentration of 2.5% (to yield a GA concentration of 2%). Finally 40 g

$MgSO_4$ is added and pH is then adjusted to between 4 and 5 with 6 M HCl. GA monohydrate: 0.75 g paraformaldehyde and 40 g $MgSO_4$ is dissolved in 75 ml phosphate buffer as above. In another solution 3 g glyoxylic acid monohydrate is dissolved in 75 ml phosphate buffer and pH is adjusted to 4.8-5.0 with NaOH pastilles. The solutions are then mixed to give a final concentration of 0.5% FA and 2% GA. pH is (if necessary) adjusted to between 4 and 5 with 6 M HCl. Sodium glyoxylate and GA monohydrate are available from Fluka (Buchs, Switzerland) and Sigma.

2. *Further processing.* Freezing, freeze-drying, FA treatment, paraffin embedding and sectioning are done as in Protocol I.

PROTOCOL III: THE GA-VIBRATOME METHOD
Source: Lindvall and Björklund (1974a). See Section 5.2.

1. *Perfusion.* The rat is perfused under barbiturate anesthesia with 150 ml of an ice-cold GA solution, using a 150 ml syringe driven by hand. The GA solution is prepared by dissolving 2% GA in a Krebs-Ringer bicarbonate buffer (initial pH = 7.0; composition in g per litre: NaCl 6.923; KCl 0.354; $CaCl_2 \times 6\ H_2O$ 0.278; KH_2PO_4 0.162; $MgSO_4\ 7\ H_2O$ 0.294; $NaHCO_3$ 2.100; with 1.8 g/l D-glucose added). The buffer is saturated with a mixture of 95% O_2 and 5% CO_2. Upon addition of GA the solution becomes acid, and the pH has therefore to be adjusted back to 7.0 with NaOH. Further addition of 0.5% paraformaldehyde will facilitate sectioning (Berger et al. 1976). The perfusion is performed manually using a 150 ml syringe. The perfusion should be rapid and completed within 0.5 - 1 min. GA monohydrate is available from Sigma, or from Fluka (Buchs, Switzerland).

2. *Sectioning.* The brains are rapidly taken out, cooled in the buffer and the desired piece (maximally 5-6 mm thick) is dissected out. The specimen is then glued to the holder of the Vibratome using an acrylic adhesive (Loctite; Loctite Corp., Newington, CT 06111, USA; or Eastman 910 adhesive). Ordinary razor blades, divided in the middle, are used; they are changed frequently (at least a new blade for every new tissue piece) in order to get optimum results. During the sectioning procedure, the tissue piece is immersed in the oxygenated, pure Krebs-Ringer bicarbonate buffer (pH about 7.0) kept at a temperature between 0 and +5°C by non-corroding metal bars, cooled to a very low temperature in a solid carbon dioxide-ethanol mixture. These metal bars are placed in the buffer trough and changed at suitable intervals. The sectioning is performed at a vibration rate of 6-7 scale units and a feeding speed of 1-3 scale units. Sections down to 20 μm can be obtained in successful cases; as a standard, sections about 30-35 μm thick should be used. The tissue piece will remain in an acceptable condition in the cool buffer for a maximum of 3-4 h, during which time 15-20 good sections are usually obtained. It is recommended to change the buffer in the trough for oxygenated buffer with regular intervals.

3. *Immersion.* The sections are transferred with a blunt glass-rod to the ice-cold 2% GA solution. During this immersion, which should be continued for about 3-5 min, the sections have to be kept below the surface. The sections are then transferred to glass microscope slides in the following way: The section is picked up on the glass rod, which is then dipped into the solution so that the section partly floats out on the surface. The slide is now put below the section and the edge of the section is allowed to attach onto the glass. The section is then spread out on the slide by gently lifting it out of the bath. In this way, folding of the sections is minimized. Excess buffer is removed from the slides with a filter paper. Care should be taken not to stretch or tear the sections on the slide.

4. *Drying.* The sections are dried in a 2-step procedure: first under the warm air stream from a hair-dryer for about 15 min and then in a dessicator in vacuo over fresh phosphorous pentoxide overnight. Omitting the first drying step, or using air of room temperature, causes diffusion of the fluorophores from the nervous structures. During the drying procedure, which thus involves a moderate heating of the sections under the warm air stream, fluorophore formation takes place. This means that sections can be examined in the fluorescence-microscope immediately after this first drying step, i.e. less than half an hour after the animal has been

killed. The fluorescence picture in these sections is of high quality, and only minor differences e.g., in fluorescence intensity, can be seen as compared to sections further processed with drying overnight, GA vapor treatment, or heating.

5. *Reaction.* To further react the sections by *heating*, they are simply put in a rack and placed in an oven at $+100°C$ for 6 min. The fluorescence yield in the catecholamine-containing structures is somewhat increased by this treatment. *GA vapor treatment* is now very seldom used for reaction of the Vibratome sections. With CNS tissue, equally good results on catecholamine-containing structures are obtained if the sections are simply heated. With peripheral tissues, when cells containing, for example, 5-HT or tryptophanyl-peptides are to be demonstrated, GA vapor treatment should be used (cf. Björklund et al. 1973b). For details on the practical performance of the GA vapor reaction, see Lindvall and Björklund (1974a).

6. *Mounting.* The slides are coverslipped with paraffin or immersion oil, Entellan or Fluoromount.

PROTOCOL IV: THE FA-VIBRATOME METHOD

Source: Hökfelt and Ljungdahl (1972), Lorén et al. (1980). See Section 5.2.

1. *Perfusion.* The rat is perfused, under brietal anesthesia, with an ice-cold 4% FA solution for 5-15 min, using a gravity perfusion system. 40 g of paraformaldehyde powder is dissolved in 1 liter 0.1 M phosphate buffer. The solution is allowed to stand in a boiling water bath until all paraformaldehyde is dissolved. The solution is cooled in crushed ice to $+4°C$ or less.

2. *Sectioning.* The sectioning is performed as in Protocol III, above.

3. *Immersion.* This is carried out in 150 ml of an ice-cold Tyrode's or Kreb-Ringer bicarbonate buffer with 2.5 g $Al_2(SO_4)_3 \times 18 H_2O$ added per 150 ml buffer. The initial pH is 7.2-7.4 and added aluminum salt adjusts the pH to lower values. The sections are kept free-floating, below the surface, and the optimal immersion time is 15-30 sec. The sections are transferred onto slides from the immersion bath, as in Protocol III. *This step can be omitted.*

4. *Drying.* The sections are dried for about 15 min in a rack under a cool or warm air stream from a hair-dryer, and then in a desiccator over fresh phosphorous pentoxide, in vacuo, for 2-24 h.

5. *FA reaction.* The sections are first pre-warmed in the $+80°C$ oven for a few minutes, and then exposed to VF vapor at $+80°C$ for 1 h as described in Protocol I. Paraformaldehyde equilibrated in 70% air humidity is usually optimal.

6. *Mounting* is done in Entellan, Fluoromont, paraffin oil or immersion oil.

PROTOCOL V: THE FAGLU METHOD

Source: Furness et al. (1977a, 1978), Blessing et al. (1978), Furness, personal communication. See Section 5.2.

1. *Perfusion.* The rat is perfused, under barbiturate anesthesia, via the ascending aorta in 2 steps, using equipment of the type shown in Figure 6. *The preperfusion* is made at 120 Torr during 10-30 sec, and consists of a 1% solution of sodium nitrate in 0.01 M phosphate buffer, pH 7.0. Alternatively isotonic NaCl, with 5000 IU/l of heparin added, can be used. The solutions have room temperature. *The main perfusion* consists of 200 ml of 0.1 M phosphate buffer containing 4% FA and 0.5% glutaraldehyde (electron-microscopy grade). The solution has room temperature and is perfused at 120 Torr over about 10 min. Dissected tissue pieces are stored in the Faglu solution at $+4°C$ until sectioned (up to 3 days).

2. *Sectioning.* The piece is glued to the Vibratome holder with acrylic adhesive and sectioned in the cold room at $+4°C$. During sectioning the surface is kept moist with the Faglu fluid while the surrounding bath is empty. Speed 6, amplitude 7-7.5 and 30 μm are commonly used. The sections are transferred to a dish with the Faglu mix, from which they are floated onto glass microscope slides.

3. *Drying.* Excess fluid is removed with a filter paper and the sections are dried over fresh P_2O_5 for 1 h in a dessicator, in vacuo.

4. Mounting is done in paraffin oil or Fluoromount.

PROTOCOL VI: THE GA-CRYOSTAT METHOD
Source: De La Torre and Surgeon (1976), De La Torre (1980). See section 5.3

1. Freezing. Pieces of nonperfused, unfixed tissue are glued to pre-cooled cryostat chucks and frozen. De La Torre (1980) recommends freezing in the −30°C cryostat chamber, but more rapid freezing may be advantageous, as discussed in Section 5.3, under 'Freezing and sectioning'.
2. Sectioning. Sections are made at 16-32 μm in the cryostat and picked up on clean room temperature glass slides.
3. Immersion. The sections are immediately dipped 3 times (about 1 dip/sec) in a 1% GA solution at room temperature. This so-called SPG solution is made by dissolving 1.5 g GA monohydrate, 10.2 g sucrose and 4.8 g monobasic KH_2PO_4 in 100 ml of distilled water. When clear, pH is adjusted to 7.4 with 1 N NaOH and distilled water is added to a final volume of 150 ml.
4. Drying. Excess fluid is wiped-off from the slides with absorbent paper. The sections are dried under the cool air stream from two hair-dryers until they are completely dry (up to 15-30 min).
5. Reaction. 1-2 drops of paraffin oil or immersion oil are placed on top of each section (this is done in order to eliminate air bubbles underneath the sections). The slides are heated in an oven set at +95°C for 2-5 min.
6. Mounting is done in paraffin oil or immersion oil.

PROTOCOL VII. THE GA-FA CRYOSTAT METHOD
Sources: Bloom and Battenberg (1976), Nygren (1976), Lorén et al. (1977). See Section 5.3.

1. Perfusion. The animal is perfused under chloral hydrate or barbiturate anesthesia with an ice-cold solution of 2% GA and 0.5% FA. The solution is made by mixing equal volumes of the following 2 solutions: *(a)* Paraformaldehyde is depolymerized in a boiling water bath in double- strength phosphate buffer (0.3 M, pH 7.4) at a concentration of 1 g/100 ml. The solution is then chilled to 2-4°C prior to use. *(b)* GA monohydrate (Sigma or Fluka) is dissolved in mammalian Ringer's solution at room temperature in a concentration of 4 g/100 ml. The two solutions are combined in equal volumes, the pH is adjusted to 7.4 with 10 N NaOH, and the solution chilled to below +4°C.
In the modification of Lorén et al. (1977), $MgSO_4 \times 7H_2O$ is added to the perfusion fluid in a concentration of 80 g/300 ml. The $MgSO_4$ is best added to the cool FA solution (Solution *a*) in double final concentration. The pH of the mixed perfusion solution is adjusted to 4.5 with 6 N HCl.
Adult rats are perfused with 150-250 ml, via the heart or the ascending aorta, during 30-90 sec.
2. Sectioning. Pieces of tissue are glued onto pre-cooled cryostat chucks and frozen in powdered dry ice. After the specimens have equilibrated with the temperature of the cryostat chamber, sections are cut at 8-36 μm. Bloom and Battenberg (1976) use temperatures of −16 to −20°C, while Lorén et al. (1977) for CNS tissue recommend the cryostat to be set at −30°C and sections to be cut at a temperature between −25 and −30°C (measured at the knife). The sections are picked up either on cold or room-tempered glass slides. On cold glass slides, the section is thawed onto the slide with finger pressure to the back of the slide.
3. Immersion. The sections are immediately immersed for 11 min in the ice-cold 2% GA solution (Solution *b*, above, diluted with an equal volume of Ringer's solution). *This step can be omitted* if FA-vapor reaction is used (cf. Lorén et al. 1977; Nygren 1976).
4. Drying. The sections are dried under the warm air stream from a hair-dryer for about 5 min. If the sections are to be reacted with FA vapor, it is recommendable to dry the sections further in a desiccator, in vacuo, over fresh phosphorous pentoxide for at least 1 h.

111

5. *Reaction.* *(a)* GA-immersed sections are reacted by heating in a 100°C oven for 6-10 min. *(b).* Non-immersed sections are reacted with FA vapor at +80°C for 1 h, as described in Protocol I, and in Section 5.1, under 'FA vapor treatment'.

6. *Mounting* is done in paraffin oil.

PROTOCOL VIII: THE GA-ALFA CRYOSTAT METHOD
Source: Lorén et al. (1980). See Section 5.3.

1. *Perfusion.* Rats are perfused in 2 steps, first with a preperfusion and then with the main perfusion (the aluminum-containing) solution. The *preperfusion* solution consists of (a) 150 ml of an ice-cold Tyrode's or equivalent buffer (pH 7.2), or (b) 150 ml of an ice-cold 2% GA solution (pH 7.0). The *main perfusion* solution consists of 300-450 ml of an ice-cold Tyrode's buffer with 30 g $Al_2(SO_4)_3 \times 18\ H_2O$, 1.14 g $Na_2B_4O_7 \times 19\ H_2O$ and 1-4% paraformaldehyde added per 300 ml. The composition of the Tyrode's buffer is given in Protocol II.

For studies on the brain and cranial spinal cord, rats are perfused with 300 ml of the main perfusion solution with the descending aorta clamped. Larger volume (450 ml) is used for spinal cord, PNS, endocrine and visceral organs. 2.5-5% sucrose can be added to each of the two perfusion solutions to improve the morphology of the sections.

2. *Freezing and sectioning.* Perfused and nonperfused tissue are rapidly dissected and glued to, or frozen onto, cryostat chucks, and frozen in powdered dry-ice. The tissue pieces are then stored in the cryostat at about −25 to −30°C (CNS tissue) or at about −15 to −20°C (PNS, endocrine and visceral organs) to equilibrate to the temperature of the cryostat. Sectioning of CNS tissue is carried out at a temperature of about −25 to −30°C. For the demonstration of catecholamines and 5-HT in neuronal and non-neuronal storage sites in, e.g. endocrine and visceral organs, it is possible to achieve a good fluorescence picture with higher sectioning temperatures, about −15 to −20°C, which makes sectioning easier. The tissue is sectioned at 15-25 μm, and the sections are then picked up and thawed on room-tempered microscope slides.

3. *Drying, FA vapor treatment and mounting.* The sections are dried under the warm air stream from a hair-dryer for 5-15 min, and then in vacuo in a dessicator over fresh phosphorous pentoxide for at least 1 h. The sections are finally reacted with FA vapor at 50-70% humidity for 1 h at +80°C, as described in Protocol I, and mounted in paraffin oil or Entellan.

10. REFERENCES

Abramovitch RA, Spencer IA (1964): The carbolines. In: Katritzky AR (Ed), *Advances in Heterocyclic Chemistry, Vol. 3,* pp. 79-207. Academic Press, New York − London.

Agnati LF, Benefati F, Cortelli P, D'Alessandro R (1978): A new method to quantify catecholamine stores visualized by means of the Falck-Hillarp technique. *Neurosci. Lett., 10,* 11−17.

Agnati LF, Andersson K, Wiesel F, Fuxe K (1979): A method to determine dopamine levels and turnover rate in discrete dopamine nerve terminal systems by quantitative use of dopamine fluorescence obtained by Falck-Hillarp methodology. *J. Neurosci. Meth., 1,* 365−373.

Ajelis V, Björklund A, Falck B, Lindvall O, Lorén I, Walles B (1979): Application of the aluminum-formaldehyde (ALFA) histofluorescence method for demonstration of peripheral stores of catecholamines and indolamines in freeze-dried paraffin-embedded tissue, cryostat sections and whole-mounts. *Histochemistry, 65,* 1−15.

Alumets J, Håkanson R, Sundler F, Chang K-J (1978): Leu-enkephalin-like material in nerves and enterochromaffin cells in the gut. An immunohistochemical study. *Histochemistry, 56,* 187−196.

Axelrod J (1971): In: Wurtman RJ (Ed), *Brain Monoamines and Endocrine Function, Neurosciences Research Program Bulletin, Vol. 9,* pp. 313−326.

Axelsson S, Björklund A, Lindvall O (1972a): Identification of bufotenin in toad brain by chromatography and mass spectrometry of its dans-derivative. *Life Sci., 10,* 745−749.

Axelsson S, Björklund A, Lindvall O (1972b): Fluorescence histochemistry of biogenic monoamines. A study of the capacity of various carbonyl compounds to form fluorophores with biogenic monoamines in gas-phase reactions. *J. Histochem. Cytochem., 20,* 435−444.

Axelsson S, Björklund A, Falck B, Lindvall O, Svensson LA (1973): Glyoxylic acid condensation: A new fluorescence method for the histochemical demonstration of biogenic monoamines. *Acta Physiol. Scand.*, 87, 57–68.

Bacopoulus NG, Bhatnagar RK, Schnute WJ, Van Orden III LS (1975): On the use of the fluorescence histochemical method to estimate catecholamine content in brain. *Neuropharmacology, 14,* 291–299.

Barter R, Pearse AGE (1953): Detection of 5-hydroxytryptamine in mammalian enterochromaffin cells. *Nature, 172,* 810.

Barter R, Pearse AGE (1955): Mammalian enterochromaffin cells as the source of serotonin (5-hydroxytryptamine). *J. Path. Bact., 69,* 25–31.

Baumgarten HG (1972): Biogenic monoamines in the cyclostome and lower vertebrate brain. *Prog. Histochem. Cytochem., 4,* 1–90.

Bentivoglio M, Kuypers HGJM, Catsman-Berrevoets CE, Dann O (1979): Fluorescent retrograde neuronal labeling in rat by means of substances binding specifically to adeninethymine rich DNA. *Neurosci. Lett., 12,* 235–240.

Berger B, Glowinski J (1978): Dopamine uptake in serotoninergic terminals in vitro: A valuable tool for the histochemical differentiation of catecholaminergic and serotoninergic terminals in rat cerebral structures. *Brain Res., 147,* 29–46.

Berger B, Thierry AM, Tassin JP, Moyne MA (1976): Dopaminergic innervation of the rat prefrontal cortex: A fluorescence histochemical study. *Brain Res., 106,* 133–145.

Berger B, Nguyen-Legros J, Thierry AM (1978): Demonstration of horseradish peroxidase and fluorescent catecholamines in the same neuron. *Neurosci. Lett., 9,* 297–302.

Bieger D, Harley C (1982): Acetylcholinesterase in pontomedullary catecholamine neurons of the adult albino rat. *Brain Res. Bull., 8,* 223–228.

Björklund A, Falck B (1968): An improvement of the histochemical fluorescence method for monoamines. Observations on varying extrability of fluorophores in different nerve fibers. *J. Histochem. Cytochem., 16,* 717–720.

Björklund A, Falck B (1973): Cytofluorometry of biogenic monoamines in the Falck-Hillarp method. Structural identification by spectral analysis. In: Sernetz M, Thaer A (Eds), *Quantitative Fluorescence Techniques as Applied in Cell Biology,* pp. 171–181. Springer-Verlag, Heidelberg.

Björklund A, Skagerberg G (1979a): Simultaneous use of retrograde fluorescent tracers and fluorescence histochemistry for convenient and precise mapping of monoaminergic projections and collateral arrangements in the CNS. *J. Neurosci. Meth., 1,* 261–277.

Björklund A, Skagerberg G (1979b): Evidence for a major spinal cord projection from the diencephalic A11 dopamine cell group in the rat using transmitter-specific fluorescent retrograde tracing. *Brain Res., 177,* 170–175.

Björklund A, Stenevi U (1970): Acid catalysis of the formaldehyde condensation reaction for sensitive demonstration of tryptamines and 3-methoxylated phenylethylamines. 1. Model experiments. *J. Histochem. Cytochem., 18,* 794–802.

Björklund A, Ehinger B, Falck B (1968a): A method for differentiating dopamine from noradrenaline in tissue sections by microspectrofluorometry. *J. Histochem. Cytochem., 16,* 263–270.

Björklund A, Falck B, Håkanson R (1968b): Histochemical demonstration of tryptamine. Properties of the formaldehyde-induced fluorophores or tryptamine and related indole compounds in models. *Acta Physiol. Scand., Suppl. 318,* 5–31.

Björklund A, Nobin A, Stenevi U (1971a): Acid catalysis of the formaldehyde condensation reaction for a sensitive histochemical demonstration of tryptamine and 3-methoxylated phenylethylamines. 2. Characterization of amine fluorophores and application of tissues. *J. Histochem. Cytochem., 19,* 286–298.

Björklund A, Falck B, Stenevi U (1971b): Microspectrofluorometric characterization of monoamines in the central nervous system: Evidence for a new neuronal monoamine-like compound. *Prog. Brain Res., 34,* 63–78.

Björklund A, Ehinger B, Falck B (1972a): Analysis of fluorescence excitation peak ratios for the cellular identification of noradrenaline, dopamine, or their mixtures. *J. Histochem. Cytochem., 20,* 56–64.

Björklund A, Falck B, Owman C (1972b): Fluorescence microscopic and microspectrofluorometric techniques for the cellular localization and characterization of biogenic amines. In: Berson SA (Ed), *Methods of Investigative and Diagnostic Endocrinology, Vol. 1: The Thyroid and Biogenic Amines,* (Eds: Rall JE, Kopin IJ), pp. 318–368. North-Holland Publ. Co, Amsterdam.

Björklund A, Lindvall O, Svensson LA (1972c): Mechanisms of fluorophore formation in the histochemical glyoxylic acid method for monoamines. *Histochemistry, 32,* 113–131.

Björklund A, Falck B, Lindvall O, Svensson LÅ (1973a): New aspects on reaction mechanisms in the formaldehyde histofluorescence method for monoamines. *J. Histochem. Cytochem., 21,* 17–25.

Björklund A, Håkanson R, Lindvall O, Sundler F (1973b): Fluorescence histochemical demonstration of peptides with NH_2- or COOH–terminal tryptophan or DOPA by condensation with glyoxylic acid. *J. Histochem. Cytochem., 21,* 253–265.

Björklund A, Falck B, Lindvall O (1975a): Microspectrofluorometric analysis of cellular monoamines after formaldehyde or glyoxylic acid condensation. In: Bradley PB (Ed), *Methods in Brain Research,* pp. 249–294. John Wiley and Sons, London.

Björklund A, Lindvall O, Nobin A (1975b): Evidence of an incerto-hypothalamic dopamine neurone system in the rat. *Brain Res., 89,* 29–42.

Björklund A, Axelsson S, Falck B (1976): Intraneuronal indolamines in the central nervous system. In: *Advances in Biochemical Psychopharmacology, Vol. 15,* pp. 87–94. Raven Press, New York.

Björklund A, Falck B, Lindvall O, Lorén I (1980): The aluminum-formaldehyde (ALFA) histofluorescence method for improved visualization of catecholamines and indolamines. 2. Model experiments. *J. Neurosci. Meth., 2,* 301–318.

Blessing WW, Chalmers JP, Howe PRC (1978a): Distribution of catecholamine-containing cell bodies in the rabbit central nervous system. *J. Comp. Neurol., 179,* 407–424.

Blessing WW, Furness JB, Costa M, Chalmers JP (1978): Localization of catecholamine fluorescence and retrograde transported horseradish peroxidase within the same nerve cell. *Neurosci. Lett., 9,* 311–315.

Blessing WW, Jaeger CB, Ruggiero DA, Reis J (1982): Hypothalamic projections of medullary catecholamine neurons in the rabbit: A combined catecholamine fluorescence and HRP transport study. *Brain Res. Bull., 9,* 279–286.

Bloom FE, Battenberg ELF (1976): A rapid, simple and sensitive method for the demonstration of central catecholamine-containing neurons and axons by glyoxylic acid-induced fluorescence. II A detailed description of methodology. *J. Histochem. Cytochem., 24,* 561–571.

Boulton AA (1976): Identification, distribution, metabolism, and function of meta and para tyramine, phenylethylamine and tryptamine in brain. In: *Advances in Biochemical Psychopharmacology, Vol. 15,* pp. 57–68. Raven Press, New York.

Bubenik GA, Brown GM, Uhlin I, Grota LJ (1974): Immunohistological localization of N-acetylindolealkylamines in pineal gland, retina and cerebellum. *Brain Res., 81,* 233–242.

Bubenik GA, Brown GM, Grota LJ (1976): Differential localization of N-acetylated indolealkylamines in CNS and the Haderian gland using immunohistology. *Brain Res., 118,* 417–427.

Caspersson T, Lomakka G, Rigler R (1965): Registrierender Fluoreszensmikrospektrograph zur Bestimmung der Primär und Sekundärfluoreszenz verschiedener Zellsubstanzen. *Acta Histochem. Suppl., 6,* 123–126.

Caspersson T, Hillarp NÅ, Ritzén M (1966): Fluorescence microspectrophotometry of cellular catecholamines and 5-hydroxytryptamine. *Exp. Cell Res., 42,* 415–428.

Chiba T, Hwang BH, Williams TH (1976): A method for studying glyoxylic acid induced fluorescence and ultrastructure of monoamine neurons. *Histochemistry, 49,* 95–106.

Corrodi H, Hillarp N-Å (1963): Fluoreszenzmethoden zur histochemischen Sichtbarmachung von Monoaminen. 1. Identifizierung der fluoreszierenden Produkte aus Modellversuchen mit 6,7-Dimethoxyisochinolinderivaten und Formaldehyd. *Helv. Chim. Acta., 46,* 2425–2430.

Corrodi H, Hillarp N-Å (1964): Fluoreszenzmethoden zur histochemischen Sichtbarmachung von Monoaminen. 2. Identifizierung des fluoreszierenden Produktes aus Dopamin und Formaldehyd. *Helv. Chim. Acta., 47,* 911–918.

Corrodi H, Hillarp N-Å, Jonsson G (1964): Fluorescence methods for the histochemical demonstation of monoamines. 3. Sodium borohydride reduction of the fluorescent compounds as a specificity test. *J. Histochem. Cytochem., 12,* 582–586.

Corrodi H, Jonsson G (1965a): Fluorescence methods for the histochemical demonstration of monoamines. 4. Histochemical differentiation between dopamine and noradrenaline in models. *J. Histochem. Cytochem., 13,* 484–487.

Corrodi H, Jonsson G (1965b): Fluoreszenzmethoden zur histochemischen Sichtbarmachung von Monoaminen. 5. Identifizierung der fluoreszierenden Produktes aus Modellversuchen mit 5-Methoxytryptamin und Formaldehyd. *Acta Histochem., 22,* 247–258.

Corrodi H, Jonsson G (1967): The formaldehyde fluorescence method for the histochemical demonstration of biogenic monoamines. A review on the methodology. *J. Histochem. Cytochem., 15,* 65–78.

Cova S, Prenna G, Mazzini G (1974): Digital microspectrofluorometry by multichannel scaling and single photon detection. *Histochem. J., 6,* 279–299.

Csilik B, Kàlmàn G (1967): Vacuumless freezing-drying: Its application in catecholamine histochemistry. *Histochemie, 9,* 275–280.

Cuello AC, Horn AS, Mackay AVT, Iversen LL (1973): Catecholamines in the median eminence: New evidence for a major noradrenergic input. *Nature (London), 243,* 465–467.

Dahlström A, Fuxe K (1964): Evidence for the existence of monoamine neurons in the central nervous system. I. Experimentally induced changes in the intraneuronal amine levels of bulbospinal neuron systems. *Acta Physiol. Scand., 62, Suppl.,* 232.

De La Torre JC (1980): An improved approach to histofluorescence using the SPG method for tissue monoamines. *J. Neurosci. Meth., 3,* 1–5.

De La Torre JC, Surgeon JW (1976): A methodological approach to rapid and sensitive monoamine histofluorescence using a modifed glyoxylic acid technique: The SPG method. *Histochemistry, 49,* 81–93.

Dreyfus CF, Gershon MD, Crain SM (1979): Innervation of hippocampus by co-cultured central adrenergic neurons from fetal mouse brainstem. *Brain Res., 161,* 431–445.

Ehinger B, Falck B (1965): Noradrenaline and cholinesterase in concomitant nerve fibres in iris. *Life Sci., 4,* 2097–2100.

Ehinger B, Falck B (1966): Concomitant adrenergic and parasympathetic fibres in the rat iris. *Acta Physiol. Scand., 67,* 201–207.

Einarsson P, Hallman H, Jonsson G (1975): Quantitative microfluorimetry of formaldehyde induced fluorescence of dopamine in the caudate nucleus. *Med. Biol., 53,* 15.

El-Badawi A, Schenk EA (1967): Histochemical methods for separate, consecutive and simultaneous demonstration of acetylcholinesterase and norepinephrine in cryostat sections. *J. Histochem. Cytochem., 15,* 580–588.

El-Badawi A, Hayashi KD, Schenk EA (1970): Histochemical demonstration of norepinephrine in postmortem tissues. *Histochemie, 21,* 21.

Ellison J-P, Olander KW (1972): Simultaneous demonstration of catecholamines and acetylcholinesterase in peripheral autonomic nerves. *Am. J. Anat., 135,* 135.

Enerbäck L, Gustafsson B, Mellbom L (1977): Cytofluorometric quantitation of 5-hydroxytryptamine in mast cells: An improved technique for the formaldehyde condensation reaction. *J. Histochem. Cytochem., 25,* 32–41.

Eränkö O (1952): On the histochemistry of the adrenal medulla of the rat, with special reference to acid phosphate. *Acta Anat., 16, Suppl.,* 17.

Eränkö O (1955a): Distribution or fluorescing islets, adrenaline and noradrenaline in the adrenal medulla of the hamster. *Acta Endocrinol., 18,* 174–179.

Eränkö O (1955b): Histochemistry of noradrenaline in the adrenal medulla of the rats or mice. *Endocrinology, 57,* 363–368.

Eränkö O (1955c): Fluorescing islets, adrenaline and noradrenaline in the adrenal medulla of some common laboratory animals. *Ann. Med. Exp. Fenn., 33,* 278–290.

Eränkö O (1961): Personal communication, quoted by Falck and Torp (1961).

Eränkö O (1967): The practical histochemical demonstration of catecholamines by formaldehyde-induced fluorescence. *J.R. Microsc. Soc., 87,* 259–276.

Eränkö O (1972): Light and electronmicroscopic histochemical evidence of granular and non-granular storage of catecholamines in the sympathetic ganglion of the rat. *Histochem. J., 4,* 213–224.

Eränkö O, Räisänen L (1965): Fibres containing both noradrenaline and acetylcholinesterase in the nerve net of the rat iris. *Acta Physiol. Scand., 63,* 505–506.

Eränkö O, Räisänen L (1966): Demonstration of catecholamines in adrenergic nerve fibres by fixation in aqueous fomaldehyde solution and fluorescence microscopy. *J. Histochem. Cytochem., 14,* 690–702.

Erös G (1932): Eine neue Darstellungsmethode der sogenannten 'gelben' argentaffinen Zellen des Magendarmtraktes. *Zentralbl. Allg. Path. Path. Anat., 54,* 385–391.

Falck B (1962): Observations on the possibilities of the cellular localization of monoamines by a fluorescence method. *Acta Physiol. Scand., 56, Suppl. 197,* 1–25.

Falck B, Owman Ch (1965): A detailed methodological description of the fluorescence method for the cellular demonstration of biogenic monoamines. *Acta Univ. Lund. Sect. 2,* No. 7.

Falck B, Torp A (1961): A fluorescence method for histochemical demonstration of noradrenalin in the adrenal medulla. *Med. Exp., 5,* 429–432.

Falck B, Hillarp N-Å, Thieme G, Torp A (1962): Fluorescence of catecholamines and related compounds condensed with formaldehyde. *J. Histochem. Cytochem., 10,* 348–354.

Falck B, Häggendal J, Owman C (1963): The localization of adrenaline in adrenergic nerves in the frog. *Q.J. Exp. Physiol., 48,* 253–257.

Furness JB, Costa M (1975): The use of glyoxylic acid for the fluorescence histochemical demonstration of peripheral stores of noradrenaline and 5-hydroxytryptamine in whole mounts. *Histochemistry, 41,* 335–352.

Furness JB, Malmfors T (1971): Aspects of the arrangement of the adrenergic innervation in guinea-pigs as revealed by the fluorescence histochemical method applied to stretched air-dried preparation. *Histochemie, 25,* 297.

Furness JB, Costa M, Blessing WW (1977a): Simultaneous fixation and production of catecholamine fluorescence in central nervous tissue by perfusion with aldehydes. *Histochem. J., 9,* 745–750.

Furness JB, Costa M, Wilson AJ (1977b): Water-stable fluorophores, produced by reaction with aldehyde solutions for the histochemical localization of catechol- and indolethylamines. *Histochemistry, 52,* 159–170.

Furness JB, Heath JW, Costa M (1978): Aqueous aldehyde (Faglu) methods for the fluorescence histochemical localization of catecholamines and for ultrastructural studies of central nervous tissue. *Histochemistry, 57,* 285–295.

Fuxe K, Jonsson G (1967): A modification of the histochemical fluorescence method for the improved localization of 5-hydroxytryptamine. *Histochemistry, 11,* 161–166.

Fuxe K, Hamberger B, Hökfelt T (1968): Distribution of noradrenaline nerve terminals in cortical areas of the rat. *Brain Res., 8,* 125–131.

Fuxe K, Hökfelt T, Jonsson G, Ungerstedt U (1970): Fluorescence microscopy in neuroanatomy. In: Nauta WJH, Ebesson SOE (Eds), *Contemporary Research Methods in Neuroanatomy,* pp. 275–314. Springer Verlag, Berlin–Heidelberg–New York.

Fuxe K, Goldstein M, Hökfelt T, Joh TH (1971): Cellular localization of dopamine-hydroxylase and phenylethanolamine-N-methyl transferase as revealed by immunohistochemistry. *Prog. Brain Res., 34,* 127–138.

Geyer MA, Dawsey WJ, Mandell AJ (1978): Fading: A new cytofluorimetric measure quantifying serotonin in the presence of catecholamines at the cellular level in brain. *J. Pharmacol. Exp. Ther., 207,* 605–667.

Grant LD, Stumpf WE (1981): Combined autoradiography and formaldehyde-induced fluorescence methods for localization of radioactively labeled substances in relation to monoamine neurons. *J. Histochem. Cytochem., 29, 1A,* 175–180.

Green AR, Koslow SH, Costa E (1973): Identification and quantitation of a new indolealkylamine in rat hypothalamus. *Brain Res., 51,* 371–374.

Håkanson R, Sundler F (1971): Formaldehyde condensation. A method for the fluorescence microscopic demonstration of peptides with NH_2-terminal tryptophan residues. *J. Histochem. Cytochem., 19,* 477–482.

Hamberger B (1967): Reserpine-resistant uptake of catecholamines in isolated tissues of the rat. A histochemical study. *Acta Physiol. Scand., Suppl. 295,* 1–65.

Hamberger B, Norberg K-A (1964): Histochemical demonstration of monoamines in fresh-frozen sections. *J. Histochem. Cytochem., 12,* 48–49.

Hamberger B, Malmfors T, Sachs C (1965): Standardization of paraformaldehyde and of certain procedures for the histochemical demonstration of catecholamines. *J. Histochem. Cytochem., 13,* 147–148.

Heene R (1968): Histochemischer Nachweis von Katecholaminen und 5-Hydroxytryptamin am Kryostatschnitt. *Histochemie, 14,* 324–327.

Hendelman WJ, Marshall KC, Ferguson R, Carriee S (1982): Catecholamine neurons of the central nervous system in organotypic culture. *Dev. Neurosci., 5,* 64–76.

Hercules DM (1966): Fluorescence and phosphorescence analysis. In: Hercules DM (Ed), *Principles and applications,* pp. 1–40. Interscience, New York–London–Sydney.

Hess SM, Udenfriend S (1959): A fluorimetric procedure for the measurement of tryptamine in tissues. *J. Pharmacol. Exp. Ther., 12,* 175–177.

Hess A, Adamo PJ, Cassady I (1976): Glycol methacrylate sections of frozen-dried tissue for histofluorescence. *Stain Technol., 51,* 63–64.

Heym Ch (1981): Fluorescence histochemistry of biogenic monamines. In: Heym Ch, Forssmann WG (Eds), Techniques in Neuroanatomical Research, pp. 139–170. Springer-Verlag, Berlin-Heidelberg-New York.

Hoffman DL, Sladek Jr JR (1973): The distribution of catecholamines within the inferior olivary complex of the gerbil and rabbit. *J. Comp. Neurol., 151,* 101–112.

Hökfelt T (1965): A modification of the histochemical fluorescence method for the demonstration of catecholamines and 5-hydroxytryptamine, using araldite as embedding medium. *J. Histochem. Cytochem., 13,* 518–520.

Hökfelt T, Ljungdahl Å (1971): Uptake of (^{3}H)-γ-aminobutyric acid in isolated tissues of the rat: An autoradiographic and fluorescence microscopic study. *Prog. Brain Res., 34,* 87–102.

Hökfelt T, Ljungdahl Å (1972): Modification of the Falck-Hillarp formaldehyde fluorescence method using the Vibratome: Simple, rapid and sensitive localization of catecholamines in sections of unfixed or formalin fixed brain tissue. *Histochemie, 29,* 325–339.

Hökfelt T, Ljungdahl Å, Johansson O, Lindblom D (1974): The Vibratome: A useful tool in transmitter histochemistry. In: Fujiwara M, Tanaka C (Eds), *Amine Fluorescence Histochemistry,* pp. 1–12. Igaku Shoin, Tokyo.

Hökfelt T, Lundberg JM, Schultzberg M, Johansson O, Skirboll L, Ånggård A, Fredholm B, Hamberger B,

Pernow B, Rehfeld J, Goldstein M (1980a): Cellular localization of peptides in neural structures. *Proc. R. Soc. London, Ser. B, 210,* 63–77.

Hökfelt T, Lundberg JM, Schultzberg M, Johansson O, Ljungdahl Å, Rehfeld J (1980b) Coexistence of peptides and putative transmitters in neurons. In: Costa E, Trabucchi M (Eds), *Neural Peptides and Neural Communication,* pp. 1–23. Raven Press, New York.

Horn AS, Coyle JT, Snyder SH (1971): Catecholamine uptake by synatosomes from rat brain: Structure- activity relationships of drugs with differential effects on dopamine and norepinephrine neurons. *Mol. Pharmacol., 7,* 66–80.

Howe PRC, Costa M, Furness JB, Chalmers JP (1980): Simultaneous demonstration of phenylethanol-amine-N-methyltransferase immunofluorescent and catecholamine fluorescent nerve cell bodies in the rat medulla oblongata. *Neuroscience, 5,* 2229–2238.

Hwang BH, Williams TH (1982): Fluorescence microscopy used in conjunction with horseradish peroxidase localization and electronmicroscopy for studying sympathetic nuclei of the rat spinal cord. *Brain Res. Bull., 9,* 171–177.

Ibata Y, Watanabe K, Kinoshita H, Kubo S, Sano Y, Sin S, Hashimura E, Imagawa K (1979): Detection of catecholamine and luteinizing hormone-releasing hormone (LH-RH) containing nerve endings in the median eminence and the organon vaculosum laminae terminalis by fluorescence histochemistry on the same microscopic sections. *Neurosci. Lett., 11,* 181–186.

Jacobowitz D, Koelle GB (1965): Histochemical correlations of acetylcholinesterase and catecholamines in postganglionic autonomic nerves of the cat, rabbit, and guinea-pig. *J. Pharmacol. Exp. Ther., 148,* 225–237.

Jennings BM (1965): Aldehyde-fuchsin staining applied to frozen sections for demonstrating pituitary and pancreatic beta cells. *J. Histochem. Cytochem., 13,* 328–333.

Johnson RP, Sar M, Stumpf WE (1979): Relationships between the catecholaminergic systems demonstrated by a combined technique of formaldehyde-induced fluorescence and immunocytochemistry. *Neurosci. Lett., 14,* 321–326.

Jonsson G (1966): Fluorescence studies on some 6,7-substituted 3,4-dihydroisoquinolines formed from 3-hydroxytyramine (dopamine) and formaldehyde. *Acta. Chem. Scand., 20,* 2755–2762.

Jonsson G (1967): Further studies on the specificity of the histochemical fluorescence method for the demonstration of catecholamines. *Acta Histochem., 26,* 379–390.

Jonsson G (1969): Microfluorimetric studies on the formaldehyde-induced fluorescence of noradrenaline in adrenergic nerves of rat iris. *J. Histochem. Cytochem., 17,* 714–723.

Jonsson G (1971): Quantitation of fluorescence of biogenic monoamines. *Prog. Histochem. Cytochem., 2,* 299–334.

Jonsson G (1973): Quantitation of biogenic monoamines demonstrated with the formaldehyde fluorescence method. In: Thaer AA, Sernez M (Eds), *Fluorescence Techniques in Cell Biology,* pp. 191–197. Springer-Verlag, Berlin–Heidelberg–New York.

Jonsson G, Sachs C (1969): Subcellular distribution of ^{3}H-noradrenaline in adrenergic nerves of mouse atrium: Effect of reserpine, monoamine oxidase and tyrosine hydroxylase inhibition. *Acta Physiol. Scand., 77,* 344–357.

Jonsson G, Einarsson P, Fuxe K, Hallman H (1975): Microspectrofluorimetric analysis of the formaldehyde induced fluorescence in midbrain raphe neurons. *Med. Biol., 53,* 25–39.

Jotz MM, Gill JE, Davis DT (1976): A new optical multichannel microspectrofluorometer. *J. Histochem. Cytochem., 24,* 91–99.

Klig V, Demirjian C, Pungaliya P (1976): Microspectrofluorometry in the study of biogenic amines: Automatic correction of excitation spectra. *J. Microsc., 107,* 173–176.

König R (1979): Consecutive demonstration of catecholamines and dopamine-β-hydroxylase within the same specimen. *Histochemistry 61,* 301–305.

Koslow SH (1974): 5-Methoxytryptamine: A possible central nervous system transmitter. In: Costa E, Gessa GL, Sandler M (Eds), *Advances in Biochemical Psychopharmacology, Vol. 10, Serotonin: New Vistas,* pp. 95–100. Raven Press, New York.

Kuypers HGJM, Catsman-Berrevoets CE, Padt RE (1977): Retrograde axonal transport of fluorescent substances in the rat's forebrain. *Neurosci. Lett., 6,* 127–135.

Kuypers HGJM, Bentivoglio M, Van der Kooy D, Catsman-Berrevoets CE (1979): Retrograde transport of bisbenzimide and propidium iodide through axons to their parent cell bodies. *Neurosci. Lett., 12,* 1–7.

Lagunoff D, Phillips M, Benditt EP (1961): The histochemical demonstration of histamine in mast cells. *J. Histochem. Cytochem., 9,* 534–541.

Laties AM, Lund R, Jacobowitz D (1967): A simplified method for the histochemical localization of cardiac catecholamine-containing nerve fibers. *J. Histochem. Cytochem., 5,* 535–541.

L'Hermite P (1969): Capture et stockage des amines catéchiques par les fibres adrénergiques du systéme nerveux et périférique. *Arch. Anat. Microsc. Morphol. Exp., 58,* 257–282.

117

Lichtensteiger W (1970): Katecholaminhaltige neurone in der neuroendokrinen steuerung. *Prog. Histochem. Cytochem., 1,* 185–276.

Lidbrink P, Jonsson G (1971): Semiquantitative estimation of formaldehyde-induced fluorescence of noradrenaline in central noradrenaline nerve terminals. *J. Histochem. Cytochem., 19,* 747–757.

Lindvall O (1975): Mesencephalic dopaminergic afferents to the lateral septal nucleus of the rat. *Brain Res., 87,* 89–95.

Lindvall O (1977): Combined visualization of central catecholamine- and acetylcholinesterase-containing neurons: Application of the glyoxylic acid and thiocholine histochemical methods to the same Vibratome section. *Histochemistry, 50,* 191–196.

Lindvall O, Björklund A (1974a): The glyoxylic acid fluorescence method for central catecholamine neurons: A detailed account on the methodology. *Histochemistry, 39,* 97–127.

Lindvall O, Björklund A (1974b): The organization of the ascending catecholamine neuron systems in the rat brains as revealed by the glyoxylic acid fluorescence method. *Acta Physiol. Scand. Suppl.,* 412.

Lindvall O, Björklund A, Hökfelt T, Ljungdahl Å (1973): Application of the glyoxylic acid method to Vibratome sections for the improved visualization of central catecholamine neurons. *Histochemistry, 35,* 31–38.

Lindvall O, Björklund A, Nobin A, Stenevi U (1974a): The adrenergic innervation of the rat thalamus as revealed by the glyoxylic acid fluorescence method. *J. Comp. Neurol., 154,* 317.

Lindvall O, Björklund A, Moore RY, Stenevi U (1974b): Mesencephalic dopamine neurons projecting to neocortex. *Brain Res., 81,* 325–331.

Lindvall O, Björklund A, Svensson L-Å (1974c): Fluorophore formation from catecholamines and related compounds in the glyoxylic acid fluorescence histochemical method. *Histochemistry, 39,* 197–227.

Lindvall O, Björklund A, Divac I (1978): Organization of catecholamine neurons projecting to the frontal cortex in the rat. *Brain Res., 142,* 1–24.

Lindvall O, Björklund A, Falck B, Lorén I (1980): New aspects on factors determining the sensitivity of the formaldehyde and glyoxylic acid fluorescence histochemical methods for monoamines. *Histochemistry, 68,* 169–181.

Lindvall O, Björklund A, Falck B, Lorén I, Svensson L-Å (1981): New fluorophore-forming reactions for histochemical visualization of N-acetylated and tertiary indolamines using glyoxylic acid, aluminum-formaldehyde and trifluoroacetic acid anhydrase as reagents. *Histochemistry, 72,* 523–543.

Ljungdahl Å, Hökfelt T, Goldstein M, Park D (1975): Retrograde peroxidase tracing of neurons combined with transmitter histochemistry. *Brain Res., 8,* 313–319.

Löfström A, Jonsson G, Fuxe K (1976a): Microfluorimetric quantitation of catecholamine fluorescence in rat median eminence. I. Aspects on the distribution of dopamine and noradrenaline nerve terminals. *J. Histochem. Cytochem., 24,* 415–429.

Löfström A, Jonsson G, Wiesel Fa-A, Fuxe K (1976b): Microfluorimetric quantitation of catecholamine fluorescence in rat median eminence. II. Turnover changes in hormonal states. *J. Histochem. Cytochem., 24,* 430–442.

Lojda Z, Gossrau R, Schiebler TH (1976): Enzymhistochemische Methoden, Springer-Verlag, Berlin–Heidelberg–New York. (English Edition 1979).

Lorén I, Björklund A, Falck B, Lindvall O (1976): An improved histofluorescence procedure for freeze-dried paraffin-embedded tissue based on combined formaldehyde-glyoxylic acid perfusion with high magnesium content and acid pH. *Histochemistry, 49,* 177–192.

Lorén I, Björklund A, Lindvall O (1977): Magnesium ions in catecholamine fluorescence histochemistry. Application to the cryostat and Vibratome techniques. *Histochemistry, 52,* 223–239.

Lorén I, Björklund A, Falck B, Lindvall O (1980): The aluminum-formaldehyde (ALFA) histofluorescence method for improved visualization of catecholamines and indolamines. 1. A detailed account of the methodology for central nervous tissue using paraffin, cryostat or Vibratome sections. *J. Neurosci. Meth., 2,* 277–300.

Lorén I, Björklund A, Lindvall O, Schmidt RH (1982): Improved catecholamine histofluorescence in the developing brain based on the magnesium and aluminum (ALFA) perfusion techniques: Methodology and anatomical observations. *Brain Res. Bull., 9,* 11–26.

Lyon H, Baeksted M, Møller M (1982): Induced fluorescence of serotonin in paraffin sections from carcinoid tumors. *Brain Res. Bull., 9,* 751–756.

Malmfors T (1965): Studies on adrenergic nerves. The use of rat and mouse iris for direct observation on their physiology and pharmacology at cellular and subcellular levels. *Acta Physiol. Scand., 64, Suppl. 248,* 1–121.

Masuoka D, Placidi G-F (1968): A combined procedure for the histochemical fluorescence demonstration of monoamines and microautoradiography of water-soluble drugs. *J. Histochem. Cytochem., 16,* 659–664.

118

Masuoka DT, Placidi G-F, Gosling JA (1971): Histochemical fluorescence microscopy and microautoradiography techniques combined for localization studies. In: Eränkö O (Ed), *Progress in Brain Research, Vol. 34, Histochemistry of Nervous Transmission,* pp. 77–86. Elsevier, Amsterdam–London–New York.

Mayer RT, Novacek VM (1974): A direct recording corrected microspectrofluorometer. *J. Microsc., 102,* 165–177.

McLean JR, Burnstock G (1966): Histochemical localization of catecholamines in the urinary bladder of the toad (Bufo Marinus). *J. Histochem. Cytochem., 14,* 538–548.

McNeill TH, Sladek Jr JR (1980): Simultaneous monoamine histofluorescence and neuropeptide immunocytochemistry: V. A methodology for examining correlative monoamine-neuropeptide neuroanatomy. *Brain Res. Bull., 5,* 599–608.

Meryman HR (1956): Mechanics of freezing in living cells and tissues. *Science, 124,* 515–521.

Meryman HT (1960): General principles of freezing and injury in cellular materials. *Ann. NY Acad. Sci., 85,* 501–734.

Nelson JS, Wakefield PL (1968): The cellular localization of catecholamines in frozen-dried cryostat sections of the brain and autonomic nervous system. *J. Neuropath. Exp. Neurol., 27,* 221–233.

Nielsen KC, Owman Ch (1967): Adrenergic innervation of pial arteries related to the circle of Willis in the cat. *Brain Res., 6,* 773–776.

Nobin A, Björklund A (1973): Topography of the monoamine neuron systems in the human brain as revealed in fetuses. *Acta Physiol. Scand., Suppl., 338,* 3–40.

Norberg K-A, Ritzén M, Ungerstedt U (1966): Histochemical studies on a special catecholamine-containing cell type in sympathetic ganglia. *Acta Physiol. Scand., 67,* 260–270.

Nygren L-G (1976): On the visualization of central dopamine and noradrenaline nerve terminals in cryostat sections. *Med. Biol., 54,* 278–285.

Olson J (1969): Intact and regenerating sympathetic noradrenaline axons in the rat sciatic nerve. *Histochemie, 17,* 349–367.

Olson L, Nygren LG (1972): A new model for fluorescence histochemical studies of central 5-hydroxytryptamine and noradrenaline nerve fibers: The filum terminale spread preparation. *Histochemie, 29,* 265–273.

Olson L, Ungerstedt U (1970a): A simple high capacity freeze-drier for histochemical use. *Histochemie, 22,* 8–19.

Olson L, Ungerstedt U (1970b): Monoamine fluorescence in CNS smears: Sensitive and rapid visualization of nerve terminals without freeze-drying. *Brain Res., 17,* 343–347.

Parker CA (1968): *Photoluminescence of Solutions,* Elsevier Publishing Company, Amsterdam–London–New York.

Pearse AGE (1968): *Histochemistry, Theoretical and Applied.* J and A. Churchill, London.

Pesce AJ, Rosén C-G, Pasby TL (1971): *Fluorescence Spectroscopy: An Introduction for Biology and Medicine.* Marcel Dekker, New York.

Pictet A, Spengler T (1911): Uber die Bildung von Isochinolinderivaten durch Einwirkung von Methylal auf Phenyl-äthylamin, Phenyl-alanin und Tyrosin. *Ber. Dtsch. Chem. Ges., 44,* 2030–2036.

Placadi GF, Masuoka DT (1968): Histochemical demonstration of fluorescent catecholamine terminals in cryostat sections of brain tissue. *J. Histochem. Cytochem., 16,* 491–492.

Ploem JS (1967): The use of a vertical illuminator with interchangeable dichroic mirrors for fluorescence microscopy with incident light. *Mikrosk., 68,* 129–142.

Ploem JS (1977): Quantitative fluorescence microscopy. In: Meek FA, Elder HY (Eds), *Analytical and Quantitative Methods in Microscopy,* pp. 55–89. Cambridge University Press, Cambridge.

Ploem JS, De Sterke JA, Bonnet J, Wasmund H (1974): A microspectrofluorometer with epi-illumination operated under computer control. *J. Histochem. Cytochem., 22,* 668–677.

Reinhold Ch, Hartwig H-G (1982): Progress in microfluorometric identification of monoamine fluorophores. *Brain Res. Bull., 9,* 97–105.

Ritzén M (1966a): Quantitative fluorescence microspectrophotometry of catecholamine-formaldehyde products. *Exp. Cell Res., 44,* 505–520.

Ritzén M (1966b): Quantitative fluorescence microspectrophotometry of 5-hydroxytryptamine-formaldehyde products in models and in mast cells. *Exp. Cell Res., 45,* 178–194.

Ritzén M (1967): *Cytochemical Identification and Quantitation of Biogenic Monoamines – A Microspectrofluorimetric and Autoradiographic Study.* M.D. Thesis, Stockholm.

Ritzén M (1973): Microfluorimetric quantitation of biogenic monoamines. In: Sernertz M, Thaer A (Eds), *Quantitative Fluorescence Techniques as Applied in Cell Biology,* pp. 183–190. Springer Verlag, Berlin–Heidelberg–New York.

Rost FWD (1974): Microspectrofluorometry. *Med. Biol., 52,* 73–81.

Rost FWD, Pearse AGE (1971): An improved microspectrofluorimeter with automatic digital data logging: Construction and operation. *J. Microsc., 94,* 93–105.

Ruch F (1973): The use of human leucocytes as a standard for the cytofluorometric determination of protein and DNA. In: Sernertz M, Thaer A (Eds), *Quantitative Fluorescence Techniques as Applied in Cell Biology,* pp. 51–55. Springer Verlag, Berlin–Heidelberg–New York.

Rundquist I (1981): A flexible system for microscope fluorometry served by a personal computer. *Histochemistry, 70,* 151–159.

Saavedra JM, Axelrod J (1976): Octopamine as a putative neurotransmitter. In: *Advances in Biochemical Psychopharmacology, Vol. 15,* pp. 95–110. Raven Press, New York.

Sachs C (1970): Noradrenaline uptake mechanisms in the mouse atrium. *Acta Physiol. Scand., Suppl.,* 341.

Sakharova AV, Sakharov DA (1971): Visualization of intraneuronal monoamines by treatment with formalin solutions. *Prog. Brain Res., 34,* 11–25.

Satoh K, Tohyama M, Yamamoto K, Sakumoto T, Shimizu N (1977): Noradrenaline innervation of the spinal cord studied by the horseradish peroxidase method combined with monoamine oxidase staining. *Exp. Brain Res., 30,* 175–186.

Schipper J, Tilders FJH (1982): Quantification of formaldehyde induced fluorescence and its application in neurobiology. *Brain Res. Bull., 9,* 69–80.

Schipper J, Tilders FJH, Ploem JS (1980): A scanning microfluorimetric study on sympathetic nerve fibres: Intraneuronal differences in noradrenaline turnover. *Brain Res., 190,* 459–472.

Schlumpf M, Shoemaker WJ, Bloom FE (1977): Explant cultures of catecholamine-containing neurons from rat brain: Biochemical, histofluorescence, and electronmicroscopic studies. *Proc. Nat. Acad. Sci. USA, 74,* 4471–4475.

Schöler J, Armstrong WE (1982): Aqueous aldehyde (Faglu) histofluorescence for catecholamines in 2 μm sections using polyethylene glycol embedding. *Brain Res. Bull., 9,* 27–31.

Schröder H, Lackner K, Heym Ch (1982): Simultaneous demonstration of catecholamines and phenylethanolamine-N-methyltransferase in the same tissue section by means of formaldehyde-induced fluorescence (FIF) and tetramethyl-rhodamine-isothiocyanate (MRITC) immunofluorescence. *J. Neurosci. Meth., 6,* 281–286.

Seiler N, Bruder K (1975): Determination of serotonin and bufotenin as their dansyl derivates. *Chromatography, 106,* 159–173.

Sernetz M, Thaer A (1973): Quantitative fluorescence analysis in microcapillaries. In: Sernertz M, Thaer A (Eds), *Quantitative Fluorescence Techniques as Applied in Cell Biology,* pp. 41–50. Springer Verlag, Berlin–Heidelberg–New York.

Sladek Jr JR, Sladek CD, McNeill TH, Wood JG (1978): New sites of monoamine localization in the endocrine hypothalamus as revealed by new methodological approaches. In: Scott DE, Kozlowski GP, Weindl A (Eds), *Neural Hormones and Reproduction, Brain-Endocrine Interaction III,* pp. 154–171. Karger, Basel.

Smith RE (1970): Comparative evaluation of two instruments and procedures to cut nonfrozen sections. *J. Histochem. Cytochem., 18,* 590–591.

Smithson KG, MacVicar BA, Hatton GI (1983): A technique compatible with immunocytochemistry, enzyme histochemistry, histofluorescence and intracellular staining. *J. Neurosci. Meth., 7,* 27–41.

Smolen AJ, Glazer EJ, Ross LL (1979): Horseradish peroxidase histochemistry combined with glyoxylic acid-induced fluorescence used to identify brain stem catecholaminergic neurons which project to the chick thoracic spinal cord. *Brain Res., 160,* 353–357.

Spriggs TLB, Lever JD, Rees PM, Graham JDP (1966): Controlled formaldehyde-catecholamine condensation in cryostat sections to show adrenergic nerves by fluorescence. *Stain Technol., 41,* 323–327.

Späth E, Lederer E (1930): Synthesen von 4-carbolinen. *Ber. Dtsch. Chem. Ges., 63,* 2102–2111.

Steinbusch HWM, Verhofstad AAJ, Joosten HWJ (1968): Localization of serotonin in the central nervous system by immunohistochemistry: Description of a specific and sensitive technique and some applications. *Neuroscience, 3,* 811–819.

Stumpf WE (1971): Autoradiographic techniques for the localization of hormones and drugs at the cellular and subcellular level. *Acta Endrocrinol., Suppl., 153,* 205–222.

Stumpf WE, Roth LJ (1969): Autoradiography using dry-mounted freeze-dried sections. In: Roth LJ, Stumpf WE (Eds), *Autoradiography of Diffusible Substances,* pp. 69–80. Academic Press, New York–London.

Stumpf WE, Sar M (1975): Autoradiographic techniques for localizing steroid hormones. In: O'Malleyand BW, Hardman JG (Eds), *Methods in Enzymology, Vol. XXXVI, Hormone Action, Part 2: Steroid Hormones.* Academic Press, New York–London.

Svendgaard NA, Björklund A, Stenevi U (1975): Regenerative properties of central monoamine neurons. Studies in the adult rat using cerebral iris implants as targets. In: *Advances in Anatomy, Embryology and Cell Biology, Vol. 51,* Fasc. 4, pp. 7–77. Springer-Verlag, Berlin–Heidelberg–New York.

Svensson LÅ, Björklund A, Lindvall O (1975): Studies on the fluorophore forming reactions of various catecholamines and tetrahydroisoquinolines with glyoxylic acid. *Acta Chem. Scand., B29*, 341–348.

Tallqvist G, Tallqvist J, Eränkö J (1967): An efficient freeze-drying apparatus. *Histochemie, 8*, 377–379.

Tilders FJH, Ploem JS, Smelik PG (1974): Quantitative microfluorimetric studies on formaldehyde-induced fluorescence of 5-hydroxytryptamine in the spinal gland of the rat. *J. Histochem. Cytochem., 22*, 967–975.

Tramu G, Pillez A, Leonardelli J (1978): An efficient method of antibody elution for the successive or simultaneous localization of two antigens by immunocytochemistry. *J. Histochem. Cytochem., 26*, 322–324.

Trump BF, Goldblatt PJ, Griffin CC, Waravdekar VS, Stowell RE (1964): Effects of freezing and thawing on the ultrastructure of mouse hepatic parenchymal cells. *Lab. Invest., 13*, 967–1002.

Ullberg S, Appelgren L-E (1969): Experiences in locating drugs at different levels of resolution. In: Roth LJ, Stumpf WE (Eds), *Autoradiography of Diffusible Substances*, pp. 279–303. Academic Press, New York–London.

Van Orden L (1970): Quantitative histochemistry of biogenic amines. A simple microspectrofluorometer. *Biochem. Pharma., 19*, 1105–1117.

Van Orden LS, Schaefer JM, Burke JP, Lodven FV (1970): Differentiation of norepinephrine storage compartments in peripheral adrenergic nerves. *J. Pharmacol. Exp. Ther., 174*, 357–368.

Victorov I, Nguyen-Legros J, Boutry J-M, Alvarez Ch, Hauw J-J (1979): The early outgrowth of catecholaminergic fibers and the development of the nucleus of the locus coeruleus in tissue culture of newborn mice in leighton tubes. *Biomedicine, 30*, 161–168.

Waris T, Rechardt L (1977): Histochemically demonstrable catecholamines and cholinesterases in nerve fibres of rat dorsal skin. *Histochemistry, 53*, 203.

Waris T, Rechardt L, Partanen S (1976): Simultaneous demonstration of cholinesterases and glyoxylic acid-induced fluorescence of catecholamines in stretch preparations. *Acta Histochem., 58*, 194–198.

Watson SJ, Barchas JD (1977): Catecholamine histofluorescence using cryostat sectioning and glyoxylic acid in unperfused frozen brain: detailed description of the technique. *Histochem. J., 9*, 183–195.

Watson SJ, Ellison JP (1976): Cryostat technique for central nervous system histofluorescence. *Histochemistry, 50*, 119–127.

Whaley WM, Govindachari TR (1951): The Pictet-Spengler synthesis of tetrahydroisoquinolines and related compounds. In: Adams R (Ed), *Organic Reactions, Vol. 6*, pp. 151–206. John Wiley, New York.

Winckler J (1970): Kontrollierte Gefriertrocknung von Kryostatschnitten. *Histochemie, 22*, 234.

Wreford NGM, Schofield GC (1975): A microspectrofluorimeter with online real-time correction of spectra. *J. Microsc., 103*, 127–130.

Wreford NGM, Smith GC (1982): Microspectrofluorometry in biogenic amine research. *Brain Res. Bull., 9*, 87–96.

Wreford NGM, Singhaniyom W, Smith GC (1982): Microspectrofluorometric characterization of the fluorescent derivatives of biogenic amines produced by aqueous aldehyde (Faglu) fixation. *Histochem. J., 14*, 491–505.

Wurtman RJ, Axelrod J (1968): The formation, metabolism, and physiologic effects of melatonin. *Adv. Pharmacol., 6A*, 141–151.

Zlotnik I (1960): The initial cooling of tissues in the freezing-drying technique. *Quart. J. Microsc. Sci., 101*, 251–254.

CHAPTER III

Ultrastructural visualization of biogenic monoamines

GRAYSON RICHARDS

1. INTRODUCTION

Cell-to-cell communication in the nervous system is generally brought about by the release of chemical messengers *(neurotransmitters)* from nerve terminals upon arrival of a nerve impulse (Iversen 1980). The monoamine transmitters, dopamine, noradrenaline and serotonin, are stored in high concentrations in membrane-bound vesicles *(synaptic vesicles)* where they are rendered inert and osmotically stable (complexed with proteins or 5'-phosphonucleotides) until released. After release of the endogenous or natural amine, its interaction at the transmitter receptor of a target neuron is terminated either by reuptake at the presynaptic neuronal membrane or by enzymatic degradation.

An important advance in the study of mechanisms of synaptic transmission in the nervous system has been the development of methods which permit the selective staining of transmitter-specific neurons. These methods have revealed that neurotransmitters, such as monoamines, are most concentrated in nerve terminals but are also present in high concentrations in dendrites although in lower quantities in neuronal perikarya and nonterminal axons.

There are several approaches which can be used to identify monoamine storage sites in the nervous system (Bloom 1973; Richards 1978). One is to convert the natural transmitter into a derivative that will fluoresce upon violet irradiation in the light-microscope *(Falck-Hillarp method)*. Another more indirect approach is to inject radioactively labelled molecules of a transmitter into an experimental animal where they are selectively taken up by the nerve terminals which synthesize and release that transmitter; the accumulated radioactivity can then be detected by placing thin sections of the tissue on radiation-sensitive film *(transmitter autoradiography)*. A third approach exploits the high-specificity of antibodies. A neurotransmitter, or an enzyme involved in its synthesis, is purified from the brain or peripheral organ and injected into an experimental animal where it induces the manufacture of antibodies that combine with it specifically. The antisera are utilized to selectively stain neurons containing the relevant antigen, i.e. the transmitter or enzyme *(transmitter immunohisto- and immunocytochemistry)*. Since these three methods are described in detail in Chapters II, IV and VII of this volume, only a few examples will be mentioned here in support of our findings using alternative methods.

Two approaches frequently used in our laboratory for the ultrastructural visualization of storage sites of biogenic monoamines are the cytochemical identification of endogenous amines using an *improved chromaffin reaction* (Tranzer and Richards 1976)

Handbook of Chemical Neuroanatomy. Vol. 1: Methods in Chemical Neuroanatomy.
A. Björklund and T. Hökfelt, editors.
© Elsevier Science Publishers B.V., 1983.

and of exogenous amines *('false' transmitters)* that are highly osmiophilic and thus easily identified by conventional fixation. In addition, monoamine storage organelles in platelets, adrenomedullary cells, sympathetic neurons and possibly also brain contain high concentrations of 5′-phosphonucleotides, such as adenosine-5′-triphosphate (ATP), which can be identified by a recently developed cytochemical method, the *uranaffin reaction* (Richards and Da Prada 1977). A wealth of information about the localization and distribution of monoamines in nervous tissue at the ultrastructural level has been gained from the application of these three methods (Richards and Da Prada 1980; Richards 1981).

Because of the complexity of neuronal networks in the brain, the development of these cytochemical methods has relied to a great extent on the use of simpler models of monoamine storage found in blood platelets, adrenomedullary cells and peripheral sympathetic neurons. Indeed, it has been possible to isolate, purify, and biochemically as well as morphologically characterize the amine storage organelles of platelets (Da Prada et al. 1981), adrenomedullary cells (Winkler 1976) and sympathetic nerves (Lagercrantz 1976; Fried et al. 1978) but not those of the brain. In the following description of the methods, therefore, emphasis will be laid on establishing their specificity in studies of these simpler models before applying them to investigations of the brain. Details of the methods can be found in the Appendix.

2. CYTOCHEMISTRY OF ENDOGENOUS AMINES

2.1. THE CHOICE OF PRIMARY FIXATIVE

Routine fixation techniques

It was early recognized that routine electron-microscopic techniques based on fixation with osmium tetroxide, with or without combination with glutaraldehyde, allow the distinction of at least two types of peripheral autonomic nerve fibers. They were characterized by the presence of synaptic vesicles with or without an electron-dense core and evidence was provided that they represented adrenergic and cholinergic nerve endings, respectively (de Robertis and Pellegrino de Iraldi 1961; Lever and Esterhuizen 1961; Richardson 1962, 1964; Wolfe et al. 1962). However, the proportion of dense core vesicles as compared to clear synaptic vesicles in such adrenergic nerve endings varied between tissues and between species. In fact, in some tissues of certain laboratory animals, such as the rat iris, it was not possible to demonstrate any dense core vesicles at all in osmium tetroxide-fixed material, in spite of the fact that noradrenergic nerves were known to be present (Nilsson 1964). This situation led to a search for novel fixation methods and in 1966 Richardson introduced potassium permanganate ($KMnO_4$) for this purpose.

Permanganate fixation method

At the time we began our cytochemical investigations, more than 15 yr ago, this fixation method of Richardson (1966) was the most frequently used technique for the identification of biogenic amines in neurons. Whereas he had used it to study amine storage sites in the peripheral nervous system, in subsequent studies by Hökfelt (1968, 1971, 1973) the method was successfully applied to the central nervous system. In the studies of Hökfelt and collaborators thin slices of tissues were immersed in the ice-cold fixative. Modifications have since been introduced: Koda and Bloom (1977) briefly perfused rats with a glyoxylic acid-formalin mixture (see, Chapter II) and then immersed tissue slices in potassium permanganate. Other examples of its use include an investigation of the fine structure of rat cerebellar noradrenaline terminals with an 'in situ perfusion' technique (Kimoto et al. 1981) and the characterization of rat brain synaptosomes (Kanerva et al. 1977b).

Potassium permanganate was first introduced by Luft (1956) as an alternative fixative to osmium tetroxide. Whereas the inability of this fixative to preserve many cellular components (it extracts proteins and lipids) and the swelling introduced in many organelles has made it unsuitable as a general fixative for electron-microscopy, it has made an important impact in monoamine cytochemistry.

Potassium permanganate is a strong oxidizing agent (redox potential 1.5) which reacts with reducing substances, such as monoamines, to produce a dark brown precipitate which is electron-dense. The phenolic hydroxyl groups are thought to be mainly responsible for the reducing capacity of the amines since β-phenylethylamine, lacking hydroxyl groups, does not precipitate with this fixative. According to model experiments (Hökfelt and Jonsson 1968), the electron-density of this precipitate might be due to metallic manganese dioxide (brownstone). The oxidized amine is probably not chemically bound to the precipitate on a molar basis but is partially retained within the precipitate (Hökfelt 1971). This interpretation has been used to explain the poor amine retention after this fixation procedure, which has led to the conclusion that the dense core in amine-storing vesicles after potassium permanganate fixation reflects the presence of amine at the moment of fixation.

The method

Hökfelt and Jonsson (1968) have made a thorough investigation of the properties of this primary fixative in monoamine cytochemistry. The potassium salt (a 3% solution) is preferred to the zinc or barium salts although a 9% solution of either the lithium or sodium salt has also been successfully used. The freshly made-up solution with or without a buffer, is used to fix small (1 mm^3) pieces of tissue for 30 min to 2 h at 4°C. Often, staining en bloc with uranyl acetate during rinsing in Ringer's solution after fixation is sufficient to obtain acceptable contrast. An improved ultrastructural detail in tissues fixed with potassium permanganate was recently reported by Todd and Tokito (1981) using physiological saline as the vehicle for all solutions and very rapid dehydration before embedding. The fact that amine-storing vesicles contain extremely high concentrations of the amine (approximately 10^{-4} pg/vesicle, i.e. >0.2 M) leads to the formation of an intense precipitate with the fixative although other cell organelles are also stained.

That monoamines of the rat adrenal medulla (and carotid body) do not form the expected electron-dense precipitate with potassium permanganate (Kanerva et al. 1977a) might be due to the higher solubility of the amine-protein (chromogranin) complex in adrenomedullary granules compared with the amine storage complex of neuronal vesicles.

Although the potassium permanganate fixation method applied to the peripheral nervous system has been very successful, in the brain reliable detection of monoamines is possible only in those amine-rich areas which contain mainly noradrenaline (e.g. periventricular hypothalamus) but not dopamine or serotonin. For other monoamine containing brain areas the visualization of the amine-storing vesicles can be facilitated by increasing the intraneuronal and intragranular amine content with exogenous amines such as α-methyl noradrenaline (i.c.v. or in vitro).

Conditions for optimal cytochemical method

Although the permanganate fixation method has its merits, the chromaffin reaction (Hopwood 1971) for the ultrastructural visualization of biogenic amines (Wood and Barnett 1964; Wood 1966) has certain advantages. When systematically investigated by Tranzer and Snipes (1968), it was found to be greatly improved in terms of specificity, sensitivity and tissue preservation. The results of their studies on the effects of numerous fixation parameters on amine localization have been summarized by Tranzer and Richards (1976).

As for all cytochemical methods, optimum results are only achieved when certain criteria are fulfilled, namely: (1) retention and insolubilization of all the amine during the fixation in its in vivo location; (2) easy recognition of the amine, by strong and selective contrast — the more selective the contrast is for the amine the better the cytochemical reaction and the stronger the contrast, the better the sensitivity (both selectivity and sensitivity can be checked by well established specific pharmacological treatments); and (3) good preservation of all other tissue components so that their relationships with the amine storage sites can be determined.

It is essential to cross-link the amine with tissue proteins in order to retain, i.e. fix, sufficient quantities for cytochemistry. This is best illustrated by the failure of osmium tetroxide, as a primary fixative, to visualize the amine storage organelles of platelets, whereas after primary fixation with glutaraldehyde followed by osmium tetroxide, highly electron-dense organelles in platelets can be observed (Fig. 1). The fact that reserpine selectively depletes these organelles of their electron-dense content (Figs 2 and 3) and the platelets of their serotonin content, is clear proof of the presence of an amine (serotonin) in these organelles. Moreover, platelets of carcinoid patients (whose serotonin levels are at least three-times those of healthy individuals) contain much more prominent osmiophilic organelles (Fig. 4) compared to controls.

Thus, the excellent cross-linking properties of glutaraldehyde make it the primary fixative of choice (Hayat 1981). Its covalent reaction, on the one hand, with free amino groups of terminal amino acids in proteins, such as lysine, and on the other, with the amino groups of neurotransmitter amines, forms Schiff bases (Fig. 5). These are the substrates for further cross-linking with other proteins and amines. The reaction product is stable to the dehydration and embedding procedures which follow fixation.

2.2. VISUALIZATION OF THE FIXED AMINE

Electron-dense heavy metals are used to stain the amines that are cross-linked with tissue proteins. The most commonly used stain, osmium tetroxide, achieves both a postfixation and staining. In the fixed amine, e.g. noradrenaline (Fig. 6), the two hydroxyl groups of the aromatic ring become oxidized leaving an insoluble, highly electron-dense reaction product called osmium black which is a cyclic osmium ester. During the formation of osmium black, the cross-linked amine becomes oxidized to a quinone and ultimately to a melanin-like reaction product. The ease with which the sympathomimetic amine 5-hydroxydopamine can be visualized, may be attributed to the additional hydroxyl group for oxidation on the aromatic ring (Richards 1981).

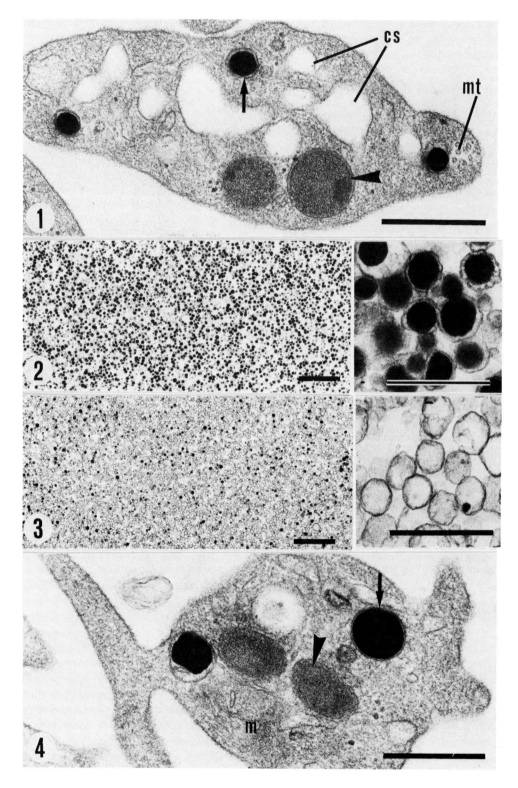

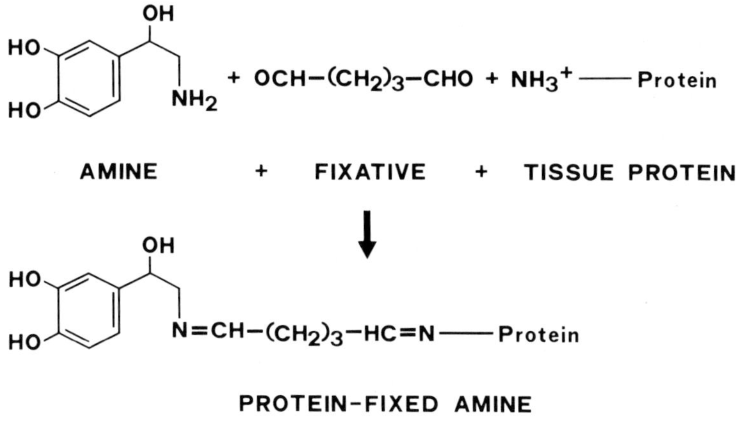

AMINE   +   **FIXATIVE**   +   **TISSUE PROTEIN**

PROTEIN-FIXED AMINE

Fig. 5. Fixation of amines to tissue proteins.

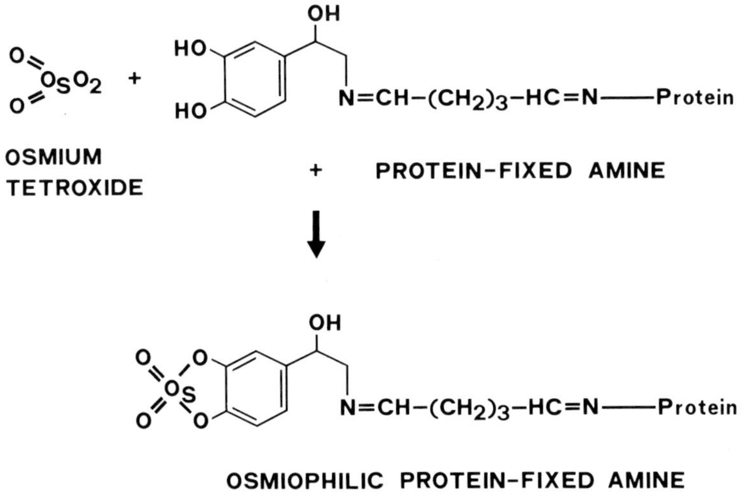

OSMIUM TETROXIDE   +   **PROTEIN-FIXED AMINE**

OSMIOPHILIC PROTEIN-FIXED AMINE

Fig. 6. Electron-dense (osmiophilic) reaction product.

Fig. 1. Rabbit platelet. Glutaraldehyde-osmium tetroxide fixation; section stained with lead citrate. Note the highly electron-dense, osmiophilic organelles (→) which are easily distinguished from α-granules (►). cs = canalicular system; mt = microtubules. Bar = 0.5 μm.

Fig. 2. Isolated amine-storing organelles of rabbit platelets. Glutaraldehyde-osmium tetroxide fixation; lead citrate stain. The almost pure fraction of highly osmiophilic organelles was prepared by density gradient centrifugation. The inset shows the same fraction in greater detail. Bar = 2 μm (inset: 0.5 μm).

Fig. 3. Isolated amine-storing organelles of reserpinized rabbit platelets. Glutaraldehyde-osmium tetroxide fixation; lead citrate stain. Note the virtual absence of electron-dense cores in these organelles. Bar = 2 μm (inset: 0.5 μm).

Fig. 4. Human platelet from a patient with a carcinoid syndrome. Glutaraldehyde-osmium tetroxide fixation; lead citrate stain. Amine-storing organelles (→) are, for human platelets, unusually prominent, i.e. virtually filled to capacity with a highly electron-dense, osmiophilic core. α-granules (►) appear normal. m = mitochondrion. Bar = 0.5 μm.

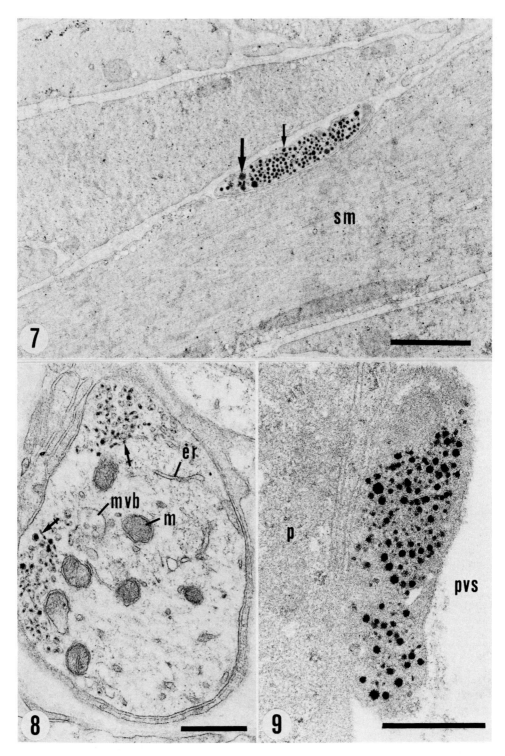

Since osmium tetroxide also stains proteins and unsaturated lipids, there is a need for a cytochemical reaction which renders the amine storage sites selectively electron-dense. The chromaffin reaction, without osmium postfixation, meets this requirement.

2.3. IMPROVED CHROMAFFIN REACTION: A CRITICAL APPRAISAL

The original method of Wood and Barrnett (1964) has been modified so that the primary fixative contains an electron-dense stain, namely the dichromate ions which form the buffer (for details, see Appendix). In this way, both fixation and staining are initiated simultaneously leading to an optimal retention and visualization of the endogenous amine. The chromaffin reaction identifies dopamine, noradrenaline, and serotonin (Hopwood 1971) but does not differentiate between these amines.

The primary fixation step is carried out in the following solution at 0–4°C: 1% glutaraldehyde + 0.4% formaldehyde in 0.1 M sodium chromate/potassium dichromate buffer at pH 7.2. The tissue is either excised from the anesthetized animal and fixed as small pieces by immersion and rotation (to improve the penetration of the fixative) or the anesthetized animal is fixed by vascular perfusion of the primary fixative via the heart. After the initial fixation, which, because of the detrimental effects that aldehydes have on the reaction product, should not exceed 20 min, the excised immersion- or perfusion-fixed tissues are immersed with rotation for up to 24 h in the slightly acidic buffer alone at 0–4°C. Postfixation (optional) is carried out by immersion in chromate/dichromate-buffered 2% osmium tetroxide for 1 h.

Bloom (1970) has outlined the requirements for an ideal electron-histochemical reaction for biogenic amines. In a critical appraisal of the improved chromaffin reaction presented here, a few examples will serve to illustrate its qualities in meeting these requirements.

a. Optimum amine visualization with good tissue preservation is best achieved by vascular perfusion fixation. In the rat vas deferens, for example, small and large vesicles in sympathetic nerve varicosities contain a highly electron-dense reaction product in well preserved tissue (Fig. 7). Differences in the amount of reaction product, frequently observed in the large vesicles, probably reflects the physiological state of amine loading in these organelles. Differences between organs might also be expected if their amine turnover differs (Fillenz and Pollard 1976).

b. A third amine-storing organelle, a tubular reticulum first described by Tranzer (1973), is also visualized by the chromaffin reaction. In dendrites of sympathetic ganglion neurons (Fig. 8) these organelles are present in clusters with small dense-cored vesicles, frequently in association with a multivesicular body. This association

---

Fig. 7. Rat vas deferens. Chromaffin reaction by perfusion fixation; lead citrate stain. Note the selective electron-density of a nerve varicosity surrounded by well preserved smooth muscle cells (sm). Both small (→) and large (→) dense core vesicles are present in the varicosity. Bar = 1 μm.

Fig. 8. Rat superior cervical ganglion. Chromaffin reaction by perfusion fixation; lead citrate stain. A dendritic profile contains 2 clusters of a tubular reticulum (+>) with some small dense-core vesicles (→) in which the cytochemical reaction can be observed. er = endoplasmic reticulum; m = mitochondrion; mvb = multivesicular body. Bar = 0.5 μm.

Fig. 9. Rat pineal gland. Chromaffin reaction (without osmium tetroxide) by perfusion fixation; lead citrate stain. Note the selective electron-density of small and large cores of amine-storing organelles of a nerve varicosity, in a perivascular space (pvs), adjacent to a pinealocyte (p). In the absence of osmium the membranes are only poorly stained, if at all. Bar = 0.5 μm.

and the occasional presence of chromaffin-positive vesicles within multivesicular bodies (Richards and Da Prada 1980) suggests their involvement in the formation (or breakdown) of amine-storing organelles in neurons. The proliferation of a tubular reticulum in sympathetic ganglion neurons of rats 24 h after injection of 6-hydroxydopamine is a possible indication of its role in the formation of new vesicles (Richards and Da Prada 1980).

c. The cytochemical reaction product is also visible in the absence of postfixation (and staining) with osmium tetroxide (Fig. 9). In this case, the vesicle and cell membranes, ribosomes, glycogen particles and mitochondrial granules are left unstained even when the sections are contrasted with lead citrate. Böck and Gorgas (1976) have suggested that the lead stain forms a highly electron-dense, insoluble complex with the protein-fixed amine. Osmium and, to a greater extent, lead increase the selective contrast of the reaction product for which chromium is mainly responsible.

d. In cholinergic nerve terminals, for example those frequently found adjacent to adrenergic nerve terminals in rat iris (Fig. 10), the vesicles are devoid of a chromaffin reaction.

e. Although amine-storing organelles are most concentrated in nerve terminals and dendrites, they can also be visualized in myelinated and unmyelinated axons (Figs 11 and 12) as well as in neuronal perikarya (Richards and Tranzer 1975); large dense-cored vesicles and clusters of small dense-cored vesicles with a tubular reticulum are chromaffin-positive. The chromaffin reaction, combined with autoradiography, has been recently used to identify amine-storing vesicles in the ligated sciatic nerve of the rat (Lascar 1981).

f. Drugs known to affect the storage or metabolism of biogenic amines can be used to check the specificity of the chromaffin reaction. As already mentioned, amine-storing organelles in platelets are selectively depleted of their electron-dense cores by reserpine. Jaim-Etcheverry and Zieher (1974) have extended their studies on the amine cytochemistry of platelets to investigations on the pineal sympathetic nerves which store both noradrenaline and serotonin. Pharmacological manipulation of these amine stores combined with a modified chromaffin reaction have lead to the development of a technique (formaldehyde-glutaraldehyde-dichromate reaction) for the selective demonstration of serotonin in these nerves. McClung and Wood (1982) have recently demonstrated that whereas paraformaldehyde blocks the glutaraldehyde-chrome reaction with noradrenaline in the rat adrenal medulla, it did not block it for serotonin-containing argentaffin cells of the gut. Reserpine depletes both the small and large vesicles of their amine-specific chromaffin reaction by irreversibly binding to the vesicle membrane and thus interfering with amine storage (Richards et al. 1979). However, it should be remembered that the electron-dense (osmiophilic) proteinaceous matrix of the large cores is reserpine resistant and is therefore no indication per se of the presence of an amine (Jaim-Etcheverry and Zieher 1974).

Fig. 10. Rat iris. Chromaffin reaction by immersion fixation; lead citrate stain. Whereas an aminergic nerve varicosity is cytochemically reactive, an adjacent varicosity (c, probably cholinergic) is not. m = mitochondrion; s = Schwann cell sheath. Bar = 0.5 μm.

Figs 11 and 12. Rat superior cervical ganglion. Chromaffin reaction by perfusion fixation; lead citrate stain. In myelinated (Fig. 11) as well as unmyelinated nerves (Fig. 12), vesicles (→) and a reticulum (↦) contain a distinct cytochemical reaction. m = mitochondrion; my = myelin sheath; nf = neurofilaments; nt = neurotubules; s = Schwann cell sheath. Bar = 0.5 μm.

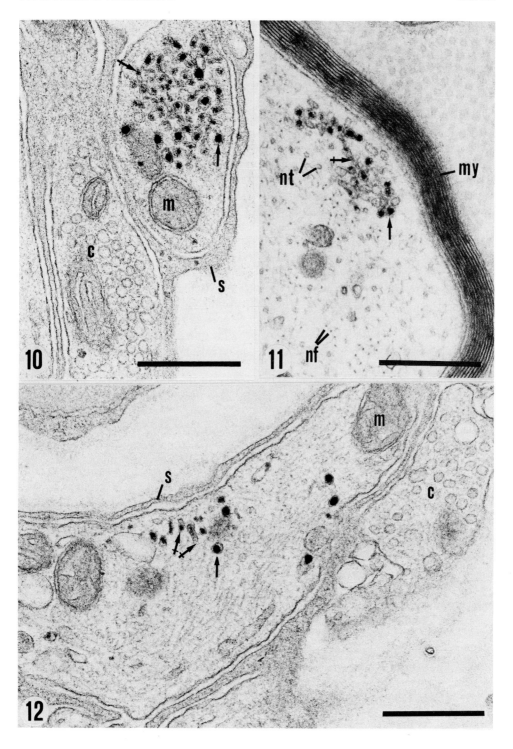

The sympathomimetic amine metaraminol, like reserpine, depletes amine stores. However, it achieves this by replacing the endogenous amine as a 'false' transmitter. Since metaraminol is chromaffin-negative (the availability of only one hydroxyl group of the aromatic ring probably restricts the number of sites at which chromium ions can react) the amine stores appear empty, i.e. electron-translucent. Treating animals with nialamide with or without reserpine (to increase extravesicular amine) does not result in an extravesicular chromaffin reaction.

g. There are not many regions of the central nervous system where the improved chromaffin reaction has been particularly successful. Among the exceptions, however, are varicose supra-ependymal axons which are efferent fibers now known to be purely serotoninergic throughout the cerebroventricular system (Lorez and Richards 1982; Richards and Guggenheim 1982). The chromaffin reaction of the small and large vesicles in these axons (Figs 13 and 14) is sensitive to both reserpine and p-chlorophenylalanine (a specific inhibitor of the rate-limiting enzyme tryptophan hydroxylase) but is resistant to α-methylparatyrosine (a specific inhibitor of tyrosine hydroxylase). This is a clear indication of the exclusive presence of serotonin (Richards and Tranzer 1974). The fact that supra-ependymal nerves become selectively labelled with [3H]serotonin (Richards 1977) and [3H]reserpine (Richards et al. 1979) confirms their serotoninergic nature. Although the immunoreactive substance P and serotonin have been shown to be present in the same dense-core vesicles in the anterior horn of the rat spinal cord (Pelletier et al. 1981), a co-transmitter for serotonin in supra-ependymal nerves has not yet been found (Richards et al. 1981).

The palisade zone of the lateral median eminence is another brain region in which amine storage sites (probably for dopamine) can be visualized with the reaction (Fig. 15).

Compared to peripheral organs, the compact nature of the brain probably delays fixation and staining in deeper, less vascularized regions leading to inconsistent results due to leakage of the amine. The small size and water-soluble nature of biogenic amines, their release by depolarization during fixation and changes in permeability of the vesicular or nerve terminal membrane during fixation might be contributory factors. As a consequence, the visualization of amine-storing sites in the brain has relied more on the use of exogenous amines, frequently in combination with the chromaffin reaction, to augment the reaction product (this approach will be discussed in Section 4).

Figs 13 and 14. Rat fourth ventricle floor. Chromaffin reaction by perfusion fixation; lead citrate stain. Note the amine-specific reaction of dense-cores in large (→) and small vesicles (→) of a supra-ependymal varicosity (*). In the absence of osmium tetroxide postfixation (Fig. 14), only the dense-cores are clearly visible. c = cilium; e = ependyma; m = mitochondrion; mv = microvilli; v = fourth ventricle. Bars = 0.5 μm.

Fig. 15. Rat median eminence. Chromaffin reaction by perfusion fixation; lead citrate stain. Two nerve profiles (*) adjacent to a perivascular space (pvs) contain amine-specific dense core vesicles. nsn = process of a neurosecretory neuron. Bar = 0.5 μm.

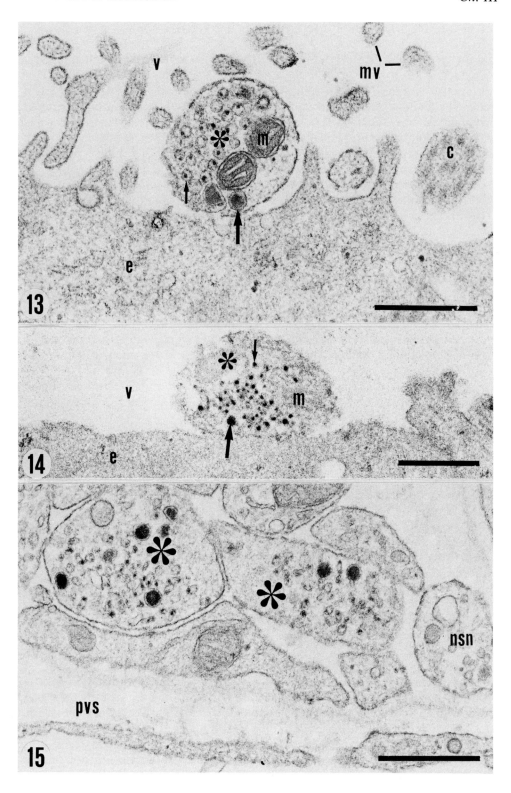

3. CYTOCHEMISTRY OF 5'-PHOSPHONUCLEOTIDES

3.1. URANAFFIN REACTION OF AMINE-STORING ORGANELLES

Just over 10 yr ago, Tranzer (1971a) observed that the amine-storing organelles of platelets became intensely stained with uranyl acetate when the reaction was carried out after glutaraldehyde fixation but before dehydration (Fig. 16). Uranyl ions also had an extremely high affinity for similar organelles in megakaryocytes (platelet stem cells), adrenomedullary cells, sympathetic ganglion cells, SIF cells and adrenergic nerves. These observations were the basis for the development of the uranaffin reaction for 5'-phosphonucleotides which are highly concentrated in amine-storing organelles and which are probably the substrates for the reaction (Richards and Da Prada 1977).

The uranaffin reaction is carried out in three steps: primary fixation in ice-cold 3% glutaraldehyde in 0.1 M sodium cacodylate buffer is followed by three 15-min rinses in 0.9% NaCl, then staining in saturated (4%) aqueous uranyl acetate pH 4 for up to 48 h with rotation at 0–4°C. Tissues are rinsed again before dehydrating and embedding.

Uranyl acetate is a well known stain and fixative in electron-microscopy. Nucleic acid (phosphonucleotide)-containing structures in a variety of tissues are intensely and preferentially stained with uranyl salts. In the uranaffin reaction, the acid pH of the uranyl acetate results in the formation of uncomplexed uranyl ions (UO_2^{2+}). These ions probably bind at the phosphate loci, according to studies of the infrared spectra of the deoxyribonucleic acid (DNA)-uranyl complex. At acid pH, one uranyl ion binds to each phosphate group in the DNA. The complexing of uranyl ions with 5'-phosphonucleotides in amine-storing organelles may occur through interactions similar to those with DNA.

3.2. PLATELETS AS MODELS

Proof that the uranaffin reaction demonstrates ATP- and ADP-rich organelles of platelets but not serotonin itself came from the following observation: isolated or in situ amine-storing organelles of rabbit platelets, depleted of their serotonin by pretreatment with reserpine, contain no cytochemically demonstrable amine but, nevertheless, have a strong affinity for uranyl ions. This results in the appearance of highly electron-dense organelles (Fig. 16). Since both the granule matrix and membrane are intensely stained by the uranaffin reaction, it was concluded that nonmetabolic ATP (and ADP) is present in high concentrations not only in the matrix but also in the membrane, possibly bound to the Mg^{2+}-dependent ATPase. Furthermore, electron-probe microanalysis of platelets stained with the uranaffin reaction (Richards and Da Prada 1980) has demonstrated extremely high contents of phosphorus and uranium in the amine-storing organelles. The formation of aggregates between serotonin and ATP, in the presence of bivalent cations, has been proposed to account for the osmotic stability of platelet amine-storing organelles.

The observation that human platelets contain only occasional chromaffin-positive organelles but several uranaffin-positive organelles (Fig. 17) confirms earlier findings which revealed that many more organelles become visible with the chromaffin reaction after loading human platelets with serotonin (Da Prada et al. 1981).

Circulating platelets originate by fragmentation of their stem cells, the megakaryocytes. In contrast to platelets, however, megakaryocytes do not contain typical highly osmiophilic amine-containing organelles but are, nevertheless, uranaffin-

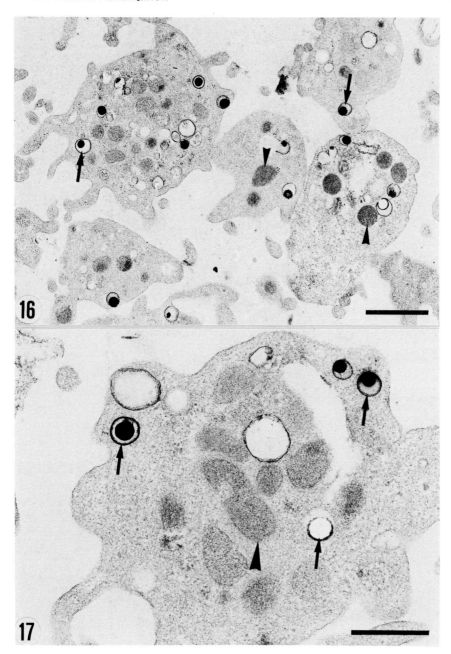

Fig. 16. Rabbit platelets. Uranaffin reaction; lead citrate stain. Both the matrix and membrane of numerous amine-storing organelles (→) have a high affinity for uranyl ions. α-granules (►) are only moderately stained. Bar = 1 μm.

Fig. 17. Human platelet. Uranaffin reaction; lead citrate stain. Several uranaffin-positive organelles (→) are present. Some of these have lost their cores during the sectioning for electron-microscopy. ► = α- granule. Bar = 0.5 μm.

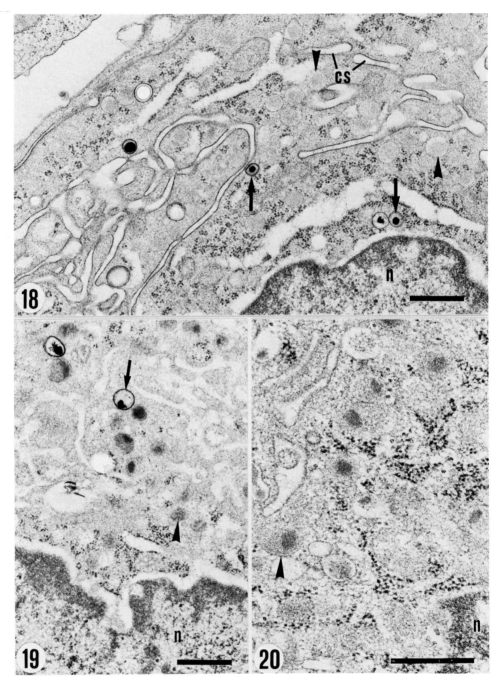

Fig. 18. Rabbit megakaryocyte. Uranaffin reaction; lead citrate stain. Cytochemically reactive organelles (→) are present throughout the cytoplasm. α-Granules (►) are uranaffin-negative. cs = canalicular system; n = nucleus. Bar = 0.5 μm.

Figs 19 and 20. Human megakaryocytes. Uranaffin reaction; lead citrate stain. Note the presence of uranaffin-positive organelles (→) in a megakaryocyte of a healthy individual (Fig. 19) but their absence in that of a patient with a storage pool disease (Hermansky-Pudlak syndrome) (Fig. 20). α-Granules (►) appear normal in both cases. n = nucleus. Bar = 0.5 μm.

positive (Fig. 18). This would suggest that specific subcellular organelles in these cells, probably containing nucleotide-metal aggregates, are the precursors of the amine-storing organelles of the platelets (Richards and Da Prada 1977). A similar uranaffin reaction is also observed in human megakaryocytes as well as in platelets of healthy individuals but not in those of patients with Hermansky-Pudlak syndrome, a storage pool disease (Figs 19 and 20) (Lorez et al. 1979). This condition of inherited bleeding disorders is characterized by a pronounced deficiency of platelet serotonin and ADP (Da Prada et al. 1981).

3.3. VISUALIZATION OF ATP IN SYNAPTIC VESICLES

The storage of serotonin in platelets appears to resemble amine storage in various other cells and tissues, e.g. adrenal medulla, sympathetic neurons and, possibly, central monoaminergic neurons in which ATP is also believed to be part of the storage complex.

Indeed, sympathetic nerve varicosities in the rat vas deferens and pineal (Figs 21 and 22) as well as sympathetic ganglion neurons and splenic nerve (Richards and Da Prada 1980) also display an uranaffin reaction. Moreover, Wilson et al. (1979) have observed a unique population of uranaffin-positive intrinsic nerve endings in the small intestine of guinea-pigs. As reported by these authors, we were also unable to detect a reaction in the so-called 'p' type (purinergic) nerve profiles which characteristically contain extremely large osmiophilic organelles. However, Iijima (1981) has recently described the occurrence of uranaffin-positive synaptic vesicles in both adrenergic and nonadrenergic (purine-rich?) nerves of the rat anococcygeus muscle.

The fact that such a reaction has not yet been observed in the brain, not even in supra-ependymal nerves storing serotonin, suggests that either another storage mechanism, possibly involving a binding protein (Tamir and Gershon 1981), operates or that the concentration of vesicular ATP in central monoaminergic neurons is too low to be detected.

4. CYTOCHEMISTRY OF EXOGENOUS AMINES

4.1. INTERSPECIFIC AMINE UPTAKE MECHANISMS

The high affinity amine uptake mechanisms for terminating the action of endogenous amines can be used to transport a number of 'false' transmitters, some of which are highly osmiophilic and some neurotoxic, into nerve terminals from the extracellular space. The phenylethylamines 5-hydroxydopamine and 6-hydroxydopamine and the hydroxylated serotonin analogues 5,6- and 5,7-hydroxytryptamine (Fig. 23) are the most well-known exogenous amines to have been used for selectively labeling or lesioning monoaminergic nerve terminals (Malmfors and Thoenen 1971; Thoenen and Tranzer 1971; Baumgarten et al. 1981).

4.2. VISUALIZATION OF NORADRENALINE AND SEROTONIN ANALOGUES

All the above mentioned amines augment the chromaffin reaction in the peripheral and central nervous systems (Figs 24–26). Since they do not penetrate the blood-brain barrier for monoamines, however, in studies of the CNS they have to be injected intracerebroventricularly or used for experiments in vitro.

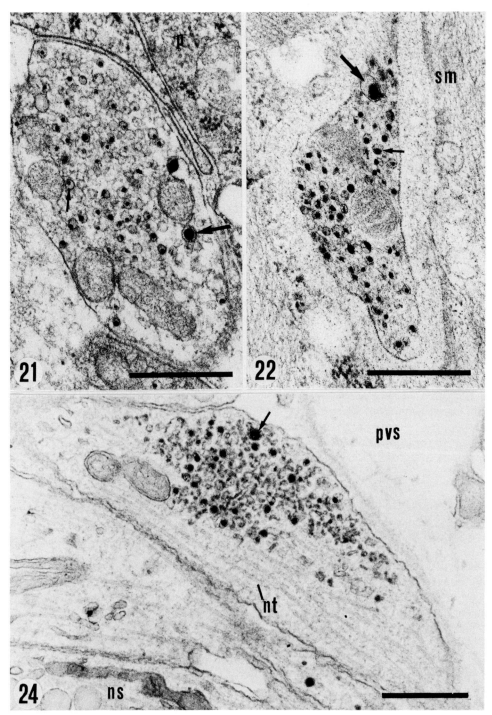

Figs 21 and 22. Rat pineal gland (Fig. 21) and vas deferens (Fig. 22). Uranaffin reaction; lead citrate stain. In both organs the small (→) and large (→) vesicles are cytochemically reactive, i.e. both the matrix and membrane of these organelles are highly electron-dense. p = pinealocyte; sm = smooth muscle cell. Bars = 0.5 μm.

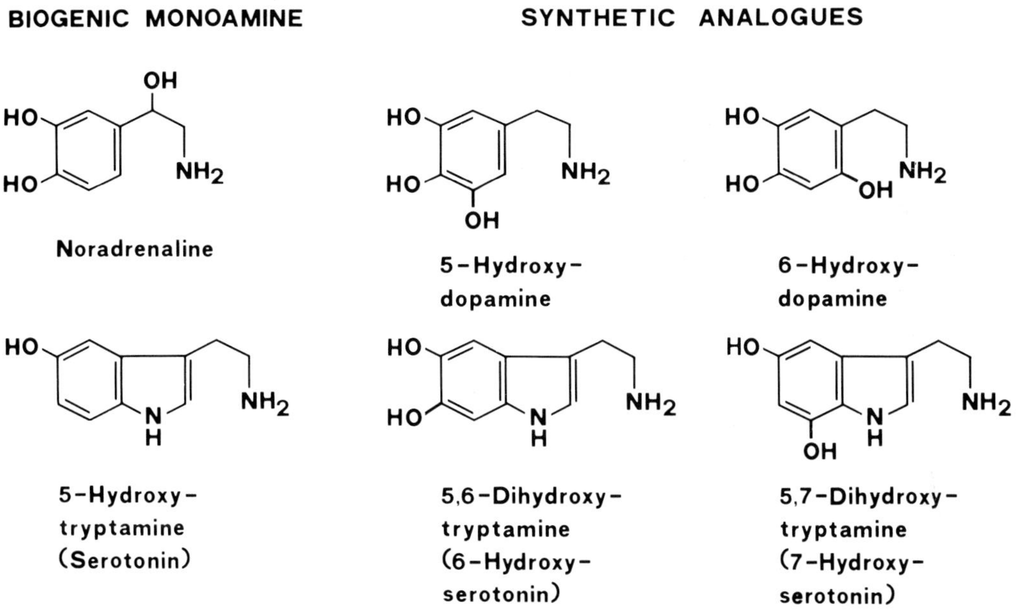

BIOGENIC MONOAMINE   **SYNTHETIC ANALOGUES**

Fig. 23. Endogenous monoamines and their synthetic analogues.

The selectivity of the various amines differs markedly. Thus, whereas 5-hydroxydopamine is rather nonselective for monoaminergic nerves, 6-hydroxydopamine is accumulated mainly by catecholaminergic nerves, 5,6-dihydroxytryptamine by serotoninergic nerves and 5,7-dihydroxytryptamine by serotoninergic and noradrenergic nerves. A simple guide to the drug source, dose, survival time, drug specificity and tissues investigated appears in the Appendix. The specificity of these compounds can be increased by the co-incubation or co-injection of natural amines with the exogenous amine. For example, in the presence of an excess of dopamine and noradrenaline, 5-hydroxydopamine will selectively label storage sites for serotonin since the physiological uptake and storage mechanisms for the catecholamines will be saturated. Likewise, the labelling by 5,7-dihydroxytryptamine of serotoninergic nerves can be studied if animals are pretreated with a noradrenaline uptake inhibitor, e.g. desmethylimipramine. From our studies and several more recent reports (Tennyson et al. 1974; Nojyo and Sano 1978; Arluison et al. 1978; Beaudet and Descarries 1978) on the use of exogenous amines for the ultrastructural identification of monoaminergic nerve terminals, it is striking that typical monoaminergic synapses are notably rare. The supra-ependymal nerves are no exception (Richards et al. 1981).

Whether nonsynaptic release of monoamines is an indication of their role as a neurohormone, which interacts with more distant target sites, has yet to be determined (Dismukes 1979).

Fig. 24. Rat pituitary (pars intermedia). 5-Hydroxydopamine (10 mg base/kg i.v., 1 h before killing). Chromaffin reaction by perfusion fixation; lead citrate stain. A varicose nerve profile contains numerous vesicles with augmented amine-specific dense cores (→). A profile of a neurosecretory cell (ns) contains large opaque granules. nt = neurotubule; pvs = perivascular space. Bar = 0.5 μm.

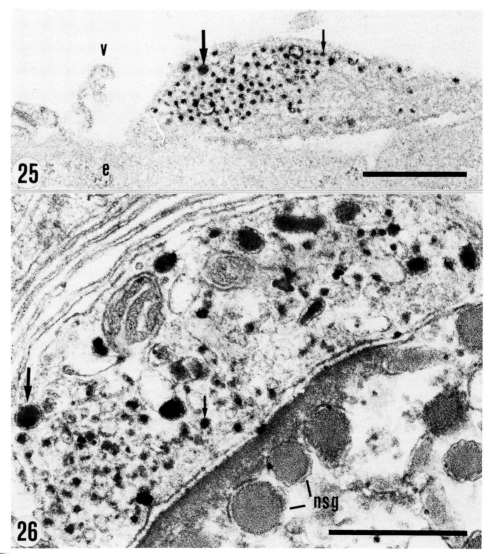

Fig. 25. Rat lateral ventricle. 5-Hydroxydopamine (200 μg in 20 μl i.c.v. by slow infusion). Chromaffin reaction (without osmium tetroxide) by perfusion fixation; lead citrate stain. A supra-ependymal varicose nerve profile contains large (→) and small (→) chromaffin-positive cores. e = ependyma; v = lateral ventricle. Bars = 0.5 μm.

Fig. 26. Rat paraventricular hypothalamus. 5-Hydroxydopamine (200 μg in 20 μl i.c.v. by slow infusion). Glutaraldehyde-osmium tetroxide fixation; lead citrate stain. Note the cytochemical reaction in large (→) and small (→) vesicles of a nerve terminal synapsing on a neurosecretory neuron. The latter contains characteristic neurosecretory granules (nsg). Bar = 0.5 μm.

4.3. NEUROTOXICITY OF ANALOGUES

Apart from 5-hydroxydopamine, all the exogenous amines mentioned above are neurotoxic once a certain intraneuronal concentration is reached. 5,6-Dihydroxytryptamine, for example, induces a degeneration of supra-ependymal nerves (Lorez

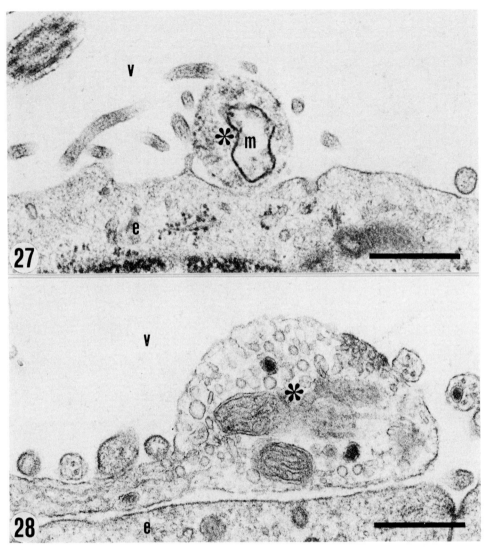

Figs 27 and 28. Rat fourth ventricle floor. 5,6-Dihydroxytryptamine (5 μg base, Fig. 27) and 6-hydroxy-dopamine (50 μg base, Fig. 28) were injected i.c.v. 2 days before killing. Glutaraldehyde-osmium tetroxide fixation; lead citrate and uranyl acetate stain. 5,6-Dihydroxytrypamine has a neurotoxic action leaving supra-ependymal serotoninergic nerves in various states of degeneration (*). However, 6-hydroxydopamine is without effect on these nerves (*). e = ependyma; m = mitochondrion; v = fourth ventricle floor. Bar = 0.5 μm.

and Richards 1976). Whereas as little as 5 μg of this amine (i.c.v.) is required to abolish the formaldehyde-induced fluorescence specific for indolamines and to lesion these nerves (Fig. 27), 50 μg 6-hydroxydopamine is ineffective (Fig. 28).

The precise mechanism of action of these neurotoxic amines is not known (Rotman 1977). The first stage in degeneration is thought to be brought about by nonenzymatic autoxidation to a 1,4-paraquinone. This either binds covalently to polymerize and denature essential cell proteins or it produces a local concentration of peroxides (e.g. in mitochondria) which are highly toxic (Baumgarten et al. 1981).

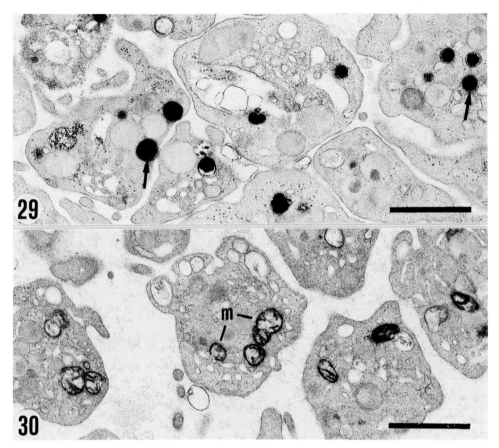

Figs 29 and 30. Platelets of controls (Fig. 29) and reserpinized rats (Fig. 30) incubated in 5,6-dihydroxytryptamine (10^{-3}M) in plasma for 1 h at 37°C. Glutaraldehyde-osmium tetroxide fixation; lead citrate stain. Reserpine (5 mg/kg i.p.) was injected 18 h before platelet incubation. Note the augmented highly electron-dense amine-storing organelles (→) in the control platelets and the lytic mitochondria (m) in the reserpinized platelets. Bars = 1 μm.

Tranzer (1971b) proposed that once a critical concentration of the amine was reached (perhaps upon saturation of storage sites), one of the first organelles to be affected might be the mitochondria since these organelles contain the major bulk of the enzymes involved in oxido-reduction reactions. In studies of rat platelets in vitro, we have observed that whereas control platelets accumulate 5,6-dihydroxytryptamine until typical amine-storage organelles become clearly visible, i.e. osmiophilic (Fig. 29), this did not occur with platelets of reserpinized or Fawn-Hooded rats (with a storage pool disease). Instead, their mitochondria appear highly electron-dense and degenerate (Fig. 30). The neurotoxicity of these compounds might be mediated by a similar mechanism.

Until more convincing methods become available, the augmentation of amine storage sites in the brain by the administration of exogenous amines, in combination with the chromaffin reaction, remains the method of choice for their visualization.

5. APPENDIX
(Materials and Methods for the ultrastructural visualization of biogenic amines)

5.1. CHROMAFFIN REACTION

1. Primary fixative:		ice-cold 1% glutaraldehyde + 0.4% paraformaldehyde in 0.1 M sodium chromate/potassium dichromate at pH 7.2
composition:	4 ml	25% glutaraldehyde solution (Merck-Schuchardt)
	0.4 g	paraformaldehyde powder (Merck) suspended in 10 ml distilled water and heated to 60°C before adding 1N NaOH dropwise until the milky solution clears
	50 ml	0.2 M sodium chromate/potassium dichromate at pH 7.2 (47.5 ml 0.2 M sodium chromate + 2.5 ml 0.2 M potassium dichromate)
	40 ml	distilled water
2. Chrome buffer stain:		ice-cold 0.2 M sodium chromate/potassium dichromate buffer at pH 6.0
composition:	22.5 ml	0.2 M sodium chromate
	75.0 ml	0.2 M potassium dichromate.
3. Chrome-buffered osmium tetroxide:		ice-cold 2% osmium tetroxide in 0.1 M sodium chromate/potassium dichromate pH 7.2
composition:	25 ml	4% osmium tetroxide in distilled water
	25 ml	0.2 M sodium chromate/potassium dichromate buffer at pH 7.2 (23.75 ml 0.2 M sodium chromate + 1.25 ml 0.2 M potassium dichromate).

5.2. URANAFFIN REACTION

1. Primary fixative:		ice-cold 3% glutaraldehyde in 0.1 M sodium cacodylate buffer at pH 7.2
composition:	12 ml	25% glutaraldehyde solution (Merck-Schuchardt)
	88 ml	0.1 M sodium cacodylate at pH 7.2 (pH adjusted with 0.1 N HCl).
2. Rinse:		ice-cold 0.9% NaCl.
3. Uranyl acetate stain:		4% aqueous uranyl acetate solution at pH 3.9; filter this saturated solution immediately before use.
4. Rinse:		repeat Step 2.

5.3. ADMINISTRATION OF EXOGENOUS AMINES

A simple guide to the dose and route of administration for a variety of tissues is given below. All compounds can be obtained from Regis Chemicals Co. Short survival times (30–60 min) should be chosen to label (augment) monoamine storage sites and long survival times (24–48 h) to lesion monoaminergic nerves.

Drug	Recommended dose	Post-injection survival time	Amine specificity	Tissues investigated
5-Hydroxy-dopamine·HCl	50 mg/kg i.p. 10 mg/kg i.v. 100 µg i.c.v.	2 h 30 min 1 h	noradrenaline serotonin	vas deferens, iris, heart, mesenteric artery, pituitary, pineal, median eminence supra-ependymal nerves, neo-striatum, peri-ventricular hypothalamus
6-Hydroxy-dopamine·HCl	50 mg/kg i.p. 10 mg/kg i.v. 200 µg i.c.v.	2 h 30 min 1 h	noradrenaline dopamine	pineal, median eminence, supra-ependymal nerves, neostriatum
5,6-Dihydroxy-tryptamine·creatinine sulfate monohydrate	10 mg/kg i.v. 200 µg i.c.v.	30 min 1 h	serotonin	pineal, median eminence, supra-ependymal nerves, neostriatum, periventricular hypothalamus
5,7-Dihydroxy-tryptamine·creatinine sulfate	10 mg/kg i.v. 200 µg i.c.v.	30 min 1 h	serotonin noradrenaline	

6. REFERENCES

Arluison M, Agid Y, Javoy F (1978): Dopaminergic nerve endings in the neostriatum of the rat. 1. Identification by intracerebral injections of 5-hydroxydopamine. *Neuroscience, 3,* 657–673.

Baumgarten HG, Jenner S, Klemm HP (1981): Serotonin neurotoxins: Recent advances in the mode of administration and molecular mechanism of action. *J. Physiol. (Paris), 77,* 309–314.

Beaudet A, Descarries L (1978): The monoamine innervation of rat cerebral cortex: Synaptic and nonsynaptic relationships. *Neuroscience, 3,* 851–860.

Bloom FE (1970): The fine structural localization of biogenic monoamines in nervous tissue. *Int. Rev. Neurobiol., 13,* 27–66.

Bloom FE (1973): Ultrastructural identification of catecholamine-containing central synaptic terminals. *J. Histochem. Cytochem., 21,* 333–348.

Böck P, Gorgas K (1976): Alkaline lead citrate: A selective stain for glutaraldehyde precipitates of indolamines and primary catecholamines in electron-microscopy. *Histochemistry, 47,* 59–62.

Da Prada M, Richards JG, Kettler R (1981): Amine storage organelles in platelets. In: Gordon JL (Ed), *Platelets in Biology and Pathology 2,* pp. 107–145. Elsevier/North-Holland, Amsterdam.

De Robertis E, Pellegrino de Iraldi A (1961): Plurivesicular secretory processes and nerve endings in the pineal gland. *J. Biophys. Biochem. Cytol., 10,* 361–372.

Dismukes RK (1979): New concepts of molecular communication among neurons. *Behav. Brain Sci., 2,* 409–448.

Fillenz M, Pollard RM (1976): Quantitative differences between sympathetic nerve terminals. *Brain Res., 109,* 443–454.

Fried G, Lagercrantz H, Hökfelt T (1978): Improved isolation of small noradrenergic vesicles from rat seminal ducts following castration. A density gradient centrifugation and morphological study. *Neuroscience, 3,* 1271–1291.

Hayat MA (1981): *Fixation for Electron-microscopy.* Academic Press, New York.

Hökfelt T (1968): In vitro studies on central and peripheral monoamine neurons at the ultrastructural level. *Z. Zellforsch. Mikrosk. Anat., 91,* 1–74.

Hökfelt T (1971): Ultrastructural localization of intraneuronal monoamines. Some aspects on methodology. *Prog. Brain Res., 34,* 213–222.

Hökfelt T (1973): Neuronal catecholamine storage vesicles. In: Usdin E, Snyder SH (Eds), *Frontiers in Catecholamine Research,* pp. 439–446. Pergamon Press, New York.

Hökfelt T, Jonsson G (1968): Studies on reaction and binding of monoamines after fixation and processing for electron-microscopy with special reference to fixation with potassium permanganate. *Histochemie, 16,* 45–67.

Hopwood D (1971): The histochemistry and electron-histochemistry of chromaffin tissue. *Prog. Histochem. Cytochem., 3,* 1–66.

Iijima T (1981): Occurrence of uranaffin-positive synaptic vesicles in both adrenergic and nonadrenergic nerves of the rat anococcygeus muscle. *Cell Tissue Res., 220,* 427–433.

Iversen LL (1980): The chemistry of the brain. *Sci. Am., 241,* 134–149.

Jaim-Etcheverry G, Zieher LM (1974): Localizing serotonin in central and peripheral nerves. In: Schmitt FO, Warden G (Eds), *The Neurosciences Third Study Program,* pp. 917–924. The MTP Press, Cambridge MA.

Kanerva L, Hervonen A, Rechardt L (1977a): Permanganate fixation demonstrates the monoamine-containing granular vesicles in the SIF cells but not in the adrenal medulla or mast cells. *Histochemistry, 52,* 61–72.

Kanerva L, Tissari AH, Suurhasko BVA, Hervonen A (1977b): Ultrastructural characterization of synaptosomes from neonatal and adult rats with special reference to monoamines. *J. Comp. Neurol., 174,* 631–658.

Kimoto Y, Tohyama M, Satoh K, Sakumoto T, Takahashi Y, Shimizu N (1981): Fine structure of rat cerebellar noradrenaline terminals as visualized by potassium permanganate in situ perfusion fixation method. *Neuroscience, 6,* 47–58.

Koda LY, Bloom FE (1977): A light- and electron-microscopic study of noradrenergic terminals in the rat dentate gyrus. *Brain Res., 120,* 327–335.

Lagercrantz H (1976): On the composition and function of large dense-cored vesicles in sympathetic nerves. *Neuroscience, 1,* 81–92.

Lascar G (1981): Ultracytochemical identification of catecholamine-containing vesicles in the ligated sciatic nerve of the rat. Comparison with sympathetic nerve terminals. *Cell Tissue Res., 209,* 433–454.

Lever JD, Esterhuizen AC (1961): Fine structure of arteriolar nerves in the guinea pig pancreas. *Nature (London), 192,* 566–567.

Lorez HP, Richards JG (1976): Effects of intracerebroventricular injection of 5,6-dihydroxytryptamine and 6-hydroxydopamine on supra-ependymal nerves. *Brain Res., 116,* 165–171.

Lorez HP, Richards JG (1982): Supra-ependymal 5-HT nerve fibres in mammalian brain: Morphological, pharmacological and functional studies. *Brain Res. Bull., 9,* 727–741.

Lorez HP, Richards JG, Da Prada M, Picotti GB, Pareti FI, Capitanio A, Mannucci PM (1979): Storage pool disease: Comparative fluorescence microscopical, cytochemical and biochemical studies on amine-storage organelles of human blood platelets. *Brit. J. Haematol., 43,* 297–305.

Luft JH (1956): Permanganate - A new fixative for electron-microscopy. *J. Biophys. Biochem. Cytol., 2,* 799–801.

Malmfors T, Thoenen H (1971): *6-Hydroxydopamine and Catecholamine Neurons.* North-Holland Publ. Co., Amsterdam.

McClung RE, Wood JG (1982): Analytical electron-microscopic evaluation of the effects of paraformaldehyde pretreatment on the reaction of glutaraldehyde with biogenic amines. *J. Histochem. Cytochem., 30,* 481–486.

Nilsson O (1964): The relationship between nerves and smooth muscle cells in the rat iris. I. The dilator muscle. *Z. Zellforsch. Mikrosk. Anat., 64,* 166–171.

Nojyo Y, Sano Y (1978): Ultrastructure of the serotoninergic nerve terminals in the suprachiasmatic and interpeduncular nuclei of rat brains. *Brain Res., 149,* 482–488.

Pelletier G, Steinbusch HWM, Verhofstad AAJ (1981): Immunoreactive substance P and serotonin present in the same dense-core vesicles. *Nature (London), 293,* 71–72.

Richards JG (1977): Autoradiographic evidence for the selective accumulation of [3H]5-HT by supra-ependymal nerve terminals. *Brain Res., 134,* 151–157.

Richards JG (1978): Cytochemistry and autoradiography in the search for transmitter-specific neuronal pathways. In: Coupland RE, Forssmann WG (Eds), *Peripheral Neuroendocrine Interaction,* pp. 1–14. Springer, Berlin.

Richards JG (1981): Ultrastructural histochemistry of nervous tissue. In: Heym Ch, Forssmann WG (Eds), *Techniques in Neuroanatomical Research*, pp. 277–292. Springer, Berlin.

Richards JG, Da Prada M (1977): Uranaffin reaction: A new cytochemical technique for the localization of adenine nucleotides in organelles storing biogenic amines. *J. Histochem. Cytochem., 25*, 1322–1336.

Richards JG, Da Prada M (1980): Cytochemical investigations on subcellular organelles storing biogenic amines in peripheral adrenergic neurones. In: Eränkö O, Sonila S, Paivaruta H (Eds), *Histochemistry and Cell Biology of Autonomic Neurons, SIF Cells and Paraneurons: Adv. Biochem. Psychopharmacol. Vol. 25*, pp. 269–278. Raven Press, New York.

Richards JG, Guggenheim R (1982): Serotoninergic axons in the brain: A bird's-eye view. *Trends In Neurosci., 5*, 4–5.

Richards JG, Tranzer JP (1974): Ultrastructural evidence for the localization of an indolalkylamine in supra-ependymal nerves from combined cytochemistry and pharmacology. *Experientia, 30*, 287–289.

Richards JG, Tranzer JP (1975): Localization of amine storage sites in the adrenergic cell body. A study of the superior cervical ganglion of the rat by fine structural cytochemistry. *J. Ultras. Res., 53*, 204–216.

Richards JG, Da Prada M, Würsch J, Lorez HP, Pieri L (1979): Mapping monoaminergic neurons with [^{3}H]reserpine by autoradiography. *Neuroscience, 4*, 937–950.

Richards JG, Lorez HP, Colombo VE, Guggenheim R, Wu JY (1981): Demonstration of supra-ependymal 5-HT nerve fibres in human brain and their immunohistochemical identification in rat brain. *J. Physiol. (Paris), 77*, 219–224.

Richardson KC (1962): The fine structure of autonomic nerve endings in smooth muscle of the rat vas deferens. *Am. J. Anat., 96*, 427–442.

Richardson KC (1964): The fine structure of the albino rabbit iris with special reference to the identification of adrenergic and cholinergic nerves and nerve endings in its intrinsic muscles. *Am. J. Anat., 114*, 173–206.

Richardson KC (1966): Electron-microscopic identification of autonomic nerve endings. *Nature (London), 210*, 756.

Rotman A (1977): The mechanism of action of neurocytotoxic compounds. *Life Sci., 21*, 891–900.

Tamir H, Gerschon MD (1981): Intracellular proteins that bind serotonin in neurons, paraneurons and platelets, *J. Physiol. (Paris), 77*, 283–286.

Tennyson VM, Heikkila R, Mytilineon C, Coté L, Cohen G (1974): 5-Hydroxydopamine 'tagged' neuronal boutons in rabbit neostriatum: Interrelationship between vesicles and axonal membrane. *Brain Res., 82*, 341–348.

Thoenen H, Tranzer JP (1971): Functional importance of subcellular distribution of false adrenergic transmitters. *Prog. Brain Res., 34*, 223–236.

Todd ME, Tokito MK (1981): Improved ultrastructural detail in tissues fixed with potassium and permanganate. *Stain Technol., 56*, 335–342.

Tranzer JP (1971a): Fixation et apport de contraste par les ions UO$_2^{++}$ et Pb^{++} en l'absence de O$_s$O$_4$. *Experientia, 27*, 24.

Tranzer JP (1971b): Discussion of the mechanism of action of 6-hydroxydopamine at a fine structural level. In: Malmfors T, Thoenen H (Eds), *6-Hydroxydopamine and Catecholamine Neurons*, pp. 257–264. North-Holland Publ. Co., Amsterdam.

Tranzer JP (1973): New aspects of the localization of catecholamines in adrenergic neurons. In: Snyder S, Usdin E (Eds), *Frontiers in Catecholamine Research*, pp. 453–458. Pergamon Press, London.

Tranzer JP, Richards JG (1976): Ultrastructural cytochemistry of biogenic amines in nervous tissue: Methodologic improvements. *J. Histochem. Cytochem., 24*, 1178–1193.

Tranzer JP, Snipes RL (1968): Fine structural localization of noradrenaline in sympathetic nerve terminals: A critical study of the influence of fixation. In: Bocciarelli DS (Ed), *Proceedings, Fourth European Regional Conference on Electron Microscopy, Rome*, pp. 519–520. Tipografia Poliglotta Vaticana, Rome.

Wilson AJ, Furness JP, Costa M (1979): A unique population of uranaffin-positive intrinsic nerve endings in the small intestine. *Neurosci. Lett., 14*, 303–308.

Winkler H (1976): The composition of adrenal chromaffin granules: An assessment of controversial results. *Neuroscience, 1*, 65–80.

Wolfe DE, Axelrod J, Potter ILT, Richardson KC (1962): Localization of tritiated norepinephrine in sympathetic axons by electron-microscope autoradiography. *Science, 138*, 440–442.

Wood JG (1966): Electron-microscopic localization of amines in central nervous tissue. *Nature (London), 209*, 1131–1133.

Wood JG, Barnett RS (1964): Histochemical demonstration of norepinephrine at a fine structural level. *J. Histochem. Cytochem., 12*, 197–209.

CHAPTER IV

Methods for immunocytochemistry of neurohormonal peptides*

LARS-INGE LARSSON

1. INTRODUCTION

This review deals with the application of immunocytochemical techniques to the study of neuronal and hormonal peptides at the light- and electron-microscopical level. Particular attention is paid to interpretation and evaluation of immunocytochemical results. Theoretical discussions of different methods for tissue preparation and staining are followed by a practical appendix containing details for some of the recommended methods. Since the review is limited in scope, some alternative methods that either are rarely used or are of little use for the study of secretory peptides have been omitted. A full discussion of these latter methods can be found in several recent texts (Larsson 1981a; Sternberger 1979). Due to their potential great use, particular emphasis has instead been placed on cytochemical model systems, monoclonal antibody methods and combination techniques. For further aspects of the preparation of antibodies and the specificity of antibodies used for immunocytochemistry, the reader is referred to Chapter V by Sofroniew et al.

2. ANTISERA AND ANTIBODIES

2.1. THE ANTIBODY MOLECULE

Most antibodies used in immunocytochemistry belong to the IgG class. IgG molecules are large ($4 \times 5 \times 8$ nm, $M_w = 160\,000$ d) glycoproteins, consisting of two heavy and two light chains, joined by disulfide bridges (Nisonoff et al. 1975). They contain two identical Fab fragments and one Fc fragment. Each of the Fab fragments contains a region capable of binding antigen. Thus, each complete IgG molecule possesses two (identical) antigen-combining sites. The crystalline fragment (Fc) is capable of binding to a larger number of different molecules, including complement. Protein A – a staphylococcal protein – reacts specifically with the Fc fragment of a large number (but not all!) of mammalian immunoglobulins. Therefore, protein A, labelled with a variety of markers (fluorescence, enzymes, colloidal gold, ferritin) has been frequently employed for detecting tissue-bound antibody (Batten et al. 1978; Notani et al. 1979; Roth et al. 1978a). Additionally, protein A – coupled to Sepharose (Pharmacia) – has

*Original work by the author reported herein was supported by the Danish Medical Research Council and Cancer Society.

Handbook of Chemical Neuroanatomy. Vol. 1: Methods in Chemical Neuroanatomy.
A. Björklund and T. Hökfelt, editors.
© Elsevier Science Publishers B.V., 1983.

been used for purifying antibodies and it has also been employed as a 'link' antibody in the peroxidase-antiperoxidase (PAP) technique of Sternberger (1979) (Notani et al. 1979).

Digestion of IgG with pepsin results in the liberation of the Fc fragment and of an F(ab')$_2$ fragment, consisting of the two joined Fab fragments. Mild reduction liberates two F(ab') fragments, each containing one antigen-combining site. Two F(ab') fragments, even if differing in specificity, can subsequently be made to rejoin upon oxidation – a feature exploited when making so-called hybrid antibodies (e.g. anti-cholecystokinin-anti-ferritin hybrids (reviewed in Sternberger 1979).

2.2. SOURCE

Antibodies are either obtained as sera from immunized animals (rabbits, goats, guinea pigs etc.) or as ascites fluid or culture fluid from hybridoma cells (see Chapter V). The former group of antibodies are generally referred to as 'polyclonal' (i.e. produced by several distinct clones of plasma cells), whereas the latter group is referred to as 'monoclonal' (Cuello et al. 1980; Köhler and Milstein 1975). These designations will, for practical purposes, be retained throughout our discussion, although it should be pointed out that the efficiency of the cloning procedure is what determines the monoclonal nature of hybridoma antibodies. A third term, 'monospecific', is operational and implies that under certain conditions the antiserum only reacts with one type of molecule. Hence, a polyclonal antiserum may sometimes, for practical purposes, be regarded as 'monospecific', whereas a monoclonal antibody may react with multiple structurally similar antigens and be 'polyspecific'.

Polyclonal antibodies are produced by immunizing animals with antigens (immunogens) emulsified in an adjuvant. Peptide antigens must often (but not invariably) be conjugated to a carrier protein, to evoke significant immune responses (Sofroniew et al. 1978, and Chapter V). Such immunogens are then used for immunization of suitable animals (rabbits, guinea pigs, goats for polyclonal antibodies; mice for later production of monoclonal antibodies). The immunogen, emulsified in a suitable adjuvant (to increase the immune response), is injected subcutaneously or intracutaneously. Also the intramuscular or intrasplenic routes have been employed (Shelley et al. 1973; Sofroniew et al. 1978; Thorell and Larsson 1978). Although different workers seem to prefer different routes of administration, clearcut superiority of one or the other route has yet to be convincingly demonstrated. We prefer injecting the immunogen subcutaneously on 2—4 places on the back of the animals. There is no reason to inject the animals in painful places, like the footpads, since this has never been shown to increase the success rate.

The dose of immunogen varies greatly between different laboratories. Low-dose immunization (range: 50—150 μg of peptide antigen) has, however, often given as good or better antisera as high-dose immunizations. Immunized animals frequently benefit from repeated immunizations (e.g. given at monthly or bimonthly intervals). Useful antibody titers are often not obtained until after the third to fifth immunization, sometimes later.

The main problem with immunizing is the need for adequate animal housing facilities. Apart from this, immunization takes no great toll on either time or skill. Immunocytochemists should be encouraged to try producing their own antisera in order to have complete control over the purity and history of their reagents. Reasons for this will be apparent from the following considerations.

Polyclonal antibodies

Many immunocytochemists benefit considerably from the generosity of their radioimmunoassayist colleagues, who very often donate appreciable quantities of antisera (sometimes with the returned benefit of co-authorship on immunocytochemical publications). Additionally, some workers buy their antisera from commercial radioimmunoassay firms. The possible drawback with this is that the immunocytochemist does not know what has happened with the antiserum prior to delivery. The antisera are often received along with a note stating that 'this antiserum reacts only with the C-terminal portion of peptide X and not at all with peptides Y and Z'. This statement may be perfectly true in a radioimmunoassay system, but when the antiserum is tested at the immunocytochemical level it may react not only with peptide X, but also with Y and Z. The explanation to such discrepancies between radioimmunoassay (RIA) and immunocytochemical test results is straightforward. Thus, in RIA a radiolabelled tracer of high purity (X*) is used. This tracer will be bound by anti-X antibodies, but not by anti-Y or anti-Z antibodies. Addition of increasing doses of unlabelled X will decrease the per cent binding of labelled X* to the antibodies. Addition of even huge quantities of Y or Z will in no way affect the binding of X* to the anti-X antibodies. Hence, in the radioimmunoassay system, the presence of possible anti-Y or anti-Z antibodies will not be detected and will not have any bearing on the assay results. However, in conventional immunocytochemistry (with the exception of labelled antigen detection techniques, to be discussed below) all antibodies that react with tissue will be detected. Hence, conventional immunocytochemistry, unlike RIA and labelled antigen detection techniques, does not discriminate between wanted and unwanted antibody populations. Moreover, since the labelling procedure (usually radioiodination with ^{125}I), necessary for preparing the tracer (X*) for RIA, may result in sufficient structural changes in the molecule to render it undetectable to certain antibodies directed towards the modified (labelled) portion, the radioimmunoassayist may not detect antibodies directed against that portion, since these will be unable to interact with the tracer. Conversely, the fixation and tissue treatment necessary for immunocytochemistry may modify (denature) the antigen in other ways, making other portions undetectable by antibodies. Thus, in extreme cases, the anti-X serum, so excellent for RIA measurements of X, may immunocytochemically detect only Y and Z, whereas tissue-bound X has been rendered undetectable by the fixation!

Thus, radioimmunoassays and immunocytochemistry differ sufficiently to make any specificity comparisons between the two unjustified. These lines, I hope, should be sufficient to discourage any immunocytochemist from citing RIA data as the sole proofs of immunocytochemical specificity. Nevertheless, the 1981 Neuroscience literature is littered with such mistakes. It is hoped that this situation will improve in the future.

Since, as we saw above, the purity of the tracer largely determines the specificity of RIA systems, many RIA workers are content by immunizing their animals with very impure (and, hence, cheap) peptide preparations. This does in no way matter in RIA, as long as the tracer is prepared from highly purified peptide and since cross-reacting antibodies (i.e. antibodies reading a non-unique portion of the intended antigen, vide infra) may as well be elicited from pure antigens. Since, however, conventional immunocytochemistry detects all antibodies that react with tissue-bound antigens, such antisera are disastrous to the immunocytochemist! It is therefore necessary to know the purity of the immunogen and also the life history of the immunized animal (e.g. previous immunizations with other antigens).

Monoclonal antibodies

A single antibody-producing cell fabricates only one species of antibody. Hence, monoclonal antibodies, originating from the offspring of a single antibody-producing cell hybrid, are structurally identical and possess the same specificity. The first step in their production consists of the immunization of mice or rats. The animals are screened for antibody production somewhat later. Subsequently, their spleens are removed and spleen cells are fused (hybridized) with mouse myeloma cells, e.g. with polyethylene glycol (Cuello et al. 1980; Köhler and Milstein 1975; Chapter V). Subsequently, the cell suspension is cultured. Spleen cells, themselves, cannot grow in culture and unfused spleen cells therefore die. The myeloma cells grow excellently in culture but belong to a mutant strain deficient in a specific enzyme (hypoxanthine guanidine phosphoribosyl transferase; HGPRT), which is present in the spleen cells. Thus, when grown on specific substrates (aminopterin, hypoxanthine; HAT medium), unfused myeloma cells also die and, consequently, only spleen cell-myeloma cell hybrids, containing HGPRT, survive. These hybrids can be cloned (using different methods; dilution techniques, semisolid media etc.) so that one single cell is the progenitor of a clone of daughter cells. Often 'recloning' is performed to substantiate the vital claim that only one single cell hybrid is the parent (Cuello et al. 1980; Chapter V). Culture fluid from each clone is subsequently tested until (hopefully) one or more clones producing the desired antibodies (usually of IgG or IgM class) is found. After its identification, the clone can be further propagated in culture or may be injected into the peritoneal cavity of a mouse, where the hybridoma cells will grow as an ascites tumor and produce ascites fluid rich in monoclonal antibodies. Culture fluid or ascites fluid may be used for immunocytochemical staining after purification (e.g. ammonium sulphide fractionation) and dilution (Cuello et al. 1980; Chapter V).

Monoclonal antibodies are in many ways ideal, pure reagents for immunocytochemistry, since they consist of only one species of antibody. It must be remembered, however, that use of a monoclonal antibody in no way guarantees immunocytochemical specificity. Thus, as will be discussed in more detail below, antibodies only recognize a limited portion of their antigen and may therefore cross-react with structurally related antigens. Hence, while eliminating the risk with contaminating antibodies, seen with the polyclonal antisera, it is important to note that monoclonal antibodies still are associated with the risk of immunological cross-reactivity (i.e. they are not monospecific by definition).

Monoclonal antibodies are superior when impure or contaminated preparations of proteins or peptides have to be used as immunogens. They will probably serve as valuable tools for the characterization, localization and purification of numerous molecules, which otherwise could not be obtained in pure form. A further advantage is that monoclonal antibodies can be mass-produced and used as universal standardization reagents.

With antigens already available in pure or synthetic form, monoclonals may, at first sight, not offer so great an advantage. Thus, strictly speaking, tracers used in RIA techniques and in labelled antigen detection techniques already select desired specific antibody populations and discriminate between wanted and unwanted antibodies (Larsson 1979; Larsson and Schwartz 1977). Moreover, the monoclonal antibodies we hitherto have worked with have been of low binding energy (avidity), resulting in that relatively high concentrations of antibodies have been necessary to use. This results in quite a heavy unspecific absorption of proteins onto tissue sections and less clear definition of immunoreactive structures than seen with many rabbit or guinea pig antibodies. Nevertheless, I feel that these drawbacks are childhood problems. What may be hoped from the future is that the low avidity of monoclonals will turn out not to be so much an intrinsic property of mouse immunoglobulins as a reflection of the unsuitability of current methods for screening for them. Such methods are often very laborious and when perhaps 200 different clones have to be screened, many workers have been content with finding one producing the desired antibody. What is needed is a method that not only identifies antibodies as such, but also provides information of their titer, avidity and region-specificity. Such a system has been developed and consists of paper models containing immobilized antigens (Larsson 1981b). These models can be stained immunocytochemically, using, in one run, harvest fluid from over 200 clones. Positive clones can then be further defined in this system with respect to minimum amount of detectable antigen, titer, cross-reactivity and region-specificity.

2.3. REGION-SPECIFICITY OF THE ANTIBODIES

The size of an antigen-combining site on an antibody is limited. Thus, an antibody will only bind to a limited portion of most antigens. Theoretical calculations and direct experiments show that, with proteins and peptides, antigenic sites vary between 3 and 8 amino acids in size. Amino acid residues outside the antigenic site are not bound by the antibody, but may affect its reactivity through steric or ionic interactions. An antigenic site may be either continuous, consisting of a linear amino acid sequence, or may be discontinuous, consisting of two or more parts of a sequence that are brought together for steric reasons (Atassi and Smith 1978).

Since the size of the antigenic site is limited, its relative uniqueness will determine the specificity of the antigen-antibody interaction. However, even if we know exactly to what amino acid sequence a given antibody binds, it is impossible to determine whether this sequence is unique among all known and unknown proteins and peptides. Therefore, strictly speaking it is futile to discuss anti-gastrin, anti-VIP etc. antibodies, when, in fact, the antibodies only recognize a part of the sequences of these peptides. With only one antiserum (monoclonal or polyclonal) we can never identify accurately the source of immune-staining in tissue!

The situation is much improved, however, if we have access to multiple antibodies, detecting multiple, well-characterized parts of an amino acid sequence. Thus, with the 20 natural amino acids, Nature can build a tripeptide unit in 8000 (20^3) ways, a tetrapeptide unit in 160000 (20^4) ways a.s.o. Thus the larger a portion of a sequence that can be recognized specifically, the smaller the chances are that the same results will be obtained with other antigens. This simple reasoning lies behind the introduction of region-specific immunocytochemistry (Larsson and Rehfeld 1977b).

With increasing numbers of region-specific antibodies we may ultimately attain the final goal; the identification of a single species of molecule. Region-specific antibodies may be obtained from several sources: (a) fortuitously: immunization of an animal frequently results in different antibody populations recognizing different parts of the antigen. These can be detected by cytochemical models incorporating different fragments of the antigen, and can be purified by affinity chromatography or directly exploited in the labelled antigen detection techniques; (b) fragment immunizations: synthetic fragments of many neurohormonal peptides are available. These can be conjugated to a carrier protein and directly used for immunization; (c) conjugation strategy: it is frequently found that the method of hapten (peptide) conjugation to a carrier protein may affect the specificities of the antibodies obtained. Thus, peptides conjugated to the carrier via their α-amino groups (e.g. via glutaraldehyde) frequently elicit antibodies to their non-attached (C-terminal) end and the same applies to C-terminally conjugated peptides (e.g. with carbodiimides), which often elicits production of antibodies of N-terminal specificity. This is, however, not invariably true and fragment immunizations are generally preferable.

Neurohormonal peptides are synthesized from larger precursors, which undergo a sequence of proteolytic cleavages and sometimes also derivatizations (amidations, acetylations, sulfations). Usually, the peptides that we have at hand are the most abundant, biologically active, end products. Antibodies raised against these may require that they are derivatized or that they possess a free N- or C-terminus. Hence, such antibodies may not always react with precursor forms. In the case of the pro-piomelanocorticotropin neurons of the arcuate nucleus of the hypothalamus, we have shown that, in normal rats, these cell bodies are filled with precursor-like peptides, but contain very little of end-products, like αMSH (Larsson 1980). End products are, instead, accumulated in the nerve terminals. It is possible that this also applies to many other neurons and that the, in many cases bemoaned, inability to detect cell bodies in normal brains may be due to the use of antibodies specific for cleaved and/or derivatized end products. It might therefore be worthwhile to preliminary scan multiple antisera for their reactivity to precursors before relying upon colchicin injections for defining sites of synthesis of peptides.

3. TESTING ANTISERA FOR SPECIFICITY AND SENSITIVITY

From what has been discussed above, it is evident that, whatever the source of a poly- or monoclonal antiserum, the immunocytochemist must test the antiserum under the conditions of his method. This point cannot be stressed enough. Thus, test results from other systems, particularly radioimmunoassays, are applicable only to the conditions of that test and not to immunocytochemistry. Also pH, buffer strength, temperature, dilution and time of incubation may have profound effects on specificity. Recently, using monoclonal antibodies to chicken erythrocytes, Mosmann et al. (1980) produced compelling evidence that these parameters also profoundly affect the specificity of single species of antibody molecules, presumably by affecting charge and conformation of potentially cross-reacting antigens.

Immunocytochemical model systems therefore have gained increased importance. An ideal model system should fulfill the following criteria:
1. It should allow primary and convenient screening of sera to reveal whether desired antibodies are present.
2. It should allow immunocytochemical staining to be performed in exactly the same way as in tissue sections.
3. It should permit the study of the influences of different fixatives on immunoreactivity.
4. It should allow parallel staining of a large number of antigens to check for cross-reacting and contaminating antibodies.
5. It should preferably be as sensitive as possible in order to save precious or rare antigens.
6. It should be quantitative in order to define the minimum detectable amounts of antigens using different antisera, fixations and staining procedures.

7. It should allow testing of multiple peptide fragments in order to assess the region-specificity and, possibly, heterogeneity of the antiserum.

Many model systems fulfill one or more of these criteria. These include peptides coupled to Sepharose (agarose) beads or to polyacrylamide or diffused into protein gels (Avrameas and Ternynck 1969; Beutner 1971; Brandtzaeg 1972; Capel 1974; Knapp and Ploem 1974; Pachmann and Leibold 1976; Streefkerk 1975). The simplest and most efficient system seems, however, to be the recently developed paper model system (Larsson 1981b).

In this system, peptides or proteins are applied as 2 μl droplets onto strips of suitable filter paper, dried, immobilized and, subsequently, immunocytochemically stained. In the case of small peptides, which chromatograph on paper, it is necessary to immobilize them by a suitable vapour fixation (using formaldehyde, glutaraldehyde, diethylpyro-carbonate, parabenzoquinone or osmic acid vapours) (Larsson 1981b). Larger polypeptides and proteins, which do not chromatograph on paper in water (as can be easily tested), do not need to be vapour-fixed, but may be stained unfixed or after aqueous fixation in any desired formula.

We have by now 2 years of experience with this method and employ it increasingly to many problems. It has proven very useful for screening for both monoclonal and polyclonal antibodies, for assessing region-specificity and cross-reactivity of antibodies and has also been exploited for methodological studies testing the effects of different fixatives, buffers and pH conditions. The system has also demonstrated that different antisera have very different sensitivities, as defined as minimum detectable amount of antigen (this may vary 100-1000-fold) (Larsson 1981b). Tests with various radiolabelled small peptides have shown that the vapour-fixation with formaldehyde is highly efficient in immobilizing them and that less than 5% of the peptide comes off in subsequent washings.

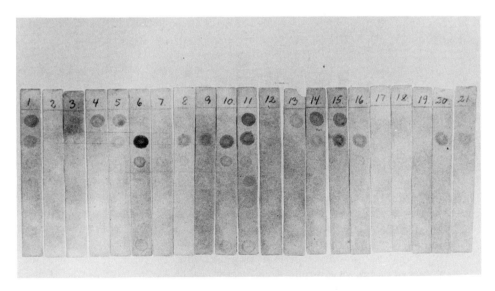

Fig. 1. Cytochemical paper models. Each paper strip (numbered 1—21) has been loaded with 2 μl droplets of different peptide fragments and then stained immunocytochemically using the PAP method and development in diaminobenzidine. The 21 antisera tested are shown to have different specificities for the different peptide fragments.

The system is used with the PAP, peroxidase-labelled antibody or radioimmunocyto-chemical methods (Fig. 1). Immunofluorescence techniques are less suitable due to background fluorescence of the filter papers. Details of the method are found in the Appendix.

4. FIXATION AND TISSUE PRETREATMENT

Most neurohormonal peptides are soluble in water and must therefore be fixed before being amenable to immunocytochemical studies. The fixatives commonly used for these purposes introduce intra- and intermolecular cross-links. They may therefore modify antigenicity as well as create dense cytoplasmic networks of cross-linked proteins, making antibody permeability difficult. Thus, the immunocytochemist is struggling with four, mutually contradictory, requirements:
1. Retention of the antigen.
2. Preservation of tissue structure.
3. Preservation of antigenicity.
4. Preservation of antigen accessibility (antibody permeability).
The obvious difficulties with satisfying all four requirements are well known from other provinces of histochemistry, particularly enzyme histochemistry, to which immunocytochemistry owes a great debt. However, it is indeed possible to arrive at workable compromises between the four criteria. In the earlier days of ultrastructural immunocytochemistry, the trend was to preserve antigenicity at the expense of structure. Consequently, much erroneous information was collected from micrographs of badly preserved cells. Modern immunocytochemistry, assisted by better conditions of microscopy, more sensitive and precise immunocytochemical methods and improved techniques for fixation and microtomy, no longer suffers seriously from these shortcomings.

4.1. FIXATION

Peptides and proteins differ in their physicochemical properties and, hence, in their behavior to different fixatives. Thus, it is not possible to design a fixative which will work well with all antigens. Moreover, it is equally impossible to state that a particular fixative will always work well with the same antigen! Hence, antibodies only recognize a small part of the antigen (3—8 amino acid residues in the case of peptides and proteins). Consequently, some fixatives may have adverse effects on one part of an antigen and destroy the antigenicity of that part, while simultaneously preserving the antigenicity of another part. It is therefore vital to be aware of the chemical properties of the peptides studied and to be ready to modify fixation conditions when need arises.

Fixatives most popular for light- and electron-microscopy include the aldehyde fixatives, above all formaldehyde and glutaraldehyde. Unfortunately, the chemical reactivities of these fixatives under histotechnical conditions are not much known (Hopwood 1969). It may be considered certain, however, that the aldehyde fixatives react with amino groups, sulphydryl groups, and possibly also with aromatic groups (Bowes and Cater 1966; Habeeb and Hiramoto 1968; Ohtsuki et al. 1978). Use of formaldehyde for a short time at low temperature (4°C) has earned a good reputation for preserving the antigenicity of a wide range of molecules (Larsson 1981a). Since commercial 'formalin' solutions contain contaminants, including methanol, that may harm antigenicity or extract peptides, it is essential to use formaldehyde prepared from paraformaldehyde a.m. (Pease 1962) (e.g. a 4% solution in 0.1 M sodium phosphate buffer, pH 7.3-7.4) (Hökfelt et al. 1975; Larsson 1981a).

Formaldehyde fixation is partially reversible and much of the formaldehyde attached to fixed tissue can be washed away by prolonged exposure to buffer.

Glutaraldehyde, a dialdehyde, is a much stronger cross-linker than formaldehyde and is frequently blamed for destroying antigenicity. While formaldehyde is an excellent choice for light-microscopic immunocytochemistry, glutaraldehyde fixation is almost invariably necessary for ultrastructural studies. In older days, it was sought to avoid the deleterious influences of glutaraldehyde on antigenicity by using weak solutions (0.1-0.3%) applied for prolonged time. As can be seen from the 1965-1975 literature, the results were often less than acceptable. Thus, some loss of antigenicity always occurred, but what was worse was that this was paired with a very poor preservation of tissue structure. Later it was found that mixtures of fixatives, e.g. formaldehyde-glutaraldehyde mixtures of the Karnovsky type (Karnovsky 1965), as well as the parabenzoquinone-formaldehyde-glutaraldehyde (PFG) mixtures (Larsson 1977) produced much better structural preservation, while retaining antigenicity for many (but not all) peptides.

Presently, the best procedure appears to be the use of a 2% formaldehyde : 3% glutaraldehyde mixture in 0.1 M sodium phosphate buffer pH 7.3 for perfusion-/immersion-fixation at 4°C for 15-30 min, followed by an overnight rinse in 0.1 M sodium cacodylate buffer pH 7.3. This brief and cold fixation produces an optimal ultrastructure and a very good preservation of the antigenicity of many peptides (Larsson 1981a). With other, more difficult antigens, attempts may be made using the PFG mixture (Larsson 1977) or the paraformaldehyde-lysine-periodic acid mixture of McLean and Nakane (1974).

Apart from aldehyde fixatives alternative formulas include carbodiimides (Kendall et al. 1971), imidates (Hassel and Hand 1974; McMillan and Luftig 1975), benzoquinone and diethylpyrocarbonate (Pearse and Polak 1975). The two latter fixatives, the chemistry of which is unknown, are sometimes applied in vapor-form to freeze-dried specimens. Used alone, most of these fixatives are not suitable for ultrastructural studies. Recently, a novel fixative combination of glutaraldehyde and carbodiimide was introduced by Willingham and Yamada (1979). This mixture is said to be useful for preserving both structure and antigenicity.

Osmic acid (OsO_4) is a well-known and indispensable fixative for electron-microscopy. It is usually applied after primary fixation in aldehydes, but is sometimes also used as a primary fixative. Although mainly thought of as a fixative for lipids, there is now much evidence that it also reacts with peptides and proteins and may form peptide-protein or peptide-lipid cross-links (Beauvillain et al. 1975; Hayat 1970; Li et al. 1977; Nielson and Griffith 1979). Additionally, recent chemical information suggests that osmic acid may cleave polypeptide chains at specific residues (Deetz and Behrman 1981). Osmic acid has earned quite a bad reputation for destroying all antigenicity. Recently, however, many studies have shown that, even as a primary fixative, osmic acid may preserve antigenicity of growth hormone and other polypeptides (Li et al. 1977). Due to the light- and electron-absorbing abilities of the osmic acid reaction products, it is, however, necessary to remove it before immunocytochemical staining is commenced. At the light-microscopical level osmic acid is usually removed by periodic acid (1% in distilled water) (Beauvillain et al. 1975) and, at the ultrastructural level, by hydrogen peroxide (Sternberger 1979). Use of osmic acid is almost indispensable for many ultrastructural studies in order to define membranes. It should be noted, however, that the agent itself is capable of cleaving polypeptide chains and that the oxidants used for removing its reaction products are potentially harmful to antigenic sites containing methionine, tryptophan and sulphydryl groups.

4.2. TISSUE PREPARATION

Although loss of antigenicity most often is blamed on the fixative, it is often due to the method of tissue preparation used. We shall therefore briefly discuss several different methods of preparing fixed or unfixed tissues for staining.

Isolated cells, imprints and tissue fragments

The main problems with these preparations relates to antigen accessibility (i.e. antibody permeability). Thus, before as well as after fixation, membranes and matrix constitute efficient diffusion barriers to antibodies. Several permeabilization techniques have been tried, including detergents like triton X-100, nonidet NP-40, acetone and freezing and thawing (Hartman et al. 1972; Bohn 1978; Laurilla et al. 1978; Ohtsuki et al. 1978; Pickel et al. 1976; Seman and Nairn 1977). In our hands, the first-choice method consists of a dehydration-rehydration sequence in graded ethanols up to xylene and down to buffer again (Larsson 1981a). This sequence corresponds to the dehydration sequences used for preparing electron-microscopical specimens and has no more untoward effects on tissue structure than these. We have successfully used this method for imprints of pituitary cells, tumour cells, cells grown on cover slips and isolated antropyloric glands (Fig. 2). Moreover, we and others have employed the method for staining isolated strips of longitudinal gastrointestinal muscle containing adherent myenteric plexus (Costa et al. 1980) (Fig. 3). So far, this method has been successful with most peptides tested. However, if problems should arise, trials with the detergent techniques may be worthwhile.

The sizes of antibodies with attached marker molecules (Table 1) have a large impact on antigen accessibility. It is always advisable to use as small a marker as possible. In our hands, the above method has worked well with the indirect immunofluorescence, PAP, and radioimmunocytochemical techniques. Electron-microscopical techniques, like the gold granule marker systems, are theoretically feasible to use (particularly since these markers can be made smaller than e.g. PAP complexes) but have not yet been tested.

Vibratome sections

In the vibrating-knife-type microtomes, sections of unfixed or fixed, unfrozen tissues can be cut down to about 30-40 μm. Antibody penetration of such sections is not uniform and generally limited to the surface area. Addition of triton X-100 to antibody solutions (0.3%) and to washing solutions (1.0%) increases the permeability of the tissue (Pickel et al. 1976). Primary formaldehyde fixation and vibratome sectioning has preserved antigenicity of all peptides so far studied by us. The method is superior for peptidergic neurons in brain and spinal cord, and parallel or identical sections can be used for studies of monoaminergic systems (see Chapter II). At the electron-microscopical level, the preservation of structure is reasonable, but with evidence of what most likely is leakage of peptides from subcellular organelles. Electron-

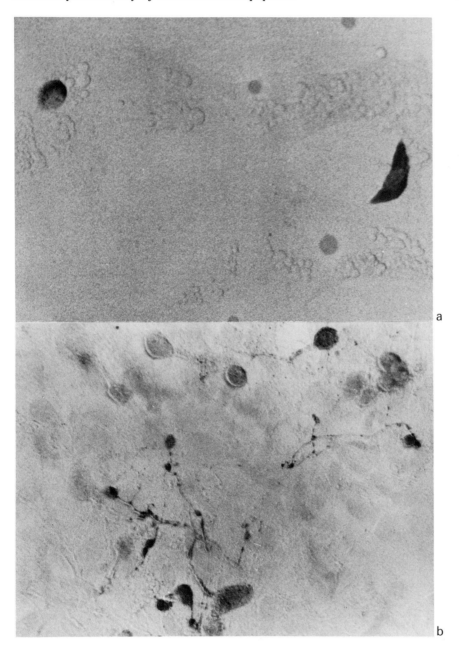

Fig. 2. Permeabilization of monolayer cultures for immunocytochemistry using the dehydration-rehydration technique. In (a) is shown a culture of newborn rat antropyloric epithelial cells stained for gastrin immunoreactivity using the PAP method and in (b) is shown a spinal cord culture (prepared by Dr. J. Lambert, Dept. of Physiology, Univ. of Aarhus) stained for enkephalin immunoreactivity (PAP method). The antropyloric culture is photographed in ordinary bright field, whereas the spinal cord culture is photographed under differential interference contrast (Nomarski) optics.

microscopy is usually carried out on osmicated and reembedded prestained vibratome sections. Due to difficulties with obtaining identical control sections (especially con-

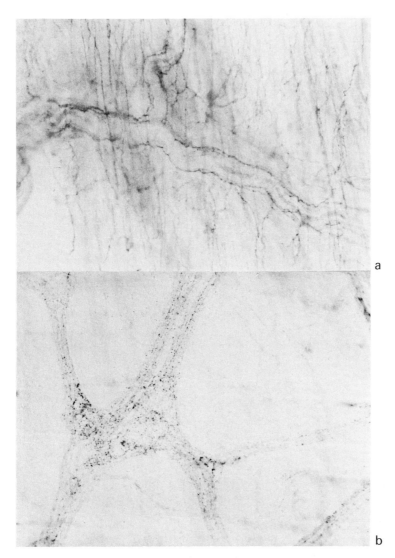

Fig. 3. Whole mount preparations of cat duodenal circular muscle layer (a) and longitudinal muscle layer with adherent myenteric plexus (b), permeabilized with the dehydration-rehydration method and immunocytochemistry stained for enkephalin-like immunoreactivity using the PAP method. Note in (a) that enkephalin immunoreactive fibers run in parallel with the (circular) muscle fibers and also surround an intramural blood vessel in an innervation-like manner. In (b) is shown that enkephalin immunoreactive fibers are abundant in the ganglia and interganglionic strands of the myenteric plexus but sparse in the outer, longitudinal muscle layer.

sidering antibody permeability in adjacent vibratome sections), we prefer to support our ultrastructural data by independent means.

Cryostat sections

Following primary fixation, specimens are soaked in a cryoprotectant (sucrose, glycerol, dimethylsulfoxide), frozen rapidly in melting Freon-22 or in a propane-

TABLE 1. *Sizes of reporter molecules*

Molecule	Size/Activity area	Molecular weight	Electron density
IgG	4 × 5 × 8 nm	160 000	—
IgM	—	900 000	—
Avidin	—	68 300	—
Biotin	—	244	—
Protein A	—	41 000	—
Horseradish Peroxidase (HRP)	Enzyme activity area ~ 40—50 nm	40 000	(enzyme activity)
PAP complexes	~ 22 nm (cf. HRP)	400 000 −429 000	(enzyme activity)
Colloidal gold particles	5—150 nm	—	+
Silica spheres	7—25 nm	—	+
Ferritin	electron dense core: 5 nm total size: 12 nm	650 000	+
Hemocyanin	30 × 50 nm	—	+
Virus particles	around 30 nm	—	+
Polyethyleneimine particles	10 nm	40 000	(osmiophilic)
Radioiodine (^{125}I)	With an L_4 emulsion developed after gold latensification in Elon ascorbic acid, 50% of autoradiographic grains are within an 80 nm circle	125	(radioactivity)

propylene mixture (cooled by liquid nitrogen) and submitted to cryostat sectioning (Dorling et al. 1976; Hökfelt et al. 1975; Isobe et al. 1977; Webb et al. 1972). Along with the vibratome technique, cryostat sectioning represents one of the most universally applicable methods for studying neurohormonal peptides, which, by now, has been used for well over 100 antigens with little evidence for losses of antigenicity. For most problems in immunocytochemistry, a combination of a cold 4% formaldehyde fixation for 3-4 hours, overnight soaking in 20% sucrose and cryostat sectioning represents a worthwhile first choice. Nakane and co-workers have employed their PLP fixative (vide supra) along with a more gradual exposure to cryoprotectants in order to apply the technique at the electron-microscopical level (Isobe et al. 1977; McLean and Nakane 1974; Tabucchi et al. 1976). In my laboratory we have slightly modified this method and have obtained very worthwhile ultrastructural results (Larsson 1981a) (details in appendix). The single most important aspect is to avoid formation of large ice crystals. This is obtained (a) by using efficient cryoprotection and (b) by quick freezing of the tissue in e.g. melting Freon-22. Freezing on solid carbon dioxide or directly in liquid nitrogen is unsuitable. Thus, in liquid nitrogen an insulating gas mantle is rapidly formed around the specimens, preventing rapid freezing.

Freeze-drying and freeze-substitution

In these techniques, which are reviewed in further detail in Chapter II by Björklund, unfixed small specimens are frozen directly in a suitable medium (Freon-22, propane-propylene mixtures, cooled by liquid nitrogen) in order to avoid as much ice crystal formation as possible. Specimens for freeze-substitution are then exposed to organic solvents (and fixatives) at low temperature to exchange the tissue water for the solvent. After such fixation and substitution, the now dehydrated specimens are embedded in paraffin or in resins (Silverman 1976; Van Leeuwen 1977).

Alternatively, specimens may be freeze-dried in special tissue freeze-driers, where the water is sublimated through gradual increases in temperature onto a cold finger or into a phosphorous pentoxide trap (Björklund et al. 1972; Larsson 1981a; Pearse and Polak 1975). The completely dried specimens can then be vapour-fixed (with paraformaldehyde, osmic acid, glutaraldehyde, diethylpyrocarbonate or parabenzoquinone vapours) and embedded in paraffin in vacuo.

The main importance with these methods is that the tissue never is exposed to aqueous solvents that may extract or modify tissue-bound molecules. The freeze-drying technique has earned its fame chiefly due to its combination with the Falck-Hillarp formaldehyde condensation technique for inducing fluorescence with catecholamines and indoleamines (see Chapter II).

Incidentally, a few years ago we found that the same type of formaldehyde vapour treatment is also a suitable fixative for many neurohormonal peptides (for review see Larsson 1981a). Combinations of the Falck-Hillarp method and immunocytochemistry has given information on the co-localization of biogenic monoamines and fluorogenic or immunoreactive peptides (Larsson et al. 1975, 1976).

Conventional dehydration-paraffin embedding

Although successful with some antigens, many cannot be demonstrated in material prepared by this technique. Still, material from e.g. pathological laboratories is often treated in this way and the clinically oriented immunocytochemist must, hence, try to cope with it.

Interestingly, if two specimens are fixed in the same way (e.g. in 4% paraformaldehyde) and then processed for cryostat sectioning and paraffin sectioning, respectively, a larger variety of peptide antigens will be demonstrable in the cryosections. Thus, in this case, the embedding in paraffin and not the fixation per se seems to damage the antigenicity. Such damage may relate to the dehydration, xylene treatment and the embedding in hot (50-60°C) paraffin. In fact, low temperature embedding in plastic resins is known to result in less losses of antigenicity. For these reasons, whenever we have a choice, we refrain from using paraffin embedding (although, truthfully, it does preserve a few antigens to an excellent degree). When working with clinical material of this type it is usually advisable to dewax sections, hydrate them and then rinse them for 12-24 hours in running tap water or buffer, before staining, as this seems to restore some of the antigenicity (Larsson 1981a).

Apart from formalin, many other fixative combinations are used with paraffin sections. Of these, certain picric acid-based formulas have earned a certain reputation for preserving antigenicity. These include Bouin's, Stefanini's (or Zamboni's) fluid and the Bouin-Hollandé-Sublimé mixtures.

An alternative to paraffin embedding is to use water-soluble polyethylene glycol (PEG). PEG has been used by Nakane and co-workers for preembedding staining for electron-microscopy of pituitary endocrine cells, but has not been much compared to other techniques with respect to retention of antigenicity (Nakane 1973).

Plastic embedding

Electron-microscopical immunocytochemistry can be performed as preembedding staining (using either isolated cells and tissues, vibratome, cryostat or polyethylene glycol sections) or as postembedding staining using plastic sections (ultracryotomy, cf. following section). Apart from this, plastic sections are very useful at the light-microscopical level, since they may be cut so thin that adjacent sections, containing parts of the same cells or nerve terminals, can be stained with different antisera (adjacent section technique) (Lange 1971).

Many different resins have been employed for this purpose. Water-soluble resins include the metacrylates, but difficulties with cutting ultrathin sections from such resins has resulted in the development of many alternative polymers, including glutaraldehyde/formaldehyde polymers of serum albumins, gelatin and urea (Hayat 1970; Kraehenbuhl 1977). With recent promising developments in ultracryotomy, it seems reasonable to assume that this technique will make water-soluble plastics less important.

For ultrastructural purposes, resins of interest include non-water-miscible plastics like Epon, Araldite and Spurr's (Sternberger 1979). Again, the temperature of polymerization may have an importance on the preservation of antigenicity and these resins should preferably be polymerized at 45°C or below. Unfortunately, embedding in resin, as in paraffin, is often associated with losses of antigenicity. Takamiya et al. (1978) recently suggested that resin monomers may interact with amino groups in tissue and, hence, modify or destroy antigenicity. In model experiments it was shown that controlled proteolytic treatment of the sections restored antigenicity (Takamiya et al. 1978). Interestingly, also with paraffin sections many workers have reported that assorted proteolytic enzymes may restore antigenicity (Curran and Gregory 1977; Donk et al. 1977; Finley et al. 1978; Huang et al. 1976; Reading 1977).

Prior to staining, plastic must be removed from the sections. This can be brought about by a variety of methods. Thus, semithin ($\sim 0.3\ \mu$m) sections can be deplasticized in sodium methoxide (Mayer et al. 1961) or in a concentrated solution of potassium hydroxide in water-free ethanol (Lane and Europa 1965, Maxwell 1978). With ultrathin sections, brief etching in 5% hydrogen peroxide has been much used (Sternberger 1979). However, in numerous experiments we have found that removal of plastic is not necessary with ultrathin sections. Thus, in a quantitative evaluation of the gold-labelled antigen detection (GLAD) method, sections from non-osmicated tissues showed the same intense labelling with or without hydrogen peroxide treatment (Larsson 1981a). This seems also to hold true for the PAP method. With osmicated tissue, however, hydrogen peroxide treatment still seems to be necessary. This probably relates to the ability of the agent to remove some of the osmium stain that otherwise would prevent or obscure the immune-reactions (Sternberger 1979).

Ultracryotomy

A few years ago, this technique would not seriously have been considered an alternative to plastic sections. However, recent developments, above all with respect to positive contrasting of the specimens (Tokuyasu 1978), make ultracryotomy a very desirable weapon in the arsenal of immunocytochemists. A few reliable devices for freezing and cutting are now available and may, if properly managed, produce sections almost on par with plastic sections. The potential value of this technique is enormous, since it may be made as universally applicable as the light-microscopical cryostat technique. Recent work on immunocytochemistry using ultracryotomy sections include that of Geuze et al. 1979, 1981) and Painter et al. (1973).

5. IMMUNOCYTOCHEMICAL DETECTION SYSTEMS

A wide variety of immunocytochemical methods are available, including fluorochromed antibodies (direct and indirect immunofluorescence), enzyme-conjugated antibodies (direct and indirect immunoenzyme, e.g. immunoperoxidase, methods), unlabelled peroxidase methods (the peroxidase-antiperoxidase or PAP method), radioactively labelled antibody and antigen detection methods, and a wide variety of particulate markers for transmission and scanning electron-microscopy (ferritin, colloidal gold, hemocyanin, silica etc.). Additionally, some methods exploit the complement-fixing properties of antibodies and still others make use of the high binding avidity between biotin and avidin. Basically, all these different techniques may be divided into two groups: labelled and unlabelled antibody detection methods and labelled antigen detection methods (Larsson 1981a).

5.1. ANTIBODY DETECTION METHODS

These can be divided into direct and indirect techniques (Fig. 4). In the direct techniques the primary (for example 'antineuropeptide') antibody is labelled, whereas in the indirect techniques the primary antibody is unlabelled and detected by a second labelled antibody, recognizing IgG molecules of the species producing the primary antibody (e.g. fluorescence-labelled goat anti-rabbit IgG). There are several advantages with the indirect methods: firstly, they circumvent the need for labelling the often scarce and precious primary antibodies; secondly, they are more sensitive because secondary

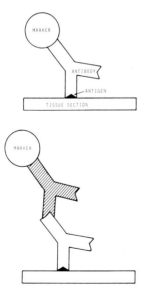

Fig. 4. Principles for direct (top) and indirect (bottom) immunocytochemistry (cf. text).

labelled antibodies may attach to multiple sites of the primary antibody (Goldman 1968; Sternberger 1979). Generally, it is conceived that indirect methods are 5-10-fold more sensitive than direct methods.

Immunofluorescence (Fig. 5)

Antibodies are usually labelled with fluorescein isothiocyanate (FITC; excitation maximum at 490 nm) producing a green fluorescence or with tetramethylrhodamine isothiocyanate (TRITC; excitation maximum at 546 nm), producing a red fluorescence. Alternative labels are numerous, but have not come into widespread use (Goldman 1968; Nairn 1976). The fluorescence colors of FITC and TRITC contrast well, which has been much exploited in double-staining studies. Procedures for fluorochroming antibodies are exemplified in the Appendix. Purification of the fluorochromed antibodies is best performed by gel filtration on a Sephadex G25 column, eluted with phosphate-buffered saline (pH 7.4-8.2) or with tris-buffered saline (0.1 M Tris buffer pH 7.4, containing 0.15 M NaCl; TBS) (cf. Appendix). Alternatively, a fluorochrome scavenger (e.g. lysine-Sepharose) may be used. Since the isothiocyanates bind to amino groups on antibodies, overlabelling may result in acidic conjugates that react non-specifically with tissue. These will have to be removed by ion-exchange chromatography (Goldman 1968; Nairn 1976; Sternberger 1979).

Workers using indirect immunofluorescence rarely prepare their own conjugates, since excellent FITC- and TRITC-labelled anti-rabbit and anti-guinea pig antibodies are available commercially. A number of companies also prepare good FITC-labelled anti-mouse IgG or IgM for use with monoclonal antibodies. When receiving a new batch of fluorochromed antiserum in the laboratory, it is, however, advisable to pass it through a Sephadex G25 column to remove free fluorochromes. Fluorochromed an-

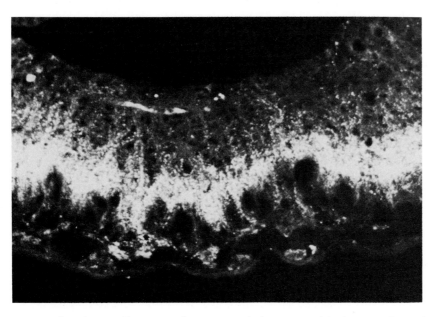

Fig. 5. Indirect immunofluorescence for somatostatin immunoreactivity in rat median eminence. Section prepared from formaldehyde-perfused and cryosectioned rat brain and stained with somatostatin antiserum R 213/3 and FITC-labelled goat anti-rabbit IgG.

163

tibodies pass rapidly through the column and appear in the volume excluded by the gel beads (void volume), whereas the low molecular weight free fluorochromes pass slowly through the column and appear at, or after, the total volume. Thus, as seen with a fluorescence lamp, samples containing free fluorochromes rapidly divide into two distinct bands, the first of which contains the desired labelled antibodies.

Immunofluorescence techniques have earned an unjustified reputation for low sensitivity. Although it is true that immunoenzymatic techniques are more sensitive, this reputation is chiefly caused by the fact that many workers use very suboptimal conditions for microscopy.

For optimal visualization of FITC it is desirable to use a xenon lamp which has a high emission at 490 nm. Preferably, this should be combined with selective interference filters and an epi-illumination system (Nairn and Ploem 1974). A mercury lamp is much less desirable for FITC since this lamp actually has a drop in its emission at the excitation peak of FITC. A mercury arc, however, does admirably well for TRITC, because of a sharp increase in its emission at about the excitation maximum (540-550 nm) of this fluorophore. The major microscope companies now sell excellent packages with interference filters and dichroic mirrors for epi-excitation of FITC and TRITC. Although costly, these systems represent a well-spent investment for the cytochemist who intends to base much of his work on immunofluorescence. Points of concern are primarily the choice of light source (xenon, mercury or halogen), the length of the light path (which is unnecessarily long in some microscopes, with ensuing losses of light) and proper objectives (preferably of the oil, water or glycerine immersion types, particularly at low magnifications).

Immunoperoxidase and peroxidase-antiperoxidase methods (Fig. 6)

Nakane and Avrameas pioneered the techniques whereby enzymes like horseradish peroxidase or alkaline phosphatase could be conjugated to antibodies without great losses of enzyme or antibody activity (for review, see Nakane 1978). Many different conjugation methods have been devised, including one-step and two-step conjugations. Additionally, periodate oxidation of sugar groups on the molecules has been used to create aldehyde groups for subsequent conjugations (Murayama et al. 1978; Nakane 1973; Sternberger 1979). Unfortunately, many enzyme-antibody conjugates may contain large aggregates of antibodies and markers with accompanying impairment of penetration and specificity (Sternberger 1979). Nevertheless, many conjugates (also commercially available) show excellent staining properties and have found widespread use in immunocytochemistry and in enzyme-linked immunosorbent assays (ELISA).

It was felt that immunologic, rather than covalent attachment of enzyme to antibodies would result in less impairment of enzyme and antibody activities. Hence, unlabelled immunoenzyme techniques were created (Petrusz et al. 1975; Sternberger et

Fig. 6. Peroxidase-antoperoxidase (PAP) staining as visualized in bright field (a), dark field (b), differential interference contrast (c) and in the electron-microscope (d). In (a) and (b), mouse cerebral cortex (formaldehyde-perfusion, cryosectioning) has been stained with vasoactive intestinal polypeptide (VIP) antibody 5603 using the PAP method. In (c), a similarly stained section of rat retina is shown, illustrating a VIP immunoreactive amacrine-like cell. In (d) is shown an electron-micrograph of a pancreatic polypeptide (PP) cell process in feline pancreas (specimen fixed in formaldehyde-glutaraldehyde, embedded in Epon and cut in an ultramicrotome, whereafter ultrathin sections were stained on grids directly). Note the presence of numerous immunocytochemically stained secretory granules in the PP cell process which separates two non-immunoreactive pancreatic zymogen cells.

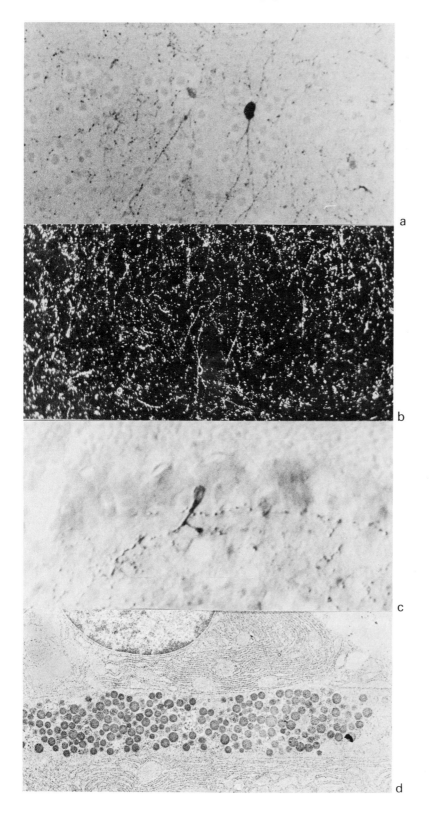

al. 1970). The principle of the best known of these modifications, the peroxidase-antiperoxidase (PAP) technique of Sternberger (Sternberger et al. 1970; Sternberger 1979) is schematically outlined in Fig. 7 and details are given in the Appendix. The technique relies on the use of three layers of antibodies. The first layer consists of rabbit antibodies directed against the tissue antigen under investigation. The second layer consists of unlabelled (e.g. sheep or pig) antibodies to rabbit immunoglobulins and is applied in excess, so that only one of the two antigen-combining sites on the anti-rabbit IgG antibodies binds to the antibodies of the first layer. The remaining antigen- combining sites are, hence, free to react with any type of added rabbit IgG and react with the third layer, consisting of an immunocomplex between horseradish peroxidase and rabbit anti-horseradish peroxidase antibodies. As mentioned in our discussion of indirect immunofluorescence, the anti-rabbit IgG molecules used as the second layer may attach to several sites on the primary antibody and, subsequently, each of these antibodies may bind a PAP complex, consisting of three peroxidase molecules and two rabbit anti-horseradish peroxidase molecules. The amplification of the reaction is significant and the PAP method possesses a detection efficiency superior to that of most other techniques. Earlier variants of the unlabelled immunoperoxidase or immunoglobulin bridge techniques consisted of the sequential application of antiperoxidase antibodies as a third layer and of horseradish peroxidase as a fourth layer. However, as indicated by Sternberger (1974), the preparation of preformed PAP complexes produces an important increase in detection efficiency. The anti-rabbit IgG ('link') antibody may be replaced by the staphylococcal protein A, which is polyvalent with respect to IgG molecules (cf. Sternberger 1979 and Notani et al. 1979). Introduction of this bridging molecule would probably be advantageous when non-rabbit antibodies have to be used as the first antibody layer. In cases where primary guinea pig antibodies have to be used, it is, however, possible to find anti-rabbit IgG antisera which cross-react with guinea pig IgG, and to use these as link antibodies (Erlandsen et al. 1975).

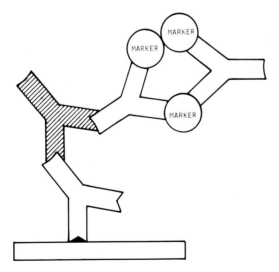

Fig. 7. Principle of the peroxidase-antiperoxidase (PAP) method. Note that the hatched anti-rabbit IgG molecule bridges the tissue-bound (rabbit) primary antibody to the subsequently applied PAP complex (marker = peroxidase) by its two (anti-rabbit IgG) combining sites.

Hybrid antibody techniques

An interesting and useful modification of the immunocytochemical technique has been the introduction of hybrid antibodies. In this technique $F(ab')_2$ fragments are formed by pepsin digestion. Subsequent mild reduction results in the liberation of $F(ab')$ fragments, containing only one antigen-combining site. Reassociation to $F(ab')_2$ fragments containing two antigen-combining sites can be brought about by oxidation. Since the reassociation is not dependent upon the antibody specificity, $F(ab')$ fragments of e.g. peptide antibodies can be made to reassociate with $F(ab')$ fragments of e.g. anti-ferritin or antiperoxidase antibodies (Sternberger 1974; Williams and Chase 1976). By mixing varying proportions of different $F(ab')$ fragments, reassociation of the desired hybrids can be directed. Thus formed hybrid antibodies may be purified by affinity chromatography and used for staining with the desired marker, immunologically bound to one of the antigen-combining sites. Since reassociated non-hybrid antiperoxidase or antiferritin $F(ab')_2$ fragments do not interfere with localization studies, it may, in selected instances, not be necessary to remove them. In contrast, reassociated non-hybrid antipeptide $F(ab')_2$ fragments may mask antigenic sites for the hybrid antibodies and have to be removed by affinity absorption.

Particulate markers and radioactivity

Both enzyme-labelled antibodies, unlabelled immunoenzyme techniques and hybrid antibodies have successfully been applied for the electron-microscopical localization of tissue antigens. In addition to enzymes, antibodies used for electron microscopical localization of antigens have been marked with ferritin (cf. Kraehenbuhl and Jamieson 1972; Painter et al. 1973), derivatized silica spheres (Peters et al. 1978), colloidal gold particles (Batten and Hopkins 1978, 1979; Faulk and Taylor 1971; Roth et al. 1978; Romano et al. 1974, 1977), polyethyleneimine (Schurer et al. 1977), and chloromercuriferrocene (Yasuda and Yamamoto 1975). Electron-dense virus particles, uranium (Sternberger 1974) and radiolabels (cf. Paiement and Kopriwa 1978; Paiement and Leblond 1977) have also been employed. The application of so many different techniques at the electron-microscopical level may reflect the difficulties in ultrastructurally localizing antigens. An interesting development with monoclonal antibodies is the possibility to add radioactive amino acids to cloned hybridoma cells. These radioactive amino acids will then be incorporated into the antibody protein synthesized by the cells and, hence, internally labelled radioactive antibodies are obtained (Cuello et al. 1980).

Avidin-biotin techniques

The extremely high binding affinity of the egg white protein, avidin, for biotin (10^{15} l/mole) has recently been exploited for immunocytochemistry. Biotin can be converted into a hydroxysuccinimide ester and this ester can easily be conjugated to antibodies or other proteins ('biotinylation') (Bayer et al. 1979). Biotinylated antibodies are then allowed to react with tissue sections and are detected e.g. by use of FITC-labelled avidin, which binds to the biotin on the antibodies (Heggeness and Ash 1977). Alternative possibilities are offered by the fact that avidin is multivalent and can bind several biotinyl groups. Thus, in a sandwich method, it is possible to apply unlabelled avidin and then to proceed by applying e.g. biotinylated enzyme, which binds to the residual sites on the avidin molecule (Guesdon et al. 1979). Avidin is a very basic molecule (pI

$\simeq$ 10.5) and may consequently bind unspecifically to tissue. Guesdon and colleagues (1979) have found that partial blocking of the amino groups of avidin decreases its non-specific binding. In my own experience, fluoresceinated avidin, as well as the biotinyl-antibody-avidin-biotinyl-peroxidase sandwich, are versatile and useful probes for immunocytochemistry.

Protein A techniques

Protein A, obtained from certain strains of *Staphylococcus aureus* attaches to the Fc portion of antibodies from many (but not all!) species. Consequently, it has gained some popularity as a replacement for the second antibody in indirect immunocytochemical techniques. Its one obvious advantage is that it is not species-specific to the same extent as a normal second antibody, but may be used as a second 'link' antibody between immunoglobulins of several species in the PAP method (vide supra). Protein A has also been labelled with and conjugated to almost all of the popular markers of the day, including FITC, ferritin, colloidal gold, peroxidase and several others (Bächi et al. 1977; Batten and Hopkins 1979; Bergh and Solheim 1978; Dubois-Dalg et al. 1977; Notani et al. 1979; Romano 1977; Roth et al. 1978). I find it a useful marker, although associated with more background staining than second antibodies. When used with the colloidal gold techniques, we find a distinct advantage of anti-rabbit IgG (Romano et al. 1974) over protein A in terms of sensitivity as well as lack of unspecific background staining.

Monoclonal antibody detection

With their proven and anticipated usefulness, it is not strange that many methods have been devised for performing immunocytochemistry with monoclonal antibodies. Apart from the ingenious strategy of permitting hybridoma cells to synthesize radioactive antibodies from tritiated amino acids (Cuello et al. 1980), many alternatives exist. Thus, fluorochromed and peroxidase-labelled anti-mouse IgG preparations are available commercially, as are unlabelled rabbit anti-mouse IgG preparations. The latter can be used in the PAP method, featuring as subsequent layers: (1) mouse monoclonal antibody (IgG or IgM); (2) rabbit anti-mouse IgG (or IgM); (3) anti-rabbit IgG in surplus; and (4) rabbit PAP complex. Additionally, mouse PAP complexes are now available and monoclonal antibodies may also be directly labelled with fluorochromes, or enzymes or absorbed onto colloidal gold particles or employed in the biotin-avidin or protein A techniques.

5.2. LABELLED ANTIGEN DETECTION TECHNIQUES

All previously described immunocytochemical methods depend on the demonstration of all antibodies that attach themselves to tissue sections. Not all of these antibodies may be specific, however. Various controls, involving above all antisera preabsorbed with the appropriate antigen, are used to document immunocytochemical specificity. Theoretical and practical considerations have, however, recently emphasized that the large body of available controls may be insufficient for documenting specificity. Thus, complement-mediated binding of IgG molecules to tissue may not always be detected by adsorption controls since the absorptions may deplete antisera of complement (Buffa et al. 1979). This, however, probably only occurs in cases where immunoprecipitates or larger immune complexes are formed. Further, absorption of antisera with too large excesses of pure antigen may produce falsely positive absorption controls. Since ultrasensitive methods, like the PAP procedure, are now able to detect extremely low concentrations of IgG, the purity of the primary antiserum is of critical importance. Three different techniques for obtaining pure antibodies are available, including monoclonal antibodies, synthesis of polypeptides, mimicking the antigen-combining site of antibodies (Atassi and Zablocki 1977), and affinity chromatography. The latter technique has the advantage that it can be used in all laboratories and will, indeed, produce antibodies of selected specificity. Unfortunately, high-avidity antibodies will often bind so strongly to the affinity columns that they cannot be eluted successfully. Thus, many antisera that have been affinity-purified are relatively enriched in low-avidity antibodies. Use of such antibodies introduces the risk of dissociation or dislocation during immunocytochemical staining procedures. Hence, low-avidity antibodies may, at worst, produce erroneous of falsely negative results. Synthesis of peptides mimicking antibody combining sites still represents only an attractive theoretical possibility and use of monoclonal antibodies for all problems we wish to study will not be possible yet in several years.

The problem of detection of unspecific antibodies never occurs in radioimmunoassay (RIA) systems, simply because these employ a radiolabelled tracer (= labelled antigen), capable of reacting only with specific antibodies. It is true that unspecificity may occur also in RIA systems, but this is then usually due to the fact that the antibody reads a non-unique portion of the antigen and is never due to antibodies uncapable of recognizing the labelled antigen (cf. the discussion of region-specific antibodies). In an attempt to overcome the above-mentioned difficulties with immunocytochemistry, we introduced the so-called labelled antigen detection techniques (Larsson and Schwartz 1977; Larsson 1979, 1981a) (Fig. 8). These techniques take advantage of the fact that IgG molecules possess two equivalent antigen-combining sites. If such antibodies (or, for that matter, their F(ab')$_2$ fragments) are allowed to react with antigen in the zone of antibody surplus, a preponderance of complexes between one antibody and one antigen molecule is formed. The remaining antigen-combining sites in such complexes will, hence, remain free to react with subsequently added antigen molecules. In its original form – the radioimmunocytochemical (RICH) method – the technique was carried out by reacting surplus amounts of antibodies with their corresponding radioiodinated antigen (Larsson and Schwartz 1977; Rappay et al. 1979). The RICH complexes thus formed consisted of antibodies which bound radioiodinated antigen with only one of their two antigen-combining sites and, hence, had the remaining site

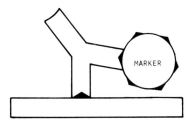

Fig. 8. Principle of labelled antigen detection methods. Antibodies are allowed to react with tissue-bound antigen with one of their two antigen-combining sites and with marker-bound pure antigen with the remaining site. Since unspecific antibodies will fail to react with pure marker-bound antigen they will remain undetected.

free to react with tissue-bound antigen. The site of reaction between the RICH complex and tissue was then revealed by autoradiography (Figs. 9 and 10). Since unspecific (unrelated) antibodies, by definition, would be unable to bind specific (radiolabelled) antigen they would remain undetected. Since only specific antibodies are demonstrated by this method, it also allows the pretreatment of the tissue with high concentrations of normal serum from the same species as the one producing the primary antiserum. This pretreatment will block sites that otherwise could have bound specific IgG molecules by non-immunologic mechanisms, like Fc binding, ionic attraction or complement-mediated binding. Although its ability to pick out only specific antibodies without selecting against high-avidity antibodies was our main reason for developing the RICH method, additional advantages became apparent: (1) Since surplus amounts of antibodies were used, the method was actually selected for high-avidity antibodies. (2) The dilutions of antisera used were of the same order of magnitude as those used

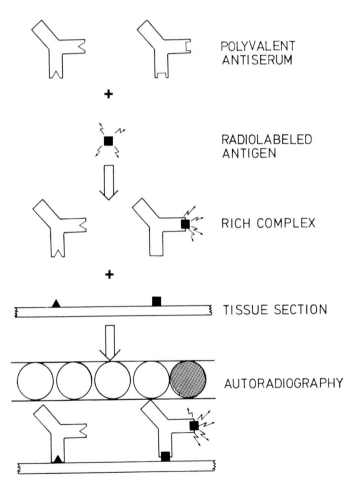

POLYVALENT
ANTISERUM

RADIOLABELED
ANTIGEN

RICH COMPLEX

TISSUE SECTION

AUTORADIOGRAPHY

Fig. 9. Principle of the radioimmunocytochemical (RICH) method. In this variant of the labelled antigen detection technique antibodies are first allowed to react with radiolabelled antigen molecules in such a way that one of their antigen-combining sites will remain free (cf. text). This site will subsequently react with tissue-bound antigen corresponding to the radiolabelled antigen. Unspecific antibodies may well bind to tissue but will not have bound radioiodinated antigen and will hence not be autoradiographically detected.

in the ultrasensitive PAP procedure and could, in fact, be increased with increasing times of autoradiographic exposure (the half-life of ^{125}I is about 60 days). (3) The autoradiographic silver grains were easily detected, even in sections that were stained with a variety of conventional histological methods. (4) The RICH technique could be used in conjunction with the PAP technique on the same tissue section, allowing simultaneous light-microscopical detection of multiple antigens.

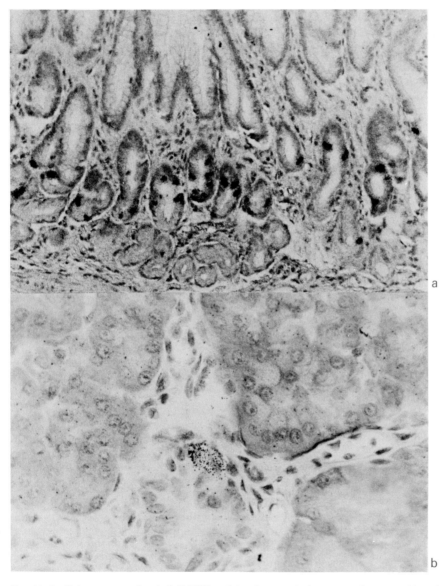

Fig. 10. Radioimmunocytochemical (RICH) staining for gastrin in rat antral mucosa (a) and pancreatic polypeptide (PP) in cat pancreas (b). Note the presence of numerous gastrin cells covered with autoradiographic silver grains (indicating the site of reaction between the RICH complex, made from antigastrin antibodies and monoiodinated synthetic human gastrin, and tissue) in (a), and of a discrete PP cell in a ductule in the cat pancreas (demonstrated by a RICH complex made from antihuman PP antibodies and ^{125}I-labelled bovine PP).

A particularly amusing detail was that the specificity of the antisera was influenced by the use of a radiolabelled tracer. Thus, an antiserum raised to synthetic human gastrin-17 (As. 2604), was known to be specific for this hormone in radioimmunoassay systems employing ^{125}I-labelled synthetic human gastrin-17 as a tracer. However, when used for immunocytochemistry, employing immunofluorescence or PAP procedures, this antiserum reacted equally well with cholecystokinin (CCK) and gastrin. CCK possesses a COOH-terminal pentapeptide sequence in common with gastrin-17 and we therefore initially classified this antiserum as COOH-terminus-specific. This, however, failed to explain why As. 2604 showed only negligible cross-reactivity with CCK in a radioimmunoassay system. Use of As. 2604 together with ^{125}I-labelled synthetic human gastrin-17 in the RICH method revealed, that, in this method, the antiserum reacted only with gastrin-containing cells and not with CCK cells. We interpret these observations to indicate that use of trace quantities of ^{125}I-labelled gastrin picked out a population of antibodies with high avidity to gastrin and low avidity to CCK. Since the selected antibodies were of low avidity to the latter hormone, they may, to a slight degree, have reacted with it during incubation with tissue, but have since been washed away during the rinsing procedures. These results point to the fact that labelled antigen detection systems tend to select those antibodies which are of the highest avidity to the selected antigen. Such high-avidity antibodies are likely to interact less potently with related molecules and will, hence, give more specific localizations.

Despite these advantages, certain drawbacks were associated with the RICH method. Firstly, it was associated with the use of radioiodine and autoradiography, which made many workers hesitant to use it. Secondly, contrary to our initial expectations and results, it proved very difficult to use at the electron-microscopical level, since i.a. long autoradiographic exposures were necessary. We therefore decided to introduce an alternative technique, based on the principle of labelled antigen detection, but developed primarily for use at the electron-microscopical level (Larsson 1979). This method, the gold-labelled antigen detection (GLAD) technique, employs specific antigen absorbed to the surfaces of colloidal gold particles as a tracer. Sections are allowed to react with surplus amounts of antibodies, which results in the binding of only one of the two antigen-combining sites per antibody to tissue-bound antigen. The remaining site is, hence, free to react with specific antigen absorbed on the surfaces of colloidal gold granules. The site of the bound colloidal gold granules will identify the site of reaction between tissue-bound antigen and specific antibody (Figs. 11–13). Unspecific antibodies, being unable to bind specific antigen on the gold granules, will remain undetected. As in the RICH method, non-immunologic binding of specific antibodies to the sections is prevented by pretreatment with large excesses of normal serum from the same species as the one delivering the immune serum.

Colloidal gold granules may be manufactured in several, narrowly determined, sizes from 5 nm and upwards (Baigent and Müller 1980; Faulk and Taylor 1971; Frens 1973; Horrisberger 1979; Horrisberger and Rosset 1977; Zsigmondy 1889). By comparison, the size of the IgG molecule is $8 \times 5 \times 4$ nm (Nisonoff et al. 1975) and that of the PAP complex 22 nm (Sternberger 1974). Since several sizes of gold granules can be made, differently sized gold granules can be coated with different antigens and thus provide opportunities for the simultaneous localization of multiple antigens or of multiple antigenic regions at the electron-microscopical level.

Whereas proteins, antibodies and large antigens are directly absorbable to gold granules (cf. Faulk and Taylor 1971; Geoghegan and Ackerman 1977; Horrisberger and Rosset 1977; Romano et al. 1974, 1977; Schwaab et al. 1978), this is not possible

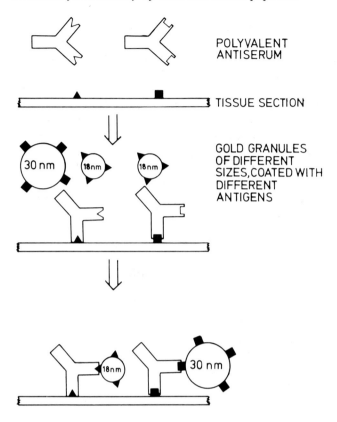

Fig. 11. Principle of the gold-labelled antigen detection (GLAD) method (cf. text).

with smaller antigens like peptide hormones. In the latter case it has, however, proven possible to conjugate the peptides to inert proteins like bovine serum albumin via glutaraldehyde or carbodiimide and thus make them absorbable to gold granules (Larsson 1979, see also Horrisberger et al. 1977). Provided appropriate controls are undertaken, this practice does not create problems since, firstly, virtually all peptide antisera are raised against the immunogen covalently coupled to an inert protein and, secondly, since the tissue material to be studied usually has been fixed in glutaraldehyde solutions. It is essential, however, to exclude cross-reactivity between the antibodies and the inert protein used for conjugation. This can be done by preabsorbing the antisera with excess amounts of the protein, preferably coupled to a solid support, like Sepharose. In addition, we have employed control gold granules, coated with glutaraldehyde-treated BSA alone or with irrelevant peptides coupled to BSA with glutaraldehyde, and have never found any unspecific staining.

The GLAD method has been used for direct staining of ultrathin sections, briefly etched in hydrogen peroxide. As mentioned above, plastic removal by hydrogen peroxide is not invariably necessary. Sections are first reacted with large amounts of normal serum from the same species as the one producing the antiserum and then with appropriate dilutions of the desired antisera. If desired, the antiserum may be diluted in normal (but hormone-free!) serum instead of buffer. After a short rinse in Tris-buffered saline, pH 7.4, the sections are floated on drops of antigen-coated gold

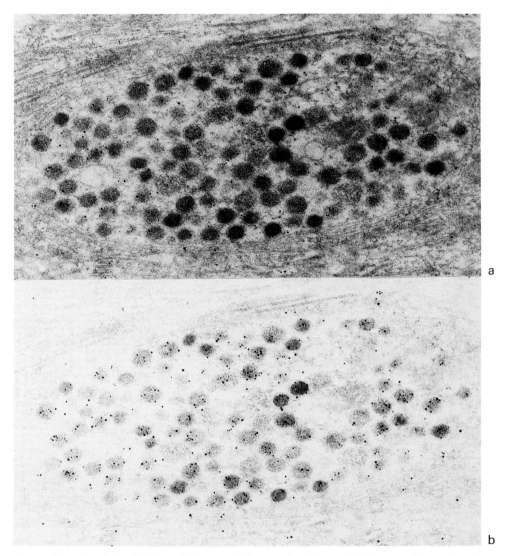

Fig. 12. Example of the GLAD method as applied to osmicated material. Electron-micrographs of an enkephalin immunoreactive nerve terminal of cat stomach stained with an enkephalin antiserum (cross-reacting with both met- and leu-enkephalin) and with leu-enkephalin-coated 12 nm colloidal gold particles. The micrograph has been reproduced in both a normal (a) and a light version (b) to illustrate both the excellent preservation of the enkephalin immunoreactive granular vesicles and the membranes, as well as the dense accumulation of gold particles (indicating sites of met-/leu-nekephalin immunoreactivity) over the granular vesicles. The specimen used was perfusion-fixed in formaldehyde-glutaraldehyde, postfixed in OsO_4 and embedded in Epon. Ultrathin sections, collected on Ni-grids, were etched for 10 min on H_2O_2 (cf. text) and stained according to the GLAD method. The postfixation in OsO_4 was necessary to obtain a clear ultrastructural definition of the granular vesicles and membranes.

granules, rinsed and postfixed with glutaraldehyde. Dried sections are finally contrasted with lead citrate and uranyl acetate – a practice which is not possible with immunoenzyme procedures. Technical details of the entire procedure are given in the Appendix.

We recommend the use of several controls in conjunction with the GLAD procedure:

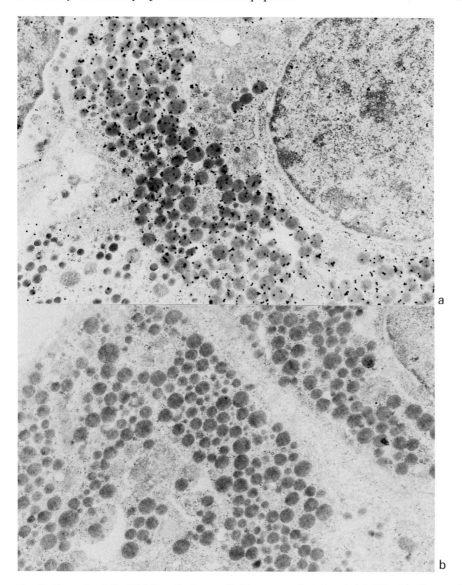

Fig. 13. Example of the GLAD method as applied to non-osmicated material. Ultrathin Epon sections of formaldehyde-glutaraldehyde-fixed rat pituitary were stained with anti-human growth hormone (HGH) antiserum and HGH-coated 18 nm colloidal gold particles (a) or, as a control, with HGH-preabsorbed antiserum and HGH-coated 18 nm colloidal gold particles (b). Note that most growth hormone immunoreactivity resides in the secretory granules of the somatotrophs and that preabsorption of the antiserum with HGH virtually eliminates staining.

1. use of antigen-coated colloidal gold granules, alone and in combination with irrelevant antisera;
2. use of antigen-inactivated antisera;
3. use of a blocking test: sections reacted with the primary antiserum are exposed to varying concentrations of free antigen (1-100 μg/ml) for 2 hours at room temperature before application of the antigen-coated gold granules.

Use of the first control is necessary, not least since recent studies have indicated that receptors for peptide hormones may survive processing for electron-microscopy. Such receptors may already have bound endogenous hormones or may bind hormone bound to antibodies or to colloidal gold granules. Such receptors will interfere in all immunocytochemical systems since, even in unabsorbed antisera, some antibodies will bind hormone that is either of endogenous origin or derived from the immunogen. Often rather elaborate procedures, involving i.a. the use of affinity-purified antisera, have to be used to detect such receptors. In the GLAD procedure, receptors may easily be detected by permitting the sections to react with peptide-coated gold granules alone. Conceivably, mixtures of peptide-coated gold granules and related free peptide fragments may be used to determine the specificity and degree of competition for such receptor sites. So far, we have not detected any receptors for the peptide hormones with which we have worked (ACTH, gastrin, caerulein, βendorphin, αMSH and βMSH). This may indicate that the tissues studied are devoid of receptors, that the receptors are destroyed during tissue processing or that they are unable to bind the peptides when conjugated to albumin. It should be noted that we have used the term 'receptor' in a rather loose sense in the above discussion. What we are dealing with could, more appropriately, be named 'binding sites' for peptides, since, so far, no correlation between the binding and a biological effect has been established. Recent elegant studies by Sternberger and colleagues on the binding of LH-RH to pituitary LH cells, has, however, provided compelling evidence for the existence of true receptors in at least these cells (see Sternberger 1979 and also Kurzon and Sternberger 1978).

The second recommended control is the equivalent to the absorption control in conventional immunocytochemistry. Since the specificity is probably better defined by the ability of the antibodies to bind the appropriate antigen-coated gold granules, this control may prove superfluous with time.

The third control is of great practical and theoretical value. It shows that free peptides may compete with peptides attached to colloidal gold granules for binding to the free antigen-combining sites. Depending upon the concentrations of free antigen and the time of exposure, reductions to total abolishment of binding of antigen-coated colloidal gold granules may be achieved. Incidentally, this control also forms an attractive way for testing the region-specificity of the antibodies. Thus, various synthetic peptide fragments may be allowed to compete with the antigen-coated gold granules for binding to the antibodies.

It would perhaps be expected that the dilutions of the primary antibodies would have to be low, in order to allow them to react with only one of their two antigen-combining sites. Practice showed us, however, that the dilutions are equal or better than those of conventional enzyme-labelled procedures and only slightly inferior to those of the PAP procedure. This economizes the use of antisera and leads to the suspicion that even in conventional immunocytochemistry many antibodies bind to tissue-bound antigen with only one of their two combining sites. Since, in ultrathin sections, tissue-bound antigens are in a fixed position, this may indicate that, for conformational reasons, many antibodies may actually be prevented from reacting with both of their combining sites.

By including trace amounts of radioiodinated peptide in the peptide solutions used for conjugation with BSA and, subsequently, for absorption to gold granules, the overall yield of peptide molecules per gold granule can be determined. Experiments involving the coupling of 'cold' (200 nmoles) and ^{125}I-labelled (100,000 cpm) ACTH (1–39) to BSA (60 nmoles) and then to 18 nm gold granules (100 ml suspension) showed that each gold granule was substituted with about 70 ACTH (1–39) molecules (Larsson

1979). Thus, theoretically, each gold granule could react with 70 antigen-combining sites. This is, however, not the case, since the size of the IgG molecule is $8 \times 5 \times 4$ nm (Nisonoff et al. 1975). Thus, for sterical reasons the reaction is restricted to only a few antigens per gold granule. Accordingly, we have prepared gold granules containing fewer antigen molecules (down to 10 per granule); these do not yield results inferior to those using more highly substituted gold granules.

It is likely that one single IgG molecule is sufficient to 'bridge' a gold granule to the section, but that at sites of high antigen concentrations more IgG molecules may bind one single gold granule. The size of the IgG molecules makes the reaction between one granule and more than a few IgG molecules unlikely.

Since the efficiency with which gold granules can be detected is much higher than that of e.g. enzyme-reaction products, the GLAD method may be used in conjunction with optimally fixed and contrasted electron-microscopy sections. The easy recognition of each gold granule, paired with the exceedingly low background, makes it probable that sites containing only single antigen molecules may be demonstrable.

Since each single gold granule is easily detected, it is possible to evaluate the degree of unspecific staining versus specific staining by counting gold granules. Thus, different cytoplasmic areas may be counted in stained sections and in control sections and, hence, this technique will allow a specificity discrimination.

It could be hypothesized that sites containing an abundance of densely packed antigen molecules would require lower dilutions of antibodies, since they would bind proportionately more antigen-combining sites than areas of lower antigen-desity. Practical results, however, have failed to confirm this. Firstly, cytoplasmic hormone-storing granules of endocrine cells store densely packed peptides and in such cells the appropriate GLAD method always results in the deposition of the largest number of gold granules over the cytoplasmic granules. Secondly, we have tried to study this potential problem by making preformed complexes between antigen-coated gold granules and their corresponding antibodies in such a way that free (residual) antigen-combining sites will stick out from the gold granules. Results with such preformed complexes would not be affected by variations in antigen-density. The preformed complexes, however, have yielded results equivalent to those of the sequential method in every instance so far tested.

Colloidal gold particles represent very attractive tracers for ultrastructural immunocytochemistry and related techniques. The mechanism whereby they absorb proteins and conjugates is not yet fully understood although some correlation to both the molecular weight (Horisberger et al. 1977) and to the isoelectric point of the protein (Geoghegan and Ackerman 1977) exists. Many proteins absorb best at a pH roughly equivalent to their isoelectric points and it may therefore be necessary to perform pH isotherm studies of the type suggested by Geoghegan and Ackerman (1977). Apart from peptide-albumin conjugates (Larsson 1979) a large variety of molecules have been absorbed to gold particles (protein A: Batten and Hopkins 1978, 1979; Geuze et al. 1981; Romano and Romano 1977; Roth et al. 1978; Slot and Geuze 1981; FITC-labelled protein A: Roth et al. 1980; immunoglobulins: Faulk and Taylor 1971; Geoghegan and Ackerman 1977; Horisberger 1979; Romano et al. 1974; tetanus toxin: Schwaab and Thoenen 1978; horseradish peroxidase: Geoghegan et al. 1977; lectins: Horisberger and Rosset 1977; Horisberger 1979; and several other molecules cf. Geoghegan and Ackerman 1977; Horisberger 1979 for reviews).

6. CONTROLS AND EVALUATION OF RESULTS

It is convenient to subdivide immunocytochemical staining results into three categories: wanted, specific staining; unwanted, specific staining and unspecific staining. The first of these categories refers to staining of the intended antigen, the second to staining of other antigens by contaminating antibodies and the third category to non-immunologic staining of tissue structures by e.g. Fc binding, complement-mediated binding, overlabelled conjugates, protein absorption etc.

Immunologic cross-reactivity hence enters the first category. As pointed out earlier, antibodies only recognize between 3 and 8 amino acid residues of polypeptide antigens. If the sequence and conformation of these residues are not unique to that peptide, the antibodies will ('cross'-)react with other molecules containing the same structure. Nevertheless, the antibodies are highly specific for the structure they bind to. Thus, antibodies reacting with the C-terminal pentapeptide portion of gastrin will also react with cholecystokinin (CCK), which contains the identical C-terminal sequence. All work on localization of CCK neurons in the brain, spinal cord and periphery is actually based on the use of such 'cross-reacting' antibodies. Not only would it be unfair to CCK neuroimmunocytochemists to refer to their results as 'unwanted, specific', but also scientifically incorrect. No antiserum can be assumed to be specific to anything but the structure it binds to. This truism seems to be the hardest lesson to learn in immunocytochemistry. Antisera raised against e.g. leu-enkephalin (Tyr-Gly-Gly-Phe-Leu) are, hence, customarily referred to as leu-enkephalin antisera and the structures they demonstrate as 'leu-enkephalin-like immunoreactivity'. If proper tests of many of these antisera were carried out, it would be found that the term 'leu-enkephalin-like immunoreactivity' may include everything from β-endorphin, α-neoendorphin, dynorphin and met-enkephalin to leu-enkephalin. Common to all these peptides is the sequence Tyr-Gly-Gly-Phe and properly the antibodies should therefore be referred to as 'anti-Tyr-Gly-Gly-Phe antibodies'. Such designations, of course, are entirely impractical, but on the other hand, the designation of so many different molecules as leu-enkephalin-like immunoreactive will create misunderstandings among the many scientists who are not daily exposed to the traumas of immunological nomenclature. A reasonable compromise for the immunocytochemist is to spell out in his paper the uncertainty of the specificity of the localization. As a frequent reviewer of immunocytochemical papers, I wish to emphasize that such statements are looked upon with much more sympathy than are boasting declarations of 'specificity', unsupported by sufficient experimental data.

Instead of the above, sometimes necessary, compromise, it is, of course, better to narrow the possible spectrum of molecules that might contribute to the '-like immunoreactivity'. This can be achieved by: (a) testing antisera against all possibly reactive peptides in cytochemical models and by differential absorption controls and (b) by the use of multiple antisera having specificities to different regions of the molecule to be studied (region-specific antisera) (Larsson and Rehfeld 1977; Larsson 1981a). Combined use of well-characterized region-specific antisera may clearly identify tissue-bound immunoreactivity. Hence, no antibody in itself can be assumed to be specific for a given antigen, but combined use of many antisera recognizing different parts of the antigen may very closely approximate the truth.

6.1 FIRST LEVEL (SPECIFICITY) CONTROLS

These controls aim at examining the specificity of interaction between the antigen-combining sites of the antibodies and tissue-bound antigens. Thus, if an antiserum contains two antibody populations, anti-X and anti-Y, absorption of the antiserum with highly purified or synthetic X will block staining of antigenic site X in the tissue, while Y will remain stained. Now imagine a third antigen, Z, which also binds ('cross-reacts') to the anti-X antibodies. Also this antigen will be stained if present in the tissue sections and undamaged by fixation and tissue processing. If the anti-X antibodies are of homogeneous specificity, absorption of the antiserum with either X or Z will block staining of both X and Z in tissue (whereas Y will remain stained). If, on the other hand, only a subpopulation of the anti-X antibodies will bind Z, absorptions against this peptide will block staining of sites containing Z, but not of sites containing X, whereas absorptions against X will block sites of both X and Z immunoreactivity. Thus, by multiple absorptions of the type outlined, the specificity of an antiserum can be determined. This stategy, however, requires that the antigens in question are known and available in pure, preferably synthetic, form. The reliability of absorption or specificity controls (like that of RIA) stands and falls with the purity of the peptides available!

Imagine a fourth binding site (C) in the tissue. This site is not an antigen, but can fix antibodies e.g. by Fc binding, protein absorption etc. Absorption of the above antiserum with X + Y will eliminate staining of sites X and Y. Staining of C will, however, remain unperturbed, since staining of this site occurs through sites different from the (occupied) antigen-combining sites on the antibodies. Hence, absorption controls will identify staining of C as unspecific staining or as contributed by an unknown antibody population. Staining (second level) controls must be carried out to determine whether staining of C is caused by contaminating antibodies or by other mechanisms.

Pitfalls of first level controls are in reality few, as long as we remember the rule that, with a given antigen-antibody system, these controls only aim at showing that the antibodies specifically recognize an antigenic site common to the tissue-bound antigen and the antigen used for absorption and do not necessarily imply identity between these two. A few possible sources of error have, however, been reported to occur. Foremost of these is the presence of receptors for the peptides used for absorption (Sternberger and Hoffman 1978; Sternberger and Petrali 1975). Such receptors may, hence, in selected instances, bind the peptide while attached to the antibodies and produce false negative absorption controls. This can be circumvented by using the peptides coupled to a solid phase, like Sepharose beads, prior to absorption. These beads will specifically extract the antibodies from the immune serum and will, hence, not give problems with receptor-binding. Additionally, many immune sera contain proteolytic enzymes that may degrade peptides used for absorptions. This too, may result in false negative outcomes and can also be circumvented by using solid-phase absorptions and addition of protease inhibitors (Larsson and Stengaard-Pedersen 1981). Usually, this mechanism is of little significance, but has been noted with enkephalins which may be degraded by serum enzymes both during absorption and during incubations with tissue sections. Other possible, but less well proven shortcomings of absorption controls have been reported elsewhere (reviewed in Larsson 1981a). These shortcomings, however, are in practice very few and often insignificant and should not be used as an excuse for not performing specificity controls. If doubt arises, additional controls that may support or refute the results of absorption controls are (a) cytochemical model systems and (b) extraction and chemical characterization of the antigen investigated.

Absorption controls are customarily carried out by adding varying concentrations of the peptide(s) to be tested (e.g. 0.1, 1, 10 and 100 μg per ml diluted antiserum) and incubate for, at least, 24–48 hours at 4°C before use (in order to attain binding equilibrium). Solid-phase absorptions are carried out with the peptides covalently linked to Sepharose 4B beads (cyanogen bromide-activated, Pharmacia, Uppsala, Sweden) and to incubate an excess of Sepharose-bound peptide (5-100 μg/ml) with diluted antiserum for 24–48 hours at 4°C. Thereafter the depleted antiserum is harvested by centrifugation and removal from the beads (from which affinity-purified antibodies can be regained). Use of one or the other type of control depends on what problem is to be studied. However, in the case of monoclonal antibodies, liquid-phase absorptions are most desirable, since extractions of specific antibodies with the solid phase method will leave only pure buffer! Thus, such 'buffer controls' will not tell us whether the binding of the monoclonals to tissue was due to specific or unspecific reactions with the antibodies.

6.2. SECOND LEVEL (STAINING) CONTROLS

Apart from absorption controls, several types of second level controls are necessary to perform. These include:
1. omission of the first antibody layer (primary or 'peptide' antiserum);
2. omission of the second antibody layer (in indirect methods);
3. omission of the third antibody layer (in e.g. the PAP method);
4. omission of all antibodies;
5. replacement of the first antibody layer with non-immune (or pre-immune) serum or with another unrelated antiserum;
6. in direct techniques; application of unlabelled antibodies first, followed by the labelled antibodies ('blocking test').

Second level controls provide us with no information about the specificity of interaction between the primary antibodies and tissue-bound antigens, but are essential for evaluating the quality of the immunocytochemical systems. They, hence, assess the quality of the tissue preparations (presence of autofluorescence and endogenous enzyme activity) and evaluate the performance of the detection systems (presence of e.g. free fluorescent dyes, overlabelled conjugates, cross-reactivity between second and third layer antibodies with tissue constituents). Without negative second level controls, reliable immunocytochemistry is impossible. These controls may, however, never replace the use of first-level controls, although this has been the practice also of recent investigators.

In the case of monoclonal antibodies, replacement of specific antibodies with the same concentration of non-sense antibodies (e.g. anti-DNP) represents a valuable control. Nevertheless, since different antibodies differ in physicochemical properties, it is advisable also to perform (liquid phase) absorption controls (vide supra).

6.3. HOW TO DEAL WITH UNWANTED STAINING

As mentioned introduction-wise, unwanted staining can result either from immunological or non-immunological (absorption) phenomena. In the case of immunological unwanted staining, the strategy must be to: (a) use as pure (synthetic) antigens as possible for immunization; (b) use as highly diluted antisera as possible (in the hope that the titer of the wanted antibodies is much higher than that of the unwanted ones); and (c) if necessary, determine the specificities of the unwanted antibodies and remove these by affinity absorption. Obviously, these strategies are not applicable to all antisera. In these instances, use of the labelled antigen detection (RICH and GLAD and variants thereof) methods is strongly recommended, since these methods select only specific, desired antibodies out of a soup of unwanted antibodies, irrespective of titers and specificities of the latter. Monoclonal antibodies will not give rise to immunological unwanted staining, but may produce cross-reactivity (vide supra) or non-immunological unwanted staining.

Quite often, it is found that antisera to a given peptide contain multiple subpopulations of antibodies, reacting with different regions of the same antigen. If synthetic peptide fragments are available, this can easily be determined by the above-mentioned paper cytochemical model system (Larsson 1981b). Such antisera can be depleted of one or the other subpopulation by differential absorption against the corresponding peptide fragment and, hence, be employed as excellent region-specific detection reagents.

Non-immunological staining may arise from multiple types of interactions including protein absorption, Fc binding, complement-mediated binding, overlabelled conjugates etc. Additionally, tissue autofluorescence and endogenous peroxidase activity may obscure the staining results. The second level controls outlined will disclose whether the tissue properties (autofluorescence, enzymes) or the first, second (or third) layer of antibodies is the cause of such unspecificity. Since many neuroimmunocytochemists employ the same second and/or third layer reagents on the same tissue for years, it is often found that the primary antiserum is the cause.

Many primary antisera differ so much in their properties that, even at the same IgG concentration, one may yield strong unspecific staining, whereas another does not give unspecific staining at all. This invalidates the use of a pre-immune or 'non-immune' serum control as the only specificity control! This also makes it naïve to state that over a certain dilution (e.g. 1:5000), only immunological staining is seen. Although, admittedly, the degree of unspecific staining decreases with dilution, this varies too much between antisera to allow setting of dilution limits.

Strategies to avoid or reduce non-immunological staining include:

1. To exclude presence of autofluorescence or endogenous peroxidase activity in tissue. If such interference is present, changes in fixation technique, blocking of peroxidase activity or change of immunocytochemical detection system (fluorescence/peroxidase/radioactivity) should be attempted.
2. Counter-staining. This is mainly used in immunofluorescence to mask weaker 'background' staining and autofluorescence. Unfortunately, counterstaining can also mask specific staining and should usually be refrained from. For preparation of spectacular colour-slides, counter-staining of FITC-specimens with Evans blue produces a vivid red background that emphasizes histological detail. This should, however, only be used for illustrative, as opposed to investigative, purposes.
3. Dilution. As mentioned above, antisera should be used at as high dilution as possible without sacrificing sensitivity.
4. Detergents. As introduced by Hartman et al. (1972), use of Triton X-100 (Sigma) in antisera (0.3—0.4%) and washing solutions (1% strongly reduces unspecific staining. We only add triton to washing solutions and not to the antisera, since this seems to produce as good results. An exception is vibratome sections, where addition of triton to the antisera apparently assists penetration as well (Pickel et al. 1976).

5. Preconditioning of sections. All sections, particularly Epon sections, strongly absorb all types of proteins (Sternberger 1974; Moriarty 1976). If the sections are first exposed to inert protein, absorption of later applied proteins is reduced. It is therefore advisable to precondition sections with exposure to 10-30% normal serum or to serum albumin (Moriarty 1976; Sternberger 1974; see also Zehr 1978). In selected instances, albumin is preferred since serum is much richer in proteolytic enzymes that may modify and destroy tissue-bound antigens. In indirect methods (including PAP), serum from the same species as that producing the second layer of antibodies can be used. In labelled antigen detection techniques, serum from the same species as that producing the primary antibodies is used (Larsson and Schwartz 1977; Larsson 1979). Pretreatment with serum, apart from quenching unspecific protein absorption, may also reduce Fc and complement-mediated binding.

6. Differential avidity elution. A common characteristic to all antigen-antibody reactions is their high avidity (i.e. binding energy), usually in the 10^{10}—10^{15} l/mol range. It is therefore often almost impossible to elute antibodies from already immunocytochemically stained sections by reagents like urea or glycine-HCl buffers (cf. the section on double-staining). In contrast, unspecific non-immunological staining is of much lower avidity. We (Larsson and Eriksen: to be published) have therefore recently developed a technique, in which sections after staining are exposed to 2 M urea (in distilled water) for 30 min. Subsequently, they are thoroughly rinsed in buffer and mounted (immunofluorescence) or developed (immunoperoxidase, RICH). With 14 different antisera, urea concentrations could be increased up to 8 M and the time to 2 hours without loss of staining. With one antiserum to somatostatin, however, 8 M urea for 2 hours produced some loss of fine nerve terminals in rat cerebral cortex. As tested on the paper cytochemical models, the urea treatment did not increase the minimal detectable amount of peptide (varying from 100 pg to 10 ng with the antisera tested). Treatment of the sections with 2 M urea for 30 min completely eliminated background staining even with low antiserum dilutions and this concentration was therefore selected.

We believe that the differential avidity elution method is a useful method when problems with unspecific staining have arisen. Since some cross-reactive antibodies have low avidities, these may also be washed away by graded urea treatment. In the case of some CCK antibodies, we have experimental data supporting this notion. Urea treatment should always be used with great care and results be compared to results obtained with non-urea-treated sections!

7. ASSOCIATED TECHNIQUES

7.1. DEMONSTRATION OF MULTIPLE ANTIGENS

It is often desirable to demonstrate more than one antigen within the same cell or nerve terminal (cell identification, transmitter coexistence). Numerous methods are available for this, but we will concentrate on a few well-documented techniques here (for a more complete review see Larsson, 1981a).

Adjacent section technique

With the aid of an ultramicrotome it is possible to cut serial adjacent plastic sections that are thin enough to contain parts of the same cell or nerve terminal (Lange 1971). Section thickness is usually at 0.3—1.0 μm, but, if immunofluorescence is used, ultrathin sections can be used. Sections are mounted on glass slides and subsequently stained as desired. Adjacent ultrathin sections can be cut simultaneously, mounted on grids and contrasted for electron-microscopical identification of immunoreactive structures (Fig. 14). With non-osmicated plastic sections mounted on glass slides, plastic (Epon or Araldite) may be removed by a concentrated solution of KOH in absolute ethanol (aged until it attains a cognac-like colour) (Lane and Europa 1965; Maxwell 1978). With osmicated sections, this is followed by exposure to periodic acid (1%, 5—10 min) to remove osmium stain (Beauvillain et al. 1975). Details for staining Epon/Araldite sections are given in the Appendix.

Double-staining procedures

Only three methods will be discussed: (a) Indirect immunofluorescence. If the primary antisera are raised in different animals (e.g. rabbit and guinea pig or mouse) and if species-specific fluorochromed second layer antibodies are available (e.g. TRITC-labelled anti-rabbit IgG and FITC-labelled anti-guinea pig IgG), this method is one of the most simple and best double-staining procedures. Note that second layer antibodies frequently not are species-specific. Unknown batches must always be cross-tested (e.g.

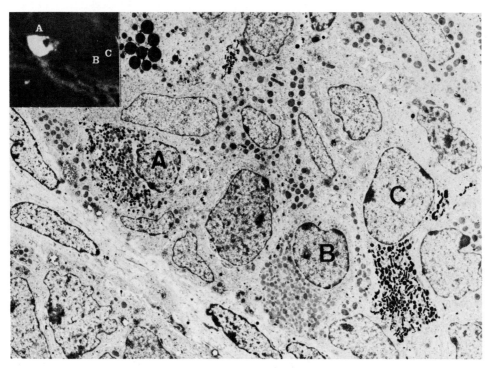

Fig. 14. Adjacent section technique for ultrastructural identification of immunoreactive structures. Of two serial adjacent sections of fetal human duodenum, the first was immunocytochemically stained for gastrin/CCK immunoreactivity using the CCK[30-33]-specific antibody 4562 and FITC-labelled goat anti-rabbit IgG (inset). The second section was conventionally contrasted after mounting on a Cu-grid. One immunofluorescent cell (A) corresponds to a characteristically granulated cell in the electron-micrograph, whereas two other types of granule-containing cells (B, C) are devoid of immunoreactivity.

test primary guinea pig IgG against FITC-labelled anti-rabbit IgG and vice versa). Sometimes, second layer antibodies may be rendered species-specific by differential absorption (absorb FITC-labelled anti-guinea pig IgG with rabbit IgG and vice versa). Unfortunately, most primary antisera are raised in the same species, necessitating use of alternative methods.

(b) Mixed sensitivity staining (Fig. 15). Since the PAP method is more sensitive than indirect immunofluorescence, it is possible to dilute primary antibodies more for PAP detection than for immunofluorescence (by a factor 5—10). This means, that at optimal dilutions, primary antibodies used in the PAP procedure are below the detection limit of indirect immunofluorescence. It is, hence, possible to stain a section first with the PAP procedure and then with indirect immunofluorescence (Larsson 1981a). This method is extremely useful when the two antigens occur in separate structures (cells, terminals or granules). It can also be used with antigens occurring in the same structure, but then requires reversal of the staining sequence and multiple controls. Its main use is, hence, for demonstrating relationships between different immunoreactive structures.

(c) Peroxidase double-staining methods: Antigen A is demonstrated by immunoperoxidase or PAP techniques. Subsequent to development with diaminobenzidine (DAB), antibodies (but not the reaction product) are eluted from the section. Many different elution methods have been described, but, in our experience, the only reliable is that of Tramu et al. (1978). Note, however, that this method may damage some antigens (e.g. antigenic sites containing tryptophan, methionine and disulfide groups) (Larsson 1981a). Subsequent to elution, the sections are exposed to anti-rabbit IgG and PAP complexes (or peroxidase-conjugates, depending upon what is to be used in the second step). Peroxidase activity is now developed with a substrate giving another colour than DAB (4-Cl-1-naphtol or 3-amino-9-ethylcarbazole). No peroxidase activity should be demonstrable in successfully eluted sections. If negative, sections are now stained for antigen B by the desired (PAP or immunoperoxidase) procedure and development with 4-Cl-1-naphtol (Vandesande et al. 1975, 1976) or 3-amino-9-ethylcarbazole (Graham et al. 1965). This method demonstrates two antigens in different colours. Again, difficulties may arise with antigens occurring in the same structures. Such antigens are best studied by sequential staining.

Fig. 15. Double-staining for met- and leu-enkephalin immunoreactivity in cat stomach using the mixed sensitivity method. A cryosection from gastric muscle wall of a formalin-perfused cat was first stained for met-enkephalin immunoreactivity using leu-enkephalin-preabsorbed met-enkephalin antiserum and the PAP method (a and b) and was thereafter stained for leu-enkephalin immunoreactivity using indirect immunofluorescence (c). The result shows clearly that some leu-enkephalin immunofluorescent cell bodies (arrow) and terminals are not stained in the preceding PAP procedure and, hence, are devoid of detectable met-enkephalin immunoreactivity. It is, however, not possible to tell from this picture whether the met-enkephalin immunoreactive (PAP stained) cell bodies and terminals contain leu-enkephalin or not, since the peroxidase reaction product may mask immunofluorescence of the PAP stained structures. In other experiments, however, reversal of the staining sequence (staining for leu-enkephalin with the PAP method and then for met-enkephalin with indirect immunofluorescence) showed that some neurons were met-enkephalin immunoreactive and leu-enkephalin unreactive. Hence, these results allowed the conclusion that the gut contained some exclusively met-enkephalin immunoreactive neurons and some exclusively leu-enkephalin immunoreactive neurons. However, the possible occurrence of neurons containing both met- and leu-enkephalin immunoreactants cannot be confirmed or refuted by this technique, but requires sequential staining procedures (see Fig. 16).

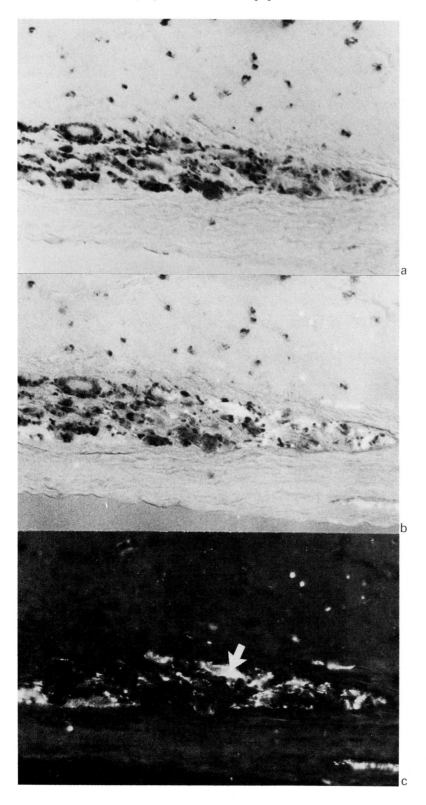

Sequential-staining procedures

Antigen A is demonstrated by any desired procedure (indirect immunofluorescence, immunoperoxidase, PAP; with the latter two methods an ethanol-soluble peroxidase reaction product should be formed, e.g. by use of the substrates 4-Cl-1-naphtol or 3-amino-9-ethylcarbazole). Staining results are documented by photography and, subsequently, antibodies are eluted by the procedure of Tramu et al. (1978). If a peroxidase procedure has been used, the ethanol-soluble reaction product is eluted after or simultaneously with the antibodies (e.g. by exposure to 70%, 96% and absolute ethanol). Subsequently, the sections are exposed to the second (and, if applicable, third) layer antibodies that are to be used in the second staining step. These reagents should not produce staining (fluorescence/peroxidase) of successfully eluted and destained sections. If completely negative, the sections may now be stained for antigen B using the desired method and results compared to the previously taken photographs (Fig. 16). Note again that the elution procedure may destroy or modify certain antigens. This can be tested on cytochemical paper models, but it is always useful to run parallel sections (e.g. one first stained for antigen A and the second first stained for antigen B).

Double-staining at the ultrastructural level

We have for some years employed the GLAD method for this purpose. Differently sized gold particles (e.g. 5 nm, 12 nm, 18 nm and 30 nm) can be fabricated and coated with different antigens (Larsson 1979). Ultrathin sections are stained by the desired antisera (in sequence or as mixture) and are then exposed to the corresponding gold particles (in sequence or as a mixture). Since only specific antibodies will react with their corresponding antigen on the gold particles, the staining can be carried out in only two steps. Controls are the same as those recommended for the GLAD method (vide supra). It is imperative for the success of this method that the gold particles used are of a very narrow size range and easily can be distinguished under the electron-microscope. This must be determined by mixing varying proportions of the two sizes of gold particles that are to be used and check the mixtures by counting in the electron-microscope. Recently, Slot et al. (1981) devised a very worthwhile method for sizing gold particles on sucrose or glycerol gradients.

7.2. COMBINATIONS WITH FORMALDEHYDE-INDUCED FLUORESCENCE METHODS

It is often desirable to combine results from formaldehyde-induced fluorescence of biogenic monoamines and fluorogenic peptides with immunocytochemistry. Thus, relations between monoaminergic and peptidergic pathways can be studied and coexistence of monoamines and peptides in neurons and endocrine (APUD) cells may be revealed.

Since the isoquinoline or β-carboline structures formed from the reaction between formaldehyde and monoamines are small and easily soluble, it is very hard to preserve these in sections that are sufficiently affixed to slides to allow subsequent immunocytochemical staining. Thus, sections which in any way come into contact with water will immediately loose fluorophores formed from the formaldehyde reaction. Previously, we have circumvented this problem by using a hyperosmolar solution of

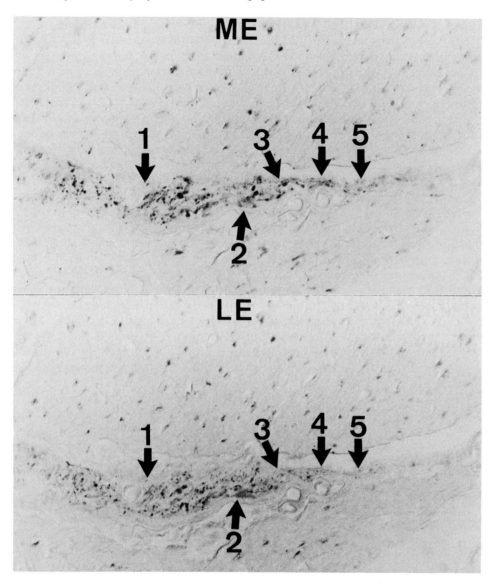

Fig. 16. Sequential staining for met-enkephalin (ME) (a) and leu-enkephalin (LE) (b) immunoreactivity in a cryosection of cat stomach wall. Careful comparisons between the two pictures show that several met-enkephalin immunoreactive terminals are also leu-enkephalin immunoreactive, but that, in addition, some exclusively met-enkephalin immunoreactive (e.g. regions 1, 3, 4, 5) and exclusively leu-enkephalin immunoreactive terminals (e.g. region 2) exist. This section was stained by selective immunocytochemical procedures for detecting met- and leu-enkephalin, respectively, using the PAP method and development in 3-amino-9-ethylcarbazole. Antibodies were eluted by the procedure of Tramu et al. (1978) (cf. text).

glycerine and gelatine in buffer to affix sections to slides. This resulted in very little diffusion of formaldehyde-induced fluorophores which therefore could be photographed prior to immunocytochemical staining (Larsson et al. 1976). Some diffusion was, however, often noticed. We have therefore started using an improved technique (Larsson, unpublished):

Tissues are freeze-dried and exposed to formaldehyde vapours according to the classical Falck-Hillarp method or variations thereof (Björklund et al. 1972, Chapter II). After embedding in paraffin in vacuo, sections are cut at 3—10 μm and floated out on slides coated with glycerin-gelatin. For flotation and stretching of sections, a mixture of 3% glutaraldehyde and 2% formaldehyde (see Appendix) is used. Sections are stretched on this solution by holding them against a hot-plate (40—45°C). Subsequently, they are allowed to lie on the slides for 5 min and are then blotted by a filter paper moistened with water. After exposure to formaldehyde gas (80°C, 1 hr in a closed one l jar containing 5—7 g of paraformaldehyde), sections are mounted in Entellan® (Merck), xylene or paraffin oil and are photographed in the fluorescence microscope. This affixing method results in no diffusion of monoamines from neurons or endocrine cells, which can be checked easily by comparisons to sections not affixed to slides. Subsequently, cover slips and mounting media are removed in xylene, sections hydrated in descending ethanols and buffer and immunocytochemically stained. All immunocytochemical staining procedures can be employed. Immunofluorescence, however, necessitates use of TRITC-labelled antibodies, since some of the formaldehyde-induced fluorophores are so firmly fixed to cells and neurons that they will withstand even the prolonged washing necessary for immunocytochemistry. It is possible that the glutaraldehyde-formaldehyde mixture used for stretching the sections acts by cross-linking the isoquinolines/β-carbolines already formed (by the reaction between formaldehyde and monoamines) to tissue proteins. No novel fluorophores seem to be formed in the sense that the spectral properties of the formaldehyde-induced fluorophores are the same in affixed and non-affixed sections (this, however, is as yet only based on visual impressions and filter changes!).

It is advisable to use a fume cupboard for stretching sections on slides since the vapours formed from the warmed glutaraldehyde-formaldehyde mixture are hazardous.

7.3. MODIFICATIONS OF TISSUE-BOUND ANTIGENS

Peptide chemists have access to a large arsenal of reagents which specifically modify certain amino acid residues in peptides and proteins (see Becker 1975 for review). Conceivably, these could be employed as very useful reagents for confirming specificity in peptide immunocytochemistry. We have thus employed cyanogen bromide and oxidation-induced destruction of methionine residues to differentiate between sites of leucine- and methionine-enkephalin immunoreactivities using cross-reactive antisera (Larsson et al., 1979). This strategy may be applicable also to other problems where closely related antigenic sites must be differentiated.

Most hormonal and neuronal peptides are synthesized as larger precursors which subsequently undergo multiple proteolytic cleavages to yield terminal secretory products. Most of our antisera are raised to the terminal products and often require a free N- or C-terminal amino acid or a specific derivatization for reaction. Consequently, they may be unable to react with precursor peptides. To some extent proteolytic enzymes have been employed for making such precursors demonstrable by specific antisera (Ravazzola and Orci, 1980). Additionally, assorted proteolytic enzymes have been used for making antigens 'masked' by formaldehyde and paraffin/resin embedding demonstrable (Curran and Gregory 1977; Denk et al. 1977; Finley et al. 1978; Huang et al. 1976; Reading 1977). The scientific foundation of the latter practice is uncertain although recent work indicates that such methods work by (1) splitting reaction products between plastic monomers and protein antigens (Takamiya 1978) or (2) releasing antigenic sites caught in antigenically uncomfortable conformations induced by fixation and embedding.

7.4. CORRELATION TO CHEMICAL AND PHYSIOLOGICAL INFORMATION

Since antibodies only recognize limited portions of their corresponding antigen, the specificity of an immunocytochemical reaction is always open to doubt. Although the situation is much improved by use of region-specific antibodies it is highly commendable to correlate the data obtained with chemical and physiological information. It needs emphasizing, however, that the 'immunocytochemical despair', i.e. the feeling that immunocytochemical results are notoriously uncertain, is totally unfounded. Critical immunocytochemical studies using sets of region-specific antibodies, well-proven techniques and well-founded interpretations of the results have probably more than any other type of studies provided us with outstanding novel and, sometimes, controversial information, It may be sobering to undertake a cost-benefit analysis of immunocytochemistry in order to realize that many of the controversial results reported 5—10 years ago now are part of the general biological knowledge and form the basis for numerous subsequent biochemical and physiological studies. Provided established methods and appropriate controls are undertaken, the only worthless immunocytochemical results are the negative ones. Thus, since so many factors (fixation, embedding, mounting, buffers, antibody specificity, sensitivity, dilutions etc.) can influence an immunocytochemical reaction only positive results can be considered. Immunocytochemistry, hence, by definition, cannot exclude the presence of a given molecule.

Another shortcoming of immunocytochemistry is its inability to determine the size and charge of antigens. Although certain region-specific antibodies may be specific for certain N- or C-terminal amino acids or for derivatized amino acids, it is often impossible to tell whether a precursor or a terminal secretory product is present at a certain site.

These shortcomings may be overcome by combining immunocytochemistry with chemical techniques. In the past, radioimmunoassay techniques have often been employed for supplementing immunocytochemical data. These techniques have allowed extracted antigens to be separated by gel filtration, electrophoresis, ion-exchange chromatography and, more recently, by high performance liquid chromatography and have thus provided a better chemical information. Due to their high sensitivity, radioimmunoassay techniques will no doubt continue to be a useful adjunct to immunocytochemistry.

Recent developments, above all with respect to cytochemical paper models (Larsson 1981b), have, however, provided the immunocytochemist with a new tool for characterizing extractable antigens. Thus, chromatographical fractions can be immobilized on filter paper strips that later are immunocytochemically stained. In our hands, these procedures have, with the best antisera available, a sensitivity down to 100 pg per spot. Additionally, methods for staining polyacrylamide gels (SDS gels, gradient gels and isoelectric focussing gels) have been devised using either staining of the gel per se or of replicas thereof (Adair et al. 1978; Van Raamsdonk et al. 1977).

8. APPENDIX

1. Carbodiimide coupling of peptide to carrier protein (Sofroniew et al. 1978)

a. 2.4 mg synthetic ACTH[1-23] and 15 mg bovine thyroglobulin are dissolved in 450 μl water.
b. 150 μl of freshly prepared 1-ethyl-3-(3-dimethyl-aminopropyl)carbodiimide (23 mg/5ml water) is added (gives a molar ratio peptide:thyroglobulin:carbodiimide of 60:1:112). Incubate for 18 h at room temperature.
c. add 600 μl 1.0 M hydroxylamine and incubate for 5 h at room temperature:
d. for immunization, emulsify the conjugate in 2 ml Freund's adjuvant: for the first 8 injections use complete adjuvant, thereafter incomplete. Give multiple intradermal injections and let the first injection be accompanied by BCG- and pertussis-vaccine. Give pertussis-vaccine also for the 2nd-4th injection.

Note: the method is said to produce a conjugation efficiency of 15-40%. It has been documented to be highly successful for raising antibodies to arginine-vasopressin and ACTH and has also given high-quality antisera to LHRH, oxytocin and secretin. Many modifications of the method are possible, including conjugation to other proteins like bovine serum albumin; dialysis of the conjugate prior to point 4 and omission of the vaccines. The outcomes of these modifications have not been tested. The author immunized his animals with 2 week intervals with 3 month pauses between the 4th and 5th and 8th and 9th injection. All animals surviving beyond the 4th injection produced antisera. The authors ascribe the success to the high antigenicity of thyroglobulin paired with their use of repeated multiple intradermal injections of low doses of antigen. The conjugate prepared was divided among 6 rabbits.

2. Glutaraldehyde coupling of peptide to carrier protein (Clement-Jones et al. 1980)

a. Dissolve 500 μg met-O-enkephalin and 5 mg bovine thyroglobulin in 2.5 ml 0.05 M sodium phosphate buffer pH 7.4.
b. Add 12 μl 20 per cent glutaraldehyde; incubate at room temperature for 30 min.
c. Dialyze for 48 hr against 2 changes of distilled water; freeze-dry if necessary to reduce volume.

3. Purification of IgG by affinity chromatography and preparation of F(ab)$_2$ fragments (after Goding 1976)

a. Swell protein A-Sepharose (Pharmacia, Uppsala, Sweden) in phosphate buffered saline (PBS; 0.02 M phosphate, 0.13 M NaCl, 0.05% merthiolate, adjust pH to 7.4) to obtain 5 ml swollen gel (1 g dry gel gives 3—3.5 ml swollen gel).
b. Pack the gel in a 10 ml disposable syringe, containing a nylon net at its bottom (to support the gel beads); when not in use store column at 4°C equilibrated with PBS. Connect polyethylene tubing to the tip of the syringe.
c. Attach a UV-absorption monitor to the column.
d. Wash column with 20 ml PBS; allow the buffer to reach the surface of the gel; then stop the column by a clamp.
e. Apply 10 ml rabbit antiserum and allow it to run into the column (at about 50 ml/hr) by removing the clamp; when the last serum has reached the top of the gel wash the sides of the column above the gel with 5 ml PBS and allow the column to run until the buffer surface reaches the top of the gel.
f. Wash the column with PBS until the UV monitor does not register any more protein coming out from the column. The wash is generally complete after 40 ml PBS.
g. Allow the washing buffer to reach the top of the gel and elute IgG with 0.58% (v:v) glacial acetic acid in 0.15 M NaCl. When elution is complete (as seen by the fall of the protein peak

on the UV monitor), wash the column with 20 ml PBS. The IgG eluate (typically 10 ml, containing ~ 6.0 mg IgG/ml) is dialyzed overnight at 4°C against pH 9.3 carbonate/bicarbonate buffer (17.3 g $NaHCO_3$ plus 8.6 g Na_2CO_3 in 1 l distilled water).

Note: The above procedure is very helpful when preparing IgG for fluorescent or enzyme labelling. Note that IgG of all species will not bind to protein A*. The same 5 ml column is said to be reusable for 50 times with no noticeable deterioration. The column may also be used for obtaining pure IgG for preparation of $F(ab)_2$ fragments; in this case the eluate is dialyzed overnight against 0.2 M acetate buffer, pH 4.5 (37 ml 0.2 M sodium acetate plus 63 ml 0.2 M acetic acid) instead of against carbonate buffer. After dialysis pepsin is added at a ratio of 10 mg pepsin per gram IgG. Digest at 37°C for 12 hr and terminate by dialysis against PBS. Apply the digest to the protein A column; since protein A binds the Fc fragment the $F(ab)_2$ fragments will pass through the column and can be collected. Undigested IgG and Fc fragments can then be eluted with acetic acid as in point g to regenerate the column (Goding 1976).

4. Fluorescein isothiocyanate-labelling and rhodamine isothiocyanate-labelling of proteins (modified from Nairn 1976 and Sternberger 1974)

a. IgG (e.g. from point 3) or other protein to be labelled is dissolved in 0.2 M Na_2HPO_4.
b. Fluorescein isothiocyanate (FITC) is dissolved immediately prior to use in 0.1 M Na_2HPO_4. For IgG use 12.5 μg FITC/mg IgG and for avidin (Mw = 68 300) use 30 μg FITC/mg. Thus, for 1 mg avidin, dissolved in 1 ml 0.2 M Na_2HPO_4, 30 μg FITC, dissolved in 1 ml 0.1 M Na_2HPO_4, is prepared. The FITC must be dissolved by vigorous crushing until a clear solution is obtained.
c. The FITC solution is added to the protein solution dropwise while stirring under 2-3 min.
d. Measure pH and adjust to pH 9.5 by dropwise addition of Na_3PO_4 (0.1 M). Wrap the container in foil to protect from light.
e. Incubate for 30 min—1 hr at room temperature and check pH intermitently (e.g. by placing a drop of the reaction mixture on pH paper). Continuously adjust pH to 9.5 as above; adjustment is frequently needed at the beginning of coupling.
f. Centrifuge if a precipitate forms, and then terminate coupling and simultaneously purify conjugate by Sephadex G-25 chromatography. When small volumes (2 ml) are available, disposable, prepacked Sephadex G-25 columns (Pharmacia), eluted with PBS (point 3a), are very conveneint. Alternatively, Sephadex G-25 fine is swollen in PBS as indicated in point 3a and is packed in a glass column or 20 ml disposable plastic syringe with the bottom supported by a nylon net. The conjugate mixture rapidly dissolves itself into 2 bands upon elution with PBS; the first, rapidly moving, band is the conjugated protein, which is easily detected by holding a fluorescence lamp against the column. This band is collected when it reaches the tip of the column. The second band represents residual free FITC and is much delayed on the column.

Note: The chromatographical purification on G-25 columns is very convenient and is also recommended when new batches of fluorochromed antibody are tested. This procedure reliably removes all free dye which otherwise will interfere with staining procedures and with determination of FITC/protein ratios (vide infra). When low molecular weight materials (MW < 5000) are labelled, Sephadex chromatography is not able to remove free dye. In this case, lysine-Sepharose (lysine coupled to cyanogen bromide-activated Sepharose 4B) is a useful FITC scavenger that will bind free fluorochrome on its surplus amino groups. Since FITC reacts with primary amino groups it will decrease the basicity of the labelled molecule. Overlabelling of IgG may result in very acidic conjugates that will contribute to unspecific staining. Therefore, determination of FITC/protein ratios is very important. Occasionally, ion-exchange chromatography

*Protein A binds to human IgG (subclass 1, 2, 4), IgA (subclass 2), IgM, mouse IgG (subclass 2a, 2b, 3), rat IgG (subclass 1, 2c), guinea pig IgG (subclass 1, 2), rabbit IgG, sheep IgG (subclass 2), goat IgG (subclass 2), dog IgG (subclass A, B, C, D) and cow IgG (subclass 2).

on DEAE-Sephadex is needed to remove over-labelled conjugate as well as unlabelled IgG (Goding 1976). Overlabelling of avidin may be less of a problem since the very basic nature of the native molecule necessitates blocking of some of its amino groups to prevent unspecific staining (Guesdon et al. 1979). According to Sternberger (1979) a FITC/protein ratio of 1—2 is most desirable. FITC/protein ratios of fractions from DEAE-Sephadex or DEAE-cellulose chromatography can be determined by measuring their optical densities at 280 and 490 nm (OD_{280} = protein; OD_{490} = FITC) (Sternberger 1979):

$$\frac{(OD_{490}\ of\ conjugate)\cdot 0.244\cdot 150\ 000}{\left[(OD_{280}\ of\ conjugate) - \dfrac{(OD_{490}\ of\ conjugate)\cdot(OD_{280}\ of\ fluorescein\ diacetate)}{(OD_{490}\ of\ fluorescein\ diacetate)}\right]\cdot 0.62\cdot 374}$$

using a molecular weight of 374 for fluorescein and 150 000 for igG.

A similar procedure may be used for tetramethylrhodamine isothiocyanate- (TRITC-)-labelling. IgG is dissolved at a concentration of 6 mg/ml in 0.01 M carbonate buffer pH 9.3 and TRITC is dissolved in dimethylsulfoxide (1 mg/ml). The TRITC-solution is added dropwise to the protein solution to give 5 μg TRITC per mg IgG. The mixture is incubated in the dark for 2 hrs and subsequently purified by gel chromatography on Sephadex G-25 and, if necessary, by DEAE-Sephadex chromatography (optical density now being measured at 550 and 280 nm).

5. Coupling of proteins or peptides to cyanogen bromide-activated Sepharose 4B (from the booklet Affinity Chromatography, principles and methods, Pharmacia Fine Chemicals, Uppsala, Sweden)

a. Weigh out the required amount of CNBr-activated Sepharose 4B.

b. Wash and reswell the gel on sintered glass filter using 1 mM HCl (200 ml/g). 1 g dry gel gives approximately 3.5 ml swollen gel. Swelling is complete in about 15 minutes; then wash the gel with the residual 1 mM HCl.

c. Dissolve the peptide or protein in coupling buffer (0.1 M $NaHCO_3$ buffer pH 8.3 containing 0.5 M NaCl). Up to 10 mg protein may be coupled per ml gel. With small peptides (met-enkephalin) we generally use 1 mg per 3.5 ml gel. Use a gel:buffer ratio of 1:2.

d. Rotate the peptide or protein solution with the gel suspension overnight at 4°C. Do not use magnetic stirrer as this will destroy the beads.

e. Remove supernatant and add 1 M ethanolamine pH 8.0 to block surplus active groups. Do not use amino acids for this purpose since these will introduce surplus acidic (carboxyl) groups in the gel. Allow to stand for 2 hrs at room temperature.

f. Wash away excess absorbed protein by frequent changes between coupling buffer and acetate buffer (0.1 M, pH 4, containing 0.5 M NaCl). Alternate between buffers five times (removes non-covalently bound peptide or protein).

g. Wash thoroughly in coupling buffer, store at 4—8°C after addition of sodium azide or mer-thiolate (0.005%).

Note: The affinity gel can now be used as an immunosorbent for purification of antisera or for affinity chromatography. The gel beads can also be attached to chrome-alum-gelatin-coated slides and immunocytochemically stained (Streefkerk et al. 1975, Larsson, Childers and Snyder 1979). CNBr-activated Sepharose 4B binds proteins and peptides covalently through interaction with their primary amino groups. Alternative gels with spacer arms and with the ability to bind proteins through carboxyl groups are avialable (Pharmacia).

6. Cytochemical models for assaying antibody specificity, method sensitivity and for screening for monoclonal antibodies (Larsson 1981b, and unpublished data)

Peptide antigens:

a. Peptides are dissolved at varying concentrations (0.02—20 μM) in suitable volatile buffers or in distilled water.

b. 2 μl droplets are applied to strips of Whatman no. 1 filter papers (or other brands of filter paper). Usually we cut the papers 1-2 cm broad and 10-20 cm long. Each strip may therefore accommodate 8-20 spots (2 μl droplets give even spots, whereas 10 μl and larger droplets give a peripheral, more concentrated halo).

c. After drying, the paper strips are exposed to paraformaldehyde vapours in a 1 l jar kept in a fume cupboard at 80°C for 1 hr (put 5-7 g paraformaldehyde powder (Merck) in the bottom of the jar). Other fixatives (glutaraldehyde, benzoquinone, osmic acid, DEPC) may be tested instead of formaldehyde.

d. The paper models are now stained after an initial rinse in Tris-buffered saline (TBS: 0.05 M Tris buffer with 0.15 M NaCl, pH 7.4). We usually stain with PAP or peroxidase-labelled methods since papers give a high fluorescence background in immunofluorescence techniques. The strips are supported on glass slides and stained in exactly the same way as tissue sections. They are developed with diaminobenzidine or 3-amino-9-ethyl-carbazol (vide infra).

Other antigens:

Peptides usually chromatograph on paper with water or aqueous buffers. It is therefore necessary to immobilize them by vapour fixation. Many other antigens (e.g. proteins) do not chromatograph on paper and can therefore easily be stained without fixation. This property can be exploited for testing influences of different aqueous fixatives on protein immunoreactivity. Experimenters are encouraged to test primarily whether their antigens chromatograph on paper; if not vapour fixation is not necessary.

Note: With our best antisera we could detect down to 100 pg of peptide (enkephalin, αMSH) per spot on the papers. Addition of a carrier protein (e.g. serum albumin) to the peptides prior to immobilization and vapour fixation increased sensitivity further.

7. Fixatives

a. 4% paraformaldehyde in 0.1 M sodium phosphate buffer, pH 7.3 (Pease 1962). Add paraformaldehyde powder to the buffer; warm to 65° until the powder completely dissolves. Usually the powder dissolves completely; should problems arise a few drops of dilute sodium hydroxide will clear the solution.

This is an excellent fixative, especially for light microscopical studies. Preferably, animals are perfusion-fixed whereafter specimens are post-fixed for 1—24 h. In combination with cryostat sectioning or vibratome sectioning this fixative is one of the most universally applicable. Even though it not per se destroys immunoreactivity of many peptides, subsequent embedding in paraffin may lead to substantial losses of antigenicity. Therefore the cryostat technique is strongly recommended (Hökfelt et al. 1975).

b. Bouin's fluid (150 ml saturated aqueous solution of picric acid + 50 ml 40% formalin + 10 ml glacial acetic acid). Fix by perfusion and postfix for 1-24 h. The fixative is exclusively used for light microscopy.

c. Zamboni's (Stefanini's) fixative. Paraformaldehyde (20 g) is dissolved in 150 ml saturated aqueous solution of picric acid. The solution is warmed to 60°C and 2.52% sodium hydroxide is added dropwise until a clear solution results. Filter and cool. Dilute to 1 l with phosphate buffer (3.31 g $NaH_2PO_4 \cdot H_2O$ and 33.77 g $Na_2HPO_4 \cdot 7H_2O$ to 1 l distilled water). Fix for 8 hrs and wash in phosphate buffer. The solution is used for both light and electron microscopy, sometimes in conjunction with cryotomy. Like the PLP fixative (7d), it is said to produce a better ultrastructure than pure formaldehyde.

d. PLP (periodic acid-lysine-paraformaldehyde; McLean and Nakane 1974). To 0.2 M lysine-HCl in distilled water add 0.1 M dibasic sodium phosphate until pH is 7.4. Dilute to a concentration of 0.1 M lysine with 0.1 M sodium phosphate buffer pH 7.4. Dissolve paraformaldehyde in distilled water. Just before use mix 3 parts of lysine-phosphate buffer with 1 part paraformaldehyde and add solid sodium metaperiodate. Periodate concentrations can be varied up to 0.1 M and formladehyde concentrations op to 4%. The pH of the fixative may decrease down to 6.2 upon addition of paraformaldehyde and tissues are fixed without readjusting pH. McLean and Nakane (1974) found the best mixture to consist of 0.01 M periodate, 0.075 M lysine, 2% paraformaldehyde and 0.037 M phosphate buffer. Small pieces are fixed under shaking for 3 hrs at 4°C. Specimens are then soaked in 0.05 M sodium phosphate buffer pH 7.2, containing 7% sucrose for 4 hrs, then in the same buffer with 15% sucrose for 4 hrs and finally in buffer with 25% sucrose and 10% glycerol for 2 hrs. Tissues are then embedded in Ames O.C.T. compound and frozen for cryostat sectioning. The fixative is thought to act by oxidation of carbohydrate moieties in tissue (by m-periodate) to form aldehyde groups. Lysine then cross-links the carbohydrate components by reacting bivalently with such aldehydes and formaldehyde is added to stabilize protein and lipid moieties. The fixative gives quite good preservation of ultrastructure and preserves antigenicity of many molecules.

e. Formaldehyde-glutaraldehyde mixtures of the Karnovsky type (modified from Karnovsky 1965). A mixture of 3% paraformaldehyde and 2% glutaraldehyde in 0.1 M sodium phosphate buffer pH 7.3 is prepared by dissolving the paraformaldehyde in the buffer and then adding the glutaraldehyde. Fixation, preferably by perfusion followed by immersion, is from 10—30 minutes at 4°C, whereafter specimens are rinsed in buffer for Epon-embedding or in sucrose-solutions (point 7d) for cryosectioning. A short and cold fixation in formaldehyde-glutaraldehyde mixtures represents a better alternative for preserving structure and antigenicity than a long fixation in weak glutaraldehyde formulas.

8. Freeze-drying and vapour-fixation (see also Björklund, Chapter II)

The tissue material is rapidly dissected out from anaesthesized animals, frozen in melting Freon-22 and then transferred to liquid nitrogen (freezing directly in liquid nitrogen produces a protective gas mantle of gaseous nitrogen, which effectively insulates the tissue and causes slow freezing with ice crystal formation). Care must be taken in preventing the frozen tissue from thawing. Frozen specimens may be stored either in a liquid N_2 container or in a −80°C freezer. The specimens may be freeze-dried in any of a number of commercial freeze-driers. 'Rapid' overnight freeze-drying is to be avoided since this most often results in poor morphology. Two types of traps for the sublimated water are employed: either a 'cold finger' trap or a container with phosphorous pentoxide. Following completed freeze-drying, which in the more reliable contraptions takes from 4 days to 1 week, the specimens are very hygroscopic and must rapidly be fixed (see below) and embedded in paraffin in vacuo.

Freeze-drying was originally introduced for the study of small and/or water-soluble molecules which, like biogenic monoamines, were easily lost from tissues treated with aqueous fixatives. Since many peptides are also easily soluble and are readily dislocated or lost from sections, freeze-drying certainly defends its place in peptide immunocytochemistry.

Fixation (i.e. immobilization) takes place before embedding and before the tissue comes into contact with any solvent. Usually the freeze-dried specimens are exposed to formaldehyde vapours generated by heating paraformaldehyde at 80°C for 1 hr. Such formaldehyde vapour treatment also results in the formation of fluorescent derivatives of i.a. catecholamines and 5-hydroxytryptamine. These fluorescent derivatives, however, possess distinct spectral properties and are, furthermore, largely dissolved out of the sections during the processing in aqueous media necessary for immunocytochemical studies.

Another, quite useful vapour fixation is the diethylpyrocarbonate (DEPC, diaethylpyrokohlensäure esther) method introduced by Pearse and Polak (1975). DEPC (0.5 ml) is placed in a small beaker in the bottom of a 1 l jar containing the specimens, which subsequently are incubated at 60°C for 3 h. With paraformaldehyde, it is sufficient to cover the bottom of the jar with a spoonful (~ 7 g) of the paraformaldehyde powder (which, hence, always is present in excess) and incubating the jar with the specimens for 1 hr at 80°C.

Following completion of the fixation the specimens are rapidly embedded in paraffin in vacuo. Following embedding the specimens are protected from atmospheric water and can be stored as other paraffin blocks. For further details on freeze-drying procedures the reader is referred to Chapter II by Björklund.

9. Isolated cells, glands, tissues and monolayer cultures

The size of the antibody molecules makes effective penetration of the diffusion barriers, created by previous fixation, very difficult. As discussed in the text, various more or less elaborate procedures involving i.a. detergent treatment have been constructed to overcome these difficulties. We and others (E. Solcia and R. Buffa personal communication; Larsson 1981a; Costa et al. 1980) have, however, found that a much simpler method may suffice.

Cells or tissues, primarily fixed in e.g. paraformaldehyde solutions, are spread out and attached to a glass slide. For light microscopy, fixed cells may be allowed to dry onto the slide. Monolayer cultures, grown on coverslips, are directly fixed in 4% paraformaldehyde and are then rinsed. The slide (which may be albuminized) is carried up through ascending ethanols (50%, 70%, 80%, 96% and absolute; 2 × 10 min in each) to xylene (2 × 10 min) and then carried down to water through the ethanols. This dehydration-rehydration treatment results in efficient breaking of diffusion barriers and allows many intracellular antigens to be immunocytochemically demonstrated. Since an analogous dehydration sequence is used for embedding tissues for electron microscopy, it is conceivable that the technique may also be used for ultrastructural preembedding staining.

10. Cryostat sectioning

As mentioned above standard embedding in paraffin and plastic often causes losses in antigenicity of many peptides. Several workers have had considerable success with procedures combining primary perfusion-fixation in Pease's 4% paraformaldehyde solution (see 7a) with cryostat sectioning. An optimal procedure is as follows (modified from Hökfelt et al. 1975):
a. Perfusion- and subsequent immersion-fixation in 4% paraformaldehyde in 0.1 M sodium phosphate buffer, pH 7.3 as described in 7a.
b. The immersion-fixed specimens are transferred into a solution of 20% sucrose in 0.1 M sodium phosphate buffer pH 7.3. They initially float in this dense solution and may at the very earliest be taken out when they have reached the bottom of the container. Preferably they should be soaked overnight.
c. The now cryo-protected specimens (sucrose diminishes the size of the ice crystals formed upon freezing) are frozen in melting Freon-22, transferred to liquid nitrogen and subsequently sectioned in a cryostat (cabinet temperature around −20°C). They must not be allowed to thaw during transport to the cryostat since this will lead to reformation of ice crystals.

Cryoprotection with sucrose probably represents the cheapest and easiest method. Ordinary cane sugar may well be used. Alternative methods include treatment of sections with increasing concentrations of glycerol or dimethyl sulfoxide (DMSO). In the case of specimens which are to be used for subsequent EM studies it is advisable to soak in an ascending series of sucrose concentrations (e.g. 5%, 10% and 20%) before freezing. The freezing method employed (Freon-22) results in minimal ice crystal formation and permits EM studies of the material. For purely light microscopical studies it is possible that simpler methods of freezing suffices.

This method of tissue pretreatment has proven eminently suitable for demonstrating many types of peptide antigens. At present the technique is probably the closest we may approach a universally applicable method. This again reflects the severe negative effects of tissue embedding in paraffin or plastic on many antigens which are not overtly affected by the primary fixative.

11. Preembedding staining for electron microscopy

A method used in our laboratory (slightly modified from Nakane 1973) is as follows:
a. Animals are perfusion-fixed with a Karnovsky-type fixative, Pease's 4% paraformaldehyde, Stefanini's fixative or the PLP fixative as indicated under point 7.
b. Following postfixation by immersion for 1—24 hrs, as deemed optimal by experiments, the blocks are soaked in a succession of 10%, 12%, and 15% sucrose solutions in 0.1 M sodium

phosphate buffers. Addition of 4×10^{-5} M digitonin to the sucrose solutions may improve membrane structure (Nakane 1973). The specimens are allowed to stay for at least 2 h in the 10%, 12%, and 15% sucrose and are then soaked overnight in a 20% sucrose + 5% glycerol solution.

c. Specimens are frozen in melting Freon-22 and transferred to liquid nitrogen. They are cut in a cryostat at 20—40 μm.

d. Staining of the sections is performed according to the PAP method or with peroxidase or colloidal gold-labelled antibodies.

e. Postfixation of the stained specimens in 2% osmic acid in Veronal or phosphate buffer for 30 min-1 hr. Rinsing in water, dehydration in ethanols (or acetone) and clearing in propylene oxide.

f. An Epon-filled capsule is inverted over the specimen. Polymerization is allowed to proceed at 45—60°C.

g. After the Epon is polymerized, the slide is warmed to 90°C–100°C for 15 min. Subsequently, the capsule with the adherent section can easily be broken off, trimmed and cut in an ultramicrotome.

Note: The method has two major disadvantages: Firstly, penetration of antibodies through the thick cryostat section may be sufficient to produce a clear, light microscopical staining, but insufficient to give enough contrast in ultrathin EM sections. This may, to some degree, be improved by the addition of 0.3% triton X-100 (Sigma) to the antisera and of 1% triton X-100 to the rinsing solutions during staining (vide infra). Secondly, it is difficult to obtain appropriate staining and specificity controls since these always have to be performed on adjacent (thick) cryostat sections. It is, hence, often difficult to be sure whether absorbed antisera have penetrated adjacent sections as efficiently as the unabsorbed antisera. Nevertheless, despite these difficulties, the method is helpful in ultrastructurally identifying antigen-rich areas. In the case of specimens where the antigen occurs only in few and scattered structures we usually refrain from using preembedding staining due to difficulties in obtaining appropriate and reliable controls.

By similar methodologies preembedding staining can also be carried out on tissue slices, Vibratome[R] sections and on isolated cells and tissues.

12. Postembedding staining

This method has its advantage in that ultrathin sections are directly stained. Hence, there are no problems with antibody penetration and controls may be carried out on the very same cells and other structures in adjacent sections. The main drawback with the technique is that the fixation and embedding procedures may adversely affect the antigenicity of the peptides to be studied. To some extent, the popular embedding media, Epon 812 and Araldite, have therefore been replaced by water-soluble media like methacrylates, albumin and urea. These media have, however, much inferior sectioning properties. Recently, ultracryotomy has been introduced, offering a very worthwhile alternative to embedding procedures (Geuze et al. 1979; Tokayasu 1978).

Despite the drawback with Epon 812 and Araldite, these media have served well in a large number of postembedding staining procedures. One should, however, always remember that these resins may partially or totally destroy antigenicity of some peptides.

For electron microscopy, the fixation usually consists of a primary aldehyde (formaldehyde, glutaraldehyde) and a secondary osmic acid fixation. Standard fixation schedules may well be compatible with retained antigenicity of many peptides. Recent data have even emphasized that a primary osmic acid fixation may preserve antigenicity of many peptides. As a routine procedure we usually employ:

a. Perfusion-fixation at 4°C with a mixture of 3% formaldehyde and 2% glutaraldehyde in 0.1 M sodium phosphate buffer pH 7.3 (point 7e).

b. Postfixation in the above mixture for 10-30 min at 4°C.

c. Rinsing 3 h in 0.1 M sodium phosphate buffer pH 7.3, whereafter half of the specimens are postfixed in 1% osmic acid for 1 hr while the rest remains in the rinsing buffer.

d. Standard dehydration and clearing in propylene oxide.

e. Embedding in Epon 812 using polymerization at 45°C.

13. Pretreatment of sections for immunocytochemical staining

Cryostat sections and paper cytochemical models are soaked for 15—30 min in tris-buffered saline (TBS = 0.05 M Tris buffer pH 7.6, containing 0.15 M NaCl), containing 1% triton X-100 before the primary antisera are applied. Isolated cells and tissues are rehydrated-dehydrated (point 9) and subsequently soaked in triton-TBS as above. Paraffin sections can be dewaxed and hydrated according to standard histological techniques prior to treatment with triton-TBS. Many workers prefer to block endogenous peroxidase activity (e.g. the pseudoperoxidase of erythrocytes). This can be achieved through treating the sections with methanol: H_2O_2 (0.1 ml 30% hydrogen peroxide to 100 ml methanol) for 30 min during the hydration sequence. Since this oxidative treatment may also modify or destroy the reactivity of some antigens it is wise to include non-pretreated controls when working with new antisera and antigens.

Plastic sections often produce better resolution and definition of immunoreactive structures than other techniques. In addition, it is possible to cut 'semithin' ($\simeq 0.3$ μm thick) resin sections adjacent to ultrathin sections. The sections will be so thin that parts of the same cells will be represented in all sections. In this way the semithin sections may be immunocytochemically stained and the ultrastructure of the immunoreactive cells identified by electron microscopy of their adjacent ultrathin companions. Many different techniques for staining semithin sections have been suggested. In our experience, the method described gives excellent and reliable results with 0.3 μm sections of Epon 812-embedded material:

a. Adjacent 0.3 μm thick and ultrathin sections are cut from Epon 812 blocks that have been polymerized at 45°C. Higher temperatures during polymerization often destroy antigenicity although some antigens, of course, are resistant to raised temperature.

b. The 0.3 μm sections are mounted on slides by permitting them to float on a minimal drop of glycerin-gelatin jelly. The latter is formed by dissolving 1 g of gelatin in 100 ml of warmed (40°C) distilled water. The solution is filtered and 12 ml glycerin and a small amount of thymol (to prevent bacterial growth) is added. Surplus mounting medium is carefully sucked off with a filter paper (do not blot!), whereafter the sections are treated for 1 hr in paraformaldehyde vapours (conveniently obtained by placing a spoonful (~ 7 g) paraformaldehyde powder in the bottom of a 1 l jar, applying the sections in racks above the powder and incubating for 1 hr at 80°C). With this technique, which also is suitable for paraffin sections, the formaldehyde cross-links the gelatin-containing mounting medium and produces very firm attachment of the sections. When semithin sections are to be stained with routine procedures (toluidine blue, methylene blue) for light microscopy, many technicians 'burn' the sections to the slides on a hot-plate at high temperature. This 'burning' method cannot be used for immunocytochemistry, since it will destroy all antigenicity. Other standard mounting procedures often result in losses of sections during staining. We therefore strongly recommend the glycerin-gelatin-formaldehyde vapor method. Control experiments have shown that the hydrophilic formaldehyde is unable to penetrate the plastic or paraffin and, hence, no further fixation of the tissue occurs. Raising the temperature to 80°C for 1 hr does not seem to overtly affect the antigenicity of most peptides. Following attachment of the sections to slides, these may be stored protected from light for a considerable time before being stained.

c. Before staining the sections are deplasticized in a saturated solution of KOH in ethanol (Lane and Europa 1965). A saturated solution of potassium hydroxide (or NaOH) in water-free ethanol is allowed to stand for about a week or until it attains a cognac-like color at which time it is ready for use. Slides are placed in the solution in a covered jar for 30 min—1 hr, and are then removed, drained and placed in absolute ethanol for 5 min. Drain and wash with at least 4 baths of absolute ethanol that must be totally water-free. Subsequently, sections are routinely dehydrated in graded ethanols.

d. If the material has been post-fixed in osmium tetroxide, osmium must be removed since it will interfere with most immunocytochemical procedures. The deplasticized hydrated sections are placed in 1% aqueous periodic acid for 7 min (0.3 μm sections; thicker sections may take slightly longer (Beauvillain et al. 1975). Following periodic acid treatment most or all osmium is removed and the sections are rinsed in several changes of distilled water and finally in triton-TBS. Step d is, of course, unnecessary with non-osmicated tissue.

e. Sections are rinsed for 15—30 min in triton-TBS, whereafter staining is performed as for all other sections. It is noteworthy that Epon sections show a very high background absorption of proteins and that therefore the treatment of the sections with inert protein solutions, as described below, is absolutely necessary, regardless of what staining method is employed.

14. Indirect immunofluorescence

a. After soaking for 15—30 min in triton-TBS (cf. point 13) sections are exposed to an inert protein solution to block unspecific protein binding sites in the tissue. A 10% solution of normal serum from the same species as the one delivering the second (fluorescence-labelled) antibody (usually sheep, goat or swine) is often used. This is derived from the fact that the serum proteins of the 'second antibody species' are unlikely to react with the second antibody. In the case of hormone immunocytochemistry one should make sure that: (1) the serum used does not contain endogenous hormone or hormone antibodies and (2) that it will not produce proteolytic break-down of tissue hormone stores. The latter effect, caused by both 'inert' sera and antisera is probably a more common cause of artifacts than commonly appreciated. For these reasons, many peptide immunocytochemists prefer pretreating their sections with a 1% solution of an inert protein like bovine or human serum albumin or ovalbumin. It is of course imperative that such inert proteins have not been used for conjugation of the peptide during immunization!

   Whether inert protein solutions or 10% serum is used the sections are incubated with the agent in a moist chamber at room temperature for 30 min to 1 hr. The agent is conveniently applied as drops over the sections.

b. Following a brief rinse in triton-TBS (1 $\times$ 15 min), antisera are applied at their optimal dilutions as drops onto the sections. Incubation in a moist chamber for 20 hrs at 4°C plus a subsequent reequilibration period for 2 h at room temperature (Sternberger 1974) is advantageous since it allows antigen-antibody equilibrium to be reached. Occasionally, workers prefer even longer incubations (48—72 hrs), but this produces, in our hands, only marginally better results. The popular short incubation period of 30 min does not admit equilibrium to be reached and, hence, much lower dilutions of the primary antisera must be employed, (as an example we may quote our antibody 4562 which produces optimal staining at a dilution of 1:640 for 30 min and can be diluted to 1:50,000 when applied for 20 + 2 hr).

   All antisera are diluted in TBS (point 13). Some workers include 0.3% triton X-100 in their antisera as well, but we have not found any major advantages with this, provided that rinsing is performed in 1% triton-TBS as described. Possibly, addition of 0.3% triton X-100 to antisera may produce an improved penetration and may be important for staining isolated cells and Vibratome® sections.

   All antisera should be used at their optimal dilution i.e. the highest dilutions at which they produce optimal staining. With 20 + 2 h of incubation we usually scan antisera using doubling dilutions from 1:100, 1:200, 1:400 a.s.o. If an antiserum then produces good staining at 1:400 and moderate or weak staining at 1:800 we go on by testing the optimal dilution in this interval (1:400, 1:500, 1:600, 1:700 and 1:800). It is important to determine the optimal dilutions of the antisera, not only for economical reasons but also since a high dilution will produce lower background staining.

c. After incubation with the primary antisera sections are thoroughly rinsed in triton-TBS (at least 3 $\times$ 10 min) at room temperature. In these and all subsequent steps, different jars must be used for sections incubated with different antisera.

d. Sections are coated with optimally diluted (in TBS) fluorescence-labelled antiserum to the IgG of the species contributing the primary antiserum. Thus, in most cases, fluorescence-labelled anti-rabbit IgG or anti-guinea pig IgG antisera will be used. There are many excellent commercial preparations labelled with either fluorescein isothiocyanate (FITC) or tetramethylrhodamine isothiocyanate (TRITC). The commercial antisera are usually produced in goat, sheep or swine. When new sources of fluorochromed antisera are tested, it is advisable to run the antisera on a Sephadex G-25 fine column equilibrated in TBS (or phosphate buffer) (cf. point 4). Labelled antibodies are applied for 30 min at room temperature (although, conceivably, longer incubation times could increase sensitivity). Optimal dilutions should be determined for every new lot to be tested. For 30 min incubations the dilutions most commonly range 1:10—1:50.

e. Rinse (at least 3 × 10 min) in triton-TBS. If desired, the specimens stained with FITC-labelled antisera may be counterstained with a solution of Evans blue in TBS. A very small amount of the dye may be dissolved in TBS to produce a light blue solution. Following rinsing the sections are immersed in this solution until they attain a light blue coloration. The staining is progressive, but can be differentiated by immersing over-stained sections in TBS. Experience is the best guide to optimal staining and the technique is easily mastered. Evans blue produces a clear red fluorescence at the wave-length used for FITC excitation (490 nm). It may mask some specific antigenic sites and should be used with care.

f. Sections are mounted in a 9:1 mixture of glycerol and TBS, cover-slipped and observed in the fluorescence microscope using exciting light of 490 nm for FITC and of 546 nm for TRITC.

15. Peroxidase-antiperoxidase (PAP) procedure (Sternberger 1974, 1979)

a. As in point 13—14 sections are first soaked in triton-TBS and then exposed to an inert protein solution (either an albumin solution or inert serum). The inert serum is derived from the species producing the second layer or 'link' antibody. The same precautions as stated under point 14 also apply to the PAP procedure.

b. Rinse briefly (or not at all!) in triton-TBS and apply the primary antiserum at its optimal dilution for 20 h at 4°C plus for an additional 2 h at room temperature (longer times may also be tried, particularly with low-avidity antisera). The optimal dilutions are higher in the PAP procedure than in the indirect immunofluorescence procedure and antisera should be titrated as in point 14. Dilutions are made in TBS with or without 0.3% triton X-100.

c. Sections are rinsed (at least 3 × 10 min) in 1% triton-TBS.

d. Apply antiserum to the IgG of the species producing the primary antibody. Since these antibodies will form a 'link' between the primary antibodies and the subsequently applied PAP complex, their specificity is dictated by the species producing both the primary antibodies and the antibodies of the PAP complex. The PAP complex is almost invariably built up of rabbit antibodies and, hence, the second (link) antibody should be anti-rabbit IgG and consequently the primary antibody should be produced in rabbit. Erlandsen and co-workers (1975) found, however, that many anti-IgG antibodies are not totally species-specific. Thus, with some efforts, anti-rabbit IgG antibodies cross-reacting with e.g. guinea pig IgG can be found. Such antibodies wil allow the use of a primary guinea pig antibody, a link antibody to rabbit IgG (cross-reacting with guinea pig IgG) and a rabbit PAP complex. Subsequently, the use of protein A instead of a link antibody has been suggested since protein A will cross-link IgG's from many different species (Notani et al. 1979). It seems possible that use of protein A (Pharmacia Fine Chemicals, Uppsala, Sweden) will widen the spectrum of species from which the primary antibody can be obtained for PAP staining. Very recently, mouse PAP complexes have become available for use with monoclonal antibodies.

The function of the second antibody is to provide a link between the primary antibody and the PAP complex. It should therefore be applied in excess so that only one of its two antigen-binding sites will bind to the primary antibodies. With most commercial link antibodies optimal dilutions vary from 1:10—1:50 for a 30 min-1 h incubation at room temperature.

e. Rinse (at least 3 × 10 min) in triton-TBS.

f. Apply the peroxidase-antiperoxidase complex at its optimal dilution for 30 min at room temperature in the moist chamber. Link antibodies, which have reacted with primary an-

tibodies with only one of their antigen-combining sites will react with the rabbit IgG component of the PAP complex with their remaining site, and, hence, link the complex to the site
of the primary antigen-antibody reaction.

PAP complexes may be fabricated according to the detailed instructions of Sternberger
(1974, 1979). Alternatively, excellent commercial PAP complexes are available. We routinely
use one from Dakopatts A/S (Copenhagen, Denmark) at a dilution of 1:70 for 30 min at
room temperature. Contrary to claims, we find that the quality of commercial PAP complexes slowly deteriorates upon storage at either 4°C or −20°C. Consequently, upon receipt
of new lyophilized PAP complexes we dissolve the contents, dilute to 1:70 and store aliquots
at −80°C. With these precautions, excellent stability of both home-made and commercial
preparations has been obtained whereas storage at higher temperature, and, in particular,
repeated freezing and thawing, leads to a striking, gradual loss of activity as manifested by
slowly decreasing titers.

g. Rinse (at least 3×10 min) in 1% triton-TBS.
h. Rinse twice in Tris buffer pH 7.6 without triton.
i. Peroxidase activity is demonstrated by the diamino-benzidine-hydrogen peroxide method of
   Graham and Karnovsky (1966; cf. Steinberger 1974). Diamino-benzidine-tetrahydrochloride
   (50 mg) is dissolved in 100 ml 0.05 M Tris buffer. The solution is filtered and 30% H_2O_2 is
   added to a final concentration of 0.01%. Sections are incubated for 30 min. Some authors
   prefer to initially soak their sections in the diaminobenzidine solution for 10—30 min and
   subsequently to add the hydrogen peroxide for a final incubation of 10—20 min. Following
   development the sections may be routinely dehydrated, cleared and embedded in Permount.
   Alternatively, the 4-Cl-1-naphtol procedure of Nakane (1968), as modified by Vandesande
   and Dierickx (1975, 1979) may be used:

   100 mg 4-Cl-1-naphtol is dissolved in 10 ml absolute ethanol whereafter 190 ml Tris-buffer
   (0.05 M pH 7.6) is added. A white precipitate forms − contrary to others we prefer not to
   remove it since stronger staining is obtained in its presence. Finally, 30% H_2O_2 is added to a
   final concentration of 0.005%. Sections are developed for 15—20 min. They may not be
   dehydrated in ethanol since this dissolves the reaction product.

   It is the experience of many workers that the 4-Cl-1-naphtol procedure is much less sensitive than the DAB procedure. An alternative, quite sensitive, procedure is offered by the use
   of 3-amino-9-ethylcarbazole (modified from Graham et al. 1965): 20 mg of 3-amino-9-
   ethylcarbazole (90% pure, Sigma) is dissolved in 2.5 ml dimethylformamide and added to 50
   ml 0.05 M acetate buffer pH 5.5. Immediately before use 25 μl 30% H_2O_2 is added. Filter.
   Develop sections for 5-20 min. A dark red reaction product ensues that contrasts well with a
   haematoxylin or light green counterstain. Mount in glycerin as the reaction product is water-
   soluble.
j. Many workers post-treat sections developed with the DAB or 4-Cl-1-naphtol procedure with
   a 1% osmic acid solution in distilled water or in various buffers. This technique makes the
   polymerization product electron dense and must be used in cases where the reaction product
   is to be visualized in the electron microscope. For light microscopy, postosmification is not
   generally necessary since enough contrast is produced by the reaction product itself. Due to
   its ability to produce a quite heavy staining of background details, postosmification is better
   avoided altogether at the LM level. It may often be advantageous to counter-stain the
   preparations weakly with haematoxylin (in the case of DAB and 3A9EC) or with Kernechtrot
   (in the case of 4-Cl-1-naphtol). Alternatively, the sections may be observed under differential
   interference contrast a.m. Nomarski or in darkfield. Phase contrast is less suitable since the
   DAB polymer produces an amorphous, lucent image.
h. In selected instances it may be desirable to further increase the intensity of PAP staining. This
   may be achieved by repeating steps d-f after the rinse (step g) (Sternberger and Joseph, 1979).
   Since the PAP complexes contribute novel rabbit IgG molecules to the section, a repetition
   of these steps will lead to the attachment of more link antibodies and subsequently of more
   PAP complexes to the sections. Conceivably, this rerun could be repeated many times. The
   high sensitivity of the PAP method, however, makes this practice unnecesssary in most cases

and we have no personal experience with it. It does, however, represent a most interesting way of further increasing PAP sensitivity and deserves further testing.

16. Radioimmunocytochemistry (RICH)

This method requires access to radioiodinated antigen and autoradiographic procedures.

a. The peptide to be studied is radiolabelled with carrier-free $Na^{125}I$ by any of a number of available iodination procedures (chloramine T, lactoperoxidase, iodogen, Bolton-Hunter reagent etc.). Various iodination procedures are variously successful with different antigens and the radioimmunoassay literature should be consulted for finding optimal conditions for labelling and purification of various antigens. A good introduction is given in the book of Thorell et al. (1978).

b. The iodinated antigen (tracer) is mixed with the antibody in varying proportions. Preferably, graded amounts of tracer are added to aliquots of a constant dilution of antibody (in TBS). Following incubation of the mixtures for the preferred time (24—72 h) antibody-bound tracer is separated from free tracer by a suitable technique (like second antibody precipitation, dextran-coated charcoal or ethanol precipitation, depending upon the system studied, cf. Thorell et al. 1978). The precipitate and supernatant are counted in a γ-counter and the per cent bound tracer is calculated. It will be found that the binding per cent falls with increasing concentrations of tracer. A graph is constructed with the binding per cent on the y-axis and the amount of tracer (cpm) on the x-axis. The tracer concentration at which all or nearly all tracer is bound is sought. At this point there will be a preponderance of antibodies which bind labelled antigen with only one of their two antigen-combining sites. If lower concentrations of tracer are added, most antibodies will not bind tracer at all (zone of antibody surplus). If higher concentrations are added, most antibodies will bind tracer with both of their combining sites (zone of antigen (= tracer) surplus).

Using the results of this experiment a larger pool of RICH complexes can be made by allowing a larger volume of diluted antiserum to react with the optimal concentration of tracer as shown on the diagram. When larger amounts of RICH complexes have been mixed it is always advantageous to take a small aliquot for separation and determination of binding per cent as an internal control.

The antibody dilution used for preparing RICH complexes will depend upon the quality of the antibody, the amount of tracer added and the desired length of autoradiographic exposure (cf. Larsson and Schwartz, 1977). As a rule of thumb, with 1 week of autoradiographic exposure, the optimal dilution of the antibody roughly equals the dilution in the PAP procedure. With lower dilutions, shorter autoradiographic exposures should be used (dilutions for 1 day of exposure roughly equals the dilutions for indirect immunofluorescence).

Of course the single most important factor governing the time of exposure and, hence, the antibody dilution is the total amount of radioactivity added. In our experience it has been highly advantageous to use tracer concentrations varying between $2 \times 10^4 - 2 \times 10^5$ counts per minute (cpm) per ml. Some workers may, hence, prefer to decide upon using e.g. 10^5 cpm/ml and to add this constant amount of tracer to graded concentrations of antibody. In this case the graph will be constructed from the binding per cent versus antibody dilution. Again, it will be found that with excess antibodies, all tracer molecules will be bound (B% = 100) and that with high antibody dilutions, progressively less tracer molecules will be bound (B% → 0). As before, the point on the curve where the highest dilution of antibody still gives total binding of added tracer is sought. At this point the highest number of antibody molecules binding antigen with only one combining site (= RICH complexes) is found (for details cf. Larsson and Schwartz, 1977).

c. Tissue sections from specimens fixed, embedded and cut according to the methods described in point 13 are used. Following an initial rinse for 15—30 min in triton-TBS (point 13), the sections are exposed to a 1:10—1:30 (30 minutes-1 hr) dilution of normal rabbit serum in TBS provided that the RICH complex is made from rabbit antibodies. Note that with this technique sections are pretreated with normal serum from the same species as the one producing the primary antibodies! This practice assures that unspecific binding of specific immuno-globulins does not occur. This homologous blocking method is also employed in the GLAD method, but cannot be used with techniques, which like indirect immunofluorescence or the PAP method, relies on the detection of all antibodies that have bound to the tissue sections.

d. After pretreatment with normal serum, the RICH complexes are applied as droplets onto the sections. Incubation proceeds for 20—24 h at 4°C, in a moist chamber. The RICH complexes, binding tracer with one of their two antigen-combining sites will now react with the corresponding tissue-bound antigen with their remaining combining site.

e. Sections are rinsed 3 × 15 min in triton-TBS.

f. Fix sections in 2.5% glutaraldehyde in 0.2 M sodium cacodylate buffer, pH 7.2 for 5—15 min (optional: this postfixation is not necessary with high-avidity antibodies).

g. Rinse in distilled water (5—10 min).

h. Coat with a suitable autoradiographic emulsion (e.g. Kodak NTB-2). Alternatively, stripping film may be used.

17. Peroxidase-antiperoxidase (PAP) procedure for post-embedding staining for electron microscopy

There are no principal differences between light microscopical PAP staining (point 15) and PAP staining of ultrathin sections mounted on formvar-coated or uncoated Ni-grids (Cu-grids cannot be used). In our laboratory the detailed instructions of Sternberger (1974, 1979) have been carefully followed and have produced excellent results. We refer the reader to Sternberger's original texts (1974, 1979) for instructions in this important technique.

18. Gold-labelled antigen detection (GLAD) procedure (Larsson 1979, 1981a)

a. Preparation of colloidal gold granules (Frens 1973): 200 ml of redistilled water is brought to boiling under reflux. Subsequently, 2 ml of sodium citrate (0.5 g/l) (trisodium citrate 2-hydrate) is added under shaking, and then 0.5 ml 4 per cent trichloroauric acid ($HAuCl_4$, Merck) is added under shaking. The mixture is brought to boiling again, is allowed to boil for 30 min under reflux and is then cooled.

This procedure results in gold granules with a diameter of 18 nm. The size range is very narrow. It is advisable to check and measure the gold granules in the electron microscope.

By varying the amount of sodium citrate added, gold granules of differing diameters can be made. Thus, if 1.5 ml sodium citrate is added (instead of the 2 ml as in the example above) gold granules of 31 nm diameter result.

Recently, we have started using 12 nm gold granules, which are excellent for many purposes and tend to give a very dense labelling of immunoreactive structures. These are prepared as follows (Horisberger 1979): 10 ml 0.07% sodium ascorbate is very rapidly mixed with a solution of (1 ml 1% $HAuCl_4$ + 1.5 ml 0.2 N K_2CO_3 + 25 ml distilled water) under magnetic stirring. Rapidly, the resulting solution is diluted to 100 ml with distilled water. It is important to mix the ascorbate and gold chloride solutions very rapidly; too slow mixing may result in very variable diameters of the gold granules. It is advisable to check the diameters of the gold granules under the electron microscope, at least if they are to be used for double-staining experiments.

For double-staining at the EM level we routinely use gold granules of 12, 18 and 31 nm since these are easily distinguished, but any diameter can be manufactured. In the subsequent manipulations it is often noted that smaller gold granules tend to be more stable.

b. Preparation of peptide-albumin conjugates and their coupling to gold granules. Small peptides do not absorb well to gold granules and must therefore be conjugated to a larger protein like albumin before being absorbable to gold granules. Note that the recipe given below produces 20-40 ml working solution of gold granules. This amount greatly exceeds the needs of many investigators and can therefore easily be scaled down by a factor of 10.

b:1. 50-200 nmol of the peptide to be investigated and 60 nmol BSA are dissolved in 250 μl 0.005 M NaCl in redistilled water (with the pH adjusted beforehand to 7.0).

b:2. 50μl 0.25% glutaraldehyde (Merck) is added. The mixture is incubated for 2 h at ambient temperature (20-25°C).

b:3. The resulting conjugate is diluted using 13 ml of 0.005 M NaCl in redistilled water. The pH is adjusted to pH 4.0—4.5 (using dilute HCl).

b:4. Filter through a Millipore membrane (pore size: 0.45 μm) and mix with 100 ml of gold granule suspension (point 1), while shaking.

b:5. The mixture is incubated for 2 min, whereafter a Millipore-filtered 1% solution of polyethylene glycol (Carbowax, Mw = 20 000) is added. For every 10 ml of gold granule - conjugate mixture 1 ml of the polyethylene glycol solution is added.

b:6. The pH is adjusted to 7 using a pH-stick (not a pH-meter!) with 0.02 M K_2CO_3. Shake the solution while adding the K_2CO_3. Around 3—4 ml of the solution are usually needed.

b:7. The now coated and polyethylene glycol-stabilized gold granules are spun down at 15000 rpm (20—30 min, 4°C) and are then redispersed in 4 ml 0.05 M Tris buffer, pH 7.9, containing 0.15 M NaCl and 0.5 mg polyethylene glycol (Mw 20 000) and 0.5 mg sodium azide (as preservative) per ml.

b:8. Comments: (1) all solutions added to the gold granules should be Millipore-filtered; (2) the gold granules remain stable for at least a month, probably longer when stored at 4°C; (3) this procedure can with advantage be scaled down by a factor of 10 since a large volume of gold granules is obtained.

c. Staining of ultrathin sections.

c:1. Sections are collected on Formvar-coated or unsupported Ni-grids or Au-grids.

c:2. Grids may be 'deplasticized' with hydrogen peroxide which also removes some of the OsO_4 from osmicated specimens. As suggested by Sternberger (1974) grids from non-osmicated specimens may be allowed to float on a drop of 10% hydrogen peroxide for 6 min, whereas sections from osmicated specimens are treated for 20 min in the same solution.

All droplets on which sections are to float in this and subsequent steps can be conveniently made on small impressions in dental wax or Parafilm®.

It should be noted that hydrogen peroxide does not remove the plastic, but rather is believed to 'soften' it, thereby increasing antibody permeability.

Recently, while staining for several different antigens we have noted that this hydrogen peroxide treatment may not be necessary with non-osmicated specimens. Thus, almost the same degree of staining is obtained whether or not the treatment is included suggesting that staining of ultrathin sections is mainly a surface phenomenon. These preliminary observations, hence, suggest that plastic removal is unnecessary for EM immunocytochemistry also with other techniques. More experiments are, however, needed before we can finally recommend the exclusion of this procedure from the staining protocol.

c:3. Sections are rinsed in TBS (delivered as a stream over the grid by a pipette) and are briefly blotted by holding them with their edge against lens paper. They should never be allowed to get completely dry.

c:4. Whether or not sections have been treated with hydrogen peroxide they must be exposed to an inert protein solution before the antiserum is applied. In the GLAD method where only specific antibodies are detected this can be made by letting the sections float on droplets of a 1:10 dilution of normal serum from the same species as that delivering the immune serum for 30 min at room temperature in a moist chamber.

c:5. With (or without) a short rinse in TBS followed by blotting as in c:3, the sections are allowed to float on droplets of the immune-serum on dental wax in a moist chamber for 20 h at 4°C and for a subsequent 2 h at room temperature. The immune-serum may be diluted in TBS or in a 1:10 solution of normal rabbit serum in TBS. Optimal dilutions are as always determined by experiments. They tend to be intermediate between the optimal dilutions for indirect immunofluorescence and PAP staining.

c:6. Rinse and blot as in c:3.

c:7. Antigen-coated colloidal gold granules are centrifuged for 2 min at 700 g (in order to remove possible aggregates) and are subsequently applied to the grids (as droplets on dental wax cf. above) for 2 h at room temperature in a moist chamber. Longer times of incubation are feasible. Optimal dilutions are determined by experiments, but usually vary between 1:5—1:60 for 2 h of exposure. Dilutions are made with the solution described in point b:7. Following the incubation the grids are rinsed with a spray of this solution from a pipette 2—3 times. Finally, they are allowed to float on a drop of this solution for 1—2 hr.

c:8. Grids are fixed by floating on a drop of 1% glutaraldehyde in cacodylate buffer (0.2 M, pH 7.2) for 30 min at room temperature.

c:9. Rinse and blot with TBS as in c:3.

c:10. Contrast the sections by any desired method (e.g. uranyl acetate and lead citrate).

c:11. Rinse in distilled water and let dry in air.

19. Antibody elution technique (from Tramu et al. 1978).

a. Immunocytochemical staining of sections for antigen A:
immunofluorescence
peroxidase-labelled 2nd Ab.
PAP method
(with peroxidase/PAP method develop with 3-amino-9-ethylcarbazole or 4-Cl-1-naphtol)

b. If peroxidase-preparation: elute reaction color in dilute ethanol, rehydrate
if immunofluorescence: directly to point (c).

c. From distilled water to mixture of
1 vol 2.5% $KMnO_4$
+ 1 vol 5% H_2SO_4
+ 140 vol distilled water
treatment time: depends on section thickness, usually 1-5 min
(vibratome sections: 10 min or more!)

d. Destain in 0.5% $Na_2S_2O_5$ 30 sec.

e. Thorough rinse in tap water (running 10—20 min).

f. Distilled water 5 min.

g. Stain for antigen B.

h. *Note:*
1. The efficiency of elution must always be checked! Incomplete elution usually affects 2nd or 3rd Abs. before 1st Ab. Test for efficiency by replacing point g (2nd immune serum) with non-immune serum (or absorbed antiserum) and use detection system as desired (fluorescence/peroxidase). The stained and developed sections must be completely free of reaction product and are then stained for antigen B.
2. This elution procedure destroys antigenic sites containing methionine (and probably disulfide and tryptophan groups). We have deliberately used this property to differentiate between met- and leu-enkephalin in tissue using antibodies reactive with leu/met-enkephalin but unreactive towards sulfoxidized met-enkephalin (Larsson et al. 1979).
3. Advantages with the method are that it reliably elutes also high-avidity antibodies, which usually remain (sometimes unsuspectedly) after elution with dilute HCl, NH_3^+, glycine-HCl and other alternative methods. It is essential to remember, however, that this oxidative technique may damage antigens. This damage, however, can be tested for in advance using paper models of the desired antigens.

9. REFERENCES

Adair WS, Jurivich D, Goodenough UW (1978): Localization of cellular antigens in sodium dodecyl sulfate-polyacrylamide gels. *J. Cell Biol., 79,* 281–285.

Atassi MZ, Smith JA (1978): A proposal for the nomenclature of antigenic sites in peptides and proteins. *Immunochemistry, 15,* 609–610.

Atassi MZ, Zablocki W (1977): Can an antibody-combining site be mimicked synthetically? *J. Biol. Chem., 252,* 8784–8787.

Avrameas S, Ternynck T (1969): The cross-linking of proteins with glutaraldehyde and its use for the preparation of immunosorbents. *Immunochemistry, 6,* 53–66.

Bächi T, Dorval G, Wigzell H, Binz H (1977): Staphylococcal protein A in immunoferritin techniques. *Scand. J. Immunol., 6,* 241–246.

Baigent CL, Müller G (1980): A colloidal gold prepared with ultrasonics. *Experientia, 36,* 472–473.

Batten TFC, Hopkins CR (1978): EM immunocytochemical localization of hormones on the surface of ultrathin sections using antibody bound to a gold particle marker of specific size. Paper presented at: Secretory Biology Symposium, Guildford, Surrey, Sept. 1978.

Batten TFC, Hopkins CR (1979): Use of protein A-coated colloidal gold particles for immunoelectron microscopic localization of ACTH on ultrathin sections. *Histochemistry, 60,* 317–320.

Bayer EA, Skutelsky E, Wilchek M (1979): The avidin-biotin complex in affinity cytochemistry. *Methods Enzymol., 62,* 308–315.

Beauvillain J-C, Tramu G, Dubois MP (1975): Characterization by different techniques of adrenocorticotropin and gonadotropin producing cells in Lerot pituitary. *Cell Tissue Res., 158,* 301–317.

Becker M (1975): Active groups in proteins and their modification. *Scand. J. Immunol., 20, Suppl.3,* 11–18.

Bergh OJ, Solheim BG (1978): Detection of thrombocyte antibodies by ^{125}I labelled protein A. *Tissue Antigens, 12,* 189–194.

Beutner EH (1971): Defined immunofluorescent staining: Past progress, present status and future prospects for defined conjugates. *Ann NY Acad. Sci., 177,* 506–526.

Bigbee JW, Kosek JC, Eng LF (1977): Effects of primary antiserum dilution on staining of 'antigen-rich' tissues with the peroxidase-antiperoxidase technique. *J. Histochem. Cytochem., 25,* 443–447.

Björklund A, Falck B, Owman CH (1972): Fluorescence microscopic and microspectrofluorometric techniques for the cellular localization and characterization of biogenic monoamines. In: Berson SA (Ed), *Methods of Investigative and Diagnostic Endocrinology, Vol. 1, The Thyroid and Biogenic Amines,* Rall JE, Kopin IJ (Eds), pp. 318–368. Amsterdam, North-Holland.

Bohn W (1978): A fixation method for improved antibody penetration in electron-microscopical immunoperoxidase studies. *J. Histochem. Cytochem., 26,* 293–297.

Bowes JH, Cater CW (1966): The reaction of glutaraldehyde with proteins and other biological materials. *J. R. Microsc. Soc., 85,* 193–200.

Brandtzaeg P (1972): Evaluation of immunofluorescence with artificial sections of selected antigenicity. *Immunology, 22,* 117–183.

Buffa R, Solcia E, Fiocca R, Crivelli O, Pera A (1979): Complement-mediated binding of immunoglobulins to some endrocrine cells of the pancreas and gut. *J. Histochem. Cytochem., 27,* 1279–1280.

Capel PJA (1974): A quantitative immunofluorescence method based on the covalent coupling of protein to Sepharose beads. *J. Immunol. Methods, 5,* 165–178.

Clement-Jones V, Lowry PJ, Rees LH, Besser GM (1980): Development of a specific extracted radioimmunoassay for methionine enkephalin in human plasma and cerebrospinal fluid. *J. Endocrinol., 86,* 231–243.

Costa M, Furness JB, Lewellyn-Smith IJ, Davies B, Oliver J (1980): An immunohistochemical study of the projections of somatostatin-containing neurons in the guinea pig intestine. *Neuroscience, 5,* 841–852.

Cuello AC, Galfré G, Milstein C (1980): Development of a monoclonal antibody against a neuroactive peptide: Immunocytochemical applications. In: Pepen G, Kuhar MJ, Enna SJ (Eds), *Receptors for Neurotransmitters and Peptide Hormones,* pp. 349–363. Raven Press, New York.

Curran RC, Gregory J (1977): The unmasking of antigens in paraffin sections of tissue by trypsin. *Experientia, 33,* 1400–1401.

Deetz JS, Behrman EJ (1981): Reaction of osmium reagents with amino acids and proteins. *Int. J. Pept. Protein Res., 17,* 495–500.

Denk H, Radaszkiewicz T, Weirich E (1977): Pronase pretreatment of tissue sections enhances sensitivity of the unlabelled antibody-enzyme (PAP) technique. *J. Immunol. Methods, 15,* 163–167.

Dorling J, Kingston D, Webb JA (1976): Anti-streptococcal antibodies reacting with brain tissue: II. Ultrastructural studies. *Br. J. Exp. Pathol., 57,* 255–265.

Dubois-Dalcq M, McFarland H, McFarlin D (1977): Protein A-peroxidase: A valuable tool for the localization of antigens. *J. Histochem. Cytochem., 25,* 1201–1206.

Erlandsen SL, Parsons JA, Burke JP, Redick JA, Van Orden DE, Van Orden LS (1975): A modification of the unlabelled antibody enzyme method using heterologous antisera for the light-microscopic and ultrastructural localization of insulin, glucagon and growth hormone. *J. Histochem. Cytochem., 23,* 666–677.

Faulk WP, Taylor CM (1971): An immunocolloid method for the electron-microscope. *Immunochemistry, 8,* 1081–1083.

Finley JCW, Grossman GH, Dimeo P, Petrusz P (1978): Somatostatin-containing neurons in the rat brain: Widespread distribution revealed by immunocytochemistry after pretreatment with pronase. *Am. J. Anat., 153,* 483–488.

Frens G (1973): Controlled nucleation for the regulation of the paricle size in monodisperse gold suspensions. *Nature (Phys. Sci.), 241,* 20–22.

Geoghegan WD, Ackermann GA (1977): Adsorption of horseradish peroxidase, oromucoid and antiimmunoglobulin to colloidal gold for the indirect detection of concanavalin A, wheat germ aglutinin and goat antihuman immunoglobulin G on cell surfaces at the electron-microscopic level: A new method, theory and application. *J. Histochem. Cytochem., 25,* 1187–1200.

Geuze HJ, Slot JW, Van der Ley A, Scheffer RCT, Griffith JM (1981): Use of colloidal gold particles in double-labelling immunoelectron-microscopy of ultrathin frozen sections. *J. Cell. Biol., 89,* 653–665.

Geuze HJ, Slot JW, Tokuyasu KT, Goedemans WEJ, Griffith JM (1979): Immunocytochemical localization of amylase and chymotrypsinogen in the exocrine pancreatic cell with special attention to the golgi complex. *J. Cell. Biol., 82,* 697–707.

Goding JW (1976): Conjugation of antibodies with fluorochromes: Modifications to the standard methods. *J. Immunol. Methods, 13,* 215–226.

Goldman M (1968): *Fluorescent Antibody Methods.* Academic Press, New York.

Graham RC, Karnovsky MJ (1966): The early stages of absorption of injected horseradish peroxidase in the proximal tubules of mouse kidney. Ultrastructural cytochemistry by a new technique. *J. Histochem. Cytochem., 14,* 291–302.

Graham RC, Lundholm U, Karnovsky MJ (1965): Cytochemical demonstration of peroxidase activity with 3-amino-9-ethylcarbazole. *J. Histochem. Cytochem., 13,* 150–152.

Guesdon J-L, Ternynck T, Avrameas S (1979): The use of avidin-biotin interaction in immunoenzymatic techniques. *J. Histochem. Cytochem., 27,* 1131–1139.

Habeeb AFSA, Hiramoto R (1968): Reaction of proteins with glutaraldehyde. *Arch. Biochem. Biophys., 126,* 16–26.

Hartman BK, Zide D, Udenfriend S (1972): The use of dopamine-β-hydroxylase as marker for the noradrenergic pathways of the central nervous system in the rat. *Proc. Nat. Acad. Sci. USA, 69,* 2722–2726.

Hassell J, Hand AR (1974): Tissue fixation with diimidoesters as an alternative to aldehydes. I. Comparison of cross-linking and ultrastructure obtained with dimethylsuberimidate and glutaraldehyde. *J. Histochem. Cytochem., 22,* 223–239.

Hayat MA (1970): Principles and techniques of electron microscopy. In: *Biological Applications, Vol. 1,* pp. 5–110. Litton Educ. Publ. Inc., New York.

Heggeness MH, Ash JF (1977): Use of the avidin-biotin complex for the localization of actin and myosin with fluorescence microscopy. *J. Cell Biol., 73,* 783–788.

Hökfelt T, Fuxe K, Goldstein M (1975): Applications of immunohistochemistry to studies on monoamine cell systems with special references to nervous tissues. *Ann. NY Acad. Sci., 254,* 407–432.

Hopwood D (1969): Fixatives and fixation: A review. *Histochem. J., 1,* 323–360.

Horisberger M (1979): Evaluation of colloidal gold as a cytochemical marker for transmission and scanning electron-microscopy. *Biol. Cell., 36,* 253–258.

Horisberger M, Rosset J (1977): Colloidal gold, a useful marker for transmission and scanning electron-microscopy. *J. Histochem. Cytochem., 25,* 295–305.

Huang S-N, Minassian H, More JD (1976): Application of immunofluorescent staining on paraffin sections improved by trypsin digestion. *Lab. Invest., 35,* 383–390.

Isobe Y, Chen S-T, Nakane PK, Brown WR (1977): Studies on translocation of immunoglobulins across intestinal epithelium. I. Improvements in the peroxidase-labelled antibody method for application to study of human intestinal mucosa. *Acta Histochem. Cytochem., 10,* 161–171.

Karnovsky MJ (1965): A formaldehyde-glutaraldehyde fixative of high osmolality for use in electron-microscopy. *J. Cell Biol., 27,* 137 A.

Kendall PA, Polak JM, Pearse AGE (1971): Carbodiimide fixation for immunohistochemistry: Observations on the fixation of polypeptide hormones. *Experientia, 27,* 1104–1106.

206

Knapp W, Ploem JS (1974): Microfluorometry of antigen-antibody interactions in immunofluorescence using the defined antigen substrate spheres (DASS) system. Sensitivity, specificity and variables of the method. *J. Immunol. Methods, 5,* 259–273.

Köhler G, Milstein C (1975): Continuous cultures of fused cells secreting antibody of predefined specificity. *Nature, 256,* 495–497.

Kraehenbuhl JP, Jamieson JD (1972): Solid-phase conjugation of ferritin to Fab-fragments of immunoglobulin G for use in antigen localization on thin sections. *Proc. Nat. Acad. Sci. USA, 69,* 1771–1775.

Kraehenbuhl JP, Racine L, Jamieson JD (1977): Immunocytochemical localization of secretory proteins in bovine pancreatic exocrine cells. *J. Cell Biol., 72,* 406–423.

Lane BP, Europa DL (1965): Differential staining of ultrathin sections of epon-embedded tissues for light-microscopy. *J. Histochem. Cytochem., 13,* 579–582.

Lange RH (1971): A light and electron microscopic study including immunohistochemistry of non-β- cells in the islets of Langerhans (frog, rat), with special reference to the number of cell types. *Mem. Soc. Endocrinol., 19,* 457–466.

Larsson L-I (1977): Ultrastructural localization of a new neuronal peptide (VIP). *Histochemistry, 54,* 173–176.

Larsson L-I (1979): Simultaneous ultrastructural demonstration of multiple peptides in endocrine cells by a novel immunocytochemical method. *Nature, 282,* 743–746.

Larsson L-I (1980): Corticotropin and α-melanotropin in brain nerves: immunocytochemical evidence for axonal transport and processing. In: Costa E, Trabucchi M (Eds), *Neural Peptides and Neuronal Communication,* pp. 101–107. Raven Press, New York.

Larsson L-I (1981a): Peptide immunocytochemistry. In: *Progress in Histochemistry and Cytochemistry, Vol. 13, No. 4,* pp. 1–85.

Larsson L-I (1981b): A novel immunocytochemical model system for specificity and sensitivity screening of antisera against multiple antigens. *J. Histochem. Cytochem., 29,* 408–410.

Larsson L-I, Childers S, Snyder SH (1979): Met- and leu-enkephalin immunoreactivity in separate neurons. *Nature, 282,* 407–410.

Larsson L-I, Håkanson R, Sjöberg N-O, Sundler F (1975): Fluorescence histochemistry of the gastrin cell in fetal and adult man. *Gastroenterology, 68,* 1152–1159.

Larsson L-I, Rehfeld JF (1977): Characterization of antral gastrin cells with region-specific antisera. *J. Histochem. Cytochem., 25,* 1317–1321.

Larsson L-I, Schwartz TW (1977): Radioimmunocytochemistry – A novel immunocytochemical principle. *J. Histochem. Cytochem., 25,* 1140–1146.

Larsson L-I, Stengaard-Pedersen K (1981): Enkephalin/endorphin-related peptides in antropyloric gastrin cells. *J. Histochem. Cytochem., 29,* 1088–1098.

Larsson L-I, Sundler F, Håkanson R (1975): Fluorescence histochemistry of polypeptide hormone-secreting cells in the gastrointestinal mucosa. In: Thompson JC (Ed), *Gastrointestinal Hormones,* pp. 169–195. Univ. of Texas Press, Austin, Tex.

Larsson L-I, Sundler F, Håkanson R (1976): Pancreatic polypeptide – A postulated new hormone: Identification of its cellular storage site by light- and electron-microscopic immunocytochemistry. *Diabetologia, 12,* 211–226.

Laurilla P, Virtanen I, Wartiovaara J, Stenman S (1978): Fluorescent antibodies and lectins stain intracellular structures in fixed cells treated with non-ionic detergent. *J. Histochem. Cytochem., 26,* 251–257.

Li JY, Dubois MP, Dubois PM (1977): Somatotrophs in the human fetal anterior pituitary. *Cell Tissue Res., 181,* 545–552.

Maxwell MH (1978): Two rapid and simple methods used for the removal of resins from 1.0 μm thick epoxy sections, *J. Microsc. (Oxford), 112,* 253–255.

Mayor HD, Hampton JC, Rosario B (1961): A simple method for removing the resin from epoxy-embedded tissue. *J. Biophys. Biochem. Cytol., 9,* 909–910.

McLean I, Nakane PK (1974): Periodate-lysine-paraformaldehyde fixative – A new fixative for immuno-electron-microscopy. *J. Histochem. Cytochem., 22,* 1077–1083.

McMillan PN, Luftig RB (1975): Preservation of membrane ultrastructure with aldehyde or imidate fixatives. *J. Ultrastruct. Res. Suppl., 52,* 243–260.

Mosmann TR, Gallatin M, Longenecker BM (1980): Alteration of apparent specificity of monoclonal (hybridoma) antibodies recognizing polymorphic histocompatibility and blood group determinants. *J. Immunol., 125,* 1152–1156.

Nairn RC (1976): *Fluorescent Protein Tracing.* 4th ed. Churchill Livingstone, New York.

Nairn RC, Ploem JS (1974): Modern microscopy for immunofluorescence in clinical immunology. *Leitz Techn. Inform., 2,* 91–95.

Nakane PK (1971): Application of peroxidase-labelled antibodies to the intracellular localization of hormones. *Acta Endocrinol. Copenhagen,* Suppl. *153,* 190–202.

Nakane PK (1973): Ultrastructural localization of tissue antigens with the peroxidase-labelled antibody method. In: Wisse E, Daems WTh, Molenaar I, Van Duijn P (Eds), *Electron Microscopy and Cytochemistry,* pp. 129–143. North-Holland Publ. Co., Amsterdam.

Nielson AJ, Griffith WP (1979): Tissue fixation by osmium tetroxide. A possible role for proteins. *J. Histochem. Cytochem., 27,* 997–999.

Nisonoff A, Hopper JE, Spring SB (1975): *The Antibody Molecule.* Academic Press, New York.

Notani GW, Parsons JA, Erlandsen SL (1979): Versatility of Staphylococcus aureus protein A in immunocytochemistry. *J. Histochem. Cytochem., 27,* 1438–1444.

Ohtsuki I, Manzi RM, Palade GE, Jamieson JD (1978): Entry of macromolecular tracers into cells fixed with low concentrations of aldehydes. *Biol. Cell., 31,* 119–126.

Pachmann K, Leibold W (1976): Insolubilization of protein antigens on polyacrylic beads using poly-L-lysine. *J. Immunol. Methods, 12,* 81–89.

Paiement JM, Kopriwa BM (1978): Use of two different methods for the electron-microscope radioautographic detection of labelled antibodies bound to thin sections. *J. Histochem. Cytochem., 26,* 765–771.

Paiement J, Leblond CP (1977): Localization of thyroglobulin antigenicity in rat thyroid sections using antibodies labelled with peroxidase or ^{125}I-radioiodine, *J. Cell Biol., 74,* 992–1015.

Painter RG, Tokuyasu KT, Singer SJ (1973): Immunoferritin localization of intracellular antigens: The use of ultracryotomy to obtain ultrathin sections suitable for direct immunoferritin staining. *Proc. Nat. Acad. Sci. USA, 70,* 1649–1653.

Pearse AGE, Polak JM (1975): Bifunctional reagents as vapour- and liquid-phase fixatives for immunohistochemistry. *Histochem. J., 7,* 179–186.

Pease DC (1962): Buffered formaldehyde as a killing agent and primary fixative for electron-microscopy. *Anat. Rec., 142,* 342.

Peters K-R, Rutter G, Gschwender HH, Haller W (1978): Derivatized silica spheres as immunospecific markers for high resolution labelling in electron-microscopy. *J. Cell Biol., 78,* 309–319.

Petrusz P, Dimeo P, Ordronneau P, Weaver C, Keefer DA (1975): Improved immunoglobulin enzyme bridge method for light-microscopic demonstration of hormone-containing cells of rat adenohypophysis. *Histochemistry, 46,* 9–26.

Pickel VM, Joh TH, Reis DJ (1976): Monoamine-synthesizing enzymes in central dopaminergic, noradrenergic and serotonergic neurons. *J. Histochem. Cytochem., 24,* 792–806.

Rappay GY, Kárteszi M, Makara GB (1979): ACTH radioimmunocytochemistry (RICH) on rat anterior pituitary cells. *Histochemistry, 59,* 207–213.

Ravazzola M, Orci L (1980): Transformation of glicentin-containing L-cells into glucagon-containing cells by enzymatic digestion. *Diabetes, 29,* 156–158.

Reading M (1977): A digestion method for the reduction of background staining in the immunoperoxidase method. *J. Clin. Pathol., 30,* 88–90.

Romano EL, Romano M (1977): Staphylococcal protein A bound to colloidal gold: A useful reagent to label antigen-antibody sites in electron-microscopy. *Immunochemistry, 14,* 711–715.

Romano EL, Stolinski C, Hughes-Jones WC (1974): An antiglobulin reagent labelled with colloidal gold for use in electron-microscopy. *Immunochemistry, 11,* 521–522.

Roth J, Bendayan M, Orci L (1978): Ultrastructural localization of intracellular antigens by the use of protein A-gold complex. *J. Histochem. Cytochem., 26,* 1074–1081.

Roth J, Bendayan M, Orci L (1980): FITC-protein A-gold complex for light- and electron-microscopic immunocytochemistry. *J. Histochem. Cytochem., 28,* 54–59.

Schurer JW, Hoedemaeker PhJ, Molenaar I (1977): Polyethyleneimine as tracer particle for (immuno) electron-microscopy. *J. Histochem. Cytochem., 25,* 384–387.

Schwaab ME, Thoenen H (1978): Selective binding, uptake and retrograde transport of tetanus toxin by nerve terminals in the rat iris. An electron-microscopic study using colloidal gold as a tracer. *J. Cell Biol., 77,* 1–13.

Seman G, Nairn RC (1977): Monolayer cultures for immunofluorescent staining from tumor primary explants. *Stain Technol., 52,* 323–325.

Silverman AJ (1976): Ultrastructural studies on the localization of neurohypophyseal hormones and their carrier proteins. *J. Histochem. Cytochem., 24,* 816–827.

Skelley DS, Brown LP, Besch PK (1973): Radioimmunoassay. *Clin. Chem. (NY), 19,* 146–186.

Slot JW, Geuze HJ (1981): Sizing of protein A-colloidal gold probes for immunoelectron-microscopy. *J. Cell. Biol.,90,* 533–536.

Sofroniew MV, Madler M, Müller OA, Scriba PC (1978): A method for the consistent production of high quality antisera to small peptide hormones. *Fresenius Z. Anal. Chem., 290,* 163.

Stefanini M, De Martino C, Zámboni L (1967): Fixation of ejaculated spermatozoa for electron-microscopy. *Nature, 216,* 173–174.

Sternberger LA (1973): *Immunocytochemistry.* Prentice-Hall Inc., Englewood Cliffs, N.J.

Sternberger LA (1979): *Immunocytochemistry.* 2nd Ed., John Wiley & Sons, Inc., New York.

Sternberger LA, Hardy PH, Cuculus JJ, Meyer HG (1970): The unlabelled antibody-enzyme method of immunohistochemistry. Preparation and properties of soluble antigen-antibody complex (horseradish peroxidase-antihorseradish peroxidase) and its use in identification of spirochetes. *J. Histochem. Cytochem., 18,* 315–333.

Sternberger LA, Joseph SA (1979): The unlabelled antibody method. Contrasting color staining of paired pituitary hormones without antibody removal. *J. Histochem. Cytochem., 27,* 1424–1429.

Sternberger LA, Petrali JP (1975): Quantitative immunocytochemistry of pituitary receptors for luteinizing hormone-releasing hormone. *Cell Tissue Res., 162,* 141–176.

Streefkerk JG, Defelder AM, Kors N, Kornelis D (1975): Antigen-coupled beads adherent to slides: A simplified method for immunological studies. *J. Immunol. Methods, 8,* 251–256.

Tabuchi K, Kirsch WM, Nakane PK (1976): The fine structural localization of S-100 protein in rodent cerebellum. *J. Neurol. Sci., 28,* 65–76.

Takamiya H, Bodemer W, Vogt A (1978): Masking of protein antigens by modification of amino groups with carbobenzoxychloride (benzyl chloroformate) and demasking by treatment with non-specific protease. *J. Histochem. Cytochem., 26,* 914–920.

Thorell JI, Larsson SM (1978): *Radioimmunoassay and Related Techniques.* C.V. Mosby Co., St. Louis, Mo.

Tokuyasu KT (1978): A study of positive staining of ultrathin frozen sections. *J. Ultrastruct. Res. Suppl., 63,* 287–307.

Tramu G, Pillez A, Leonardelli J (1978): An efficient method of antibody elution for the successive or simultaneous localization of two antigens by immunocytochemistry. *J. Histochem. Cytochem., 26,* 322–324.

Vandesande F, Dierickx K (1975): Identification of the vasopressin producing and of the oxytocin producing neurons in the hypothalamic magnocellular neurosecretory system of the rat. *Cell Tissue Res., 164,* 153–162.

Vandesande F, Dierickx K (1976): Immunocytochemical demonstration of separate vasotocinergic and mesotocinergic neurons in the amphibian hypothalamic magnocellular neurosecretory system. *Cell Tissue Res., 175,* 289–296.

Van Leeuwen FW (1977): Immunoelectron-microscopic visualization of neurohypophyseal hormones: Evaluation of some tissue preparations and staining procedures. *J. Histochem. Cytochem., 25,* 1213–1221.

Van Raamsdonk W, Pool CW, Heyting C (1977): Detection of antigens and antibodies by an immunoperoxidase method applied on thin longitudinal sections of SDS-polyacryl-amide gels. *J. Immunol. Methods, 17,* 337–348.

Wachsmuth ED (1976): The localization of enzymes in tissue sections by immunohistochemistry. Conventional antibody and mixed aggregation techniques. *Histochem. J., 8,* 253–270.

Webb JA, Dorling J (1972): The use of peroxidase-labelled antiglobulin for ultrastructural localization of tissue antigens reacting with serum antibodies. *J. Immunol. Methods, 2,* 145–157.

Williams CD, Chase MW (Eds) (1976): *Methods in Immunology and Immunochemistry, Vol. 5,* pp. 375–495. Academic Press, New York.

Willingham MC, Yamada SS (1979): Development of a new primary fixative for electron-microscopic immunocytochemical localization of intracellular antigens in cultured cells. *J. Histochem. Cytochem., 27,* 947–960.

Yasuda K, Yamamoto J (1975): Metal labelled antibody method. Indirect label of chloromercuriferrocene to antibody. *Acta Histochem. Cytochem., 8,* 215–219.

Zehr DR (1978): Use of hydrogen peroxide-egg albumin to eliminate non-specific staining in immunoperoxidase techniques. *J. Histochem. Cytochem., 26,* 415–416.

Zsigmondy A (1889): Über lösliches Gold. *Z. Elektrochem., 4,* 546–549.

CHAPTER V

Immunocytochemistry: Preparation of antibodies and staining specificity

MICHAEL V. SOFRONIEW, REJEAN COUTURE AND A. CLAUDIO CUELLO

1. INTRODUCTION

Immunohistochemistry has developed into a powerful and widely used tool in neurobiology allowing direct visualization of a variety of different kinds of substances produced by and contained within neurons, including transmitter candidates, peptides, structural proteins, enzyme substrates and various types of enzymes. The principle of immunohistochemistry, as described in the previous chapter, is such that it relies upon specific recognition by an antibody of an antigen which has been fixed to the tissue. Immunohistochemistry can be conducted either with polyvalent antisera or with monoclonal antibodies generated using the hybridoma technique (Cuello et al. 1979, 1983). Polyvalent antisera can often contain several antibodies directed against different determinants on the desired antigen as well as antibodies against other unwanted antigens. Monoclonal antibodies in contrast consist of a homogenous population of antibodies directed against a single determinant. The quality and specificity of the immunohistochemical staining obtained is for the most part determined by the antibodies or antisera used. In this chapter, methods for production of antisera and for production of monoclonal antibodies for use in immunohistochemical detection of various kinds of antigens will be reviewed and summarized. We will also discuss staining specificity as it relates to the antibodies used, and as it relates to immunohistochemical procedure in general.

2. ANTIGENS

A variety of different kinds of antigens have been studied using immunohistochemical techniques in neurobiology. These range from large macromolecules purified in small amounts from biological sources, to small peptides or single aminoacids requiring conjugation to carrier proteins as haptens, to the more recent use of homogenates of crude or semi-purified material from nervous tissue to generate monoclonal antibodies against unknown antigens. Each type of antigen carries with it its own peculiarities and will be discussed separately.

2.1. MACROMOLECULES PURIFIED FROM BIOLOGICAL SOURCES

This category of antigen includes specific transmitter associated enzymes (Geffen et al. 1969; Hartman 1973; Pickel et al. 1975; Eckenstein and Thoenen 1982), enzymes involved in more general cell metabolism (Ariano et al. 1982), structural proteins (Stern-

Handbook of Chemical Neuroanatomy. Vol. 1: Methods in Chemical Neuroanatomy.
A. Björklund and T. Hökfelt, editors.
© Elsevier Science Publishers B.V., 1983.

berger et al. 1978), polypeptides and proteins such as hormones (Moriarty 1976), precursor proteins or portions thereof (Livett et al. 1971), metabolically important proteins (Bloom et al. 1979), or exogenously applied tracer proteins (Sofroniew 1983). When using antigens from biological sources to produce antisera the specificity of the antisera obtained is of course directly related to the purity of the antigen preparation used. Contaminating substances in less purified preparations can also act as antigens and may be detected immunohistochemically by the polyvalent antiserum. If total purification is impossible or extremely difficult, this problem can be circumvented to some degree by using incompletely purified preparations of an antigen to raise monoclonal antibodies and selecting a monovalent clone directed solely against the desired antigen. Nevertheless, without a reasonably purified antigen, selection of the clones and establishment of the specificity of the antibody and staining eventually obtained is not simple. Of particular interest to neurobiologists has been the production of antisera for immunohistochemical application against transmitter associated enzymes. Different polyvalent antisera have been raised against a number of such enzymes allowing relatively straightforward immunohistochemical localization of, among others, dopamine-β-hydroxylase (Hartman 1973), tyrosine hydroxylase (Pickel et al. 1975; Hökfelt et al. 1976) and glutamate decarboxylase (Saito et al. 1974). However, a certain amount of controversy has developed around the purification of the acetylcholine synthesizing enzyme choline acetyltransferase (ChAT) and around the production and immunohistochemical use of antisera and monoclonal antibodies against ChAT.

A brief discussion of the problems in this case can serve to illustrate some of the difficulties which can be encountered when producing and using antisera against purified antigens. ChAT is present in very low concentrations in nervous tissue and extensive and laborious purification is necessary to achieve even partial purification. Several polyvalent antisera have therefore been generated with partially purified preparations of ChAT and immunohistochemical studies have been conducted (Eng et al. 1974; McGeer et al. 1974). The results were in some cases not reproducible, with conflicting reports appearing even from the same group (McGeer et al. 1974; Kimura et al. 1980, 1981). Criticism was strong and the need for repetition of the studies using more reliable antisera or antibodies was emphasized (Rossier et al. 1977, 1981). Different approaches to resolving the problems are currently being employed. These are to purify the enzyme to near homogeneity prior to immunization (Cozzari and Hartman 1980; Eckenstein et al. 1981), or to prepare monoclonal antibodies from partially purified preparations (Levey and Wainer 1982). Results using these approaches are beginning to appear. Using antisera prepared against ChAT of over 95% purity (Eckenstein et al. 1981; Eckenstein and Thoenen 1982) for immunohistochemical detection (Fig. 1a), the topography of central cholinergic neurons obtained correlates reasonably well with portions of previous reports, but some marked differences to the staining reported in previous reports were also found (Sofroniew et al. 1982). Most notably, no staining described as 'cholinoceptive' by Kimura et al. (1981) was observed using these antisera. The difference in results obtained by different groups purifying the same enzyme and raising antisera for immunohistochemistry indicates that particular care must be taken in this kind of approach. Another interesting observation derived from these studies is that certain monoclonal antibodies can be exquisitely specific. One monoclonal antibody raised against ChAT from pig brain showed no cross-reactivity with ChAT of other species although it bound quite well to pig ChAT (Eckenstein and Thoenen 1982).

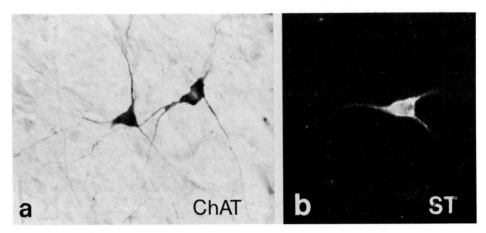

Fig. 1. (a) Immunoperoxidase staining using the PAP procedure with a polyclonal antiserum generated against choline acetyltransferase (Eckenstein and Thoenen 1982). Note the multipolar nature of the positively stained cholinergic neurons in the ventral globus pallidus of a normal rat. Antiserum courtesy of F. Eckenstein. (b) Immunofluorescence staining with FITC-labelled anti-rabbit IgG attached to polyclonal rabbit antiserum K18 780414 against somatostatin produced according to Sofroniew et al. (1978). Note the positively stained neuron in the neostriatum of a normal rat. (Photograph courtesy of J.V. Priestley)

2.2. SMALL MOLECULES REQUIRING CONJUGATION TO CARRIER PROTEINS

This category of antigen includes primarily peptides and small transmitters such as serotonin. These compounds, which are generally available synthetically in pure form, are usually too small (molecular weight of under 7000) to be effectively antigenic of themselves for various reasons. They are, therefore, conjugated as haptens to carrier proteins prior to inoculation. In this section we will consider various means of conjugation, selection of carrier proteins and conjugation strategy, i.e. proportion of hapten conjugated or exposed, hapten to carrier ratio, etc. Conjugation of haptens to carrier proteins and resultant generation of antibodies to the carrier requires attention to potential problems of staining specificity. These will be considered in Section 4.1 on staining specificity.

(a) Methods of conjugation

Conjugation involves production of a stable covalent bond between the hapten and the carrier by an activating agent. In some cases, particularly with very small antigens, it is helpful to place a spacer molecule between the hapten and the carrier. The most frequently used activating agents are carbodiimide, glutaraldehyde and formaldehyde.

Carbodiimide

This agent can be used to couple compounds containing many types of functional groups, including carboxylic acids, amines, phosphates, alcohols and thiols by the formation of amides, esters and peptide bonds (Khorana 1953; Sheehan and Hlavka 1956). The peptide bonds can be synthesized chemically in fully aqueous solutions directly from the free acid and amino components by using a water-soluble carbo-diimide (Sheehan and Hlavka 1956), the most commonly used is 1-ethyl-3(3-dimethyl-aminopropyl) carbodiimide. Carbodiimide has been used to conjugate various different haptens, both peptidic and non-peptidic, to different carriers. Some care must be taken when using carbodiimide as it may alter the aromatic ring of tyrosine to form either O-aryl isourea or N-aryl urea (Carraway and Koshland 1968). This possible tyrosine rearrangement in the presence of carbodiimide is reversed by adding hydroxyl-amine (1M) subsequent to conjugation (Carraway and Koshland 1968). Detailed conjugation procedures using carbodiimide have been described for various proteins, peptides and other compounds (see Beiser et al. 1968; Skowsky and Fisher 1972; Scherer et al. 1978; Sofroniew et al. 1978).

Glutaraldehyde

This agent reacts with the α-amino groups of amino acids, the N-terminal amino groups of some peptides and the sulfhydryl group of cysteine. The phenolic and imidazole rings of tyrosine and histidine derivatives are partially active (Habeeb and Hiramoto 1968). Glutaraldehyde conjugation proceeds via amino-amino covalent coupling with a 3-carbon fragment remaining interposed between hapten and carrier (Beiser et al. 1968). The reaction of glutaraldehyde with proteins produces 2 species: monomers and aggregates. The soluble aggregates constitute the major species and are formed through intermolecular cross-linking while the monomers constitute the minor species and are formed through intramolecular cross-linkages (Habeeb and Hiramoto 1968). Glutaraldehyde is the most effective and suitable agent for producing enzyme-protein complexes which retain part of their enzymatic and immunological specificity (Avrameas 1969). Glutaraldehyde has also been used to insolubilize proteins or to conjugate various haptens (peptidic and non-peptidic) to different carriers. Detailed conjugation procedures using glutaraldehyde have been described for peptides, proteins or enzymes (Beiser et al. 1968; Habeeb and Hiramoto 1968; Avrameas 1969).

Formaldehyde

This agent combines with the free amino groups to form amino methylol groups which then condense with other functional groups (e.g. phenol, imidazole and indole groups), to form methylene bridges. Reaction also occurs between formaldehyde and the sulfhydryl group of cysteine. Formaldehyde has been used primarily to conjugate small peptidic or aminergic haptens to different carriers. Formaldehyde is currently popular for the conjugation of transmitter candidates such as serotonin to carrier proteins (Steinbusch et al. 1978; Consolazione et al. 1981).

Other coupling agents

In some situations it may be necessary or useful to couple at sites using different reacting groups. Other less commonly used coupling agents have been described (Williams and Chase 1967; Parker 1976).

Non-covalent adsorption

Recently, useful antisera of high titer, sensitivity and specificity have been obtained against various peptides by non-covalent adsorption of the peptides to a carrier protein (Benoit et al. 1980). The procedure involves simply the adsorption of a 100-fold molar excess of the hapten to the ionized surface of methylated bovine serum albumin.

(b) Selection of carrier proteins

A wide variety of carriers has been used for attachment of haptens ranging from inorganic macromolecules such as sepharose beads (Larsson et al. 1979), to macromolecules like the synthetic polyamino acids, to naturally occurring large proteins such as serum albumin, thyroglobulin or keyhole limpet hemocyanin. Bovine serum albumin (BSA) has been frequently used because of its size, large number of reactive groups, and its solubility properties which usually permit it to remain in solution under a variety of conditions of pH, ionic strength and in the presence of organic solvents. Bovine thyroglobulin is a particularly effective protein carrier for the induction of antigenicity to small molecules and has been a useful immunogen for the production of antisera against compounds as diverse as thyroxine (Chopra et al. 1971), prostaglandin E (Scherer et al. 1978) and a large number of peptides and small proteins in 100% of the immunized animals (Skowsky and Fisher 1972; Sofroniew et al. 1978). In contrast, vasopressin and PTH failed to be antigenic when conjugated to BSA, ovalbumine and several amino acid polymers (polylysine, polyglutamic acid, multichain poly-D-, L-Ala-poly-L-Lysine) (Skowsky and Fisher 1972). It seems that the homo- and heteropolymers of polyamino acids tend to be relatively poor immunogens (Skowsky and Fisher 1972). The reason behind the ability of thyroglobulin to enhance the immune response is unclear. Current evidence suggests that the immunogenicity of a carrier protein is directly related to its stability in vivo (Sela 1969) and a large molecule like thyroglobulin (MW = 650,000 as compared with BSA MW = 70,000) has much more cross-linked peptide intramolecular bonds adding to its stability and metabolic resistance in animals. Keyhole limpet hemocyanin and limulus hemocyanin have also been used as carriers and show potent immunogenicity.

In general, it seems fair to say that best results have been obtained when using as carriers the naturally occurring large proteins thyroglobulin, hemocyanin or serum albumin. Selection of one or the other of these is often based on positive past personal experience. We have had particularly good experience with thyroglobulin which produced an extraordinarily high success ratio with over 20 different small molecule immunogens (Sofroniew et al. 1978) immunized in rabbits, rats and mice in different laboratories with numerous collaborators. Nevertheless, we have also found serum albumin a successful carrier for certain peptides (Cuello et al. 1979) and amines (Consolazione et al. 1981). With difficult or new haptens it may be useful to test several carriers.

(c) Strategy of conjugation

Ideally, attachment between a carrier and a hapten should take place in the area of the hapten that is least important for immunological recognition. Let us assume that a hapten contains several determinants A, B, C. Conjugation to the carrier through A would favor the formation of antibodies directed primarily toward B and/or C and vice versa. The choice of conjugation through A,B or C can be influenced by various factors such as the desire to distinguish between two homologous peptides different only at one site or the other. Strategies which have been employed involve conjugation of peptides at their C- or N-terminal ends, or to reactive groups on aminoacids in the center of the peptide. Met-enkephalin (H-Tyr-Gly-Gly-Phe-Met-OH) and Leu-enkephalin (H-Tyr-Gly-Gly-Phe-Leu-OH) have been distinguished with antisera generated against the C-terminal portion of enkephalins (Miller et al. 1978; Larsson et al. 1979). Glutaraldehyde was chosen in this case for its ability to react with a primary free amino group of the peptide and preferentially that of the N-terminal. Production of a specific monoclonal antibody against the C-terminal portion of SP has also been previously described (Cuello et al. 1979).

The quality of the immune response can be influenced by many factors such as carrier immunogenicity, the dose of the antigen, immunization schedule, species of animal and the incorporation ratio of hapten to carrier. A conjugate with a high molar incorporation ratio (final hapten to carrier ratio) would have multiple determinant sites exposed and might be more antigenic, although this has never been conclusively demonstrated. Selection of an intermediate incorporation of about 25-50:1 for thyroglobulin conjugate has been found to evoke excellent antibody production. During conjugation, a molar ratio of hapten:thyroglobulin:carbodiimide of about 60-120:1:200 gave an optimal final incorporation ratio of hapten onto carrier (Skowsky and Fisher 1972; Sofroniew et al. 1978). However, a variety of different molar ratios of reagents in the conjugation mixture have been successfully used in various studies using carbodiimide, glutaraldehyde or other conjugating agents in combination with other carrier proteins. Final selection of a ratio depends upon the availability of the hapten, nature of the carrier and the type of conjugating agent used. The ratios used in the studies listed have been selected empirically because of their efficacy, and when using a new hapten it is probably wise to at least initially not deviate much from these values.

2.3. CRUDE OR SEMIPURIFIED HOMOGENATES OF NEURAL TISSUES AS ANTIGENS

The application of monoclonal antibodies to immunohistochemistry in neurobiology has opened several new areas of experimental approach. Among these is the injection of homogenates of neural tissue to raise antibodies against unknown antigens and isolation of the clones producing antibodies against single determinants. The antibodies are screened immunohistochemically to determine to which structures they bind, often revealing previously unsuspected antigenic relationships between various structures. The antibodies can then also be used to isolate and characterize antigens of particular interest. Studies of this nature are just beginning to emerge and have employed unpurified homogenates of brain areas (Sternberger et al. 1982) or dorsal root ganglia (Wood et al. 1982) or of cultured peripheral neural ganglia (Vulliamy et al. 1981) as well as semipurified fractions such as synaptic plasma membranes from cerebellum (Hawkes et al. 1982). Interesting relationships that have been discovered include common antigenic determinants between sensory neurons and the parasite *Trypanosoma cruzi* (Wood et al. 1982). The common antigens may underly the degeneration of these neurons observed during Chagas' disease which is caused by this organism. In addition, common antigenic determinants between populations of neurons in different central nervous system (CNS) areas (Sternberger et al. 1982) as well as antigenic determinants restricted to specific cellular locations (Hawkes et al. 1982) and antigens specific for a CNS region (Galfré, Milstein and Cuello, in preparation) have been found. Antibodies distinguishing peripheral from central neurons

(Vulliamy et al. 1981) or antibodies recognizing glial cells (Sommer and Schachner 1981) have also been developed. This approach also promises to reveal much new and exciting information.

3. PREPARATION AND USE OF POLYCLONAL ANTISERA

The preparation of a polyclonal antiserum involves the inoculation of an animal with an antigen and, after an appropriate lenght of time, the harvesting of the animal's plasma or serum which contains antibodies against the antigen. In practice, certain antigens are only poorly antigenic or certain antigens are available only in small amounts so that it is wise to follow certain procedures which have repeatedly proven successful. The first decision is which animal to use. Rabbits have been the most common source of antisera used in immunohistochemistry. They are easy to handle, of convenient size and produce reasonably large amounts of serum. Nevertheless excellent antisera have been obtained from guinea pigs, rats, mice or goats. An obvious problem with smaller animals is the smaller amount of serum which can be harvested. Conversely, a problem with goats is their expense and the difficulty in caring for them. Today the necessary immunohistochemical developing reagents such as labelled and unlabelled 2nd antibody and PAP-complex are available to match a large number of different species of primary antibody so that this need not be a consideration in selecting a species for immunization. Next, the amount of antigen to be inoculated must be determined. Experience has shown that smaller amounts seem to produce more antibodies of higher affinity. This is, of course, valid only up to a point. Therefore, unless following a protocol known to have been successful before, it is wise to use different amounts. In general, amounts in the microgram range for unconjugated macromolecules have proven successful: in the range of 10-100 μg for mice, rats or guinea pigs or in the range of 50-300 μg for rabbits or goats per animal per inoculation. The amount of conjugated antigen is slightly more difficult to estimate but we have had very good success with amounts ranging from 0.5-2.5 mg of conjugate per inoculation per animal for rabbits (Sofroniew et al. 1978), and from 50-250 μg for rodents. Smaller amounts can also be used. As little as 3 μg of conjugate containing 3 ng of peptide has been effective in inducing antibodies to substance in P in rats (Cuello et al. 1979). The antigen should be dissolved in a small amount of water or saline and emulsified in an equal amount of Freund's complete adjuvant (procedures for this are described in many immunology texts). The next decision involves the means of inoculation. One of the most successful procedures has proven to be the intradermal injection technique (Vaitukaitis et al. 1971). In this technique small amounts (10-25μl) of antigen-emulsion are injected into the skin in muliple sites spread over the entire back of the animal (about 25-50 sites per 500 μl). Care should be taken that the injections are truly intradermal and not subcutaneous. In intradermal injections, the antigen-emulsion remains in the skin for long periods of time and provides a slow constant exposure to the antigen. This procedure may be used alone or in combination with injection into the footpads and intraperitoneally.

After the first inoculation, selecting a further inoculation schedule can depend upon the size of the antigen, the immunogenic properties of the antigen and on the animals used. There is no proven optimal schedule. Biweekly inoculations are perhaps the most common. We have had good success with 'difficult' antigens using an initial series of 3 or 4 biweekly inoculations followed by pauses of varying length followed by resumption of inoculations in rabbits (Sofroniew et al. 1978). In general, antibodies can be expected 6-10 weeks after the initial inoculation. The quality of the antiserum can in some cases improve up to 9 months following initial inoculation. Antisera are best harvested by bleeding the animals 10-14 days after inoculation. Rabbits are best bled through the ear veins, rats and mice through the tail veins. Following centrifugation, the serum is best aliquoted and stored frozen or lyophilized. Antisera may also be 'purified' to remove known unwanted antibodies, such as those against carrier proteins. This will be discussed in Section 5.1 on establishing the specificity of antisera. Polyvalent antisera are used in a number of different immunohistochemical procedures. Most commonly they are used with the indirect immunofluorescent technique of Coons (1958) (Fig. 1b), or with the unlabelled antibody enzyme PAP procedure of Sternberger (1979) (Fig. 1a). They can also be used with biotin-avidin peroxidase conjugates (Hsu et al. 1981) or with protein A-gold complex (Roth et al. 1978).

4. PREPARATION AND USE OF MONOCLONAL ANTIBODIES

Monoclonal antibodies are produced using the hybrid myeloma (hybridoma) technique developed by Köhler and Milstein (1975). This technique permits the derivation of highly specific antibodies from pure or impure immunogens. The in vitro maintenance of hybrid myeloma cells ensures a continuous supply of large quantities of the same antibody with the same binding properties. The in vitro production of antibody allows the preparation of radioactive internally labelled antibodies of high specific activities. Production of monoclonal antibodies for use in immunohistochemistry has recently been described in detail by Cuello et al. (1983). In principle, the production of monoclonal antibodies with the hybridoma technique consists of: (1) inoculating mice or rats with the desired antigen so as to produce an immune response; (2) collection of spleen immunocytes from the hyperimmune animals and fusion of these with hybrid myeloma cells; (3) isolation and culture of clones producing the desired antibodies. At present fusions can routinely be performed with mouse × mouse myeloma, rat × mouse myeloma, rat × rat myeloma. Hybridomas with other species are being explored in several laboratories. The myeloma parent cell contributes to the hybridoma its ability to grow permanently in tissue culture while the immunocytes provide the genetic information for the production of a specific antibody. The limitation of available myeloma cell lines to mice or rats necessitates that these species be used for initial immunization. The immunization of the mice or rats for eventual production of monoclonal antibodies follows the same procedures used for production of antisera as described in the previous section. It is recommended to use several different protocols, varying doses and inoculation schedules. The antisera produced by the immunized animals are tested and those animals having the best antisera are selected for fusion. The fusion is conducted preferably with a myeloma cell line of the same species, although some interspecies fusions have been successful (Cuello et al. 1979). Fusion is conducted under sterile conditions. The spleen is removed and a cell suspension made. This cell suspension is mixed with suspended myeloma cells which have been exposed to polyethylene glycol to promote fusion. Following fusion, the non-fused parental cells are eliminated from the cultures. To do this, the cultures are grown in so-called HAT (hypoxanthine, aminopterin, thymidine) selective medium (Littlefield 1964; Szybalski et al. 1962). The myeloma cell lines usually utilized are azaguanine resistant which is taken as an indication that the cells are lacking the enzyme hypoxanthine-guanine phosphoribosyltransferase (HGPRT). These mutant cells are unable to survive in 'HAT medium'. In this medium aminopterin blocks the main biosynthetic pathway for the production of nucleic acids and the cells are forced to use the so-called 'salvage pathway' of HGPRT and thymidine kinase (Ringertz and Savage 1976). The immunocytes from hyperimmune animals provide the genetic material for the production of a specific antibody and for HGPRT, allowing the hybrids to grow in HAT medium. Non-fused parental myeloma will disappear in HAT while non-fused immunocytes are overgrown by the hybrids. After the elimination of parental cells the hybrids can be grown in a normal culture medium (Dulbecco's modified Eagles medium) and antibody production tested from the spent fluid. Isolated clones are grown in individual wells in tissue cultures and the culture medium of the various clones is tested for antibody production. Positive clones are regrown in large amounts and portions frozen for future availability.

Once a clone has been selected as producing an antibody suitable for routine immunohistochemical use, there are a number of alternatives open. The supernatant containing the antibodies can be diluted and used directly in any of the conventional immunohistochemical procedures described for use with antisera. Alternatively, the clone cells can be intraperitoneally injected into an animal of the donor species and ascites collected at regular intervals. The clone cells will form a myeloma in the host abdomen and the ascites will contain the monoclonal antibodies in high concentration. The ascites can be diluted and used directly in any of the conventional two or more step immunohistochemical procedures. Monoclonal antibodies also offer a variety of means of direct, or one-step, immunocytochemical procedures. The antibodies can be directly labelled with peroxidase (Boorsma et al. 1983), colloidal gold particles (De Mey 1983), or can be internally radioactively labelled (Cuello et al. 1982) (Figs 2 and 3). Internal radioactive labelling results in an extremely sensitive marker which can effectively be combined with other immunohistochemical techniques at both the light- (Fig. 4a-c) and electron-microscopic (Fig. 4d) levels for the simultaneous visualization of more than one antigen in the same tissue section (Cuello et al. 1982).

Monoclonal antibodies can also be used as so-called developing antibodies in the immunohistochemical procedure. Developing antibodies are those involved in making visible the primary antibody bound to the tissue-fixed antigen. These developing antibodies are anti-IgG's which bind to the primary antibodies, or anti-peroxidase antibodies used in the unlabelled antibody-enzyme procedure. Rat PAP made from monoclonal antibodies has proven to be a useful reagent for use with rat primary monoclonal antibodies (Cuello, Wright, Bramwell and Milstein, in preparation). We have also recently raised a mouse monoclonal anti-rabbit-IgG for use as a developing antibody with polyvalent primary rabbit antisera (MacMillan et al. 1983). This monoclonal anti-rabbit-IgG works successfully with the conventional PAP procedure. However, more importantly, internally radioactively labelled antibody has been produced allowing the use of radioimmunocytochemistry with a wide variety of available rabbit antisera (Fig. 5), making these antisera available for use in different procedures for the simultaneous detection of several antigens.

5. STAINING SPECIFICITY

Specificity of the staining obtained using immunohistochemistry is determined to a large degree by the specificity of the antibodies or antisera used. However, specificity problems can also be caused by other aspects of the histological procedure such as fixa-

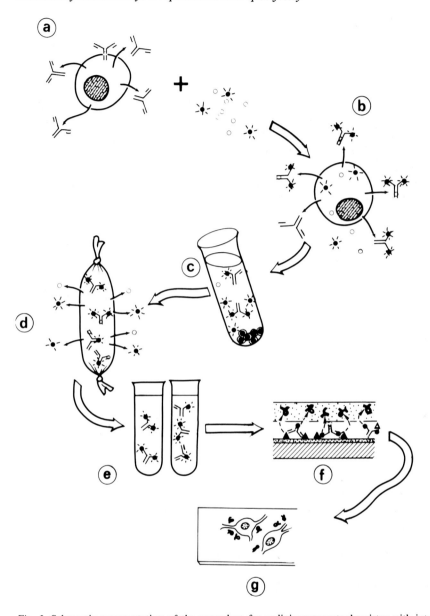

Fig. 2. Schematic representation of the procedure for radioimmunocytochemistry with internally labelled monoclonal antibodies. (a) Biosynthesis of unlabelled antibodies in tissue culture by the hybrid myeloma; (b) biosynthesis of radioactive antibodies by the addition of radiolabelled amino acids in the culture medium; (c) separation of the cells from medium by centrifugation; (d) dialysis of supernatant to eliminate non-incorporated radioactive amino acids; (e) storage of tritiated monoclonal antibodies for long periods (3H, 14C); (f) recognition of tissue antigens (dark triangles) by the internally labelled antibodies. Small arrows represent the emission of β-particles from labelled monoclonal antibodies and thick curled traces silver grain in the overlying photographic emulsion; (g) development of preparation as conventional radioautograph for light- or electron-microscopy. (From Cuello and Milstein 1981.)

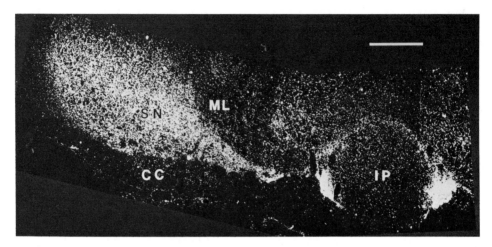

Fig. 3. Light-microscopic radioautograph (dark field) of a rat midbrain stained with internally radiolabelled monoclonal anti-substance P antibody (^{3}H-NCl/34). SN = substantia nigra; IP = interpeduncular nucleus; CC = crus cerebri; ML = medial lemniscus. Scale bar = 100 μm. (From Cuello et al. 1982.)

tion or tissue processing. These two basically different situations will be considered in separate sections.

5.1. SPECIFICITY OF ANTISERA AND MONOCLONAL ANTIBODIES

Having raised antisera or monoclonal antibodies against a defined antigen it is necessary to determine the specificity of the recognition of that antigen. Specificity problems which may be encountered include that the antibodies recognize substances closely related to the antigen or that polyvalent antisera may contain antibodies which recognize totally unrelated substances also present in the tissue sections. One of the more common means of testing the specificity of antibodies is in vitro tests such as radioimmunoassay or hemagglutination. However, these in vitro tests compare antigens and substances which have not been exposed to fixative. The antibody binding obtained under these conditions are not necessarily representative of the antibody binding obtained in fixed tissue sections and need not reflect immunohistochemical specificity. This point is clearly illustrated by the differential binding exhibited by the monoclonal antibody YC5/45 under in vitro conditions or in immunohistochemistry as demonstrated by Consolazione et al. (1981) and Milstein et al. (1983). This antibody was raised against serotonin (bound to serum albumin as a carrier) and was shown by various immunohistochemical means to react only with serotonin neurons and not with other monoamine-containing neurons in fixed tissue sections. However, in in vitro tests the antibody clearly recognizes dopamine, tryptamine and other monoamines and indeed has been shown in this type of test to have a higher affinity for several monoamines other than serotonin (see Table 1). The binding of the antibody to monoamines linked to serum albumin using paraformaldehyde was also tested in vitro. In this case the antibody recognized only serotonin (Milstein et al. 1983). This example clearly shows that fixation such as occurs in the tissue sections used for immunohistochemistry can dramatically affect the binding characteristics of antibodies to different substances. Thus it seems clear that specificity tests conducted in vitro with

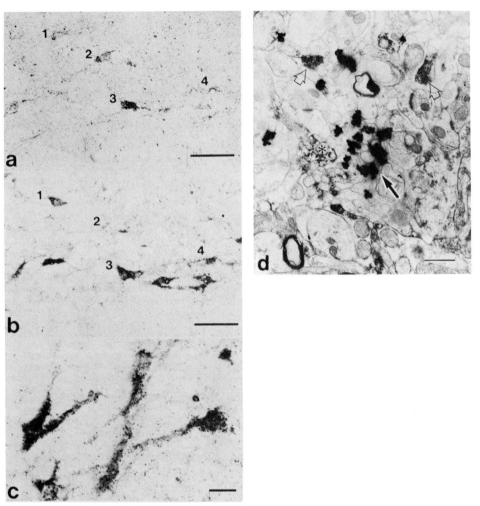

Fig. 4. Combined radioimmunocytochemistry and PAP immunocytochemistry. (a-c) Cryostat sections (10 μm thick) of the raphe magnus of the rat medulla oblongata. Antibodies were ^{3}H-NCl/34 (radiolabelled monoclonal anti-substance P antibody) and YC5/45 (anti-serotonin monoclonal antibody). *a* and *b* are consecutive serial sections. (a) Control. YC5/45 was adsorbed with excess serotonin. Note absence of immunoperoxidase reaction but intense radiolabelling over certain cell bodies (1-4), indicating the presence of substance P immunoreactivity. Scale bar = 200 μm. (b) Same preparation as *a* except that YC5/45 was not preadsorbed. Certain cells (1,3,4) observed in *a* appear in serial section and now show immunoperoxidase staining in addition to radiolabelling. This indicates that they contain serotonin as well as substance P. Scale bar = 200 μm. (c) High-magnification micrograph of a similar preparation to *b*, where silver grains (indicating substance P immunoreactivity) and homogeneous peroxidase reaction products (indicating serotonin immunoreactivity) appear over single neurons of the nucleus raphe magnus of the rat. Scale bar = 20 μm. (d) Combined radioimmunocytochemistry for substance P immunoreactivity and immunoperoxidase for Leu-enkephalin immunoreactivity in the substantia gelatinosa of the spinal nucleus of the trigeminal nerve (rat lower medulla oblongata, colchicine-treated animal). In this case the specimen has been prepared for electron-microscopy. Note clusters of silver grains over a nerve terminal in the centre of the field (solid arrow), indicating substance P immunoreactivity as revealed by ^{3}H-NCl/34. Open arrows denote the presence of Leu-enkephalin immunoreactive nerve terminals in the same field as revealed by immunoperoxidase. The asterisk indicates Leu-enkephalin immunoreactivity in a neuronal process (presumptive dendrite). Scale bar = 1 μm. (From Cuello et al. 1982.)

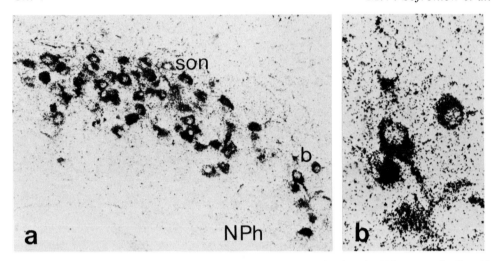

Fig. 5. Radioimmunocytochemistry using internally labelled monoclonal anti-rabbit IgG antibodies. (a) Light-microscopic autoradiograph of a paraffin section of the hypothalamic supraoptic nucleus of a Brattleboro-strain rat stained for neurophysin using a rabbit antiserum against neurophysin and an internally labelled mouse monoclonal antibody (^{3}H-RB/23) against rabbit immunoglobulin. Note the discrete accumulation of silver grains over only those neurons containing neurophysin (in this case only oxytocin neurons since the Brattleboro rat is genetically unable to produce vasopressin). (b) Detail of (*a*). (From MacMillan et al. 1983.)

unfixed antigens and other substances need not reflect immunohistochemical specificity. Although antigens exposed to fixative might prove more reliable in this sort of test, further investigation will be required to establish this.

Various sorts of immunohistochemical specificity tests have been devised generally based on the prevention of staining by absorption of the antiserum or antibodies with antigen, but not by absorption with other substances. Although these types of tests may give a general indication of specificity they do not conclusively demonstrate specificity or nonspecificity. Since absorption is conducted in vitro using unfixed substances the same objections just raised to other in vitro tests apply. Other objections may be raised

TABLE 1. *Inhibition of YC5/45 agglutination of serotonin-coupled red cells by a variety of substances*[a]

Substance	Concentration of inhibitor (10^{-6}M)
Serotonin	1200
Tryptamine	20
5-Methoxytryptamine	300
Dopamine	80
5-Hydroxyindolacetic acid	10,000
GABA	10,000
Noradrenaline	10,000
Adrenaline	10,000
5-Hydroxytryptophan	10,000
Carnosine	10,000
Melatonin	10,000
Serotonin albumin conjugate[b]	0.05

[a]The number refers to the concentration giving complete or almost complete inhibition (sample volume 50 μl).
[b]Molarity calculated as concentration of albumin. Adapted from Consolazione et al. (1981).

as well (Swaab et al. 1977). Perhaps a better system is the fixation of antigen and other substances to glass slides and investigation of staining properties on these slides (see Pool et al. 1983), but to date no optimal means of demonstrating immunohistochemical specificity has been devised.

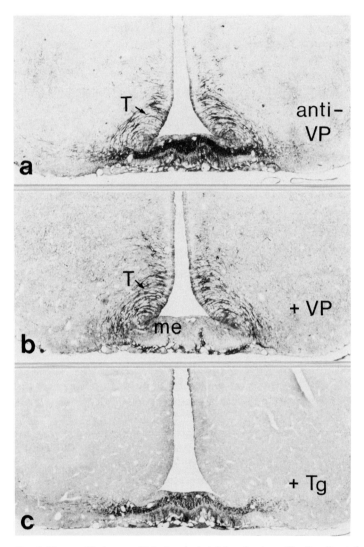

Fig. 6. Nonspecific immunohistochemical staining due to antibodies directed against a carrier protein used in producing an antiserum against a peptide. (a-c) Closely neighboring sections through the median eminence of a rat. (a) Staining with untreated anti-vasopressin antiserum Rb19. Note the positive staining not only of fibers in the median eminence (me), but also of tanycytes (T). (b) Staining with antiserum Rb19 preabsorbed with vasopressin. Note the complete absence of staining of fibers in the median eminence while the staining of tanycytes (T) is still present in full intensity. (c) Staining with antiserum Rb19 preabsorbed with the carrier protein used during immunization, bovine thyroglobulin. Note the complete absence of staining of tanycytes while the staining of fibers in the median eminence is still present in full intensity. Thus the staining of tanycytes observed with untreated antiserum Rb19 is not due to antibodies directed against the peptide vasopressin, but rather is due to antibodies directed against the carrier protein used to generate the antiserum and is therefore nonspecific.

One type of specificity problem which can be clearly demonstrated and effectively eliminated deals with polyvalent antisera which contain antibodies not directed against the desired specific antigen but which still react with and stain substances present in the tissue sections. This happens most frequently with antisera raised against haptens conjugated to carrier proteins, with the undesired antibodies being directed against a determinant on the carrier. An example of this is demonstrated by the antiserum Rb19 generated against vasopressin conjugated to thyroglobulin (Sofroniew et al. 1978). In addition to the structures known to contain vasopressin, this antiserum stained a population of tanycytes in the region of the infundibulum (Fig. 6a). The specificity of this staining was doubted and tested by absorption of the antiserum with peptide or carrier. Absorption of the antiserum with vasopressin prevented the staining of known vasopressinergic fibers, but staining of the tanycytes remained (Fig. 6b). Conversely, absorption of the antiserum with the carrier protein thyroglobulin prevented staining of the tanycytes while the staining of known vasopressinergic fibers remained (Fig. 6c). This test clearly demonstrated that a population of antibodies directed against a determinant in the carrier protein thyroglobulin was reacting with and staining the tanycytes. This possibility should always be considered when using antisera generated against antigens conjugated to carrier proteins. Excess and unwanted antibodies against carrier proteins can easily be removed from an antiserum by covalent binding of the carrier to sepharose beads, incubation of the antiserum with these beads and subsequent removal of the beads by centrifugation.

Yet another specificity problem one should consider is that the determinant on the antigen being studied, which is recognized by the otherwise specific antibodies, is shared by a different substance which is therefore also recognized by the antibody. The possibility is quite difficult to control and can ultimately only be demonstrated by simultaneous biochemical and immunological tests.

5.2. GENERAL METHOD SPECIFICITY

When considering specificity of immunohistochemical staining as determined by the antibodies or antisera used, the specificity of staining as determined by other aspects of immunohistochemical procedure should not be neglected. First and foremost among these is perhaps tissue fixation, followed by tissue processing subsequent to fixation and other aspects of immunohistochemical protocol. As we have already seen in the previous section, fixation can profoundly influence the substances recognized or not recognized by antibodies. Over or under fixation can result in false-positive or false-negative results due to alteration of molecular structure. In addition, poor fixation or delayed fixation such as that of autopsy specimens or other immersion fixed specimens, can result in the dislocation of antigens leading to the 'specific' immunohistochemical detection of substances in structures not normally containing them. Thus, attention to proper fixation is essential for correct interpretation of immunohistochemical results. Tissue processing subsequent to fixation can also affect immunohistochemical results. Many antigens will not survive dehydration in alcohol- or paraffin-embedding, leading to false-negative results. In addition, tissue processing of this nature can also occasionally result in false-positive staining for unknown reasons. Lastly, antisera and other reagents should not be used in too high concentrations as this will often result in nonspecific staining.

6. CLOSING REMARKS

Immunohistochemical techniques provide the potential to answer many pertinent neurobiological questions which cannot at present be approached by other means. The use of polyvalent antisera will continue to be of importance in this, but in particular the use of monoclonal antibodies promises to greatly enhance the impact made by immunohistochemical techniques. Nevertheless, it should never be far from mind that the identification made is immunological and subject to all the limitations that this implies. Even with monoclonal antibodies recognizing only a single determinant the true nature of the substance containing that determinant is not always certain. In addition, specificity is dertermined not only by the antibodies used but also by the fixation of the tissue and other more general histological parameters. Perhaps because of the ease with which visual observations tend to be accepted, unusual or controversial immunohistochemical findings should be supported by findings using other techniques, and the need for careful and critical interpretation of immunohistochemical findings in general deserves repeated emphasis.

7. ACKNOWLEDGEMENTS

We thank A. Barclay, J. Lloyd and B. Archer for photographic work and E. Iles and P. Campbell for editorial assistance. Grant support was provided by NINCDS (NRSA 1 F32 NS06959-1) to MVS; The MRC Canada and Conseil de la Recherche en santé du Québec to RC; and by the Wellcome and EP Abraham Cephalosporin Trusts to ACC.

8. REFERENCES

Ariano MA, Lewicki JA, Brandwein HJ, Murad F (1982): Immunohistochemical localization of guanylate cyclase within neurons of rat brain. *Proc. Nat. Acad. Sci. USA, 79,* 1316–1320.

Avrameas S (1969): Coupling of enzymes to proteins with glutaraldehyde. Use of the conjugates for the detection of antigens and antibodies. *Immunochemistry 6,* 43–52.

Beiser SM, Butler VP, Erlanger BF (1968): Hapten protein conjugate methodology and applications. In: Miescher PA, Muller Eberhard HJ (Eds). *Textbook of Immunopathology,* pp.15–23. Grune and Stratton, Inc, New York.

Benoit R, Ling N, Lavielle S, Brazeau P, Guillemin R (1980): Production of higher quality antisera against brain peptides with and without coupling. *Fed. Proc., 39,* 1166–1171.

Bloom FE, Ueda T, Battenberg E, Greengard P (1979): Immunocytochemical localization, in synapses, of protein I, an endogenous substrate for protein kinases in mammalian brain. *Proc. Nat. Acad. Sci. USA, 76,* 5982–5986.

Boorsma DM, Cuello AC, Van Leeuwen FW (1983): Direct immunocytochemistry with a horseradish peroxidase conjugated monoclonal antibody against substance P. *J. Histochem. Cytochem, 30,* 1211–1216.

Carraway KL, Koshland ED (1968): Reaction of tyrosine residues in proteins with carbodiimide reagents. *Biochem. Biophys. Acta, 160,* 272–274.

Chopra IJ, Nilson JC, Solomon DH, Fisher DA (1971): Production of antibodies specially binding triiodothyronine and thyroxine. *J. Clin. Endocrinol. Metab., 32,* 299–308.

Consolazione A, Milstein C, Wright B, Cuello AC (1981): Immunocytochemical detection of serotonin with monoclonal antibodies. *J. Histochem. Cytochem., 29,* 1425–1430.

Coons AH (1958): Fluorescent antibody methods. In: *General Cytochemical Methods.* Academic Press, New York.

Cozzari C, Hartman BK (1980): Preparation of antibodies specific to choline acetyltransferase from bovine caudate nucleus and immunohistochemical localization of the enzyme. *Proc. Nat. Acad. Sci. USA, 77,* 7453–7457.

Cuello AC, Milstein C (1981): In: Bizollon A Ch (Ed), *Physiological Peptides and New Trends in Radioimmunology,* p. 299. Elsevier/North-Holland, Amsterdam.

Cuello AC, Milstein C, Galfre G (1983): Immunocytochemistry with monoclonal antibodies. In: Cuello AC (Ed), *Immunohistochemistry. IBRO Handbook Series. Methods in the Neurosciences.* John Wiley and Sons, Inc. Chichester. In press.

Cuello AC, Priestley JV, Milstein C (1982): Immunocytochemistry with internally labeled monoclonal antibodies. *Proc. Nat. Acad. Sci. USA., 79,* 665–669.

Cuello AC, Galfre G, Milstein C (1979): Detection of substance P in the central nervous system by a monoclonal antibody. *Proc. Nat. Acad. Sci. USA., 76,* 3532–3536.

De Mey JR (1983): The preparation of immunoglobulin gold conjugates (IGS reagents) and their use as markers for light and electron microscopic immunocytochemistry. In: Cuello AC (Ed), *Immunohistochemistry IBRO Handbook Series. Methods in the Neurosciences.* John Wiley and Sons, Inc. Chichester. In press.

Eckenstein F, Thoenen H (1982): Production of specific antisera and monoclonal antibodies to choline acetyltransferase: Characterization and use for identification of cholinergic neurons. *EMBO Journal., 1,* 363–368.

Eckenstein F, Barde Y-A, Thoenen H (1981): Production of specific antibodies to choline acetyltransferase purified from pig brain. *Neuroscience, 6,* 993–1000.

Eng LF, Uyeda CT, Chao LP, Wolfgram F (1974): Antibody to bovine choline acetyltransferase and immunofluorescent localization of the enzyme in neurons. *Nature (London), 250,* 243–245.

Geffen LB, Livett BG, Rush RA (1969): Immunohistochemical localisation of protein components of catecholamine storage vesicles. *J. Physiol. (London), 204,* 593–603.

Habeeb AFSA, Hiramoto R (1968): Reactions of proteins with glutaraldehyde. *Arch. Biochem. Biophys., 126,* 16–26.

Hartman BK (1973): Immunofluorescence of dopamine-β-hydroxylase. Application of improved methodology to the localisation of the peripheral and central noradrenergic nervous system. *J. Histochem. Cytochem., 21,* 312–317.

Hawkes R, Niday E, Matus A (1982): Monoclonal antibodies identify novel neural antigens. *Proc. Nat. Acad. Sci. USA., 79,* 2410–2414.

Hökfelt T, Johansson O, Fuxe K, Goldstein M, Park D (1976): Immunohistochemical studies on the localisation and distribution of monoamine neuron systems in the rat brain. I. Tyrosine hydroxylase in the mes- and diencephalon. *Med. Biol., 54,* 427–453.

Hsu S-M, Raine L, Fanger H (1981): Use of avidin-biotin-peroxidase complex (ABC) in immunoperoxidase techniques: A comparison between ABC and unlabeled antibody (PAP) procedures. *J. Histochem. Cytochem., 29,* 577–580.

Khorana H-G (1953): The chemistry of carbodiimide. *Chem. Rev., 53,* 145–166.

Kimura H, McGeer PL, Peng JH, McGeer EG (1981): The central cholinergic system studied by choline acetyltransferase immunohistochemistry in the cat. *J. Comp. Neurol., 200,* 151–201.

Kimura H, McGeer PL, Peng F, McGeer EG (1980): Choline acetyltransferase-containing neurons in rodent brain demonstrated by immunohistochemistry. *Science, 208,* 1057–1059.

Köhler G, Milstein C (1975): Continuous culture of fused cells secreting antibody of predefined specificity. *Nature (London), 256,* 495–497.

Larsson L-I, Childera S, Snyder S (1979): Met- and Leuenkephalin immunoreactivity in separate neurones. *Nature (London), 282,* 407–410.

Levey AI, Wainer BH (1982): Cross-species and intraspecies reactivities of monoclonal antibodies against choline acetyltransferase. *Brain Res., 234,* 469–473.

Littlefield JW (1964): Selection of hybrids from masting of fibroblasts *in vitro* and their presumed recombinants. *Science, 145,* 709–716.

Livett BG, Uttenthal LO, Hope DB (1971): Localization of neurophysin II in the hypothalamo-neurohypophysial system of the pig by immunofluorescence histochemistry. *Phil Trans. Roy. Soc. Lond., B 261,* 371–378.

MacMillan FM, Sofroniew MV, Sidebottom E, Cuello AC (1983): Immunocytochemistry with monoclonal anti-immunoglobulin as a developing agent: Application to immunoperoxidase staining and radioimmunocytochemistry. Submitted for publication.

McGeer PL, McGeer EG, Singh VH, Chase WH (1974): Choline acetyltransferase localization in the central nervous system by immunohistochemistry. *Brain Res., 81,* 373–379.

Miller RJ, Chang K-J, Cooper B, Cuatrecasas P (1978): Radioimmunoassay and characterization of enkephalins in rat tissues. *J. Biol. Chem., 253,* 531–538.

Milstein C, Wright B, Cuello AC (1983): The discrepancy between the cross reactivity of a monoclonal antibody to serotonin and its immunohistochemical specificity. *Molec. Immunol., 20,* 113–123.

Moriarty GC (1976): Immunocytochemistry of the pituitary glycoprotein hormones. *J. Histochem. Cytochem., 24,* 846–851.

Parker CW (1976): *Radioimmunoassay of Biologically Active Compounds.* Prentice Hall, Inc, Englewood Cliffs, New Jersey.

Pickel VM, Joh TH, Field CG, Reis DJ (1975): Cellular localization of tyrosine hydroxylase by immunohistochemistry. *J. Histochem. Cytochem., 23,* 1–6.

Pool ChrW, Buijs RM, Swaab DF, Boer GJ, van Leeuwen FW (1983): On the way to a specific immunocytochemical localization. In: Cuello AC (Ed), *Immunohistochemistry IBRO Handbook Series. Methods in Neurosciences.* John Wiley and Sons, Inc, Chichester. In press.

Ringertz NR, Savage RE (1976): *Cell hybrids.* Academic Press, New York–London.

Rossier J (1977): Choline acetyltransferase: A review with special reference to its cellular and subcellular localization. *Int. Rev. Neurobiol., 20,* 284–337.

Rossier J (1981): Serum monospecificity: A prerequisite for reliable immunohistochemical localization of neuronal markers including choline acetyltransferase. *Neuroscience, 6,* 989–991.

Roth J, Bendayan M, Orci L (1978): Ultrastructural localization of intracellular antigens by the use of protein A-gold complex. *J. Histochem. Cytochem., 26,* 1074–1081.

Saito K, Barber R, Wu J-Y, Matsuda T, Roberts E, Vaughn JE (1974): Immunohistochemical localization of glutamate decarboxylase in rat cerebellum. *Proc. Nat. Acad. Sci. USA, 71,* 269–273.

Scherer B, Schnermann J, Sofroniew M, Weber PC (1978): Prostaglandin (PG) analysis in urine of humans and rats by different radioimmunoassays: Effect on PG-excretion by PG-synthetase inhibitors, laparotomy and furosemide. *Prostaglandins, 15,* 235–266.

Sela M (1969): Antigenicity: Some molecular aspects. *Science, 166,* 1365–1374.

Sheehan JC, Hlavka JJ (1956): The use of water-soluble and basic carbodiimides in peptide synthesis. *J. Org. Chem., 21,* 439–441.

Skowsky WR, Fisher DA (1972): The use of thyroglobulin to induce antigenicity to small molecules. *J. Lab. Clin. Med., 80,* 134–144.

Sofroniew MV (1983): Direct reciprocal connections between the bed nucleus of the stria terminalis and dorsomedial medulla oblongata: Evidence from immunohistochemical detection of tracer proteins. *J. Comp. Neurol., 213,* 399–405.

Sofroniew MV, Eckenstein F, Thoenen H, Cuello AC (1982): Topography of choline acetyltransferase-containing neurons in the forebrain of the rat. *Neurosci. Lett., 33,* 7–12.

Sofroniew MV, Madler M, Müller OA, Scriba PC (1978): A method for the consistent production of high quality antisera to small peptide hormones. *Fresenius Z. Anal. Chem., 290,* 163.

Sommer IJ, Schachner M (1981): Monoclonal antibodies (01 to 04) to digodendrocyte cell surfaces: An immunocytological study in the central nervous system. *Dev. Biol., 83,* 311–327.

Steinbusch HWM, Verhofstad AAJ, Joosten HWJ (1978): Localization of serotonin in the central nervous system by immunohistochemistry: Description of a specific and sensitive technique and some applications. *Neuroscience, 3,* 811–819.

Sternberger LA (1979): *Immunocytochemistry, 2nd Ed.,* John Wiley and Sons Inc., Chichester.

Sternberger LA, Harwell LW, Sternberger NH (1982): Neurotypy: regional individuality in rat brain detected by immunocytochemistry with monoclonal antibodies. *Proc. Nat. Acad. Sci. USA, 79,* 1326–1330.

Sternberger NH, Itoyama Y, Kies MW, Webster H de F (1978): Myelin basic protein demonstrated immunocytochemically in oligodendroglia prior to myelin sheath formation. *Proc. Nat. Acad. Sci. USA, 75,* 2521–2524.

Swaab DF, Pool ChrW, van Leeuwen FW (1977): Can specificity ever be proved in immunocytochemical staining? *J. Histochem. Cytochem., 25,* 388–391.

Szybalski W, Szybalska EH, Kagni G (1962): Genetic studies with human cell lines. *Nat. Cancer Inst. Monogr., 7,* 75–89.

Vaitukaitis J, Robbins JB, Nieschlag E, Ross GT (1971): A method for producing antisera with small doses of immunogen. *J. Clin. Endocrinol. Metab., 33,* 988–991.

Vulliamy T, Rattray S, Mirsky R (1981): Cell surface antigen distinguishes sensory and autonomic peripheral neurones from central neurones. *Nature (London), 291,* 418–420.

Williams CA, Chase MW (Eds) (1967): *Methods in Immunology and Immunochemistry, Vol. 1.* Academic Press, New York.

Wood JN, Hudson L, Jessell TM, Yamamoto M (1982): A monoclonal antibody defining antigenic determinants on subpopulations of mammalian neurones and *Trypanosoma cruzi* parasites. *Nature (London), 296,* 34–38.

CHAPTER VI

Combination of retrograde tracing and neurotransmitter histochemistry*

TOMAS HÖKFELT, GUNNAR SKAGERBERG, LANA SKIRBOLL AND
ANDERS BJÖRKLUND

1. INTRODUCTION

The origin of the recent revolution in retrograde tracing of neuronal connections dates
back to the beginning of the seventies when Kristensson, Olsson and Sjöstrand reported
that the fluorescent dye Evans blue (bound to albumin) as well as the enzyme horseradish peroxidase (HRP) are taken up by the axonal processes of neurons and are retrogradely transported to the parent cell bodies after administration into their peripheral
terminal fields (Kristensson 1970; Kristensson and Olsson 1971; Kristensson et al.
1971). Evans blue could be visualized directly by fluorescence-microscopy, and HRP
by light-microscopy after reaction with a suitable substrate such as diaminobenzidine
(DAB), according to Graham and Karnovsky (1966). The application of HRP for
anatomical tracing of neuronal pathways was developed by LaVail and LaVail in 1972
and several methodological contributions, in particular those of De Olmos (1977) and
Mesulam (1978), have further improved the applicability and sensitivity of the HRP
technique and made it the currently most commonly used method for retrograde
neuronal tracing. The use of Evans blue for the purpose of retrograde tracing of
neuronal connections was further exploited by Steward and Scoville (1976), and in 1977
Kuypers and collaborators showed that, besides Evans blue, several other fluorescent
substances of low molecular weight were efficiently taken up by axons and retrogradely
transported in the nervous system. This discovery initiated a systematic search for new
fluorescent tracers and a thorough characterization of their properties (Kuypers et al.
1977, 1979, 1980; Bentivoglio et al. 1979a, 1980). Some of these fluorescent tracers
have since been shown to be at least as efficient for retrograde tracing as HRP
(Sawchenko and Swanson 1981, Aschoff and Holländer 1982), and the combination of
different fluorescent tracers has proved to be a powerful method for anatomical studies
of neurons with branching projections (Van der Kooy et al. 1978; Bentivoglio et al.
1979b, 1981; Van der Kooy 1979; Van der Kooy and Kuypers 1979; Kuypers et al. 1980;
Van der Kooy and Hattori 1980; Huismann et al. 1981; Bentivoglio and Kuypers 1982).
For general reviews on retrograde tracing techniques in neuroanatomical research, the
reader is referred to, for example, Cowan and Cuenod (1975), Kuypers (1981), Steward
(1981), Mesulam (1982) and Kuypers and Huismann (1983).

Parallel to these developments new histochemical techniques for neurotransmitter
localization were introduced (see, Jones and Hartman 1978; Livett 1978). Thus, during

*The present studies were supported by The Swedish Medical Research Council (04X-2887; 04X-4493);
NIH-NS 06701; Magnus Bergvalls Stiftelse; and Knut och Alice Wallenbergs Stiftelse.

Handbook of Chemical Neuroanatomy. Vol. 1: Methods in Chemical Neuroanatomy.
A. Björklund and T. Hökfelt, editors.
© Elsevier Science Publishers B.V., 1983.

the seventies the immunocytochemical methodology (Coons et al. 1942; Weller and Coons 1954; Nakane and Pierce 1967; Avrameas 1969; Nairn, 1969; Sternberger et al. 1970) was applied for localization of peptides and neurotransmitter-related proteins in neurons (Geffen et al. 1969; Hartman and Udenfriend 1970; Fuxe et al. 1970, 1971; Goldstein et al. 1972; Hartman et al. 1972; Hartman 1973; Hökfelt et al. 1973, 1975a; see also, Chapter IV), and a series of improvements of the original Falck-Hillarp method for aldehyde-induced monoamine fluorescence was published (Hökfelt and Ljungdahl 1972; Lindvall et al. 1973; Lindvall and Björklund 1974; Lorén et al. 1976, 1980; Furness et al. 1978; see also, Chapter II).

A successful combination of a retrograde tracing technique with neurotransmitter histochemistry was achieved by Ljungdahl and collaborators in 1975. They used a sequential method of immunocytochemistry in combination with HRP for visualization of tyrosine hydroxylase containing (i.e. catecholamine producing) cells in the substantia nigra that projected to a site of HRP injection in the nucleus caudatus-putamen (Ljungdahl et al. 1975). Simultaneously, Warr (1975), Hardy et al. (1976) and Mesulam (1976) were able to combine retrograde HRP tracing with acetylcholinesterase (AChE) histochemistry. Another approach was tried by Satoh et al. (1977) who used HRP in combination with histochemical staining of the enzyme monoamine oxidase for the visualization of monoaminergic neurons projecting to the spinal cord. Later on, several groups independently published methods in which the HRP-technique was combined with monoamine histofluorescence (Berger et al. 1978; Blessing et al. 1978; Smolen et al. 1979). These methods were all sequential procedures in which the monoamine fluorescence was first photographed and thereafter the same section was reacted for HRP and rephotographed. Since the HRP staining quenches the monoamine fluorescence, these procedures require careful and potentially time-consuming comparisons of photographs in the search for double-labeled cells. More recently, Blessing and collaborators (1981b) have improved this technique to allow for HRP visualization with the monoamine fluorescence still retained (see also, Törk and Turner 1981), and several groups (Bowker et al. 1981c; Lechan et al. 1981; Priestley et al. 1981; Sofroniew and Schrell 1981) have introduced alternative procedures for simultaneous visualization of HRP and transmitter suspects, in which the HRP tracing is combined with the peroxidase-antiperoxidase (PAP) (Sternberger et al. 1970) or indirect HRP (Nakane and Pierce 1967; Avrameas 1969) immunohistochemical techniques in the same section (see, Section 5.2). Also wheat germ agglutinin (WGA) has been used as retrograde tracer in conjunction with PAP or fluorescence immunohistochemistry (Lechan et al. 1981).

The use of fluorescent tracers, instead of HRP, in combination with neurotransmitter specific techniques is potentially advantageous, since it eliminates the need of separate histochemical processing for the visualization of the tracer substance. In 1979 the use of fluorescent tracers in combination with immunocytochemistry was described by Hökfelt et al. (1979b) and at the same time a procedure for the combination of fluorescent tracers with aldehyde-induced monoamine fluorescence was published by Björklund and Skagerberg (1979a). Modifications of these methods have since been described by several authors (Brann and Emson 1980; Steinbusch et al. 1980, 1981; Sawchenko and Swanson 1981, 1982; Van der Kooy and Steinbusch 1980; Van der Kooy and Wise 1980; Guynet and Crane 1981; Nagai et al. 1981; Ross et al. 1981; Van der Kooy et al. 1981; Albanese and Bentivoglio 1982b; Stevens et al. 1982), and recently two groups have described the use of fluorescent tracers in combination with AChE staining (Albanese and Bentivoglio 1982a; Bigl et al. 1982; Woolf and Butcher 1982).

The combined technique has also been successfully applied in the peripheral nervous system (Helke et al. 1981; Neuhuber et al. 1981; Dalsgaard et al. 1982a,b).

All the combination methods discussed so far are, in principle, two-step procedures. The first step consists of the nonspecific uptake and retrograde transport of a tracer, be it HRP or a fluorescent substance. This first step is nonspecific in the sense that the uptake and transport of tracer probably occur in all systems regardless of the transmitter content of the neuron. The second step is then employed to verify the presence of a substance in the tracer-labeled cell body that is specifically related to a certain neurotransmitter or neuronal marker. The interpretation of the results, finally, rests on the assumption that the neurotransmitter, whose presence is indicated in the cell body, is the same as the one stored and released at its terminals. A more direct approach to transmitter-specific retrograde tracing is the use of a tracer that by itself confers the specificity by being internalized and transported only in systems utilizing a certain neurotransmitter. Many types of neurons possess a specific uptake mechanism for their particular transmitter, as is the case in monoaminergic nerve cells (see, Iversen 1967; Hökfelt and Ljungdahl 1975) and these substances are, in fact, retrogradely transported. Thus, possibilities exist to visualize with autoradiography radiolabeled transmitters which after uptake into specific nerve endings have been retrogradely transported to the cell bodies. This principle was first applied by Hunt and co-workers (Hunt and Künzle 1976; Hunt et al. 1977) and Leger et al. (1977), who worked with [^{3}H]γ-aminobutyric acid (GABA) and 5-dihydroxytryptamine (5-HT), respectively, and has since been utilized with various radiolabeled transmitter candidates, including monoamines and D-[^{3}H]aspartate (Araneda et al. 1980; Streit 1980; Wiklund et al. 1982). The specificity and application of these techniques are described in further detail in Chapter VIII.

Another 'one-step procedure' with claimed specificity for noradrenergic systems, is based on the uptake and retrograde transport of antibodies to dopamine-β-hydroxylase (Jacobowitz et al. 1975; Fillenz et al. 1976; Ziegler et al. 1976; Silver and Jacobowitz 1979; Westlund et al. 1981).

The present chapter gives a survey of available procedures, with particular emphasis on methods using fluorescent dyes or HRP as retrograde tracers.

In the Appendix (8.1) a survey of approaches for combining retrograde tracing and neurotransmitter histochemistry, indicating the different steps in the various procedures, has been given. Appendix 8.2 summarizes information on fluorescent tracers.

2. GENERAL PROPERTIES OF FLUORESCENT DYES AND HRP AS RETROGRADE TRACERS

The first fluorescent dyes used by Kuypers and collaborators for retrograde tracing in the central nervous system (CNS) were Evans blue and 4,6-diamidino-2-phenylindol (DAPI) (Kuypers et al. 1977). Subsequently, the same research group introduced several other fluorescent substances for the purpose of tracing neuronal connections (Kuypers et al. 1979, 1980; Bentivoglio et al. 1979a, 1980). All these substances are of relatively low molecular weight (some 100 Daltons) and are efficiently excited by the ordinarily used high-pressure mercury lamp (Figs. 1 and 2). Some of their basic properties, of importance with respect to their use for the tracing and neuronal connections in the CNS, are listed in Table 1, wherein their abbreviated names are also given.

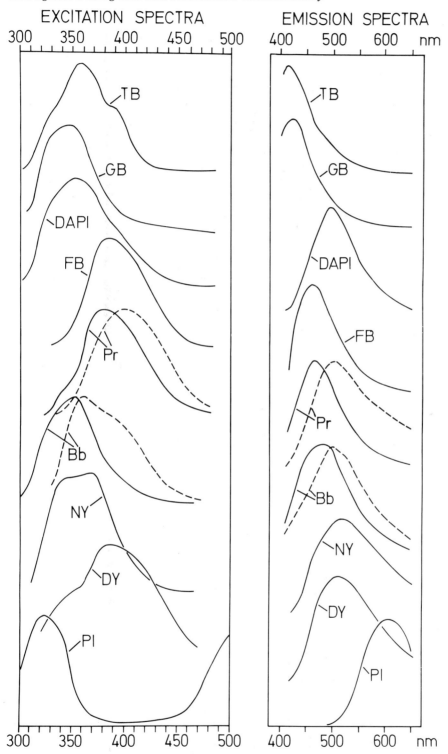

Fig. 1. Excitation and emission spectra for some fluorescent tracers in models. In the excitation spectra to the left the height of the curve indicates the efficiency of fluorescence excitation at the corresponding wavelength. The emission spectra indicate the intensity of the emitted light when the tracer is excited at its maximal excitation wavelength. Measurements were performed on the compounds enclosed in a dried protein matrix as described by Björklund and Skagerberg (1979a). For primuline and bisbenzimide the dashed lines indicate the spectra recorded in tissue processed according to the procedure described in Appendix 8.1 (from Skagerberg and Björklund 1983).

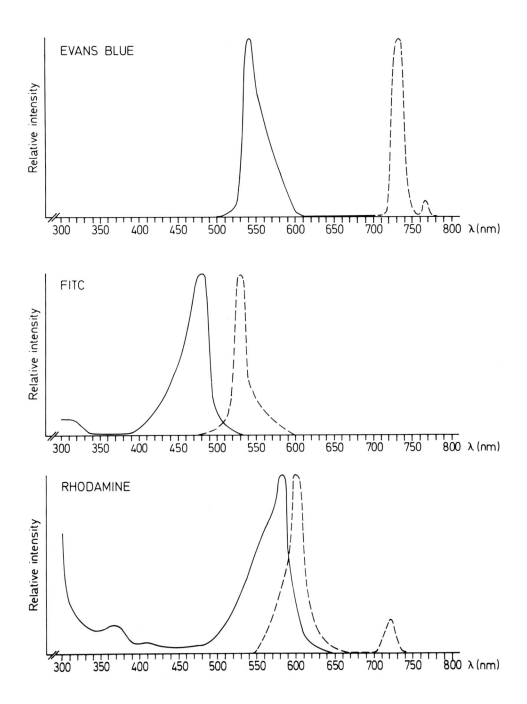

Fig. 2. Excitation (−) and emission (− − −) curves for Evans blue (EB), FITC and rhodamine (TRITC). The EB spectra show uncorrected instrumental values recorded in water solution in an Aminco-Bowman spectrofluorometer. FITC and rhodamine spectra are reproduced from Nairn (1969).

Table 1
Some basic characteristics of fluorescent tracers and other fluorophores

Compound	Conc. w/v (%)	Spread of injection site	Optimal survival time	Exc. max. (nm)	Em. max. (nm)	Neuronal localization and morphology		Glial labeling		Relative intensity in tissue (%)				
						Cryostat procedure	Freeze-dried	Cryostat	Freeze-dried	at 365 nm	at 405 nm	at 435 nm	at 546 nm	at 577 nm
Bisbenzimide (Bb)	1	++	1	360 (400)	500 (glia = 480)	N	G, C	++	+	100	65	20	0	0
Diamidinoyellow (DAY)	2	+	32	385	510	N	G, C	–	–	82	100	56	0	0
DAPI	2.5	+	16	360	490–500	G, C	G, C	+	–	100	60	30	0	0
Evans blue (EB)	10	+++	4	540	735	D, C, N	D, C, N	–	–	0	0	0	100	18
Fast blue (FB)	2	+	4	385	460	G, C	G, C	(+)	–	100	85	20	0	0
Granular blue (GB)	5	+	32	355	425	G, C	G, C	(+)	–	100	40	25	0	0
Nuclear yellow (NY)	1	++	2	370	520	N	N (G)	++	(+)	100	28	6	0	0
Primuline (Pr)	10	++	16	400	465	G, C	G, C	+	–	55	100	65	–	–
Propidium iodide (PI)	3–5	+++	6	340, 500	600–610	G, C, No	G, C, No	+	+	20	8	8	100	100
True blue (TB)	3–5	+	32	365 (390)	420–430	D, C, N	G, C	+	–	100	20	1	0	0
Catecholamines (CA)				(340) 415	490–520					30	100	70	0	0
Serotonin (5-HT)				365, 410	520–540					95	100	70	0	0
Rhodamine (TRITC)				(370) 580	610 (720)									
FITC				480	530									

Optimal survival time is given in relative *arbitrary units* to allow for comparison between different tracers. Exc. max. = excitation maxima, value in brackets indicates the position of a second smaller peak. Em. max. = emission maxima. N = nuclear labeling. G.C. = granular cytoplasmic labeling. G.C. = diffuse cytoplasmic labeling; No = labeling of the nucleolus. The CA and 5-HT spectra are recorded in specimens processed according to the ALFA procedure. From Skagerberg and Björklund (1983).

Each compound is characterized by a distinctive excitation and emission spectrum, as is shown in Figures 1 and 2. These individual spectra may be affected by such factors as variations in pH and binding to tissue proteins, but with the exception of bisbenzimide and primuline, the spectra shown for models in Figure 1 correspond closely to the spectra recorded from intraneuronally located tracers in tissue processed either by the freeze-drying technique or by the more commonly used cryostat procedure (to be described later). In the fluorescence microscope most of the tracers are activated with the 365 nm line of the mercury lamp, which results in emission of fluorescence in the blue-green-yellow range. The tracers with red fluorescence emission (i.e. Evans blue and propidium iodide) are, however, most optimally excited with the 546 and 577 lines (compare Figs 1, 2 and 3).

A particular advantage of the fluorescent tracers is that they are fluorescent in their native state and are thus visible without any further histochemical processing. In the procedure developed in Kuypers' laboratory, the injected animals are anesthetized and transcardially perfused with 4–10% formalin. Pieces of brain or spinal cord are removed and soaked in 10% sucrose in buffer (pH 7) for several hours. Tissue pieces are then frozen and cut on a cryostat at 20–30 μm, mounted on slides and directly examined in the fluorescence microscope (Kuypers 1981). This method will henceforth be referred to as the 'wet' procedure. Sections processed for immunohistochemistry have to go through several additional 'wet' steps.

The fluorescent tracers are used as water solutions or suspensions in concentrations varying from 1–10% (w/v) (Table 1). HRP is also used as a water (or saline) solution but usually at a concentration of 20–50%. The higher concentrations give in general an increased neuronal labeling but are more difficult to use because of their high viscosity. For HRP the addition of 0.1–0.5% poly-L-ornithine (Hadley and Trachtenberg 1978), 1–3% lysolecithin (Frank et al. 1980), 2% dimethylsulfoxide (Keefer 1978) or 5% of a non-ionic detergent (Lipp and Schwegler 1980) has been shown to increase the effectiveness of this tracer in some experimental situations. The effects on neuronal labeling of additives to the solutions of fluorescent tracers has so far not been extensively documented, but Kuypers' group has recommended 1% poly-L-ornithine to be used with Evans blue (Kuypers 1981) and fast blue to be dissolved in 2% DMSO (Huisman, personal communication). Illert et al. (1982) have reported increased labeling of somatic motoneurons after dissolving the blue tracers, i.e. true blue, granular blue and fast blue in ethylene glycol.

The injected tracers are taken up by axons terminating at the site of injection. In most cases uptake also seems to occur by damaged fibers at the injection site. For HRP, fast blue and bisbenzimide, uptake has also been demonstrated in the CNS into apparently intact axons traversing the injection site in the CNS (Herkenham and Nauta 1977; Sawchenko and Swanson 1981). The possibility of non-terminal uptake of tracer into either intact or damaged axons may, however, vary from one region to another as has been shown to be the case in the peripheral nervous system (PNS) (Deuschl et al. 1981; Illert et al. 1982). Recently, Schmued and Swanson (1982) have introduced a new fluorescent tracer (abbreviated SITS) which apparently is exclusively taken up at neuronal terminals, thereby avoiding the potential problem of labeling of fibers of passage.

Most of the HRP-uptake seems to be mediated by fluid-phase endocytosis (pinocytosis), a constantly ongoing process, whereby extracellular fluid is internalized inside membrane bound vesicles formed by invagination of the axonal membrane at the terminals (Zacks and Saito 1968; Teichberg et al. 1975). Most of this uptake of extra-

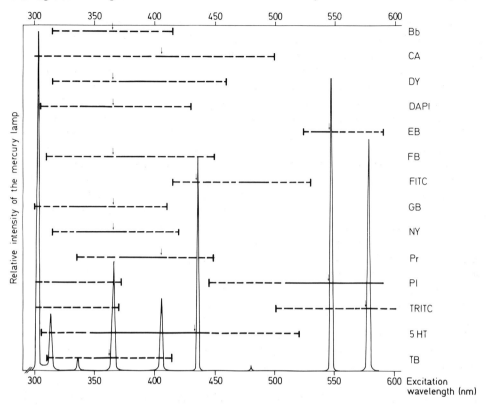

Fig. 3. In this figure the intensity of the different emission peaks of the mercury lamp, in the range between 300 and 600 nm, is indicated according to Parker (1968). The horizontal bars indicate the wavelengths at which the tracer compounds (indicated to the right) are efficiently excited. The dashed part of the bar indicates the range of 5–90% of maximum fluorescence intensity. The solid part of the bar indicates the wavelengths range at which the compound emits 90–100% of its maximum fluorescence. The arrows mark for each compound the mercury lamp peak which gives optimum excitation in the fluorescence microscope (from Skagerberg and Björklund 1983).

cellular material and its subsequent transport occur as a process which is independent of the electrical activity of the neuron or of exocytosis of synaptic vesicles, but regulated by other factors as in non-nervous tissue (Edelson and Cohn 1978; Silverstein et al. 1977). Enerbäck et al. (1980) have, however, shown that for the fluorescent tracer primuline, a minor proportion of the total tracer uptake and/or transport (in the order of 10–20%) may be directly dependent on the synaptic activity at the terminals. That the labeling of neuronal cell bodies by retrogradely transported tracers is to some extent modified by the functional activity of the neuron is further supported by studies in which various kinds of physiological stimulations have shown to increase uptake and/or transport of HRP (Eisenman and Azmitia 1982; Fryer and Maler 1982). HRP-filled endocytotic vesicles have also been observed to be formed along axons (La Vail and La Vail 1974), which could explain the phenomenon of tracer uptake by fibers of passage.

Although large molecular size and positive charge facilitate uptake by this process (Kristensson 1978), the fluid-phase endocytosis appears to be a nonspecific mechanism, whereby molecules outside the neuronal membrane are indiscriminately internalized. In this context it is interesting to note that Evans blue and primuline have been shown to bind to albumin extracellularly, which accordingly may facilitate their endocytotic uptake (Kristensson 1978; Enerbäck et al. 1980). Such protein binding may also occur with other tracer compounds, once they are deposited in the nervous tissue. The nonspecific nature of fluid phase endocytosis explains why HRP and the fluorescent substances are apparently taken up by all kinds or neurons irrespective of their functional activity or neurotransmitter content. Such an uptake mechanism is obviously quite different, e.g. from the high-affinity membrane transport system for monoamines into aminergic and other types of neurons (see, Iversen 1967; Hökfelt and Ljungdahl 1975), or from receptor mediated endocytosis of hormones or other ligands (Gonatas 1982; Pastan and Willingham 1981).

At sites of axonal injury the permeability of the plasma membrane is changed in such a way that extracellular tracer may diffuse passively into the cytoplasmic matrix (Brightman et al. 1970). HRP that has been passively internalized in this way is initially diffusely distributed but later on becomes sequestered into membrane-bound organelles (Kristensson and Olsson 1976; Chu-Wang and Oppenheim 1980).

Once the tracer has been located inside the membrane-bound vesicles, it may be transported somatopetally by the fast component of retrograde axonal transport which has a velocity of between 200 and 400 mm per day (Grafstein and Forman 1980). Upon reaching the cell body the tracer-containing vesicles tend to coalesce with one another to form bigger vesicles (La Vail and La Vail 1974; La Vail 1975), which then fuse with lysosomes (Chu-Wang and Oppenheim 1980; Sellinger and Petiet 1973), in which the tracer may be degraded or retained.

The mechanisms discussed above underlying the uptake, transport and storage of HRP may also, at least in part, apply to the various fluorescent tracers. The difference encountered between different tracers in terms of, e.g. efficiency of neuronal labeling or optimal survival time, can thus conceivably be explained largely on the basis of quantitative differences in, e.g. water solubility, protein binding, intracellular breakdown and toxicity. It seems possible, therefore, that the mechanism for HRP referred to above may be applicable to all tracer compounds dealt with in the present context. Regarding the principle of visualization of the tracers, there is of course a fundamental difference between HRP, on one hand, and the fluorescent tracers, on the other. The HRP method takes advantage of an enzymatic 'amplification' step to produce a black or brown reaction product (that is easily observed in the light microscope), while the sensitivity of the fluorescent tracers, in this respect, is dependent on the high fluorescence yield of these substances (Björklund and Skagerberg 1979a).

When working with retrograde tracers it is of great importance to determine the postinjection survival time which provides for optimal neuronal labeling. Based on the required survival times the retrograde tracers discussed here can roughly be divided into three groups:

(1) *Short survival times, i.e. less than 48 h*, are optimal when working with bisbenzimide, HRP or nuclear yellow, implying that these substances are transported fast and are efficiently visualized. If longer survival times are used, the HRP-labeling will decay, probably due to intracellular breakdown of the enzyme (La Vail 1975). For bisbenzimide and nuclear yellow another reason in favor of short survival times is the possibility of leakage of tracer out of labeled cell bodies or axons with subsequent labeling or surrounding glial cells (Bentivoglio et al. 1980). The leakage of tracers, and the associated glial labeling, is exaggerated by wet post-mortem handling of the

specimens. The in vivo leakage can to a large extent be avoided by using short survival times (Bentivoglio et al. 1980) and the in vitro leakage (during tissue processing) can be counteracted by using a freeze-drying procedure for the preparation of tissue. Since breakdown or diffusion of HRP, bisbenzimide and nuclear yellow is not restricted to labeled cell bodies, short survival times are also essential for delineation of the injection site when working with these tracers.

(2) *Intermediate survival time, i.e. 2–5 days* are optimal for Evans blue and propidium iodide and may also be used for fast blue. These slightly longer survival times probably indicate that these compounds may accumulate over a longer time period in the cell body by being somewhat less suspectible to diffusion out of the neuron or to intracellular breakdown. After about 5 days there is, however, a gradual decrease in the labeling intensity of both Evans blue and propidium iodide. Glial labeling around tracer-labeled neurons is not seen with Evans blue but may sometimes be observed when working with propidium iodide. Perhaps more importantly, there is a continuous diffusion of these tracers at the injection site, making it harder to demarcate the injection site, the longer survival time. Fast blue is often optimally visualized at these intermediate survival times, but differs from Evans blue and propidium iodide in being well retained both in labeled cells and at the injection site. The use of fast blue is therefore compatible also with extended survival times up to several weeks.

(3) *Long survival times, i.e. 5 days to several weeks*, are the most useful survival times for DAPI, primuline, granular blue, true blue and DAY. These substances are all hard to dissolve in water, a property which may cause a slow neuronal uptake, but, on the other hand, this property may be good for retention both in the labeled cells and at the injection site, leading to a gradual but marked tracer-accumulation in the cell body over time. The long-time neuronal retention of true blue, fast blue and granular blue in particular has been used advantageously in developmental studies (Innocenti 1981; Stanfield et al. 1982). For the tracers in the first two groups factors other than transport distance are the most important for determining the optimal survival time when working with small animals such as rat. In contrast, our own studies with true blue in the bulbospinal system (Skagerberg and Björklund 1983) show a positive relationship between transport distance and required survival time already at relatively moderate transport distances, such as those present in rats. This indicates that true blue is carried retrogradely, at least in part, at a much slower transport rate than most of the other tracers. For this tracer the low transport velocity may then partly explain the long survival time often required.

Thus, different factors are of importance in determining the optimal survival time for different tracers, and it should be noted that there are, in most cases, no simple relations between transport velocity and optimal survival time. In practice the optimal time will vary widely depending on the tracer used, the system and species studied, and the method of tissue processing. The relative optimal survival times given in arbitrary units for different tracers in Table 1 can serve as a general guide only.

The fluorescence microscopic appearance of cells labeled with fluorescent tracers varies depending on the technique applied for processing of the tissue. As outlined in some detail in Chapter II, water soluble compounds are easily subjected to postmortem diffusion from their in vivo storage sites. This phenomenon is best avoided by rapid freezing of the tissue to temperatures below $-30°C$ and subsequent freeze-drying at such low temperatures. At high temperatures or in the wet state, diffusion will occur unless the water soluble compounds are well bound to non-soluble tissue constitutents. The differences seen between tissue freeze-dried at low temperatures (the 'dry' pro-

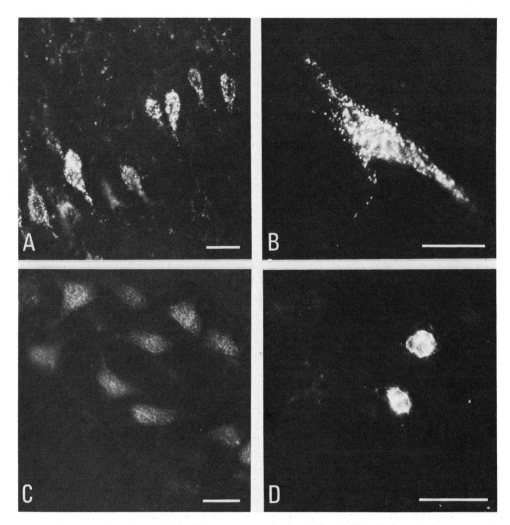

Fig. 4 A-D. Examples of the morphological appearance of retrogradely labelled cells in specimens processed by the 'dry' method. (A,B) Granular cytoplasmic labeling with granular blue (GB) and DAPI, respectively. (A) shows GB-labeled cells in rat sensorimotor cortex after injection into the cervical spinal cord, 9 days survival. (B) A cell in the rat parafascicular nucleus after tracer injection into the neostriatum, 3 days survival. (C) Diffuse labeling with Evans blue in rat substantia nigra 4 days after injection into the neostriatum. (D) Nuclear labeling by nuclear yellow in the parafascicular nucleus, 2 days after injection into the neostriatum. Bars indicate 25 μm.

cedure) (Björklund and Skagerberg 1979a) and tissue processed by cryostat sectioning and air drying (the 'wet' procedure) (Bentivoglio et al. 1980) are probably due to such post-mortem diffusion of the tracers. The main differences, listed in Table 1, are the following (Skagerberg and Björklund 1983):

(1) Some tracers, which have an exclusively granular cytoplasmic storage in freeze-dried tissue, often exhibit a diffuse cytoplasmic labeling in the 'wet' procedure. This is the case for true blue, fast blue and bisbenzimide. In the 'dry' processing all fluorescent

tracers except Evans blue and nuclear yellow have a granular cytoplasmic distribution (Fig. 4).

There is some variability with regard to the cellular compartmentalization of some of the fluorescent dyes, notably true blue and fast blue. Although these dyes have a predominantly cytoplasmic localization according to Bentivoglio et al. (1980) and Kuypers et al. (1980), a strong nuclear staining has also been described (Illert et al. 1982; Skirboll et al. 1983). This nuclear staining is particularly prominent after processing for immunofluorescence which may be due to a facilitated diffusion of the tracer from the cytoplasm to the nucleus in sections, in which the membranes have been partly dissolved with Triton X-100, a detergent used to enhance penetration of antibodies (Hartman et al. 1972).

(2) The two yellow tracers, bisbenzimide and DAY give in the 'wet' procedure an exclusive, or almost exclusive, nuclear labeling which is entirely absent in freeze-dried tissue. It seems likely that the nuclear labeling with these dyes, when exposed to the 'wet' procedure, is due to a redistribution of the tracer during processing. Thus, the tracer may in vivo be excluded from the nuclear compartment but gain access to, e.g. nuclear DNA by diffusion after death. These compounds are known to have a strong affinity for adenine- and thymidine-rich DNA (Bentivoglio et al. 1979a).

(3) Perineuronal glial labeling is less pronounced in freeze-dried tissue than in tissue processed according to the 'wet' procedure. We feel that much of the glial labelling seen with bisbenzimide and to some minor degree also with propidium iodide, reflects in vivo leakage of tracer out of labeled neurons, whereas the glial labeling that occurs with other substances in the 'wet' procedure (Table 1) is due to post-mortem translocation. For nuclear yellow the use of short survival times (up to 2 days) and the 'dry' procedure completely abolish the glial labeling around labeled neurons, although some glial labeling occurs in the proximity of large fiber bundles, whose cell bodies of origin are located close to the injection site. At the injection site heavy glial labeling is always observed with this tracer (Skagerberg and Björklund 1983).

3. FLUORESCENT RETROGRADE TRACING AND ALDEHYDE FLUORESCENCE HISTOCHEMISTRY

3.1. TISSUE PROCESSING

When using fluorescent tracers in conjunction with monoamine histochemistry the animals are, after appropriate survival time, perfused and the tissue processed according to a slightly modified protocol of the aluminium formaldehyde (ALFA) procedure, as listed in the Appendix (Protocol 8.3). In brief, this procedure involves perfusion of the animals with an ice-cold mixture of aluminum sulfate and 4% formalin in Tyrode's buffer under high pressure. The tissue is freeze-dried and reacted with formaldehyde vapor which converts the monoamines into fluorescent compounds. The specimens are then embedded in paraffin in vacuo and finally sectioned and mounted in a conventional manner. As mentioned above, this 'dry' procedure results in a different intracellular localization for some of the tracers (Table 1) as compared to the 'wet' cryostat procedure, while the spectral characteristics of the tracers are generally unaffected by the mode of processing. Thus, the principles outlined below are valid also for specimens obtained in cryostat or Vibratome procedures. For further details, the reader is referred to Chapter II.

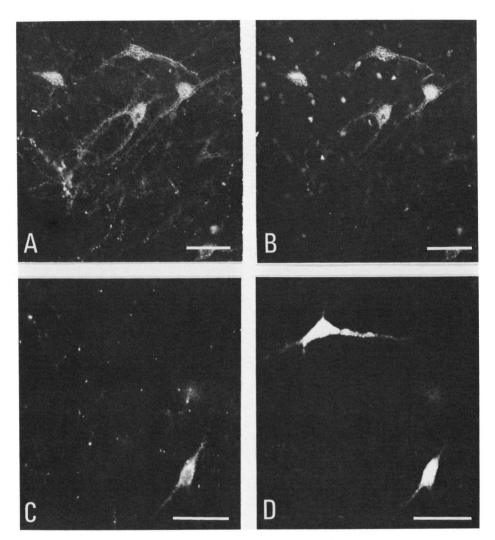

Fig. 5 A-D. (A,B) Concomitant visualization of dopamine (DA) and nuclear yellow (NY) in pars reticulata of substantia nigra after injection of NY into the neostriatum (2 days survival). In A, only the DA fluorescence is visible at 435 nm excitation. In B, both the cytoplasmic DA and the nuclear tracer labeling are visible in left and right cells at 365 nm excitation. Note also the glial NY-labeling in the pars reticulata (B), probably resulting from anterograde transport of NY. (C,D) Concomitant visualization of DA and Evans blue (EB) in pars reticulata of substantia nigra, 2 days after EB injection into the neostriatum. In C, only DA is visible at 435 nm, and in D, two EB-labeled cells, one of which is the DA-containing one in C, are visualized at 546 nm excitation. Magnifications 240× (A,B) and 290× (C,D).

3.2. MICROSCOPIC AND SPECTRAL DISTINCTION BETWEEN TRACERS AND MONOAMINE FLUOROPHORES

When working with methods using two or more fluorophores simultaneously, there are principally 3 different properties that can be used for distinguishing the different substances: (1) differences in intracellular localization; (2) differences in emission charac-

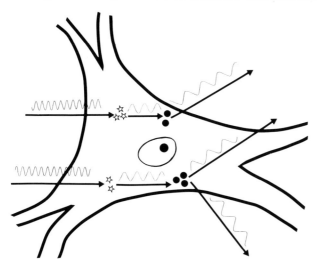

Fig. 6. The 'scintillation effect'. To the left, light of a certain wavelength excites a fluorescent compound (stars), which in turn emits light of longer wavelength. If a second fluorescent compound (filled circles) is excited by the light emitted by the first compound, the light that is finally emitted from the cell may be totally dominated by the emission of the second compound. The fluorescence color of the cell, and hence its emission spectrum, may thus not reveal the presence of the first compound. The excitation characteristics, on the other hand, which are unaffected by this phenomenon, will still detect both compounds.

teristics; and (3) differences in excitation (or activation) characteristics. Often all 3 of these distinguishing characteristics are taken advantage of.

Differences in intracellular localization have proved very useful in double-labeling studies using 'wet' procedures. Bisbenzimide, nuclear yellow and more recently DAY, have contributed a nuclear labeling while usually true blue or fast blue have been used for cytoplasmic labeling (see, e.g. Bharos et al. 1981). When using the 'dry' procedure, however, nuclear yellow is the only tracer that retains the useful characteristic of nuclear labeling (Figs 4, 5). This allows for distinction between the fluorescent tracer and the monoamine fluorophores, since the latter compounds all have an exclusive cytoplasmic localization (see Fig. 5).

Differences in emission characteristics, i.e. fluorescence colors, between the monoamine fluorophores and the tracer substances are more useful and are particularly reliable when working with the red tracers (Evans blue and propidium iodide) in combination with the blue-yellow monoamine fluorophores. The tracer compounds with blue or yellow fluorescence color, (i.e. true blue, granular blue, fast blue, DAPI and bisbenzimide) are more problematic to distinguish from the monoamine fluorophores on the basis of color impression alone. As seen in Figure 1, bisbenzimide, DAPI, DAY, fast blue and nuclear yellow have emission spectra (and hence fluorescence color) very similar to those of the catecholamines. The ice-blue color of true blue and granular blue is more different from that of the catecholamines, but with these compounds there is a risk of the so-called scintillation effect. This effect, which is illustrated in Figure 6, implies that the true blue or granular blue fluorescence light is reabsorbed by the surrounding monoamine fluorophores, which in turn give off a blue-yellow fluorescent light characteristic for the monoamines. Model experiments with true blue-catechol-

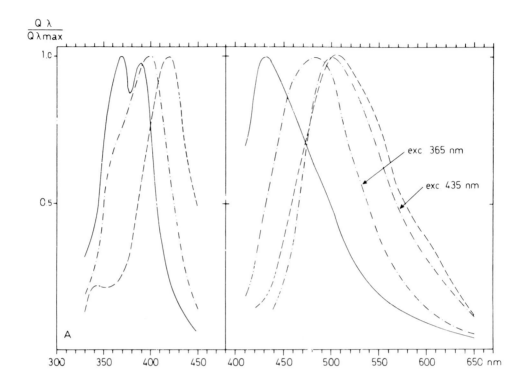

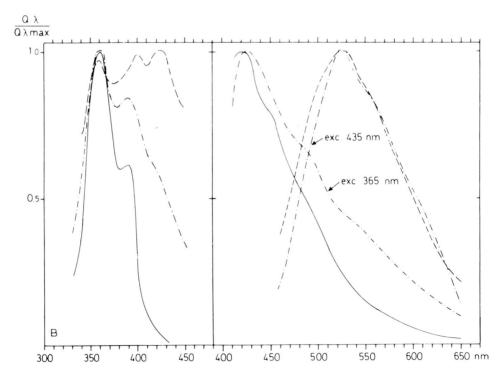

amine mixtures have shown that this effect occurs when the catecholamine to true blue ratio is relatively high (Björklund and Skagerberg 1979a).

In our experience the single most useful criterion for distinguishing between tracers and monoamine fluorophores in the fluorescence microscope is *differences in excitation characteristics*. As is evident from the excitation curves in Figures 1 to 3, there are wide differences in the excitation characteristics between different tracer compounds as well as between certain tracer compounds and the monoamine fluorophores. In particular, the differences seen between nuclear yellow, true blue, propidium iodide and Evans blue, on one hand, and the serotonin and catecholamine fluorophores, on the other, are particularly useful for their distinction in mixtures (see Figs 3, 7 and 8).

When making use of the differences in excitation characteristics for differentiation in a regular fluorescence microscope (i.e. without the aid of equipment for registration of spectra), it is important to realize that the light emitted by the mercury lamp is discontinuous. Thus, as illustrated in Figure 3, most of the light is emitted in a few bands or peaks with little light in between them. The peaks useful for activation of compounds with fluorescence in the visible range are at 365, 405, 435, 546 and 577 nm. For narrow band excitation, which is essential for selective visualization of monoamine fluorophores or fluorescent tracers, only these wavelengths provide high enough intensity to be useful.

Figures 1 to 3 also show that most of the fluorescent tracers have excitation peak maxima different from those of the monoamine fluorophores. This would make it possible to distinguish most of the available fluorescent tracers from the cellular monoamines by means of spectral recordings in a microspectrofluorometer. This also holds true for the tracers whose emission spectra are close to those of the monoamine fluorophores. For four of the tracers, i.e. Evans blue, nuclear yellow, true blue and propidium iodide, the excitation characteristics are, however, sufficiently different from those of the monoamine fluorophores to make possible reliable subjective distinction in the fluorescence microscope, without spectral recordings. Evans blue and propidium iodide are maximally activated at 500–550 nm, i.e. at a wavelength range where the catecholamines and indolamines (as well as the other tracers tested) yield no detectable fluorescence. Thus, Evans blue-labeled cells and propidium iodide-labeled cells can selectively be visualized at 546/577 nm illumination, whereas the catecholamine or indolamine content of the cells is visualized at 405 nm illumination. At this latter wavelength propidium iodide is very weakly fluorescent, while EB is not visualized at all (cf. Fig. 9).

Bisbenzimide, DAPI, granular blue, nuclear yellow and true blue yield maximum fluorescence in a wavelength range of 345–365 nm, where the monoamine fluorophores yield significant, albeit suboptimal fluorescence. Thus, when viewed under illumination from the 365 nm line of the mercury lamp both the monoamine content and the

---

Fig. 7 A,B. Fluorescence excitation spectra (left hand panels) and emission spectra (right hand panels) recorded from cell bodies in the brain stem of the rat after injection of true blue (TB) into the spinal cord. In (A) (–) = cell body containing TB only; (-----) = cell body containing noradrenaline (NA) but no TB label; (– · – · –) = cell body containing both NA and TB. In the latter case the excitation emission spectra recorded at 365 nm exhibit an intermediate profile representing the mixture of the two fluorophores. The emission curve recorded at 435 nm activation reveals the NA component exclusively. (B) (–) = cell body containing TB alone; (– – –) = cell body containing 5-hydroxytryptamine but no TB; (– · – · – ·) = cell body containing both 5-HT and TB. As in A, the emission recorded at 435 nm activation demonstrates the monoamine exclusively, since TB is not activated at this excitation wavelength (from Björklund and Skagerberg 1979a).

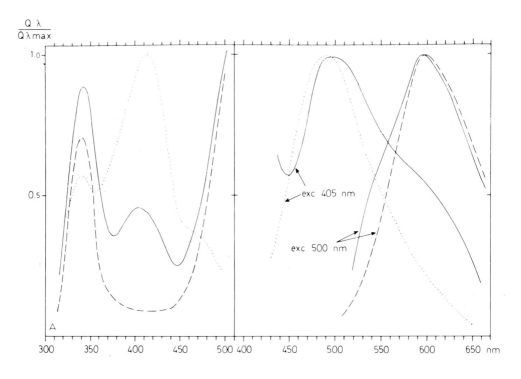

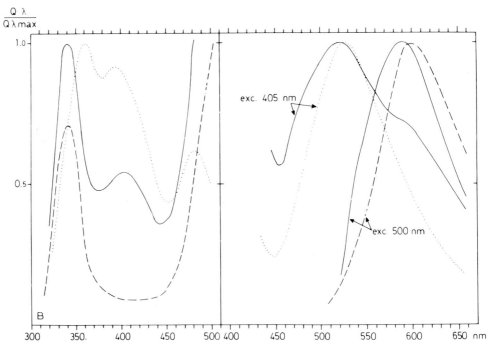

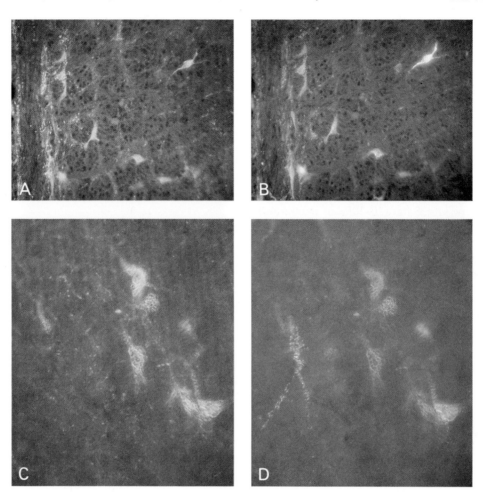

Fig. 9 A-D. Combined visualization of monoamines and the fluorescent retrograde tracer, true blue (TB), in the nuc. raphe obscurus (A and B) and in the pontine A7 cell group (C and D). In A and C, the 5-hydroxytryptamine (5-HT)-containing cell bodies and the noradrenaline (NA)-containing cell bodies, respectively, are selectively visualized at 435 nm illumination wavelength. B and D show the same fields, but now illuminated with a shorter wavelength (365 nm) which gives a bright blue fluorescence from the TB-labeled cell bodies, while the 5-HT and NA fluorescence is somewhat reduced. A and B thus reveal both labeled and non-labeled 5-HT-containing cell bodies in the nuc. raphe obscurus after an injection of TB in the thoracic spinal cord, and C and D reveal one labeled (bottom right) and a few unlabeled NA-containing bodies in the A7 cell group, plus part of one labeled, non-NA-containing cell (just medial to the lateral lemniscus) after a TB injection into the ipsilateral thoracic cord.

Fig. 8 A,B. Fluorescence excitation spectra (left hand panels) and emission spectra (right hand panels) recorded from cells in the brain stem of the rat after injection of propidium iodide (PI) in the spinal cord. (A) (····) = cell body containing noradrenaline (NA) but no PI; (– – –) = cell body containing PI but not NA; (——) = cell body containing both NA and PI. In the latter case the emission curves recorded at 405 and 500 nm activation reveal the NA and PI contents respectively. (B) (·····) = cell body containing 5-hydroxytryptamine (5-HT) but no PI; (– – – –) = cell body containing PI but no 5-HT (——) = cell body containing both 5-HT and PI. As in A activation at 405 and 500 nm reveals the monoamine and PI components, respectively (from Björklund and Skagerberg 1979a).

245

tracer will be visible. Nuclear yellow and true blue have, however, the favorable property of having practically no fluorescence at 435 nm (about 1% of the fluorescence recorded at 365 nm; see Fig. 1), while the intensity of the catecholamine and serotonin fluorophores are close to maximum at this wavelength. Thus, as illustrated in the photographs in Figures 5 and 9, illumination of a section from a nuclear yellow or true blue-labeled specimen at 435 nm will selectively visualize cells containing catecholamine or serotonin, whereas the nuclear nuclear yellow-labeling or the bright, ice-blue true blue-fluorescent cytoplasmic granules will appear in the labeled cells when the illumination is switched to 365 nm. Non-labeled monoamine-containing cells will be seen with a slightly weaker yellowish cytoplasmic fluorescence at this wavelength. Fast blue, granular blue, DAPI and bisbenzimide are clearly less well suited for this kind of subjective distinction since they yield stronger fluorescence than true blue or nuclear yellow at 435 nm (20–30% of maximum).

The highly useful properties of true blue and propidium iodide for combination with monoamines are illustrated in the spectral recordings in Figures 7 and 8, where the left hand panels give the excitation spectra and the right hand panels the emission spectra recorded from labeled and non-labeled neuronal cell bodies in the brain stem after injections into the cervical spinal cord. The spectra recorded from non-monoaminergic cells labeled with true blue or propidium iodide (solid and dashed lines, respectively) are widely different from the spectra recorded from non-labeled monoamine-containing cells (dashed and dotted lines, respectively) in both cases. In cells containing both a monoamine and the true blue or propidium iodide tracer, the excitation spectrum represents a summation of the tracer and the monoamine curves (dash-dotted line in the left panels in Fig. 7 and solid lines in the left panels in Fig. 8). In case of true blue-labeled monoamine-containing cells, activation at 365 nm gives an emission curve that is intermediary between the true blue and the catecholamine or serotonin curve (dash-dotted lines in the right hand panels in Fig. 7). With propidium iodide labeled monoamine-containing cells, activation at 500 nm gives an emission curve that is close to that of pure propidium iodide, and activation at 405 nm yields emission curves where the catecholamine or serotonin components predominate.

3.3. PRACTICAL CONSIDERATIONS

The method we now use for combination of tracers with monoamine histofluorescence is described in detail in the Appendix (Protocol 8.3). The procedure is quick and reliable and allows for convenient screening of large areas at fairly low magnification (16-25X objective).

When working with the *combination of true blue and monoamine fluorescence* (Fig. 9), the section is first examined at 435 nm excitation: all cells that are fluorescent at this excitation wavelength are monoamine containing – true blue is not at all visualized at this wavelength. When the excitation is changed to 365 nm some of the cells that were fluorescent at 435 nm will exhibit higher fluorescence intensity: these are monoamine-containing cells retrogradely labeled with true blue. Monoamine-containing cells that are not labeled with true blue will show a decrease in fluorescence intensity at 365 nm. Finally, true blue-labeled cells that do not contain monoamines will show up at 365 nm, but disappear if the excitation is again changed to 435 nm. Although an increased granularity in the cytoplasm and a more blue hue in the true blue-labeled monoamine-fluorescent cells is often helpful in distinguishing true blue-labeled cells, we have found the changes in fluorescence intensity to be the most reliable criteria for the identifica-

Table 2

Fluorescence intensity of some fluorescence tracers and other fluorophores when activated at the most commonly used wavelengths in the fluorescence microscope.

Excitation wave-length (nm)	Filter combinations			CA	EB	FB	FITC	NY	PI	5-HT	TB	TRITC
	Zeiss epi-illumination	Zeiss trans-illumination	Leitz epi-illumination									
365	01	UG 1, 44	A	+	0	+++	(+)	+++	++	++	+++	+
405	04	BG 12, 47	G	+++	0	++	+	+	+	++	+	0
435	06	BP 435, 47	E3	++	0	+	++	0	+	+++	0	0
450–490	10	–	12	+	0	+	+++	0	++	+	0	0
546	15	BP 546, 610	M2 (N2)	0	+++	0	0	0	+++	0	0	+++

0 Denotes no fluorescence and +++ maximum fluorescence. Note that the intensity ratings are valid only for comparison of one fluorophore at different wavelengths of excitation, *not* between different fluorophores. The filter-mirror combinations used in epi-illumination are given by the manufacturers' code names. For trans-illumination, the first filter (e.g. UG 1) is the primary filter while the second (e.g. 44) is the secondary (barrier) filter. From Skagerberg and Björklund (1983).

tion of this tracer in monoamine-containing cell bodies. If there is doubt about the fluorophore content of a certain cell, microspectrofluorometric analyis represents an attractive possibility for objective verification of the fluorophores contained within a cell, as shown in Figures 7 and 8.

As mentioned earlier, it is often necessary to use several days or even a few weeks survival time to get optimal labeling with true blue. In some systems, which exhibit a very intense monoamine fluorescence, it may also prove advantageous to reduce the monoamine fluorescence (by shortening the time of formaldehyde vapor exposure), since the change in fluorescence intensity that is caused by shifting between the 435 and the 365 nm-line for excitation may otherwise be obscured.

When the *combination of nuclear yellow and monoamines* (Fig. 5) is used, the change of excitation light from 435 to 365 nm will visualize the nuclear nuclear yellow-labeling in both monoamine and non-monoamine-containing cells. This nuclear labeling is then abolished as the excitation is changed back to 435 nm. When working with nuclear yellow the risk of false-positive labeling because of anterograde transport must be kept in mind (Arbuthnott et al. 1982; Aschoff et al. 1982).

When working with *propidium iodide or Evans blue in combination with mono-amine fluorescence* (Fig. 9), the section is first viewed at 405/435 nm excitation. Catecholamine- and serotonin-containing cell bodies will now show up in a greenish-yellow or yellow color. Cells with heavy propidium iodide labeling will, in addition, show a dull brown or red fluorescence, while Evans blue is non-fluorescent at this wavelength. When changing the excitation filter to 546/577 nm, the monoamine fluorescence disappears completely and the propidium iodide labeling will appear as a bright brick-red fluorescence in the cytoplasm and in the nucleolus. Switching back and forth between the 405/435 and 546/577 nm excitation light will conveniently establish which individual cells contain both monoamine and propidium iodide.

A potential pitfall in the use of propidium iodide as retrograde marker is the risk of misinterpreting autofluorescent pigment as propidium iodide fluorescence. Such lipo-fuchsin-like pigment is present in the cytoplasm of many types of neurons, and it increases markedly with age. The true fluorescence color of most pigment is more yellow-orange than the propidium iodide fluorescence, but at the 546 nm illumination the colors of the two may appear similar. The only way to avoid this confusion is to become familiar with the appearance of the autofluorescent pigment in non-injected specimens or, in the case of unilateral labeling, by comparing the injected and non-injected sides.

On the whole, it is our impression that the combination with true blue constitutes the most specific and sensitive of these methods, provided that long enough survival times are used. The use of nuclear yellow in combination with monoamine histofluorescence is very convenient to work with under the microscope but is slightly disadvantageous, since nuclear yellow seems to be a less efficient tracer (Sawchenko and Swanson 1981; Aschoff et al. 1982), and because of the potential risk for secondary uptake subsequent to its anterograde transport. Evans blue and propidium iodide have in general a lower visibility than the other tracers, and they seem to be retrogradely transported with somewhat variable efficiency. Despite this, excellent results have been obtained with these two tracers in several different systems (Swanson and Kuypers 1980; Van der Kooy and Steinbusch 1980; Bigl et al. 1982; Stevens et al. 1982).

There are now several commercially available filter sets which are well suited for working with combinations of monoamine histofluorescence and the fluorescent tracers discussed above. Table 2 lists some of these filter sets and shows how some of the tracers, and also FITC and rhodamine, behave when activated at the different excitation wavelengths provided by these sets.

4. FLUORESCENT RETROGRADE TRACING AND IMMUNOHISTOCHEMISTRY

The combination of retrograde fluorescent tracing and immunohistochemistry offers special problems as compared to the previously and subsequently described approaches. The main difference here is that the sections have to be carried through a water phase, when the incubation with antisera and rinsing procedures are performed. Against this background the fluorescent tracers can principally be divided into two groups, one of which will not be affected by the processing, i.e. they remain during this procedure more or less in the same cellular compartment without diffusion into adjacent tissues. Although fluorescent retrograde tracers can be combined with HRP/PAP immunohistochemistry (Ross et al. 1981), we will here focus on combinations with immunofluorescence, which is based mainly on two fluorescent markers, FITC and rhodamine (TRITC). Provided that these markers can be distinguished from the retrograde fluorescent tracers, this procedure allows simultaneous evaluation of both types of markers and thus an immediate decision on co-localization. The same situation is present for the concomitant visualization of fluorescent retrograde tracers and monoamine fluorophores in freeze-dried tissue (see above). For the second group of dyes, which will diffuse out from the cellular compartment, the retrograde tracers have to be photographed *before* processing for immunohistochemistry, and these photographs then have to be compared with the immunohistochemical distribution patterns. Although the latter procedure is more tedious, it also includes some advantages, since the diffusion process, at least if complete, excludes interference between retrograde and immunohistochemical markers. Using combined retrograde tracing and immunofluorescence techniques, further problems can be approached such as tracing of collaterals of transmitter identified neurons and neurons with multiple transmitter candidates. This will be discussed below and a detailed protocol is presented in the Appendix (8.4). For further details, see Skirboll et al. (1983).

4.1. ANIMALS

A basic requirement for combination of retrograde tracing and immunohistochemistry (and other types of histochemistry) is that the compounds to be investigated are present in sufficient concentrations in the cell body. Since cell bodies often contain, as compared to nerve endings, low amounts of the transmitters and peptides and sometimes also of the transmitter synthesizing enzymes, the immunohistochemical technique may not be sensitive enough to reveal such compounds in this part of the neuron. This is particularly the case for the immunofluorescence technique which is less sensitive than the PAP procedure and its modifications, especially for the visualization of peptides in cell bodies. Therefore, animals are routinely treated with colchicine or vinblastine, drugs which are mitosis inhibitors and which arrest axonal transport and in this way cause accumulation of compounds synthesized in the cell soma (Dahlström 1968, 1971; Kreutzberg 1969; Hökfelt and Dahlström 1971; Hökfelt et al. 1975b). Colchicine is mostly given intraventricularly (Barry et al. 1973; Hökfelt et al. 1977), although peripheral administration has also been used for studies on the central nervous system (see, Sar et al. 1978). Since an optimal effect of colchicine is obtained 24–48 h after injection, and since the mitosis inhibitors also arrest transport of the retrogradely transported fluorescent dye (Skirboll et al. 1983), this procedure results in certain practical consequences. Thus, the retrograde tracers have to be injected at least 36–48 h before sacrifice. This makes it difficult to use some of the dyes for the combination technique. For example, nuclear yellow, which is rapidly transported, gives glial labeling already 12–24 h after injection in the 'wet' processing used for immunofluorescence (see, Section 2). This may not allow sufficient time for the mitosis inhibitors to cause a pronounced cell body accumulation of transmitter-related compounds.

4.2. TISSUE PROCESSING

In almost all cases the immunohistochemical technique requires fixation of the tissue, not only to preserve tissue morphology but particularly in order to secure retention of the antigens at the proper storage sites. Tissues to be processed for immunohistochemistry are in most laboratories taken from animals which have been perfused with various fixatives. There are, however, possibilities to obtain good and even excellent immunohistochemical results also by immersion fixation. A prerequisite is, of course, that the fixative by itself does not interfere with or destroy the retrograde tracer (see below).

A fixative, which seems to be compatible with both immunohistochemistry and the fluorescent tracers, is formalin (prepared in various ways, e.g. according to Pease 1962) as used in many immunohistochemical studies (Hökfelt et al. 1973; see, Jones and Hartman 1978). No systematic study of the effect of various fixatives on all tracers has been carried out to our knowlegde. Sawchenko and Swanson (1981) have tested several formalin based fixatives and procedures, including Bouin's solution and the sequential 'low pH-high pH' formalin fixation of Bérod et al. (1981) with regard to compatibility with true blue and bisbenzimide. They observed a better retention of dye (true blue) after fixation with neutral buffered 10% formalin as compared to the 'Pease formalin' (10% formalin prepared from 4% paraformaldehyde) used, for example, in our own studies. The pH-change method of Bérod et al. (1981) also gave good results although a more rapid deterioration of tracer and immunofluorescence was observed.

Addition of glutaraldehyde to the fixatives, which is very common when HRP is used as tracer, improves cellular morphology but increases background fluorescence. Fixation with para-benzoquinone, which can offer advantages for immunohistochemistry of neuropeptides (Pearse and Polak 1975; Lundberg 1981), extinguishes the fluorescence of the dyes and is thus incompatible with retrograde fluorescent tracers (Skirboll et al. 1983).

A standard procedure includes perfusion for varying times ranging from a few minutes to half-an-hour, mostly followed by immersion of the tissues in the same fixative for 1–24 h and then rinsing in phosphate buffer with added sucrose (5–30%). Sucrose immersion facilitates sectioning and counteracts freezing artifacts. After fixation the tissues can either be cut on a cryostat, or be embedded in paraffin. The paraffin procedure then requires deparaffinization of the sections before immunohistochemical incubations. The tissues can also be embedded in epoxy resins, which allows cutting of thin sections, down to 1 μm as compared to a minimum of about 5 μm with the cryostat. This may be a decisive advantage, when for example attempting to study multiple antigens in one and the same cell body. When cut at a thickness of 1 μm several adjacent sections can be obtained from the same cell body which can be unequivocally identified in several consecutive sections. Embedding in plastic will require removal of the embedding medium before immunohistochemistry, mostly by etching with H_2O_2 or alcohols. Details and references on these procedures can be found in Chapter IV.

4.3. DISTINCTION BETWEEN TRACERS AND IMMUNOFLUORESCENCE MARKERS

As for fluorescent tracers and monoamine fluorophores (see, Section 3.2), several principles can be used for distinction also between retrograde tracers and immunofluorescence markers. These include differences in intracellular localization and differences in emission or excitation characteristics. We have previously pointed out that in some cases relevant to the two-step procedures, the dye will be dissolved out from the section during immunofluorescence procedure and a distinction will then not be necessary.

Immunofluorescence techniques are based mainly on two fluorophores, the green-fluorescent fluorescein isothiocyanate (FITC), and the red-fluorescent tetramethyl-rhodamine isothiocyanate (TRITC) for which the short name rhodamine is often used. The excitation and emission characteristics of FITC and TRITC are shown in Figures 2 and 3 and in Table 1, which also allow for comparisons with the characteristics of the fluorescent retrograde tracers. In the following we will briefly discuss the usefulness of the various tracers in conjunction with immunofluorescence techniques, emphasizing some aspects on their retention during the immunohistochemical procedure, an issue which is not essential in the 'dry' procedure employed for the production of monoamine fluorophores. On this basis alone several dyes can be ruled out for combined studies with immunofluorescence.

Cellular compartmentalization

Transmitter-related compounds have in principle a cytoplasmic localization, whereas some of the retrograde tracers such as nuclear yellow (and in the 'wet' procedure also DAY) have a nuclear localization, whereas others are both cytoplasmic and nuclear (Evans blue). It should therefore be possible to distinguish the two types of tracers on this difference. In reality, however, the distinction is often less clear. First, the immunofluorescence may occupy a 'nuclear position' (in addition to the cytoplasmic one), which may be due to the fact that in the section the nucleus is covered by a string of cytoplasm or that, in fact, the antigen has diffused into the nucleus. Another problem is the situation with the retrograde tracers. Since the transmitter-related compounds principally are cytoplasmic, only 'nuclear' retrograde tracers can be used for combination on basis of different cellular compartmentalization. In our experience only few dyes remain confined to their original compartment in the elaborate processing necessary for immunocytochemistry (see Table 1). Both nuclear yellow and DAY diffuse out of the nucleus during the immunohistochemical processing, but remain in sufficiently high concentrations in the nuclear compartment to allow detection and distinction from cytoplasmic immunofluorescence. Fast blue and true blue tend to diffuse during immunohistochemistry, both out of the cell and into the nucleus, and its latter localization then allows distinction from cytoplasmic immunofluorescence. In fact, the use of membrane-disrupting detergents, such as Triton X-100, in the immunohistochemical staining (Hartman et al. 1972) may very well facilitate diffusion of the tracers into the nucleus. In this context one should remember that most of the fluorescent tracers introduced by Kuypers and collaborators are characterized by their strong affinity to nucleic acids.

A further possibility exists to distinguish different markers, namely by their *cytoplasmic* compartmentalization. For example, although most neurotransmitter-related antigens have a diffuse cytoplasmic appearance in the fluorescence microscope, some compounds have, at least partly, in addition a more characteristic appearance. Thus, for example somatostatin both in the peripheral nervous system (PNS) and CNS, vaso-active intestinal polypeptide (VIP)-, avian pancreatic polypeptide (APP)- and neuro-peptide Y (NPY)-like immunoreactivities in the PNS, are mostly localized in a peri-nuclear position (Hökfelt et al. 1978), and it has been demonstrated that this compart-ment in all probability corresponds to the Golgi apparatus (Johansson 1980, 1983). This unique characteristic has so far not been explored in combined tracing studies. Furthermore, most tracer dyes exhibit a granular (lysosomal?) appearance in the cyto-plasm in contrast to the diffuse fluorescence of transmitter related compounds. How-ever, this granular appearance is most pronounced in freeze-dried material (dry pro-cedure, see above). In tissue processed for immunohistochemistry the dye may partly enter a 'diffuse' pool of the cytoplasm and the granular fluorescence becomes weaker. This is true for both fast blue and true blue. On the other hand, primuline is strictly confined to granules also after immunohistochemistry (Fig. 10A) and can therefore be used in this context. Difficulties to distinguish such primuline-containing granules from autofluorescent granules may, however, be encountered but are less obvious in young animals.

Diffusion of tracers

As discussed above the diffusion can occur at several stages: in vivo prior to sacrifice; post-mortem during fixation-sectioning; and/or in vitro during immunohistochemical processing. Diffusion occurring during the last stage is taken advantage of in the two-step combined procedure, in which photography of the retrogradely labeled cells is car-ried out before immunohistochemistry. The diffusion may, however, have several con-sequences: (a) a complete loss of the dye; (b) decrease in fluorescence intensity with perhaps complete loss of fluorescence only in some cells, leading to false-negatives; (c) diffusion into neighboring glial cells; and (d) diffusion into other surrounding neurons causing false-positives.

The previous discussion (Section 2) on diffusion of dyes can be summarized as follows: Diffusion out of the cell in vivo may be a problem mainly with bisbenzimide (and perhaps propidium iodide). The labeling of surrounding glia is generally low in freeze-dried tissue, but is markedly enhanced by a 'wet' processing suggesting a post-mortem diffusion out of the cell of dyes such as bisbenzimide and nuclear yellow. Other dyes, such as fast blue and true blue may be redistributed from a granular to a soluble compartment in the cytoplasm and then to the nuclear compartment post-mortem during the wet procedure, and also out of the cell. The fact that almost all tracers (except Evans blue and nuclear yellow) have a granular cytoplasmic distribution with the 'dry' procedure, but are more diffuse in the wet one, also points to a redistri-bution within the cytoplasm.

It is clear that processing for immunofluorescence in some cases cause additional dif-fusion, partly due to the prolonged exposure to water phase, and, as discussed above, partly due perhaps to the addition of the detergent Triton X-100 to the antisera, a pro-cedure used to enhance penetration of antibodies to intracellular antigen sites (Hart-man et al. 1972). This is examplified by the fact that with the 'wet' procedure plus im-munohistochemistry, nuclear yellow will label neighboring glia already 6 h after injec-tion (Skirboll et al. 1983) whereas with the 'dry' procedure only little diffusion out of the cells was recorded up to at least 48 h (Skagerberg and Björklund 1983). Some dyes are lost only to a certain extent. Although no systematic analysis of the diffusion of all

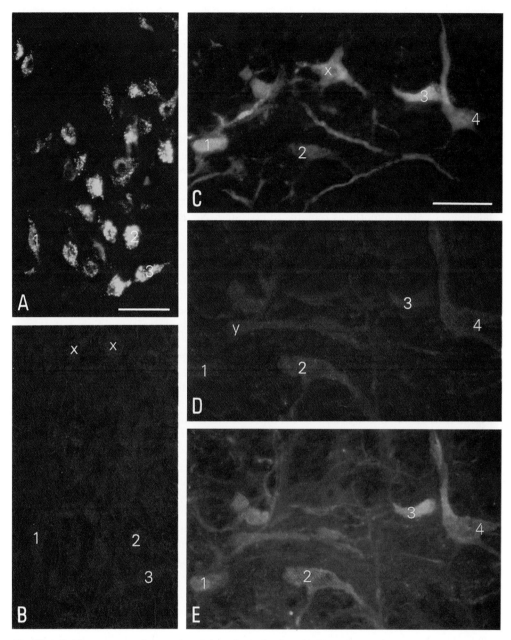

Fig. 10 A-E. Fluorescence-micrographs of the substantia nigra (A,B) nucleus raphe obscurus (C-E) after primuline (Pr) injection into the nuc. caudatus (A,B) and fast blue (FB) injection into the spinal cord (C-E) and processing for immunohistochemistry with antiserum to tyrosine hydroxylase (TH) (B) and 5-hydroxytryptamine (5-HT) (D,E) and TRITC-labeled secondary antibodies. A and B on one hand, and C-E on the other hand show the same section. (A,B) Pr-labeled cells in the substantia nigra exhibit strongly yellow fluorescent granules (A). Most TH positive cells (e.g. 1–3) contain Pr but some (x) lack the dye. (C-E) Several TB-labeled cells (C) contain 5-HT (D) (1–4): one cell is TB positive and TH negative (x); there are also TB negative and TH positive cells (y). The micrograph in E represents a double exposure taken after immunohistochemical processing, – whereby FB has first been photographed with 'blue' filters and then TRITC with 'red' filters. Bars indicate 50 μm (from Skirboll et al. 1983, unpublished).

dyes during immunohistochemistry has been performed, some data are available. In studies on the nigrostriatal system, Skirboll et al. (1983) recorded a loss of about 1/3 of all fast blue- and true blue-labeled cells during immunohistochemistry, while no effect was observed on propidium iodide and primuline. Van der Kooy and Sawchenko (1982) reported an 81% 'survival' of propidium iodide and 84% 'survival' of true blue during approximately the same procedure. Sawchenko and Swanson (1981) calculated a loss of 5% of true blue-labeled cells in a hypothalamo-spinal system during the immunohistochemical procedure. The differences between these studies may be due to survival time, fixation procedure, neuronal system studied, etc. The survival time may be of special importance. While Skirboll et al. (1983) used only short survival times, Skagerberg and Björklund (1983) favor much longer periods, up to several weeks for fast blue and especially for true blue. It may be that longer survival times result in labeling of a different pool and/or causes stronger labeling, leading to a smaller loss of labeled cells. This hypothesis remains to be tested. Nevertheless, it may be worthwhile to consider the sequential procedure for most dyes.

Even if the sequential procedure (photography before immunohistochemistry) is used, diffusion may impose a problem, namely during the mounting procedure. Mounting of sections gives a higher quality of the photography, at least at higher magnifications (25× and higher) and is in immunofluorescence studies routinely made in phosphate buffered saline (PBS)-glycerol. This step causes, however, diffusion of some dyes such as true blue, fast blue and DAY, but seemingly not of propidium iodide and primuline (Fig. 10A). Other mounting media, such as Entellan (Merck, Darmstadt, FRG) do not cause diffusion, but are less compatible with subsequent immunohistochemistry, since removal of the coverslip and subsequent processing for immunohistochemistry are difficult to carry out. Xylene is compatible with immunohistochemical staining and it does not cause diffusion of the tracers. Mounting in xylene thus allows photography of mounted sections and the coverslip to be removed for immunohistochemistry. (Care has, however, to be taken that the xylene does not evaporate, since this may 'glue' the coverslip onto the section.)

In conclusion, only few dyes resist diffusion during immunohistochemistry and are reliable for the visualization concomitantly with the immunohistochemical marker. The best ones in this respect are primuline, propidium iodide, true blue and fast blue, although losses have been observed with the latter three, suggesting that photography before immunohistochemistry should be considered. Nuclear yellow and bisbenzimide are completely washed out during the immunohistochemical procedure, whereas DAY remains in the cells but labels surrounding glial (and possibly also neuronal) cells.

Spectral differences

Examination of the spectral characteristics of the dyes and the immunofluorescence markers reveal that differences in emission and excitation characteristics exist in several cases (Fig. 1). Of the various tracers suitable for combination studies, true blue, fast blue, granular blue, primuline, DAY and propidium iodide, the blue-fluorescent ones, true blue, fast blue and granular blue, have emission characteristics clearly different from TRITC, but they are less clearly separated from FITC. Also, primuline and DAY, but not propidium iodide, can be used with TRITC. Propidium iodide is, on the other hand, the only dye which exhibits a clear spectral difference to FITC. However, differences in excitation spectra can also be used. Thus, FITC is very poorly excited below 400 nm. Thus, if FITC is excited at 450–490 nm, a separation can be obtained from the blue-fluorescent dyes. It may be emphasized that from this point of view granular blue and true blue are more favorable than fast blue, since the latter dye is excited up to about 450 nm (Fig. 1) making a distinction from FITC difficult, if they are viewed simultaneously in the same section.

4.4. PRACTICAL CONSIDERATIONS

In the following we will briefly discuss the suitability of different combinations of retrograde tracers and immunohistochemical markers on the basis of our own experiments as well as those of others (Hökfelt et al. 1979a,b, 1980; Steinbusch et al. 1980, 1981; Van der Kooy and Steinbusch 1980; Sawchenko and Swanson 1981, 1982; Van der Kooy et al 1981; Köhler et al. 1982; Sawchenko et al. 1982: Van der Kooy and Sawchenko 1982; Skirboll and Hökfelt 1983; Skirboll et al. 1983).

Several dyes can be ruled out for the present purpose. Bisbenzimide, nuclear yellow and Evans blue are easily diffusible and therefore not useful. Nuclear yellow diffusion occurs rapidly in vivo and, due to the short survival time, combination with colchicine treatment is virtually impossible. Evans blue does not, in addition, transport well in several systems. Primuline shows negligible diffusion upon perfusion and immunohistochemical processing (Fig. 10A). This dye seems to be entirely granular and can therefore be distinguished from the immunofluorescence by its specific cytoplasmic compartmentalization. Labeling with primuline is, however, strong only in some systems, and with a weak labeling it may be difficult to distinguish this fluorescence from autofluorescence. Furthermore, a strong FITC induced fluorescence tends to disguise the primuline fluorescence, but this can be circumvented either by using high dilutions of primary antisera and of the FITC conjugated antibodies and/or by fading the FITC fluorescence through prolonged exposure to UV light. A further alternative is to use TRITC as immunofluorescence marker (Fig. 10B, D). Against this background primuline may not be a retrograde tracer of primary choice, but may be used in special cases (see below). DAY is less susceptible to diffusion in vivo than nuclear yellow, but diffuses during immunohistochemistry. On spectral grounds it can be distinguished from TRITC but not from FITC. Since the DAY fluorescence is nuclear and remains there in sufficiently high concentrations during incubation with antisera, this dye can be considered for combined retrograde immunofluorescence studies using preferably TRITC, but also FITC (different compartments).

True blue, fast blue and granular blue have similar qualities. They are well transported and produce strongly labeled cells in many systems. Their fluorescence can be clearly distinguished from that of TRITC (Fig. 10C, D). All the blue-fluorescent dyes are sensitive to UV light and a decrease in fluorescence intensity (fading) can be seen during examination (and photography) in the fluorescence microscope. The fading seems most marked after mounting in buffer-glycerol mixture, possibly due to a concomitant diffusion, but occurs also clearly when unmounted sections are exposed to UV light. Interestingly, the fading seems less extensive in sections, which have passed through the immunocytochemical processing. Perhaps the dye remaining after this procedure is present in a compartment and/or pool which makes it more resistant to UV illumination? Fast blue may offer some advantage over true blue because of its better solubility and faster transport (see, Kuypers and Huisman 1983). On the other hand, there is an overlap in the excitation wavelengths of fast blue and FITC but not of true blue and FITC (Fig. 3). Thus, using proper filter combinations TB can be used together with FITC-conjugated antisera, as well as with TRITC-labeled antisera. Both dyes do, however, diffuse out of the cells during the immunofluorescence procedure to a certain extent, and some labeled cells may thus be lost. Photographic recording should therefore preferably be carried out before immunohistochemistry (Fig. 10C), at least if the labeling is weak. Since there is a diffusion of fast blue into the nuclear compartment during immunohistochemistry and since this nuclear fluorescence is retained in the nucleus, subsequent processing with TRITC-labeled antisera will reveal a red cytoplasmic immunofluorescence and a blue nuclear retrograde tracer fluorescence in double-labeled cells (Fig. 10E). Thus, the FB-TRITC combination makes possible differentiation both on the basis of different fluorescence colors and different cellular compartments (Fig. 10E).

Propidium iodide is, in our experience, the dye which is most resistant to diffusion during perfusion and immunohistochemistry, although losses have been reported (Van der Kooy and Sawchenko 1982). Since it is also insensitive to UV light and thus does not fade, and since it can be combined with FITC conjugated antisera, it seems to represent one of the most useful retrograde tracers for combination with immunocytochemistry. There is overlap in excitation wavelength between propidium iodide and FITC, and propidium iodide will shine through (as redish-yellow), when the FITC-induced immunofluorescence is analyzed. Since it shines through with a red fluorescence, there is no risk of false-positives. This may impose a problem only if the propidium iodide intensity is very high in weakly FITC-labeled cells. Addition of specific secondary filters (e.g. KP 560) can reduce the red component. It should be remembered that propidium iodide exhibits several negative characteristics – it is toxic, it does not transport well over long distances and lightly-labeled cells may be difficult to identify because of interference with autofluorescent pigment (Kuypers et al. 1981; Kuypers and Huisman 1983). References to CNS studies using combination of retrogradely transported fluorescent tracers and immunofluorescence are Hökfelt et al. (1979a,b; 1980), Brann and Emson (1980), Steinbusch et al. (1980, 1981), Sawchenko and Swanson (1981, 1982), Van der Kooy and Steinbusch (1980), Van der Kooy et al. (1981).

4.5. COLLATERAL TRACING

There are certain neuroanatomical-neurohistochemical issues, for which the fluorescent tracers offer interesting possibilities. One such possibility is the tracing of branching projections of transmitter identified neurons, i.e. a situation when two tracers and one immunohistochemical stain have to be combined. Thus, three markers have to be distinguished. Numerous combinations of fluorescent tracers have been used for studies of collateral projections, for example Evans blue and DAPI/primuline (Van der Kooy et al. 1978; Bentivoglio et al., 1979), bisbenzimide and propidium iodide (Kuypers et al. 1979), bisbenzimide and nuclear yellow (Bentivoglio et al. 1980), and fast blue and nuclear yellow (Kuypers et al. 1980; Bentivoglio et al. 1981) (for further examples and discussion see, Kuypers and Huisman, 1983). Combination of a fluorescent dye (DAPI) and HRP as retrograde tracers has also been employed (Yezierski and Bowker 1981).

The same general considerations of the suitability of the retrograde tracers for combination with immunofluorescence has, of course, to be considered. For example, Kuypers et al. (1980) have used fast blue and nuclear yellow which can be separated on the basis of cellular localization and by their different colors at identical excitation wavelength. Since nuclear yellow, as discussed above, is less suitable for combination with immunohistochemistry we have used DAY instead.

Simultaneous injection of fast blue (or true blue) and DAY in two different areas, such as the central amygdaloid nucleus and the nucleus caudatus putamen, respectively, results in cell bodies in the substantia nigra with an often granular blue fluorescent cytoplasm (fast blue) and a yellow-whitish nuclear fluorescence (DAY) (Skirboll et al. 1983). It is our opinion that photography should be carried out before immunohistochemistry, since diffusion of fast blue into the nucleus and DAY into the cytoplasm may occur, obscuring the differential localization. For immunohistochemistry TRITC should definitely be selected. A further possible combination of retrograde tracers is primuline and DAY. Using the same system as described above (nigrostriatal and nigra-amygdaloid projections), double-labeled cells can be clearly distinguished in the nigra with a granular cytoplasmic primuline-induced fluorescence and a nuclear DAY fluorescence (Skirboll et al. 1983). Both dyes are fairly well distinguishable after TRITC immunohistochemistry and all three markers can be analyzed simultaneously under the two proper filter combinations. The primuline-DAY combination may not work in all systems, since primuline, as discussed above, is often a 'weak' marker.

The two above-mentioned combinations are not the sole alternatives with respect to the fluorescent dyes so far available for the purpose of combining retrograde collateral tracing and immunohistochemistry. For example, it should be possible to combine propidium iodide and DAY with FITC immunohistochemistry, although we have not yet tested this alternative.

Studies on collaterals have not only been carried out with fluorescent markers, but also with other types of compounds, sometimes in combination with fluorescent dyes. These include HRP, tritium-labeled HRP and iron dextran (see, Steward 1981; Kuypers and Huisman 1983). It is conceivable that such markers may also be useful for combined studies with immunohistochemistry.

4.6. TRACING OF NEURONS WITH MULTIPLE TRANSMITTER CANDIDATES

It has been recognized that many neurons contain more than one putative transmitter, particularly a classical transmitter and a peptide (see, Hökfelt et al. 1980a,b, 1982); it will therefore be of interest to trace the projections of such neurons.

Several possibilities exist to establish the presence of more than one antigen in a cell. For example, thin adjacent sections, each containing a slice of the same cells can be stained with two different antisera. Alternatively, elution-restaining experiments can be used (Nakane 1968; Tramu et al. 1978) where, after photography, the first staining pattern is removed and the section reincubated with a new antiserum. These techniques have been discussed elsewhere (Hökfelt et al. 1982). When combining such methods with retrograde labeling, the principles discussed above for combinations with one labeled antibody are applicable also in combinations with two labeled antibodies. Successful studies of this type have been carried out on dopamine neurons in the ventral tegmental area containing cholecystokinin (CCK)-like peptide and projecting to the nucleus accumbens (Hökfelt et al. 1980c). True blue was used as tracer and FITC for detection of both antigens (tyrosine hydroxylase and CCK) and photography was carried out separately after each step (before and after incubation with CCK antiserum and after incubation with tyrosine hydroxylase antiserum). Furthermore, neurons in the periaqueductal central gray containing both substance P and CCK-like immunoreactivities have been shown to project to the spinal cord, using a sequential procedure with fast blue as retrograde tracer and TRITC as immunofluorescence marker (Skirboll

257

et al. 1983). If the elution-restaining technique is chosen, it should be remembered that the elution procedure may destroy or extract the dye. For example, elution with acid potassium permanganate (KMnO₄) according to Tramu et al. (1978) seems to abolish the fluorescence of all dyes tested by us (Skirboll et al. 1983). With this method it is thus necessary to photograph the retrograde tracer at the latest after the first immuno-histochemical incubation sequence. Other elution procedures such as those using acid media (Nakane 1968) or electrophoresis (Vandesande and Dierickx 1975) may, how-ever, be compatible with retention of fluorescent tracers throughout the immunohisto-chemical procedure.

The techniques mentioned in this and the previous paragraph can, of course, be com-bined. In this way collaterals of neurons containing two putative transmitters can be traced.

It may be mentioned that novel ideas for studies of multiple antigens in cells have emerged. Thus, internally radiolabeled antibodies, which are visualized by autoradio-graphy, have been used in combination with routine immunohistochemical detection of the second antigen (see, Cuello et al. 1982), but so far no studies employing this techni-que in combination with retrograde tracing have been published.

5. ALTERNATIVE TECHNIQUES FOR COMBINED RETROGRADE TRACING AND NEUROTRANSMITTER HISTOCHEMISTRY

The above-mentioned techniques represent only some of the approaches that have been taken for tracing of transmitter-identified pathways. In the following we briefly sum-marize some further succesful possibilities along these lines.

5.1. HRP RETROGRADE TRACING AND ALDEHYDE FLUORESCENCE HISTOCHEMISTRY

Combination of HRP and monoamine aldehyde histochemistry is associated with at least two methodological problems. On the one hand, HRP looses its enzymatical acti-vity if it is exposed to conventional freeze-drying with subsequent formaldehyde vapor treatment and paraffin embedding at elevated temperatures. On the other hand, the HRP method requires wet histochemical processing in solutions devoid of fixative, which may lead to marked diffusion or loss of the monoamine fluorophores. The first problem was solved by using the wet glyoxylic acid (GA) and formaldehyde-glutaral-dehyde (Faglu) techniques for visualization of monoamines (Chiba et al. 1976; Furness et al., 1978). The problem of diffusion of monoamines has been handled by using se-quential techniques so that the monoamine visualization step was performed first and the HRP reaction not started until the localization of monoamine fluorescence had been recorded (Berger et al. 1978; Blessing et al. 1978; Smolen et al. 1979). Results ob-tained with the sequential Faglu-HRP procedure of Blessing et al. (1978) are illustrated in Figure 11.

In these procedures the monoamine fluorophores are first produced by either the Faglu or GA reactions. Sections are cut on a Vibratome, mounted on glass slides and viewed in the fluorescence microscope. The exact location of cells exhibiting monoamine fluorescence is carefully documented preferably by photography or by us-ing an X-Y plotter. Extensive UV illumination (i.e. below 405 nm) should be avoided, since it may abolish the enzymatic activity of HRP (Ljungdahl et al. 1975). The

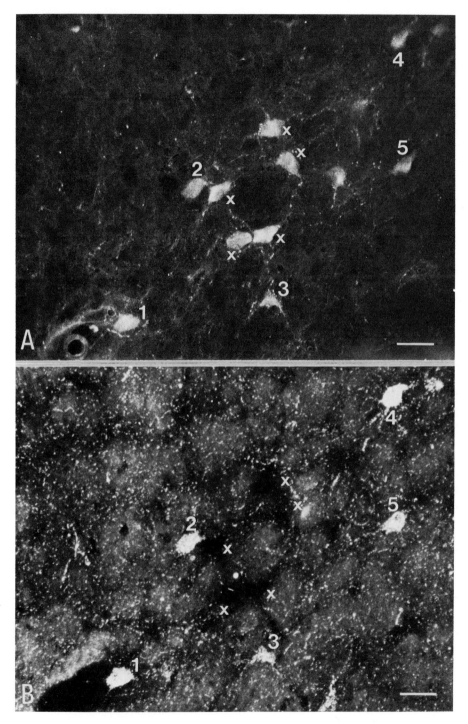

Fig. 11 A,B. Fluorescence-micrographs demonstrating formaldehyde induced catecholamine (CA) fluorescence (A) and retrogradely transported HRP (B) in the same section of the rabbit pons after intraspinal HRP injection. Cell bodies 1–5 contain both CA and HRP; cell bodies labeled with a cross in A are CA containing but not HRP positive. One HRP-labeled cell (arrow) does not seem to contain CA. Bars indicate 50 μm (from Blessing et al. 1978, with permission).

coverslip is then removed, and the slides rinsed repeatedly to wash out the remaining fixative. The sections are processed for the visualization of HRP and examined by light-microscopy in order to record the location of HRP-labeled cells. Finally, the two mappings are compared and the existence of HRP-labeled monoaminergic cells noted.

This method, which is further detailed in Protocol 8.5 in the Appendix, combines the advantage of the vast experience with the HRP technique with the relative simplicity of the GA or Faglu methods. The drawback of the method is the rather elaborate documentation procedure. The need for two subsequent mappings may however be circumvented by using a recent modification of the Faglu-HRP protocol through which the monoamine fluorescence can be retained throughout the HRP reaction (Blessing et al. 1981b). Briefly, sections from HRP injected animals are cut on a Vibratome or freezing microtome, incubated in a Faglu solution, rinsed, incubated with tetramethylbenzidine (TMB), again incubated in Faglu solution at low pH followed by Faglu at neutral pH, and mounted. Using this technique, for example, the distribution of catecholamine neurons descending to the spinal cord have successfully been mapped in the rabbit (Blessing et al. 1981b) (see Protocol 8.5 in Appendix; see also, Day et al. 1980; Blessing et al. 1981a; and Loewy and McKellar 1981).

5.2. HRP RETROGRADE TRACING AND PAP IMMUNOHISTOCHEMISTRY

Several groups have used HRP as retrograde tracer and combined this with the HRP/PAP immunohistochemical technique (Bowker et al. 1981c; Lechan et al. 1981; Priestley et al. 1981; Sofroniew and Schrell 1981; Yezierski and Bowker 1981). Although both steps use the same marker, i.e. HRP, possibilities exist to distinguish them. Thus, the retrogradely transported HRP appears as punctuate granules, whereas the HRP demonstrating immunoreactivity appears as a diffuse homogenous stain in the cytoplasm (Fig. 12). The method described by Bowker et al. (1982b) further separates the reaction product of the retrogradely transported HRP from the staining produced by the antibody-coupled HRP. This is obtained by performing the first HRP reaction (which visualizes the retrogradely transported HRP) in the presence of $CoCl_2$, resulting in a black reaction product. The second HRP reaction which visualizes the neurotransmitter related antibody is then carried out without $CoCl_2$, resulting in a brown reaction product. This color difference can easily be distinguished in the microscope, but is, of course, difficult to see in black-and-white micrographs. HRP can either be injected in pure form or conjugated to WGA. The procedure includes routine perfusion by formalin made up from paraformaldehyde powder (Pease 1962) preceeded by a body warm rinse with physiological saline. Further details on this procedure are given in the Appendix (8.6).

The advantages of this approach have been summarized by Bowker et al. (1982b), who point out that both cell markers can be demonstrated and studied simultaneously and that they are relatively permanent and not susceptible to fading. The tissue can also

---

Fig. 12. Light-micrographs demonstrating HRP-labeled (A), 5-hydroxytryptamine (5-HT)immunoreactive-PAP stained (B) and double-labeled (HRP plus 5-HT) (C) neurons in the medullary raphe complex after injection of HRP into the spinal cord. Whereas retrogradely transported HRP appears as black punctate granules (arrow heads) against a clear or unstained cytoplasm (A), 5-HT related HRP immunostaining shows a relatively homogenous staining of cytoplasm in both cell soma and processes (B). The double-labeled neuron exhibits both characteristics, i.e. black HRP granules (arrow heads) and diffuse localization of HRP (C). Bar indicates 12 μm (courtesy of R.M. Bowker, K.N. Westlund, M.C. Sullivan and J.D. Coulter).

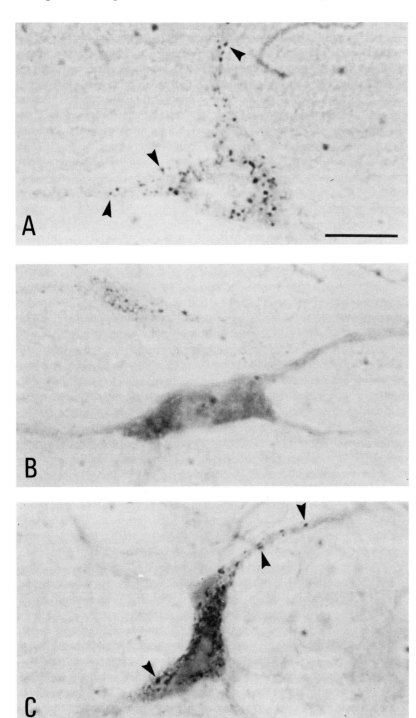

be processed for electron-microscopy. By using lectins (WGA) conjugated to HRP an increased sensitivity is obtained. The 'HRP-HRP/PAP' approach has been used to study, e.g. supraspinal descending 5-hydroxytryptamine- and peptide-containing systems. References to this work are Bowker et al. (1981a–c; 1982a–c), Priestley et al. (1981), Beitz (1982), Ritchie et al. (1982) and Yeziersky et al. (1982).

A different principle was used by Sofroniew and Schrell (1981) who studied the projections of hypothalamic oxytocin and vasopressin neurons to the spinal cord. They used inactivated HRP as retrograde tracer and the PAP technique for visualizing the peptides. The retrogradely transported, inactivated, but still antigenic HRP was detected with antibodies to HRP. Since the retrogradely transported HRP was enzymatically inactive, it did not interfere with the routine immunoperoxidase staining using diaminobenzidine (DAB) as a substrate for visualization of the neuropeptides in adjacent thin sections.

5.3. WHEAT GERM AGGLUTININ RETROGRADE TRACING AND IMMUNOHISTOCHEMISTRY

WGA is a highly sensitive retrograde tracer (Schwab et al. 1978) and Lechan et al. (1981) have used this compound in a combined procedure (see Protocol 8.7 in Appendix). This sensitive marker can be combined with immunohistochemistry and studied in the same sections. Thus, WGA injected into the striatum was detected in cell bodies in the substantia nigra of Bouin or formalin perfusion fixed brains, using antiserum to purified WGA and processing according to the PAP-technique with DAB. Free-floating Vibratome sections were used. The same sections were then processed for the indirect immunofluorescence technique using antibodies to tyrosine hydroxylase, and the occurrence of double-labeled cells could be established. Alternatively, tyrosine hydroxylase was detected with the PAP-technique using 4-chloro-1-naphtol as substrate. This dye has a blue color, which can be clearly distinguished from the WGA related brown coarse, punctate DAB reaction product reflecting retrogradely transported WGA. The avidin-biotin procedure was also employed. When tyrosine hydroxylase was visualized with FITC-labeled secondary antibodies, the coarse nonfluorescent WGA granules could be clearly seen against the background of the uniform immunofluorescence. Lechan et al. (1981) pointed out that cells containing the WGA-PAP complex exhibited a diminished immunostaining. This was interpreted as a steric hindrance to antibody penetration by the WGA accumulation (Lechan et al. 1981).

5.4. FLUORESCENT RETROGRADE TRACERS AND ACETYLCHOLINESTERASE STAINING

Retrograde fluorescent neuronal tracers have also been combined with AChE histochemistry (see, Protocols 8.8 and 8.9 in the Appendix). Butcher and collaborators (Bigl et al. 1982; Woolf and Butcher 1982) studied projections to various cortical areas and to the amygdaloid complex using Evans blue (30%) or DAPI (2.5%) mixed with primuline (10%). Albanese and Bentivoglio (1982a) used Evans blue, true blue and fast blue for studies on projections to the striatum. To increase the AChE activity in the cell bodies both groups treated the animals with di-isopropylfluorophosphate (DFP) 4–8 h before sacrifice (Butcher et al. 1974, 1975). Sections of formalin-perfused brains were cut on a freezing microtome and processed for AChE histochemistry as described by Butcher et al. (1974, 1975). Whereas the former group used sequential analysis, i.e.

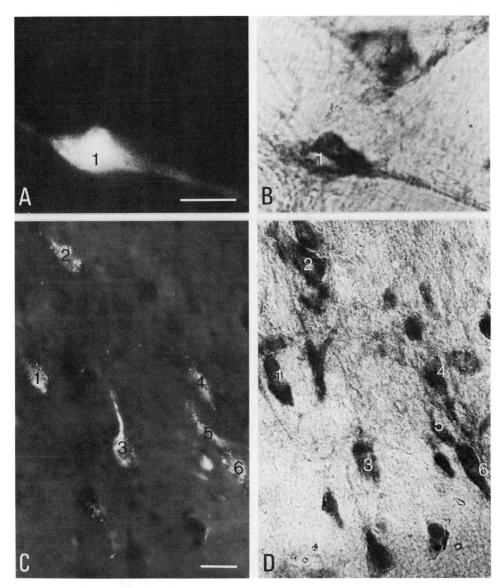

Fig. 13 A-D. Fluorescence- (A, C) and light (B, D) microscopic photographs of the substantia nigra of the rat after injection of true blue (A) and fast blue (C) into the caudate putamen and processing for AChE staining (B, D). A and B on one hand, and C and D, on the other hand show the same section. Many retrogradely labeled, fluorescent cells also contain AChE activity (compare numbers in A, B and C, D, respectively). Bars indicate 20 μm (from Albanese and Bentivoglio (1982a) (A, B) and unpublished material (C, D) from the same authors, with permission).

first photography of the retrograde fluorescent tracer and then processing for AChE histochemistry, Albanese and Bentivoglio (1982a) examined fluorescence and AChE reaction concomitantly by turning on and off the bright-field illumination of normal light during continuous UV illumination. Thus, the AChE procedure was performed without seriously affecting the fluorescence of the retrograde tracers. Our own attempts with these techniques indicate, however, that diffusion does occur with both true blue and fast blue during the AChE-staining procedure. Whether this will cause an actual loss of tracer-labeled neurons has not been carefully studied so far.

5.5. FLUORESCENT RETROGRADE TRACERS AND STEROID HORMONE AUTORADIOGRAPHY

It is now well established that some neuronal populations in the brain take up and accumulate various types of steroid hormones, as demonstrated by autoradiography (Stumpf and Grant 1975; Pfaff 1976; McEwen et al. 1979). (This methodology is reviewed in Chapter XI.) Since the steroid hormones are selectively accumulated in the nucleus of the cell body, no direct evidence on the projections of these cells can be obtained from the autoradiographic results. Morrell and Pfaff (1982) have, however, recently combined retrograde tracing, using primuline as tracer, with autoradiographic visualization of estrogen concentrating neurons in the hypothalamus. Their results demonstrated estrogen accumulating neurons in the ventromedial hypothalamic nucleus projecting to the dorsal midbrain.

6. OTHER TECHNIQUES

HRP retrograde tracing has been combined with monoamine oxidase histochemistry for studies on monoamine neurons projecting to the spinal cord (Satoh et al. 1977). The MAO-staining is, however, neither very sensitive nor a very specific marker of monoaminergic neurons. This procedure then appears to be inferior to several other techniques now available, which have been dealt with above.

Another approach for studying projections of transmitter identified systems is the use of markers which are taken up selectively into specific neuron populations. An example of this is the uptake and retrograde flow of antibodies to dopamine-β-hydroxylase, the enzyme converting dopamine to noradrenaline (Jacobowitz et al. 1975; Fillenz et al. 1976; Silver and Jacobowitz 1979), a technique which has been used by Silver and Jacobowitz (1979) and Westlund et al. (1981) to trace central noradrenergic pathways. According to these authors the uptake and transport of this enzyme is specific for noradrenergic neurons.

A related technique is the use of *labeled transmitters*, which are accumulated in neurons by specific uptake mechanisms and retrogradely transported to the cell bodies. (This is described extensively in Chapter VIII).

Azmitia and Gannon (1982) have simultaneously injected HRP and tritiated 5-HT and then compared the distribution of retrogradely labeled HRP and 5-HT cell bodies. In this case pargyline treated rats were used and the brains were fixed by perfusion with glutaraldehyde and processed for routine HRP visualization. The sections were finally processed for autoradiography according to routine principles. In this way it was possible to directly and simultaneously analyze and compare the localization of 5-HT neurons and other types of neurons (not transmitter identified) projecting to the injection site and also to study the collateralization of single 5-HT neurons.

An interesting approach has been taken by Chan-Palay and collaborators. After *injection of antibodies* to substance P and glutamic acid decarboxylase, evidence was presented for a specific uptake of these antibodies into nerve endings of substance P and GABA neurons, respectively, and a subsequent retrograde transport to the cell bodies (Chan-Palay 1979; Chan-Palay et al. 1979).

7. CONCLUDING REMARKS

In the present article we have attempted to summarize the methodology which has been developed during recent years with the aim to define retrogradely traced pathways on the basis of their transmitter, either by directly visualizing the transmitter itself or indirectly a transmitter-related compound. Most studies are based on the use of either the enzyme HRP or fluorescent compounds as retrograde tracers. The transmitter histochemistry employs aldehyde fluorescence techniques, immunohistochemistry or AChE staining. It is interesting to see how many different approaches have been successfully employed in this work (see 8.1 in the Appendix). It is at present difficult to select one particular approach as the method of choice for a particular problem. Perhaps the present article may give the reader some help in this respect, but it is clear that such decisions may depend on the previous experience of the investigator and on equipment available in the laboratory.

Most approaches included in this article may appear fairly straight forward and simple to carry out, but it should be emphasized that in our experience many problems are encountered in studies of this type. The relative success achieved in many laboratories may be due to the fact that 'favorable' systems have been studied, i.e. they transport the retrograde tracers well and their transmitters and/or related compounds can be relatively easily identified with histochemical techniques. For example, we have in part used the nigro-neostriatal dopamine system as a model (Skirboll et al. 1983). These neurons have widely divergent terminal fields and will thus take up large amounts of retrograde tracer resulting in a very strong labeling of the parent cell bodies. Furthermore, these neurons can be easily visualized both with aldehyde-induced fluorescence or immunohistochemistry. In fact, the antiserum to tyrosine hydroxylase used in our studies (Markey et al. 1980) is one of the most 'potent' antisera which we have tested for immunohistochemistry. Under these conditions combined studies can be carried out fairly easily with good results. A more advanced technology may, however, be needed when attempting to study other systems. For example, when neurons with small projection fields are studied, only small amounts of retrograde tracers can be injected and diffusion out from the injection area must be kept minimal. In this respect WGA may offer distinct advantages as compared to HRP and fluorescent dyes, since its spread in nervous tissue is limited. With regard to immunohistochemical detection of transmitter-related compounds in cell bodies, the PAP and avidin-biotin techniques may offer a higher sensitivity than immunofluorescence. In this way lower levels of transmitter-related compounds can be detected in cell bodies. Alternatively it may not be necessary to treat the experimental animals with colchicine. Although this treatment does not represent a major problem in studies on rats, it may be a distinct advantage not to have to use colchicine in larger animals such as cats and monkeys.

Under all circumstances it will be important to ensure a high quality and standard of the documentation of results from combined retrograde tracing and transmitter histochemistry. There should be a demand for convincing photographic demonstration of co-localization of retrograde tracer and histochemical marker. A problem here is that distinction often has to be made on the basis of different colors and that publication of color photographs are associated with high costs. It may therefore be worthwhile to consider the possibility to supply color prints with papers submitted for publication, (i.e. for the referees' use), even if for financial reasons only black-and-white micrographs can be published. This may be especially important if novel techniques are used and novel results are presented.

8. APPENDIX

8.1. SURVEY OF DIFFERENT METHODS FOR COMBINED RETROGRADE TRACING AND TRANSMITTER HISTOCHEMISTRY

(see pp. 268 and 269)

8.2. FLUORESCENT TRACERS

(see p. 270)

8.3. RECOMMENDED PROCEDURE FOR COMBINATION OF FLUORESCENT RETROGRADE TRACERS AND MONOAMINE HISTOFLUORESCENCE

(For further technical details see Björklund and Skagerberg 1979a and Chapter II.)

A. *Preparation of tracer suspensions.* Both TB and PI are used as 3–5% aqueous suspensions. EB is used as a 10% suspension and NY at a 1% concentration. The suspensions are sonicated for 10 min in order to reduce the particle size as much as possible. The suspensions can be stored in a freezer at $-20°C$ thawed before use and then refrozen again. These tracers can be stored in a freezer for at least a year without loss of fluorescence intensity or labeling capacity.

B. *Injections.* Injections are performed during ketamine-xylazine anesthesia (Rompun[R]-Bayer 20 mg/ml, Ketalar[R]-Parke-Davies 50 mg/ml; 1 mg Rompun + 5 mg Ketalar i.p. or i.m./100 g rat), using a 1 μl Hamilton syringe equipped with a microdrive. For small injections (0.05–0.20 μl) the syringe is affixed to a glass-capillary by surgical wax and the whole system filled with immersion oil before the volume to be injected is sucked into the capillary. The injection is administered by continuous pressure so that the suspension is delivered at a rate of 10 nl/min. The capillary is left in place for 10–20 min after the injection in order to minimize leakage along the needle-track. If larger injections are wanted, or if the purpose is to cut axon bundles at the injection site (which enhances the uptake of tracers into axons of passage), the Hamilton syringe with its attached cannula is used without a glass-capillary. Injections can also be made with a glass micropipette attached to a pressure ejection unit (Alheid et al. 1981).

C. *Survival.* The optimal survival time should be tested out for the particular system under study. For TB 1–2 weeks give optimal labeling in systems confined within the brain. For projections from the brain stem to the caudal spinal cord 3–5 weeks may be needed. When using PI it is often necessary to use shorter survival-times, since this tracer diffuses continuously and long survival times sometimes make it impossible to demarcate the injection site, and besides produce a disturbing glial labeling in the area of labeled neurons. When using EB more than 2 days survival is seldom used in the rat. After more than 5 days survival the intensity of the labeling with both EB and PI is decreased. NY is very rapidly transported and gives in our experience best labeling after 24–48 h survival time.

D. *Perfusion.* During chloralhydrate anesthesia the rat is perfused through the heart first with 150–200 ml ice cold Tyrode's buffer (8.0 g NaCl, 0.2 g KCl, 0.2 g $CaCl_2$, 0.05 g $MgCl_2$, 1.0 g $NaHCO_3$, 0.04 g NaH_2PO_4 and 1.0 g glucose per liter of distilled water) under a pressure of 0.4–0.6 bar/cm^2 (30–45 cm Hg) and secondly with

300–350 ml ice-cooled buffered ALFA solution (100 g $Al_2(SO_4)_3 \times 18\ H_2O$ is dissolved in 2% paraformaldehyde in Tyrode's buffer (see 8.4. E) 3.8 g $Na_2B_4O_7 \times 10$ H_2O is added and pH is then adjusted to about 4.7 with 100 g $CH_3COONa \times 3$ H_2O). During the ALFA perfusion the perfusion pressure is gradually increased up to 2.0 bar (150 cm Hg). Immediately after perfusion the nervous tissue are removed from their skeletal and meningeal coverings. The tissue is cut into pieces. It should be noted that the larger the pieces, the more pronounced the cracking induced by freezing.

E. *Freezing.* The tissue pieces are frozen in a two-step procedure to minimize cracking. First, the tissue is frozen for about 1 min in isopentane that has been cooled to -80 to $-90°C$ by short time immersion in liquid nitrogen. The tissue is then transferred to a 9:1 propane-propylene mixture cooled to the temperature of liquid nitrogen.

F. *Freeze-drying.* The specimens are freeze-dried at a temperature of -35 to $-40°C$ for 5 days.

G. *Formaldehyde vapor treatment.* This step induces the formation of monoamine fluorophores. The specimens are exposed to the vapor of paraformaldehyde with specified water content (equilibrated in 50–70% relative air humidity) at 80°C for 60 min.

H. *Embedding.* As soon as possible after the formaldehyde vapor treatment, the tissue are embedded in paraffin in vacuo.

I. *Sectioning and mounting.* The specimens are sectioned at 15 μm. The sections are transferred to a dry slide on a hot plate (60°) for a short time allowing the paraffin to melt and the sections to spread. The slide is removed from the hot plate and superfluous paraffin is removed. The section is then covered with a 4:1 mixture of Entellan (Merck, Darmstadt, FRG) and xylene and a coverslip added. Finally, the coverslipped slide is returned to the hot plate for 1–2 h in order to dissolve the remaining paraffin of the sections.

J. *Storing.* The mounted specimens can be stored for several months in a freezer at $-20°C$ without notable loss of fluorescence. When stored at room temperature, the background gradually increases while the monoamine fluorescence fades so that the contrast is quite low after 4–5 days. The serotonin fluorescence is especially vulnerable in this respect. At $+4°C$ the slides can be stored for 10–14 days without decreases in fluorescence quality.

K. *Microscopy.* For differentiation of the fluorophores four different lines of the mercury lamp are used for excitation (see Table 2).

L. *A simplified scheme of the appearance of the fluorophores at different excitation wavelengths*

Exc. wavelength (nm)	365	435	546/577
Catecholamines	Green-Yellow +	Green-Yellow + +	0
5-Hydroxytryptamine	Yellow +	0	0
True blue	Blue or Green + + +	0	0
Propidium iodide	Red + +	Red (+)	Red + + +
Evans blue	0	0	Red + +
Nuclear yellow	Yellow + +	0	0

Pulses denote subjective estimations of fluorescence intensity and apply only for comparison between different excitations – not between different fluorophores.

8.1. SURVEY OF DIFFERENT METHODS FOR COMBINED RETROGRADE TRACING AND TRANSMITTER HISTOCHEMISTRY

Histochemical technique	Monoamine aldehyde histochemistry		HRP		Immunohistochemistry	
Retrograde tracer	Fluorescent dyes	Fluorescent dyes	HRP	HRP	Fluorescent dyes (diffusible)	Fluorescent dyes (non-diffusible)
Fixation	ALFA perfusion + freeze-drying	GA-PF perfusion	Faglu perfusion	Faglu perfusion	Formalin perfusion	Formalin perfusion
Histochemistry I	PF vapor					
Embedding	Paraffin					
Sectioning	Microtome	Cryostat	Vibratome	Vibratome or freezing microtome	Cryostat	Cryostat
Histochemistry II						
Analysis I			Fluorescence microscope		Fluorescence microscope	
Histochemistry III		GA immersion + heating (100°C)	HRP histochemistry	Faglu immersion	Indirect immunofluorescence or PAP immunohistochemistry	Indirect immunofluorescence
Histochemistry IV				HRP histochemistry		
Analysis II	Fluorescence microscope	Fluorescence microscope	Light microscope	Fluorescence + light microscope	Fluorescence or light microscope	Fluorescence microscope
Principle procedure	Simultaneous	Simultaneous	Sequential	Simultaneous	Sequential	Simultaneous
Reference	Björklund and Skagerberg (1979a) App. 8.3.	Van der Kooy and Wise (1980)	Blessing et al. (1978) App. 8.5.	Blessing et al. (1981b)	Skirboll et al. (1983); Ross et al. (1981) App. 8.4.	Skirboll et al. (1983) App. 8.4.

Immunohistochemistry *(continued)*

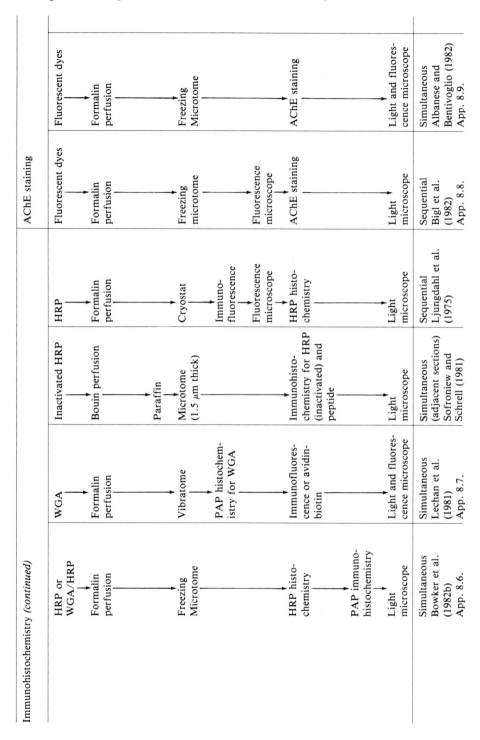

HRP or WGA/HRP	WGA	Inactivated HRP	HRP
Formalin perfusion	Formalin perfusion	Bouin perfusion	Formalin perfusion
Freezing Microtome	Vibratome	Paraffin	Cryostat
HRP histochemistry	PAP histochemistry for WGA	Microtome (1.5 μm thick)	Immunofluorescence
PAP immunohistochemistry	Immunofluorescence or avidin-biotin	Immunohistochemistry for HRP (inactivated) and peptide	Fluorescence microscope
Light microscope	Light and fluorescence microscope	Light microscope	HRP histochemistry
			Light microscope
Simultaneous Bowker et al. (1982b) App. 8.6.	Simultaneous Lechan et al. (1981) App. 8.7.	Simultaneous (adjacent sections) Sofroniew and Schrell (1981)	Sequential Ljungdahl et al. (1975)

AChE staining

Fluorescent dyes	Fluorescent dyes
Formalin perfusion	Formalin perfusion
Freezing microtome	Freezing Microtome
Fluorescence microscope	AChE staining
AChE staining	
Light microscope	Light and fluorescence microscope
Sequential Bigl et al. (1982) App. 8.8.	Simultaneous Albanese and Bentivoglio (1982) App. 8.9.

8.2. FLUORESCENT TRACERS

Code name	Code No.	Chemical name	Source
Bisbenzimide	Hoechst 33258	2-(2-(4-hydroxyphenyl)-6-benzimidazolyl)-6-(1-methyl-4-piperazyl)-benzimidazol-trishydrochloride	Hoechst Aktiengesellschaft, Postfach 8000320, 6230 Frankfurt a. M. 80, FRG. (Weisblum and Haenssler 1974; Hilwig and Gropp 1975; Latt and Stetten 1976)
DAPI	102/108 (18860)	2-(4-amidinophenyl)-indol-6-carboxamidin-dihydrochloride	Serva, Heidelberg, FRG (Dann et al. 1971; Schnedl et al. 1977)
DAY	288/26	diamidino compound; chemically related to DAPI	Prof. O. Dann, Institute of Pharmacology and Food Chemistry, Friedrich-Alexander University, Erlangen, FRG (Dann et al. 1970, 1971, 1973, 1975). Purchase: Prof Dr Illing, Warthweg 14–18, Postfach 1150, D-6114, Gross Umstadt, FRG
Evans blue	E2129		Sigma, St. Louis, USA
Fast blue	253/50	chemically related to the true blue	See DAY
Granular blue	186/134	2-(4-2(4-amidinophenoxy)phenyl)indol-6-carboxamidino-2HCl	See DAY (Dann et al. 1975)
Nuclear yellow	Hoechst S 769/12	2-(4-sulfamylphenyl)-6-(6-(4-methyl-piperazino)-2-benzimidazolyl)-benzimidazol-trishydrochloride	Hoechst (Dr H. Loewe, Hoechst Aktiengesellschaft, Postfach 800320, 6230 Frankfurt a. M. 80, FRG. (Loewe and Urbanietz 1974)
Propidium iodide	P 5264		Sigma, St. Louis, USA (Hudson et al. 1968)
True blue	150/129	(E)-2,2'-vinylendi-benzofuran-5-carboxamidin-diaceturate	See DAY (Dann et al. 1973)
Primuline	1039		Eastman, Rochester, USA

M. Some problems and their remedies

Tracer	Problem	Cause	Remedy
TB	Weak tracer-labeling	too short survival time	increase survival time
		too strong monoamine fluorescence	shorter FA treatment
NY	False-positive labeling	anterograde transport	inject kainic acid together with NY (Arbuthnott et al. 1982)
PI	No labeling	too long or too short survival time	adjust survival time
	No discernible monoamine fluorescence in PI-labeled cells	too heavy PI-labeling	adjust survival time, add KP 650 barrier filter
	Difficulties in differentiating pigment from PI-labeling	too much pigment	look for nucleolar labeling; check same region in un-injected animals; use as young animals as possible
EB	Weak or absent labeling	intracellular breakdown	decrease survival time

8.4. RECOMMENDED PROCEDURE FOR COMBINATION OF FLUORESCENT RETROGRADE TRACERS AND IMMUNOFLUORESCENCE

(For further details, see Skirboll et al. 1983.)

Of the compounds tested, FB, TB and PI and in certain cases, Pr and DAY seem to be best suited for combination with immunohistofluorescence. The two main protocols involve FB combined with TRITC-immunofluorescence and PI combined with FITC-immunofluorescence.

A. *Preparation of tracer suspension.* See Section 8.3.A.

B. *Injection.* See Section 8.3.B.

C. *Survival time.* See Section 8.3.C. Also shorter survival times, down to 2–3 days for FB and the nigrostriatal system have been used.

D. *Colchicine treatment.* To enhance visualization in cell somata, especially of several neuropeptides, the animals are pretreated with colchicine. 60–120 µg colchicine, dissolved in 0.9% sodium chloride is injected into the lateral ventricle. For studies on the lower brain stem and spinal cord, the drug can be given intracisternally (60 µg in 10 µl) and intrathecally (60–100 µg in 10 µl) (Yaksh and Rudy, 1976), respectively. The animals are sacrificed 24–48 h later. In our experience colchicine from different sources may have varying 'potency'. It is therefore recommended to test each batch before extensive use.

E. *Fixation.* The animals are anesthetized (see Section 8.3.D), ventilated by a small animal respirator (Rodent respirator, Harvard Instruments, Boston, MA, USA) and perfused via the ascending aorta. After a brief rinse with Tyrode's solution (50 ml at room temperature, followed by 50 ml of the same, icecold solution), perfusion is continued for 5–30 min with 10% ice-cold formalin, prepared according to Pease (1962) from 40 g paraformaldehyde powder in 0.1 M phosphate buffer. 80 g paraformaldehyde are dissolved in 1000 ml distilled water and heated to 60°C. Add about 8 ml NaOH until the solution is clear. Add 1000 ml of 0.2 M Sörensen phosphate buffer, pH 7.2. During the perfusion the animal is immersed in an ice-cold water bath. The brains are dissected out and immersed in the same fixative for 90 min, rinsed for at least 24 h in 0.1 M phosphate buffer with 5% sucrose added.

F. *Sectioning.* The brains are cut out on a cryostat (Dittes, Heidelberg, FRG) at 5–30 μm section thickness and thawed onto an object slide coated with chrome alum-gelatin (0.2 g chrome alum and 2 g gelatin are dissolved in 400 ml distilled water; warm until dissolved). The possibility exists to process sections for immunohisto-chemistry as free floating sections, especially when using dyes resistant to diffusion (PI, Pr). This technique has a higher 'sensitivity' than if sections are fixed on to slides.

G. *Mounting.* In the case of FB and TB the slides should be examined unmounted. If high power photographs are to be made, xylene mounting can be used, but also in this medium diffusion may occur. The sections should always be examined as soon as possible after removal from the cryostat. The sections may be exposed to a stream of dry air (or inert gas) immediately after removal from the cryostat to avoid diffusion of the dye. For PI, Pr and DAY, the section can principally be directly processed for immunohistochemistry. If sections containing these three dyes are to be photographed before immunohistochemistry, it is possible to use a mixture of PBS and glycerol (1:3) for mounting. For microscopy and photography, see below.

H. *Immunohistochemistry.* Sections are processed for the indirect immunofluores-cence procedure of Coons and collaborators (see Coons, 1958). Briefly, the sections are incubated with the primary antiserum at 4°C for 24–48 h in a humid atmos-phere. Triton X-100 (0.3%) is added to the antisera. After rinsing in PBS (30 min, several changes), the sections are incubated with FITC (PI or TB) or with TRITC (DAY, FB, Pr) conjugated antibodies for 30 min at 37°C, rinsed in PBS and mounted in PBS:glycerol (1:3).

I. *Microscopy.* The sections are examined in a Zeiss fluorescence microscope with epi- or transmitted-illumination. The excitation wavelength for the various dye and immunofluorescence markers as well as filter combinations are indicated in Table 2 (see also Appendix 8.3.L). With regard to immunofluorescence, FITC-induced fluorescence is viewed with 1 or 2 KP 500 filters for activation, possibly with the ad-dition of an LP 455 filter, which reduces brown background staining. This com-bination corresponds to Zeiss FITC 09 (BP 450-490). As stop filter an LP 520 plus a KP 560 filter can be used (Zeiss FITC 10), which is often referred to as BP 520 – 560. For TRITC-induced fluorescence a Schott BP 546 activation and an LP 590 stop filters were used. 'Blue' dyes were analyzed with a Schott UG 1 activation and a Zeiss 41 barrier filter. Tri-X-ASA 400 Kodak (Rochester, NY, USA) black and white film can be used for all markers. Scopic RPI (Gevaert, Belgium) black-and-white film is excellent for blue and green fluorescence but less sensitive to red markers (PI, TRITC). For color photography Kodak High Speed Ektachrome (160 Tungsten, artificial light) (Eastman Kodak, Rochester, NY, USA) can be used.

J. *Comments.* The use of the two basic combinations (FB or TB with TRITC and PI with FITC) offers no major problems under optimal conditions (good transport and a 'strong' antiserum). Principally it is important to achieve a good balance be-tween retrograde tracer and immunofluorescence marker. It is always advisable to work with as 'strong' antibody as possible. If too strong, it can always be diluted to avoid interference with tracer fluorescence. If FB/TB and TRITC is used, the blue fluorescence can never get too strong, since it will not shine through the red filters. If TRITC-fluorescence is too strong, it will shine through the 'blue filters' and may make it difficult to analyze FB/TB simultaneously. Remedies are to reduce antibody concentrations or photograph FB/TB before immunofluorescence. If PI is combined with FITC-immunofluorescence, a too strong PI-fluorescence will shine through the 'green filter' and may interfere with analysis of weak immunofluorescence. PI-fluorescence can hardly be reduced in intensity by prolonged exposure to UV light or extensive rinsing. It may be possible to use lower PI concentrations for the injection, to add extra stop filter (LP 560) and, perhaps, even look for a 'stronger' antibody! Spectral analysis may also be employed in critical situations.

8.5. RECOMMENDED SEQUENTIAL PROCEDURE FOR COMBINATION OF RETROGRADELY TRANSPORTED HRP AND CATECHOLAMINE HISTOFLUORESCENCE

(Protocol from Blessing et al. 1978, with permission. Details of the Faglu-HRP-procedure (simultaneous analysis) can be found in Blessing et al. 1981b.)

After HRP injection and appropriate survival time the following steps are applied.
A. *Perfusion.* Rabbits are perfused retrogradely via the abdominal aorta first with 200 ml isotonic sodium chloride containing 5000 IE heparin/l and then with 2000 ml of 4% formaldehyde plus 0.5% glutaraldehyde in 0.1 M sodium phosphate buffer, pH 7.0. Rats are preperfused for 10–30 sec with 200 ml of the Faglu solution (Furness et al. 1978).
B. *Sectioning.* After dissection sectioning is performed on a Vibratome at 30 μm.
C. *Rinsing.* The sections are washed, freefloating, in several changes of PBS, pH 7.0 over a period of about 10 min.
D. *Mounting.* With the aid of filter paper the sections are pressed onto chrome alum-coated slides (8.4.F). The sections are first dried by blowing a stream of air over the slides and then further dried over phosphorus pentoxide for 1 h. The sections are mounted in glycerine and coverslipped.
E. *Microscopy.* The specimens are examined in the fluorescence microscope at 405–435 nm activation. Care is taken to avoid exposing the preparations to UV light which abolishes the enzymatic activity of HRP. The location of catecholamine containing cells is now carefully documented.
F. *HRP histochemistry.* The coverslips are removed and the slides washed in PBS. HRP in the sections is then demonstrated according to Mesulam (1978), whereafter the location of HRP-containing cells is determined and compared with the location of catecholamine-containing cells obtained at step E.

8.6. RECOMMENDED PROCEDURE FOR COMBINATION OF RETROGRADELY TRANSPORTED HRP AND HRP IMMUNOHISTOCHEMISTRY

(Extracted from Bowker et al. 1982b, with permission.)

A. *Injections.* HRP or wheat germ agglutinin conjugated to HRP (WGA-HRP) is injected via a glass micropipette (tip diameter 50–100 μm) attached to a Hamilton syringe in anesthetized animals. The quantity of injected marker will vary depending upon the systems studied. For example, for spinal cord studies small quantities (0.1–0.2 μl) of a 25–50% solution of HRP or 0.1% solution of WGA-HRP are deposited into the spinal cord at each penetration, 6–15 times bilaterally over 2–3 spinal segments.

B. *Perfusion.* The animals are deeply anesthetized with pentobarbital and the limbs affixed to a wire grate with tape. The left ventricle of the heart is punctured with a blunt 14–18 gauge needle connected to a perfusion apparatus. For rats 300–500 ml of warm physiological saline is infused by gravity pressure for 2.5–5 min. For cats and monkeys the volume is 800–1000 ml. After rinsing cold 3.0–3.8% paraformaldehyde solution is perfused, whereby about 1200 ml are infused during 40–60 min at 5–10°C. This is followed by 1000 ml cold (5–12°C) 30% sucrose during 60–90 min. The tissues are dissected out and immersed in the sucrose solution.

C. *Sectioning.* The tissues are sectioned on a freezing microtome at 20–25 μm thickness immediately or the following day.

D. *HRP histochemistry procedure.* The sections are collected in cold phosphate buffer and rinsed 2–3 times in Tris/HCl buffer prior to incubation in 0.5% $CoCl_2$ for 5–10 min. The sections are rinsed 2–3 times in Tris/HCl buffer, 2–3 times in phosphate buffer and then reacted for HRP histochemistry. They are incubated in 0.02% DAB for 10–15 min without H_2O_2 and then 15 min in 0.22% DAB with H_2O_2. The sections are agitated during the reaction. After rinsing in 0.1 M phosphate buffer 2–3 times, the wet sections can be examined under the microscope for identification of HRP granules.

E. *Immunohistochemistry.* The sections are placed in hollow polyethylene stoppers and are incubated in an antiserum for 24–48 h at room temperature with continuous or frequent agitation. The sections are then rinsed several times and transferred to a small compartmentalized tray having a fine nylon mesh attached to its base. This permits washing and incubation of the sections in the immunocytochemical reagents during the PAP staining procedure. After 6–10 washes in 1% normal goat serum in 0.1 M PBS, the sections are incubated in 3% normal goat serum, 0.75% gelatin in PBS for 30 min to block nonspecific staining. After incubation in goat anti-rabbit IgG in 1% normal goat serum in 0.1 M PBS for 30 min, the sections are washed 6–10 times in 1% normal goat serum in 0.1 M PBS for 30 min and incubated in rabbit PAP diluted 1:80 in 1% normal goat serum in 0.1 M PBS for 30 min. After 6–10 washes in 0.1 M phosphate buffer the sections are incubated in 0.02% DAB and 0.01% H_2O_2 in 0.1 M phosphate buffer for 6 min, mounted and coverslipped in alcohols, xylene and Permount. Proper control experiments include incubation with antiserum preabsorbed with an excess of the antigen.

8.7. RECOMMENDED PROCEDURE FOR COMBINATION OF WHEAT GERM AGGLUTININ (WGA) RETROGRADE LABELING AND PAP IMMUNOHISTOCHEMISTRY

(Protocol supplied by Dr R. Lechan; see Lechan et al. 1981.)

A. *Tracer and injection.* Wheat germ agglutination (WGA) (EY Lab, Inc., San Mateo, CA) is prepared as a 0.5–0.9% solution in Tris buffered saline – HCl (TBS), pH 8.1 and administered by pressure injections with a Hamilton syringe (because of the presence of high capacity glycoprotein receptors for WGA, large injection volumes, i.e. 0.5 μl are often necessary).

B. *Colchicine treatment.* Animals are allowed to recover from anesthesia and 18–24 h later, colchicine (75 μg in 10 μl of normal saline) is administered into the lateral ventricle stereotactically or via chronic indwelling cannula. (For double-labeling of tuberoinfundibular neurons, due to limited survival time of the animals after retropharyngeal surgical approach, animals are treated with colchicine 8 h after application of WGA to the median eminence while the animal is under continuous anesthesia for a total survival time of 20–28 h.)

C. *Perfusion.* Animals are killed 20–24 h later and the brains fixed by intracardiac perfusion with Bouin's solution or 4% paraformaldehyde at 4°C for 20–30 min.

D. *WGA histochemistry.* Vibratome sections are prepared for the immunocytochemical localization of WGA based on the indirect PAP technique (Sternberger) using a rabbit antibody obtained from the EY Lab, Inc. diluted 1:600–1:1200 and diaminobenzidine as the substrate.

E. *Immunohistochemistry.* Selected tissue sections are washed in TBS and incubated with antiserum to the particular peptide sought for 24 h at 4°C. The immunostaining is visualized using the indirect immunofluorescence technique or the avidin-biotin technique (Biotinylated IgG followed by fluorescein-avidin dcs, Vector Labs, Inc., Burlingame, CA).

F. *Microscopy.* The coarse, dark staining of the WGA reaction product can often be seen through the apple-green fluorescence of double-labeled cells. Otherwise the tissue section is examined alternately under the light and fluorescence microscope. Nonspecific fluorescence must be sought in control tissue sections by omitting the primary antibody in the immunocytochemical sequence and incubating with fluorescein-labeled IgG alone.

8.8. RECOMMENDED PROCEDURE FOR COMBINATION OF FLUORESCENT RETROGRADE TRACERS AND AChE STAINING (SEQUENTIAL METHOD)

(From Bigl et al. 1982, with permission. See also Chapter I.)

A. *Fluorescent tracers.* Water solutions containing either 30% EB or 2.5% DAPI and 10% Pr are prepared immediately prior to injection.

B. *Injections.* Injections are performed using a 1 μl Hamilton syringe with its attached cannula. Tracer volumes of between 0.05–0.3 μl are injected during a 10-min period. After completed injection the cannula is left in place for 4 min and then slowly withdrawn.

C. *DFP treatment.* Rats are injected with 1.8 mg/kg di-isopropylfluorophosphate (DFP) i.m. 4 h before sacrifice. Animals which exhibit respiratory difficulties during the survival period after the DFP injection are given 10 mg/kg atropine methyl bromate.

D. *Survival time.* In the rat, optimal labeling of neurons of the basal forebrain is seen 48 h after tracer injections in the cerebral cortex.

E. *Perfusion.* Before sacrifice the animals are anesthetized with 350 mg/kg chloral hydrate i.p. and then perfused with 120 ml cold (4°C) 0.9% saline followed by 120 ml cold 10% buffered formalin (pH 7). The entire brain is then removed and further fixed in cold buffered formalin for 48 h and finally immersed in a cold 30% sucrose solution for an additional 48 h.

F. *Sectioning and mounting.* The fixed and rinsed brains are cut into 4–6 mm thick slabs, frozen with solid CO_2 and cut on a freezing microtome at 40 μm thickness.

The sections are collected in cold 0.9% saline and immediately mounted on glass slides coated with pig gelatin or chrome alum. The sections are then dried at room temperature, rinsed in distilled water, air-dried again and coverslipped under mineral oil.

G. *Microscopy*. The slides are examined in the fluorescence microscope within 48 h after mounting. For Zeiss epi-illumination microscope filter blocks 01 and 15 are well suited for visualization of DAPI-Pr and EB, respectively. The locations of tracer-labeled cells are carefully recorded.

H. *AChE visualization*. The coverslips are removed manually from the inspected slides. The slides are subsequently blotted on absorbent paper and immersed in xylene to remove the mineral oil, blotted again to remove xylene and then allowed to air-dry. The mounted sections are then rinsed in 0.9% saline for 2 min and finally processed for AChE according to the procedure of Karnovsky and Roots (1964) as modified by Butcher et al. (1974). When the reaction AChE is completed the slides are rinsed in distilled water, air dried, immersed in xylene and coverslipped under Permount.

I. *Microscope*. AChE microscopy is then performed either with dark- or brightfield illumination and the pattern of AChE-staining is compared to the previously recorded fluorescent labeling.

8.9. RECOMMENDED PROCEDURE FOR COMBINATION OF FLUORESCENT TRACERS AND AChE STAINING (SIMULTANEOUS METHOD)

(Protocol supplied by Dr M. Bentivoglio; see, Albanese and Bentivoglio 1982a.)

A. *Fluorescent tracers*. EB, TB, and FB have been used in our laboratory for this combined study. EB and TB provide the advantage that, under these experimental conditions, they do not label glial elements even after relatively long survivals. However, TB fluorescence decreases appreciably during incubation for AChE, while the decrease in EB fluorescence is much less pronounced. FB fluorescence decreases less than TB fluorescence with histochemical incubation, but a drawback with this tracer is that incubation enhances glial labeling occurring in the surroundings of the FB-labeled neural somata.

B. *Survival times*. Longer survival times are required than for simple anatomical tracing; survival time after TB injections into the rat brain is approximately 7–14 days, while after the EB and FB injections it is 5–10 days. This procedure allows build-up of the tracers into labeled somata, which compensates, at least in part, the decrease of fluorescence noted after the incubation of AChE.

C. *DFP poisoning*. DFP is usually dissolved in arachid oil (1.5%, w/v) and is then stored at 4°C for several months. This AChE inhibitor is given i.m. (1.5 mg/kg) from 4–8 h prior to the sacrifice. A 4-h survival is recommended for analysis of the areas in which darkly stained AChE neurons are found (e.g. neostriatum, basal forebrain, etc.); longer survival times are required for detailed visualization of the lightly stained AChE somata.

D. *Perfusion*. 0.9% saline followed by 10% phosphate buffered formalin (pH 7.2) is perfused transcardially.

E. *Histological procedure*. The brains are transferred into phosphate buffered (pH 7.2) 30% sucrose for 4–5 h at room temperature, and are sectioned on a freezing microtome at 20–30 μm thickness.

- Alternate sections are usually not incubated for AChE and kept as control of the fluorescent labeling. They are immediately mounted on slides from distilled water, and air-dried.
- The other sections are stained for AChE according to the following procedure:
  (a) 30 min incubation in 30 μM aqueous solution of tetra-isopropylpirophosphoramide. This step is required in order to inactivate nonspecific cholinesterases.
  (b) Two to 4 h incubation in the following solution: 50% (w/v) acetylthiocholine iodide; 65% (v/v) 0.2 M Tris maleate buffer (pH 5.7); 5% (v/v) 0.1 M sodium citrate; 10% (v/v) 30 mM copper sulfate; 10% (v/v) distilled and deionized water; 10% (v/v) 5 mM potassium ferricyanide. These incubations are carried out at room temperature (20–22°C); sections are gently shaken every 30 min.

F. *Microscopy.* Sections are studied without coverslipping, under oil immersion, by means of an epifluorescence microscope. The light conditions we use for the observation of the fluorescent dyes are: 340–380 nm light excitation wavelength and 430 nm barrier filter for the observation of FB and TB; 540–560 nm light excitation wavelength and 580 nm barrier filter for the observation of EB.

- The AChE deposits can be observed simply by turning on the bright-field while observing with epi-fluorescence, thus allowing simultaneous epi-fluorescence/ bright-field observation of both the fluorescent dye and AChE. This 'shining through' effect is not observed when EB is used, because the red (580 nm) barrier filter reduces image contrast when observing the russet-colored AChE deposits.

G. *Summary.* The main thrust of this procedure is to combine a sufficiently bright fluorescence with a sufficiently light AChE reaction. The factors influencing fluorescence of the tracers are: (a) a decrease in fluorescence during incubation for AChE, and (b) an increase in fluorescence over long survival times (especially TB and FB). The factors influencing AChE staining are: (a) an increase in the AChE deposits along with recovery from the DFP poisoning, and (b) an increase of the AChE histochemical reaction along with an increase of incubation time and temperature.

9. ACKNOWLEDGEMENTS

We would like to thank Dr M. Bentivoglio, Dr R.M. Bowker and Dr J. Furness for supplying micrographs for the present article. We express our gratitude to Dr M. Bentivoglio, Dr R.M. Bowker, Dr L. Butcher, Dr J. Furness and Dr R. Lechan for permission to include their protocols on techniques for combination of retrograde tracing and neurotransmitter histochemistry. The exact references to the work containing original micrographs and protocols including all authors are found in the text. We are most grateful to Prof M. Goldstein and Drs H. Steinbusch and A. Verhofstad for supplying antibodies to tyrosine hydroxylase and 5-hydroxytryptamine (Fig. 10B, D) and to Prof O. Dann for supplying several dyes. We thank Prof H. Kuypers for valuable advice. We thank Miss H. Olofsson for expert secretarial help.

10. REFERENCES

Albanese A, Bentivoglio A (1982a): Retrograde fluorescent neuronal tracing combined with acetyl-cholinesterase histochemistry. *J. Neurosci. Meth., 6,* 121–127.

Albanese A, Bentivoglio M. (1982b): The organization of dopaminergic and non-dopaminergic mesence-phalo-cortical neurons in the rat. *Brain Res., 238,* 421–425.

Alheid GF, Edwards SB, Kitai ST, Park HR, and Switzer RC III (1981): Methods for delivering tracers. In: Heimer L, RoBards MJ (Eds), *Neuroanatomical Tract-Tracing Methods,* pp. 91–116. Plenum Press, New York.

Araneda S, Gamrani H, Font C, Calas A, Pujol J-F, Bobillier P (1980): Retrograde axonal transport follow-ing injection of the ^{3}H-serotonin into the olfactory bulb. II. Radioautographic study. *Brain Res., 196,* 417–427.

Arbuthnott GW, Wright AK, Hamilton MH, Brown JR (1982): Orthograde transport of nuclear yellow: a problem and its solution. *J. Neurosci. Meth., 6,* 365–368.

Aschoff A, Fritz N, Illert M (1982): Axonal transport of fluorescent compounds in the brain and spinal cord of cat and rat. In: Weiss DG, Gorio A (Eds), *Axoplasmic Transport in Physiology and Pathology,* Springer, Berlin.

Aschoff A, Holländer H (1982): Fluorescent compounds as retrograde tracers compared with horseradish peroxidase (HRP). I. A parametric study in the central visual system of the albino rat. *J. Neurosci. Meth., 6,* 179–197.

Avrameas S (1969): Coupling of enzymes to proteins with glutaraldehyde: use of conjugates for the detection of antigens and antibodies. *Immunocytochemistry, 6,* 43–47.

Azmitia EE, Gannon PJ (1982): A light- and electronmicroscopic analysis of the selective retrograde transport of (^{3}H)-5-hydroxytryptamine by serotonergic neurons. *J. Histochem. Cytochem., 30,* 799–804.

Barry J, Dubois MP, Poulain P (1973): LRF-producing cells of the mammalian hypothalamus. *Z. Zellforsch. Mikroskop. Anat., 146,* 351–366.

Beitz AJ (1982): The sites of origin of brain stem neurotensin and serotonin projections to the rodent nucleus raphe magnus. *J. Neurosci., 2,* 829–842.

Bentivoglio M, Kuypers HGJM (1982): Divergent axon collaterals from rat cerebellar nuclei to diencephalon, mesencephalon, medulla oblongata and cervical cord: a fluorescent double retrograde labeling study. *Exp. Brain Res., 46,* 339–356.

Bentivoglio M, Kuypers HGJM, Catsman-Berrevoets C (1980): Retrograde neuronal labeling by means of bisbenzimide and nuclear yellow (Hoechst S 769121): measures to prevent diffusion of the tracers out of retrogradely labeled cells. *Neurosci. Lett., 18,* 19–24.

Bentivoglio M, Kuypers HGJM, Catsman-Berrevoets C, Dann O (1979a): Fluorescent retrograde neuronal labeling in rat by means of substances binding specifically to adenine-thymine rich DNA. *Neurosci. Lett., 12,* 235–240.

Bentivoglio M, Macchi G, Albanese A (1981): The cortical projections of the thalamic intralaminar nuclei, as studied in cat and rat with the multiple fluorescent retrograde tracing technique. *Neurosci. Lett., 26,* 5–10.

Bentivoglio M, Van der Kooy D, Kuypers HGJM (1979b): The organization of the efferent projections of the substantia nigra in the rat: a retrograde fluorescent double labeling study. *Brain Res., 174,* 1–17.

Berger B, Nguyen-Legros J, Thierry AM (1978): Demonstration of horseradish peroxidase and fluorescent catecholamines in the same neurons. *Neurosci. Lett., 9,* 297–302.

Bérod A, Hartman BK, Pujol JF (1981): Importance of fixation in immunohistochemistry: use of for-maldehyde at variable pH for the localization of tyrosine hydroxylase. *J. Histochem. Cytochem., 29,* 844–850.

Bharos TB, Kuypers HGJM, Lemon RN, Muir RB (1981): Divergent collaterals from deep cerebellar neurons to thalamus and tectum, and to medulla oblongata and spinal cord: retrograde fluorescent and electrophysiological studies. *Exp. Brain Res., 42,* 399–410.

Bigl V, Woolf NJ, Butcher LL (1982): Cholinergic projections from the basal forebrain to frontal, parietal, temporal occipital, and cingulate cortices: a combined fluorescent tracer and acetylcholinesterase analysis. *Brain Res. Bull., 8,* 727–749.

Björklund A, Skagerberg G (1979a): Simultaneous use of retrograde fluorescent tracers and fluorescence histochemistry for convenient and precise mapping of monoaminergic projections and collateral ar-rangements in the CNS. *J. Neurosci. Meth., 1,* 261–277.

Björklund A, Skagerberg G (1979b): Evidence for a major spinal cord projection from the diencephalic All dopamine cell group in the rat using transmitter-specific fluorescent retrograde tracing. *Brain Res., 177,* 170–175.

Blessing WW, Furness JB, Costa M, Chalmers JP (1978): Localization of catecholamine fluorescence and retrograde transported horseradish peroxidase within the same nerve cell. *Neurosci. Lett., 9,* 311–315.

Blessing WW, Furness JB, Costa M West MJ, Chalmers JP (1981a): Projection of ventrolateral medullary (A1) catecholamine neurons toward nucleus tractus solitarii. *Cell Tiss. Res., 220,* 27–40.

Blessing WW, Goodchild AK, Dampney RAL, Chalmers JP (1981b): Cell groups in the lower brain stem of the rabbit projecting to the spinal cord, with special reference to the catecholamine-containing neurons. *Brain Res., 221,* 35–55.

Bowker RM, Steinbusch H, Coulter JD (1981a): Serotonin and peptidergic projections to the spinal cord demonstrated by a combined retrograde HRP histochemical and immunocytochemical staining method. *Brain Res., 211,* 412–417.

Bowker RM, Westlund KN, Coulter JD (1981b): Origins of serotonergic projections to the spinal cord in rat: an immunocytochemical-retrograde transport study. *Brain Res., 226,,* 187–199.

Bowker RM, Westlund KN, Coulter JD (1981c): Serotonergic projections to the spinal cord from the mid-brain of the rat: an immunocytochemical and retrograde transport study. *Neurosci. Lett., 24,* 221–226.

Bowker RM, Westlund KN, Coulter JD (1982a): Origins of serotonergic projections in the lumbal spinal cord in the monkey using a combined retrograde transport and immunocytochemical technique. *Brain Res. Bull., 9,* 271–278.

Bowker RM, Westlund KN, Sullivan MC, Coulter JD (1982b): A combined retrograde transport and immunocytochemical staining method for demonstrating the origins of serotonergic projections. *J. Histochem. Cytochem., 30,* 805–810.

Bowker RM, Westlund KN, Sullivan MC, Wilber JF, Coulter JD (1982c): Transmitters of the raphe-spinal complex: immunocytochemical studies. *Peptides, 3,* 291–298.

Brann MR, Emson PC (1980): Microiontophoretic injection of fluorescent tracer combined with simultaneous immunofluorescent histochemistry for the demonstration of efferents from the caudate-putamen projecting to the globus pallidus. *Neurosci. Lett., 16,* 61–65.

Brightman MW, Klatzo I, Olsson Y, Reese TS (1970): The blood brain barrier to proteins under normal and pathological conditions. *J. Neurol. Sci., 10,* 215–239.

Butcher LL, Eastgate SM, Hodge GK (1974): Evidence that punctate intracerebral administration of 6-hydroxydopamine fails to produce selective neuronal degeneration: comparison with copper sulfate and factors governing the deportment of fluids injected into brain. *Naunyn-Schmiedeberg's Arch. Pharmacol., 285,* 31–70.

Butcher LL, Talbot K, Bilezikjian L (1975): Acetylcholinesterase neurons in dopamine-containing regions of the brain. *J. Neural Transm., 37,* 127–153.

Chan-Palay V (1979): Immunocytochemical detection of substance P neurons, their processes and connections by in vivo injections of monoclonal antibodies: light- and electronmicroscopy. *Anat. Embryol., 156,* 225–240.

Chan-Palay V, Palay SL, Wu JY (1979): Gamma-aminobutyric acid pathways in the cerebellum studied by retrograde and anterograde transport of glutamic acid decarboxylase antibody after in vivo injections. *Anat. Embryol., 157,* 1–14.

Chiba T, Hwang BH, Williams TH (1976): A method for studying glyoxylic acid induced fluorescence and ultrastructure of monoamine neurons. *Histochemistry, 49,* 95–106.

Chu-Wang IW, Oppenheim RW (1980): Uptake, intra-axonal transport and rate of horseradish peroxidase in embryonic spinal neurons of the chick. *J. Comp. Neurol., 193,* 753–776.

Coons AH, Creech HJ, Jones RN, Berliner E (1942): The demonstration of pneumococcal antigen in tissues by the use of fluorescent antibody. *J. Immunol., 45,* 455–462.

Cowan WM, Cuenod M (Eds) (1975): *The Use of Axonal Transport for Studies of Neuronal Connectivity.* Elsevier, Amsterdam.

Cuello AC, Priestley JV, Milstein C (1982): Immunocytochemistry with internally labeled monoclonal antibodies. *Proc. Nat. Acad. Sci. USA, 79,* 665–669.

Dahlström A (1968): Effect of colchicine on transport of amine storage granules in sympathetic nerves of rat. *Eur. J. Pharmacol., 5,* 111–113.

Dahlström A (1971): Effects of vinblastine and colchicine on monoamine containing neurons of the rat with special regard to the axoplasmic transport of amine granules. *Acta Neuropathol. Berlin, 5,* 226–237.

Dalsgaard C-J, Hökfelt T, Elfvin L-G, Skirboll L, Emson P (1982a): Substance P-containing primary sensory neurons projecting to the inferior mesenteric ganglion: evidence from combined retrograde tracing and immunohistochemistry. *Neuroscience, 7,* 647–654.

Dalsgaard C-J, Hökfelt T, Elfvin L-G, Terenius L (1982b): Enkephalin-containing sympathetic preganglionic neurons projecting to the inferior mesenteric ganglion: evidence from combined retrograde tracing and immunohistochemistry. *Neuroscience, 7,* 2039–2050.

Dann O, Bergen G, Demant E, Volz G (1971): Trypanocide Diamidine des 2-Phenyl-benzofurans, 2-Phenyl-indens und 2-Phenyl-indols. *Liebigs Ann. Chem., 749,* 68–99.

Dann O, Fick H, Pietzner B, Walkenhorst E, Fernbach R, Zeh D (1975): Trypanocide Diamidine mit drei isolierten Ringsystemen. *Liebigs Ann. Chem.,* 160–194.

Dann O, Hieke E, Hahn H, Miserre HH, Lurding G, Roszler R (1970): Trypanocide Diamidine des 2-Phenyl-thionaphtens. *Liebigs Ann. Chem., 734,* 23–34.

Dann O, Volz G, Demant E, Pfeifer W, Bergen G, Fick N, Welanhorst E (1973): Trypanocide Diamidine mit vier Ringen in einem oder zwei Ringsystemen. *Liebigs Ann. Chem.,* 1112–1140.

Day TA, Blessing W, Willoughby JO (1980): Noradrenergic and dopaminergic projections to the medial preoptic area of the rat. A combined horseradish peroxidase/catecholamine fluorescence study. *Brain Res., 193,* 543–548.

Deuschl G, Illert M, Aschoff A, Holländer H (1981): Single preganglionic sympathetic neurons of the cat branch intraspinally and project through different rami communicantes albi. A retrograde double label-ing study with fluorescent tracers. *Neurosci. Lett., 21,* 1–5.

De Olmos JS (1977): An improved HRP method for the study of central nervous connections. *Exp. Brain Res., 29,* 541–551.

Edelson PJ, Cohn ZA (1978): Endocytosis: regulation of membrane interactions. In: Poste G, Nicholson GL (Eds), *Membrane Fusion, Cell Surface Reviews, Vol. 5,* pp. 387–405. North Holland, Amsterdam.

Eisenman JS, Azmitia EC (1982): Physiological stimulation enhances HRP marking of salivary neurons in rats. *Brain Res. Bull., 8,* 73–78.

Enerbäck L, Kristensson K, Olsson T (1980): Cytophotometric qualification of retrograde axonal transport of a fluorescent tracer (primuline) in mouse facial neurons. *Brain Res., 186,* 21–32.

Fillenz M, Gagnon C, Stoeckel K, Thoenen H (1976): Selective uptake and retrograde axonal transport of dopamine-β-hydroxylase antibodies in peripheral adrenergic neurons. *Brain Res., 14,* 293–303.

Frank E, Harris WA, Kennedy MB (1980): Lysophosphatidyl choline facilitates labeling of CNS projections with horseradish peroxidase. *J. Neurosci. Meth., 2,* 183–189.

Fryer J, Maler L (1982): Enhanced uptake of HRP by hypophysiotropic neurons following stress and adrenalectomy. *Brain Res., 242,* 179–183.

Furness JB, Heath JW, Costa M (1978): Aqueous aldehyde (Faglu) methods for the fluorescence histochemical localization of catecholamines and for ultrastructural studies of central nervous tissue. *Histochem., 57,* 285–295.

Fuxe K, Goldstein M, Hökfelt T, Joh TH (1970): Immunohistochemical localization of dopamine-β-hydroxylase in the peripheral and central nervous system. *Res. Commun. Chem. Pathol. Pharmacol., 1,* 627–636.

Fuxe K, Goldstein M, Hökfelt T, Joh TH (1971): Cellular localization of dopamine-β-hydroxylase and phenylethanolamine-N-methyl transferase as revealed by immunohistochemistry. *Prog. Brain Res., 34,* 127–138.

Geffen LB, Livett DG, Rush RA (1969): Immunohistochemical localization of protein components of catecholamine storage vesicles. *J. Physiol. (London), 204,* 593–605.

Goldstein M, Fuxe K, Hökfelt T (1972): Characterization and tissue localization of catecholamine synthesiz-ing enzymes. *Pharmacol. Rev., 24,* 293–309.

Gonatas NK (1982): The role of the neuronal Golgi apparatus in a centripetal membrane vesicular traffic. *J. Neuropathol. Exp. Neurol., 41,* 6–17.

Grafstein B, Forsman DS (1980): Intracellular transport in neurons. *Physiol. Rev., 60,* 1168–1283.

Graham RC, Karnovsky MJ (1966): The early stage of absorption of injected horseradish peroxidase in the proximal tubules of mouse kidney: ultrastructural cytochemistry by a new technique. *J. Histochem. Cytochem., 14,* 291–302.

Guyenet PG, Crane JK (1981): Non-dopaminergic nigrostriatal pathway. *Brain Res., 213,* 291–305.

Hadley RT, Trachtenberg MC (1978): Poly-L-ornithine enhances the uptake of horseradish peroxidase. *Brain Res., 158,* 1–14.

Hardy H, Heimer L, Switzer R, Watkins D (1976): Simultaneous demonstration of horseradish peroxidase and acetylcholinesterase. *Neurosci. Lett., 3,* 1–5.

Hartman BK (1973): Immunofluorescence of dopamine-β-hydroxylase: application of improved methodolo-gy to the localization of the peripheral and central noradrenergic nervous system. *J. Histochem. Cytochem., 21,* 312–332.

Hartman BK, Udenfriend S (1970): Immunofluorescent localization of dopamine-β-hydroxylase in tissues. *Mol. Pharmacol., 6,* 85–94.

Hartman BK, Zide D, Udenfriend S (1972): The use of dopamine-β-hydroxylase as a marker for the noradrenergic pathway of the central nervous system in rat. *Proc. Nat. Acad. Sci. USA, 69,* 2722–2726.

Helke CI, Goldman W, Jacobowitz D (1981): Demonstration of substance P in aortic nerve afferent fibers by combined use of fluorescent retrograde neuronal labelling and immunocytochemistry. *Peptides, 1,* 359–364.

Herkenham M, Nauta WJH (1977): Afferent connections of the habenular nuclei in the rat: a horseradish peroxidase study, with a note on the fiber-of-passage problem. *J. Comp. Neurol., 173,* 123–146.

Hilwig J, Gropp A (1975): pH-dependent fluorescence of DNA and RNA in cytological staining with 33258 Hoechst. *Exp. Cell Res., 91,* 457–460.

Hökfelt T, Dahlström A (1971): Effects of two mitotic inhibitors (colchicine and vinblastine) on the distribution and axonal transport of noradrenaline storage particles, studied by fluorescence- and electron-microscopy. *Z. Zellforsch. Mikroskop. 119,* 460–482.

Hökfelt T, Elde R, Johansson O, Ljungdahl A, Schultzberg M, Fuxe K, Goldstein M, Nilsson G, Pernow B, Terenius L, Ganten D, Jeffcoate SL, Rehfeld J, Said S (1978): Distribution of peptide-containing neurons. In: Lipton MA, DiMascio A, Killam KF (Eds), *Psychopharmacology: A Generation of Progress,* pp. 39–66. Raven, New York.

Hökfelt T, Fuxe K, Goldstein M (1975a): Applications of immunohistochemistry to studies on monoamine cell systems with special references to nervous tissues. *Ann. N.Y. Acad. Sci., 254,* 407–432.

Hökfelt T, Fuxe K, Goldstein M, Joh TH (1973): Immunohistochemical localization of three catecholamine synthesizing enzymes: aspects on methodology. *Histochemie, 33,* 231–254.

Hökfelt T, Johansson O, Ljungdahl A, Lundberg J, Schultzberg M (1980a): Peptidergic neurons. *Nature (London), 284,* 515–521.

Hökfelt T, Kellerth JO, Nilsson G, Pernow B (1975b): Experimental immunohistochemical studies on the localization and distribution of substance P in cat primary sensory neurons. *Brain Res., 100,* 235–252.

Hökfelt T, Ljungdahl Å (1972): Modification of the Falck-Hillarp formaldehyde fluorescence method using the Vibratome: simple, rapid and sensitive localization of catecholamines in sections of unfixed or formalin fixed brain tissue. *Histochemie, 29,* 325–339.

Hökfelt T, Ljungdahl Å (1975): Uptake mechanisms as a basis for the histochemical identification and tracing of transmitter-specific neuron populations. In: Cowan WM, Cuenod M (Eds), *The Use of Axonal Transport for Studies of Neuronal Connectivity,* pp. 249–286. Elsevier, Amsterdam.

Hökfelt T, Ljungdahl Å, Terenius L, Elde RP, Nilsson G (1977): Immunohistochemical analysis of peptide pathways possibly related to pain and analgesia: Enkephalin and substance P. *Proc. Nat. Acad. Sci. USA, 74,* 3081–3085.

Hökfelt T, Lundberg JM, Schultzberg M, Johansson O, Ljungdahl Å, Rehfeld J (1980b): Coexistence of peptides and putative transmitters in neurons. In: Costa E, Trabucchi M (Eds), *Neural Peptides and Neuronal Communication,* pp. 1–23. Raven Press, New York.

Hökfelt T, Lundberg JM, Skirboll L, Johansson O, Schultzberg M, Vincent SR (1982): Coexistence of classical transmitters and peptides in neurones. In: Cuello EC (Ed.) *Co-transmission,* pp. 77–125. MacMillan, London and Basingstoke.

Hökfelt T, Phillipson O, Goldstein M (1979a): Evidence for a dopaminergic pathway in the rat descending from the All cell group to the spinal cord. *Acta Physiol. Scand., 107,* 393–395.

Hökfelt T, Skirboll L, Rehfeld JF, Goldstein M, Markey K, Dann O (1980c): A subpopulation of mesencephalic dopamine neurons projecting to limbic areas contains a cholecystokinin-like peptide: evidence from immunohistochemistry combined with retrograde tracing. *Neuroscience, 5,* 2093–2124.

Hökfelt T, Terenius L, Kuypers HGJM, Dann O (1979b): Evidence for enkephalin immunoreactive neurons in the medulla oblongata projecting to the spinal cord. *Neurosci. Lett., 14,* 55–60.

Hudson B, Upholt WB, Devinny J, Vinograd J (1968): The use of ethidium analogue in the dye-buoyant density procedure for the isolation of closed circular DNA: the variation of the superhelix density of mitochondrial DNA. *Proc. Nat. Acad. Sci. (USA), 62,* 813–820.

Huisman AM, Kuypers HGJM, Verburgh CA (1981): Quantitative differences in collateralization of the descending spinal pathways from red nucleus and other brain stem cell groups in rat as demonstrated with the multiple fluorescent retrograde tracer technique. *Brain Res., 209,* 271–286.

Hunt SP, Künzle H (1976): Selective uptake and transport of label within three identified neuronal systems after injection of (^{3}H)-GABA into the pigeon optic tectum: an autoradiographic and Golgi study. *J. Comp. Neurol., 170,* 173–190.

Hunt SP, Streit P, Künzle H, Cuenod M (1977): Characterization of the pigeon isthmo-tectal pathway by selective uptake and retrograde movement of radioactive compounds and by Golgi-like horseradish peroxidase labelling. *Brain Res., 129,* 197–212.

Illert M, Fritz A, Aschoff A, Holländer H (1982): Fluorescent compounds as retrograde tracers compared with horseradish peroxidase (HRP). II. A parametric study in the peripheral motor system of the cat. *J. Neurosci. Meth., 6,* 199–218.

Innocenti GM (1981): Growth and reshaping of axons in the establishment of visual callosal connections. *Science, 212,* 824–826.

Iversen LL (1967): *The Uptake and Storage of Noradrenaline in Sympathetic Nerves.* Cambridge University Press, Cambridge.

Jacobowitz DM, Ziegler MG, Thomas JA (1975): In vivo uptake of antibody to dopamine-β-hydroxylase into sympathetic elements. *Brain Res., 91*, 165–170.

Johansson O (1978): Localization of somatostatin-like immunoreactivity in the Golgi apparatus of central and peripheral neurons. *Histochemistry, 58*, 167–176.

Johansson O (1983): Localization of vasoactive intestinal polypeptide- and avian pancreatic polypeptide-like immunoreactivity in the Golgi apparatus of peripheral neurons. *Brain Res., 262*, 71–78.

Jones EG, Hartman BK (1978): Recent advances in neuroanatomical methodology. *Ann. Rev. Neurosci., 1*, 215–296.

Karnovsky MJ, Roots L (1964): A direct coloring thiocholine method for cholinesterases. *J. Histochem. Cytochem., 12*, 219–221.

Keefer DA (1978): Horseradish peroxidase as a retrogradely-transported detailed dendritic marker. *Brain Res., 140*, 15–32.

Köhler C, Chan-Palay V, Steinbusch H (1982): The distribution and origin of serotonin-containing fibers in the septal area: a combined immunohistochemical and fluorescent retrograde tracing study in the rat. *J. Comp. Neurol., 209*, 91–111.

Kreutzberg G (1969): Neuronal dynamics and flow. IV. Blockage of intra-axonal enzyme transport by colchicine. *Proc. Nat. Acad. Sci. USA, 62*, 722–728.

Kristensson K (1970): Transport of fluorescent protein tracer in peripheral nerves. *Acta Neuropath. (Berlin), 16*, 293–300.

Kristensson K (1978): Retrograde transport of macromolecules in axons. *Ann. Rev. Pharmacol. Toxicol., 18*, 97–110.

Kristensson K, Olsson Y (1971): Retrograde axonal transport of protein. *Brain Res., 29*, 363–365.

Kristensson K, Olsson Y (1976): Retrograde transport of horseradish peroxidase in transected axons. III. Entry into injured axons and subsequent localization in perikaryon. *Brain Res., 115*, 201–213.

Kristensson K, Olsson Y, Sjöstrand J (1971): Axonal uptake and retrograde transport of exogenous protein in the hypoglossal nerve. *Brain Res., 32*, 399–406.

Kuypers HGJM (1981): Procedure for retrograde double labeling with fluorescent substances. In: Heimer L, Robards MY (Eds), *Neuroanatomical Tract Tracing Methods*, pp. 299–303. Plenum Press, New York.

Kuypers HGJM, Huisman AM (1983): Fluorescent retrograde tracers. *Adv. Neurobiol.*, in press.

Kuypers HGJM, Bentivoglio M, Van der Kooy D, Catsman-Berrevoets CE (1977): Retrograde transport of bisbenzimide and propidium iodide through axons to their parent cell bodies. *Neurosci. Lett., 12*, 1–7.

Kuypers HGJM, Bentivoglio M, Van der Kooy D, Catsman-Berrevoets CE (1979): Retrograde axonal transport of fluorescent substances in the rat's forebrain. *Neurosci. Lett., 6*, 127–135.

Kuypers HGJM, Bentivoglio M, Catsman-Berrevoets CE, Bharos AT (1980): Double retrograde neuronal labeling through divergent axon collaterals, using two fluorescent tracers with the same excitation wavelength which label different features of the cell. *Exp. Brain Res., 40*, 383–392.

Lasek R, Joseph BS, Whitlock DG (1968): Evaluation of a radioautographic neuroanatomical tracing method. *Brain Res., 8*, 319–336.

Latt SA, Stetten G (1976): Spectral studies on 33258 Hoechst and related bisbenzamidazole dyes useful for fluorescence detection of deoxyribonucleic acid synthesis. *J. Histochem. Cytochem., 24*, 24–33.

LaVail JH, LaVail MM (1972): Retrograde axonal transport in the central nervous system. *Science, 176*, 1416–1417.

LaVail JH, LaVail MM (1974): The retrograde intraaxonal transport of horseradish peroxidase in the chick visual system: A light- and electronmicroscopic study. *J. Comp. Neurol., 157*, 303–358.

LaVail JH (1975): The retrograde transport method. *Fed. Proc., 34*, 1618–1624.

Lechan DM, Nestler J, Jacobson SJ (1981): Immunohistochemical localization of retrogradely and anterogradely transported wheat germ agglutinin (WGA) within the central nervous system of the rat: application to immunostaining of a second antigen within the same neuron. *J. Histochem. Cytochem., 29*, 255–262.

Leger L, Pujol JF, Bobillier P, Jouvet M (1977): Transport axoplasmique de la sérotonine par voie retrograde dans les neurons monoaminergiques centraux. *C.R. Acad. Sci. (Paris), 285*, 1179–1182.

Lindvall O, Björklund A (1974): The glyoxylic acid fluorescence method for central catecholamine neurons: a detailed account on the methodology. *Histochemie, 39*, 97–127.

Lindvall O, Björklund A, Hökfelt T, Ljungdahl Å (1973): Application of the glyoxylic acid method to vibratome sections for the improved visualization of central catecholamine neurons. *Histochemie, 35*, 31–38.

Lipp H-P, Schwegler H (1980): Improved transport of horseradish peroxidase after injection with a nonionic detergent (nonidet P-40) into mouse cortex and observations on the relationship between spread at the injection site and amount of transported label. *Neurosci. Lett., 20*, 49–54.

Livett BG (1978): Immunohistochemical localization of nervous system-specific proteins and peptides. *Int. Rev. Cytol., Suppl., 7,* 53–237.

Ljungdahl A, Hökfelt T, Goldstein M, Park D (1975): Retrograde peroxidase tracing of neurons combined with transmitter histochemistry. *Brain Res.,* 313–319.

Loewy AD (1981): Raphe pallidus and raphe obscurus projections to the intermediolateral cell column in the rat. *Brain Res., 222,* 129–133.

Loewy AD, McKellar S (1981): Serotonergic projections from the ventral medulla to the intermediolateral cell column in the rat. *Brain Res., 211,* 146–152.

Loewy H, Urbanietz J (1974): Basisch substituierte 2,6-Bisbenzamidazolderviate eine neue chemotherapeutisch aktive Körperklasse. *Arzneim. Forsch., 24,* 1927–1933.

Lorén I, Björklund A, Falck B, Lindvall O (1976): An improved histofluorescence procedure for freeze-dried paraffin-embedded tissue based on combined formaldehyde-glyoxylic acid perfusion with high magnesium content and acid pH. *Histochemie, 49,* 177–192.

Lorén I, Björklund A, Falck B, Lindvall O (1980): The aluminium-formaldehyde (ALFA) histofluorescence method for improved visualization of catecholamines and indoleamines. I. A detailed account of the methodology for central nervous tissue using paraffin, cryostat or Vibratome sections. *J. Neurosci. Meth., 2,* 277–300.

Lundberg JM (1981): Evidence for coexistence of vasoactive intestinal polypeptide (VIP) and acetylcholine in neurons of cat exocrine glands. *Acta Physiol. Scand., 112,* 1–57.

Markey KA, Kondo S, Shenkman L, Goldstein M (1980): Purification and characterization of tyrosine hydroxylase from a clonal pheochromocytoma cell line. *Mol. Pharmacol., 17,* 79–85.

McEwen BS, Davis PG, Parsons B, Pfaff DW (1979): The brain as a target for steroid hormone action. *Ann. Rev. Neurosci., 2,* 65–112.

Mesulam M-M (1976): A horseradish peroxidase method for the identification of the efferents of acetyl cholinesterase-containing neurons. *J. Histochem. Cytochem., 12,* 1281–1286.

Mesulam M-M (1978): Tetramethyl benzidine for horseradish peroxidase neurohistochemistry: a non-carcinogenic blue reaction-product with superior sensitivity for visualizing neural afferents and efferents. *Histochem. Cytochem., 26,* 106–117.

Mesulam M-M (Ed.) (1982): Tracing Neural Connections with Horseradish Peroxidase. In: Smith AD (Gen Ed), *IBRO Handbook Series: Methods in the Neurosciences.* John Wiley and Sons, London.

Morrell JI, Pfaff DW (1982): Characterization of estrogen-concentrating hypothalamic neurons by their axonal projections. *Science, 217,* 1273–1275.

Nagai T, Satoh K, Imamoto K, Maeda T (1981): Divergent projections of catecholamine neurons of the locus coeruleus as revealed by fluorescent retrograde double labeling technique. *Neurosci. Lett., 23,* 117–123.

Nairn RC (1969): *Fluorescent Protein Tracing.* Livingstone, Edinburgh.

Nakane PK (1968): Simultaneous localization of multiple tissue antigens using the peroxidase labeled antibody method: a study on pituitary glands of the rat. *J. Histochem. Cytochem., 16,* 557–560.

Nakane PK, Pierce GB (1967): Enzyme-labeled antibodies for the light- and electronmicroscopic localization of tissue antigens. *J. Cell. Biol., 33,* 307–318.

Neuhuber W, Groh V, Gottshall I, Celio MR (1981): The cornea is not innervated by substance P-containing primary afferents neurons. *Neurosci. Lett., 22,* 5–9.

Parker CA (1968): *Photoluminescence of Solutions.* Elsevier, Amsterdam.

Pastan IH, Willingham MC (1981): Receptor-mediated endocytosis of hormones in cultured cells. *Ann. Rev. Physiol., 43,* 239–250.

Pearse AGE, Polak JM (1975): Bifunctional reagents as vapour- and liquid-phase fixatives for immunohistochemistry. *Histochem. J., 7,* 179–186.

Pease DC (1962): Buffered formaldehyde as a killing agent and primary fixative for electronmicroscopy. *Anat. Rec., 142,* 342.

Pfaff DW (1976): The neuroanatomy of sex hormone receptors in the vertebrate brain. In: Kumar TCA (Ed.), *Neuroendocrine Regulation of Fertility,* pp. 30–45. Karger, Basel.

Priestley JV, Somogyi P, Cuello C (1981): Neurotransmitter specific projection neurons revealed by combined immunohistochemistry with retrograde transport of HRP. *Brain Res., 220,* 231–240.

Ritchie TC, Westlund KN, Bowker RM, Coultier JD, Leonard RB (1982): The relationship of the medullary catecholamine containing neurones to the vagal motor nuclei. *Neuroscience, 7,* 1471–1482.

Ross CA, Armstrong DM, Ruggiero DA, Pickel VM, Joh TH, Reis DJ (1981): Adrenaline neurons in the rostral ventrolateral medulla innervate thoracic spinal cord: A combined immunocytochemical and retrograde transport demonstration. *Neurosci. Lett., 25,* 257–262.

Sar M, Stumpf WE, Miller RJ, Chang KJ, Cuatrecasas P (1978): Immunohistochemical localization of enkephalin in rat brain and spinal cord. *J. Comp. Neurol., 182,* 17–38.

Satoh K, Tohyama M, Yamamoto K, Sakumoto T (1977): Noradrenaline innervation of the spinal cord studied by horseradish peroxidase method combined with monoamine oxidase staining. *Exp. Brain Res., 30,* 175–186.

Sawchenko PE, Swanson LW (1981): A method for tracing biochemically defined pathways in the central nervous system using combined fluorescence retrograde transport and immunohistochemical techniques. *Brain Res., 210,* 31–41.

Sawchenko PE, Swanson LW (1982): Immunohistochemical identification of neurons in the paraventricular nucleus of the hypothalamus that project to the medulla or to the spinal cord in the rat. *J. Comp. Neurol., 205,* 260–272.

Sawchenko PE, Swanson LW, Joseph SA (1982): The distribution and cells of origin of ACTH (1-39)-stained varicosities in the paraventricular and supraoptic nuclei. *Brain Res., 232,* 365–374.

Schmued LG, Swanson LW (1982): SITS: a covalently bound fluorescent retrograde tracer that does not appear to be taken up by fibers-of-passage. *Brain Res., 249,* 137–141.

Schwab ME, Javoy-Agid F, Agid Y (1978): Labeled wheat germ agglutinin (WGA) as a new, highly sensitive retrograde tracer in the rat brain system. *J. Histochem. Cytochem., 152,* 145.

Sellinger OZ, Petiet PD (1973): Horseradish peroxidase uptake in vivo by neuronal and glial lysosomes. *Exp. Neurol., 38,* 370–385.

Silver MA, Jacobowitz DM (1979): Specific uptake and retrograde flow of antibody to dopamine-β-hydroxylase by central nervous system noradrenergic neurons in vivo. *Brain Res., 167,* 65–75.

Silverstein SC, Steinman RM, Cohn ZA (1977): Endocytosis. *Ann. Rev. Biochem., 46,* 669–722.

Skagerberg G, Björklund A (1983): Neurotransmitter specific retrograde tracing based on fluorescent tracers and aldehyde induced monoamine histofluorescence: a methodological review, in preparation.

Skirboll L, Hökfelt T (1983): Transmitter specific mapping of neuronal pathways by immunohistochemistry combined with fluorescent dyes. In: Cuello AC (Ed.), *IBRO Handbook Series: Methods in the Neurosciences. Immunohistochemistry*, John Wiley and Sons, Chichester. In press.

Skirboll L, Hökfelt T, Norell G, Kuypers HGJM, Bentivoglio M, Catsman-Berrevoets C, Goldtein M, Steinbusch H, Verhofstad A, Phillipson O, Brownstein M (1983): A method for specific transmitter identification of retrogradely labeled neurons: immunofluorescence combined with fluorescence tracing. To be submitted.

Smolen AJ, Glazer EJ, Ross LL (1979): Horseradish peroxidase histochemistry combined with glyoxylic acid-induced fluorescence used to identify brain stem catecholaminergic neurons which project to the chick thoracic spinal cord. *Brain Res., 160,* 353–357.

Sofroniew MV, Schrell U (1981): Evidence for a direct projection from oxytocin and vasopressin neurons in the hypothalamic paraventricular nucleus to the medulla oblongata: immunohistochemical visualization of both the horseradish peroxidase transported and the peptide produced by the same neurons. *Neurosci. Lett., 22,* 211–217.

Stanfield BB, O'Leary DM, Fricks C (1982): Selective collateral elimination in early postnatal development restricts cortical distribution of rat pyramidal tract neurons. *Nature (London), 298,* 371–373.

Steinbusch HWM, Nieuwenhuys R, Verhofstad AAJ, Van der Kooy D (1981): The nucleus raphe dorsalis of the rat and its projection upon the caudate-putamen: a combined cytoarchitectonic and immunohistochemical and retrograde transport study. *J. Physiol. (Paris), 77,* 157–174.

Steinbusch HWM, Van der Kooy D, Verhofstad AA, Pellegrino A (1980): Serotonergic and non-serotonergic projections from the nucleus raphe dorsalis to the caudate-putamen complex in the rat, studied by a combined immunofluorescence and fluorescence retrograde axonal labeling technique. *Neurosci. Lett., 19,* 137–142.

Stevens RT, Hodge CJ Jr, Apkavian AV (1982): Kölliker-Fuse nucleus: the principal source of pontine catecholaminergic cells projecting to the lumbar spinal cord of cat. *Brain Res., 239,* 589–594.

Steward O (1981): Horseradish peroxidase and fluorescent substances and their combination with other techniques. In: Heimer L, Robards MJ (Eds) *Neuroanatomical Tract-Tracing Methods*, pp. 279–310. Plenum Press, New York.

Steward O, Scoville SA (1976): Retrograde labeling of central nervous pathways with tritiated or Evans blue-labeled bovine serum albumin. *Neurosci. Lett., 3,* 191–196.

Sternberger LA (1979): *Immunocytochemistry*, 2nd ed. John Wiley and Sons, New York.

Sternberger LA, Hardy PH Jr, Cuculis JJ, Meyer HG (1970): The unlabeled antibody enzyme method of immunohistochemistry: preparation and properties of soluble antigen-antibody complex (horseradish peroxidase-antihorseradish peroxidase) and its use in identification of spirochetes. *J. Histochem. Cytochem., 18,* 315–333.

Streit P (1980): Selective retrograde labeling indicating the transmitter of neuronal pathways. *J. Comp. Neurol., 191,* 429–463.

Stumpf WE, Grant LD (Eds.) (1975): *Anatomical Neuroendocrinology.* Karger, Basel.

Swanson LW, Kuypers HGJM (1980): The paraventricular nucleus of the hypothalamus: Cytoarchitectonic subdivions and the organization of projections to the pituitary, dorsal vagal complex and spinal cord as demonstrated by retrograde fluorescence double labeling methods. *J. Comp. Neurol., 194,* 555–570.

Teichberg S, Holtzman E, Crain SM, Peterson ER (1975): Circulation and turnover of synaptic vesicle membrane in cultured fetal mammalian spinal cord neurons. *J. Cell. Biol., 67,* 215–230.

Törk I, Turner S (1981): Histochemical evidence for a catecholaminergic (presumably dopaminergic) projection from the ventral mesencephalic tegmentum to visual cortex in the cat. *Neurosci. Lett., 24,* 215–219.

Tramu G, Pillez A, Leonardelli J (1978): An efficient method of antibody elution for the successive or simultaneous localization of two antigens by immunocytochemistry. *J. Histochem. Cytochem., 26,* 322–324.

Van der Kooy D (1979): The organization of the thalamic, nigral and raphe afferents to the medial versus lateral caudate-putamen in rat. A fluorescent retrograde double labeling study. *Brain Res., 169,* 381–387.

Van der Kooy D, Coscina DV, Hattori T (1981): Is there a non-dopaminergic nigrostriatal pathway? *Neuroscience, 6,* 345–357.

Van der Kooy D, Hattori T (1980): Dorsal raphe cells with collateral projections to the substantia nigra and caudate-putamen. A fluorescent retrograde double labeling study in rat. *Brain Res., 186,* 1.

Van der Kooy D, Hunt SP, Steinbusch HM, Verhofstad A (1981): Separate populations of cholecystokinin and 5-hydroxytryptamine containing neuronal cells in the rat dorsal raphe, and their contribution to the ascending raphe projections. *Neuroscience, 26,* 25–30.

Van der Kooy D, Kuypers HGJM (1979): Fluorescent retrograde double labeling: axonal branching in the ascending raphe and nigral projections. *Science, 204,* 873–875.

Van der Kooy D, Kuypers HGJM, Catman-Berrevoets CE (1978): Single mammillary body cells with divergent axon collaterals: demonstration by a simple, fluorescent retrograde double labeling technique in the rat. *Brain Res., 158,* 189–196.

Van der Kooy D, Sawchenko PE (1982): Characterization of serotonergic neurons using concurrent fluorescent retrograde axonal tracing and immunohistochemistry. *J. Histochem. Cytochem., 30,* 794–798.

Van der Kooy D, Steinbusch HWM (1980): Simultaneous fluorescent retrograde axonal tracing and immunofluorescent characterization of neurons. *J. Neurosci. Res., 5,* 479–584.

Van der Kooy D, Wise RA (1980): Retrograde fluorescent tracing of substantia nigra neurons combined with catecholamine histofluorescence. *Brain Res., 183,* 447–452.

Vandesande F, Dierickx K (1975): Identification of the vasopressin producing and of oxytocin producing neurons of the hypothalamic magnocellular neurosecretory system of the rat. *Cell Tiss. Res., 164,* 153–162.

Warr WB (1975): Olivocochlear and vestibular efferent neurons of the feline brain stem: their location, morphology and number determined by retrograde axonal transport and acetylcholinesterase histochemistry. *J. Comp. Neurol., 161,* 159.

Weisblum B, Haenssler E (1974): Fluorometric properties of the bisbenzimidazole derivative Hoechst 33258, a fluorescent probe specific for AT concentration in chromosomal DNA. *Chromosoma (Berlin), 46,* 255–260.

Weller TH, Coons AH (1954): Fluorescent antibody studies with agents of varicella and herpes zoster propagated in vitro. *Proc. Soc. Exp. Biol. (N.Y.), 86,* 789–794.

Westlund KN, Bowker RM, Ziegler MG, Coulter JD (1981): Origins of spinal noradrenergic pathways demonstrated by retrograde transport of antibody to dopamine-β-hydroxylase. *Neurosci. Lett., 25,* 243–249.

Wiklund L, Toggenburger G, Cuenod M (1982): Aspartate: possible neurotransmitter in cerebellar climbing fibers. *Science, 216,* 78–80.

Woolf NJ, Butcher LL (1982): Cholinergic projections to the basolateral amygdala: a combined Evans Blue and acetylcholinesterase analysis. *Brain Res. Bull., 8,* 751–763.

Yaksh TL, Rudy TA (1976): Analgesia mediated by a direct spinal action of narcotics. *Science, 192,* 1357–1358.

Yezierski RP, Bowker RM (1981): A retrograde double label tracing technique using horseradish peroxidase and the fluorescent dye 4',6-diamidino-2-phenylindole 2HCl (DAPI). *Neurosci. Meth., 4,* 53–62.

Yezierski RP, Bowker RM, Kevetter GA, Westlund KN, Coulter JD, Willis WD (1982): Serotoninergic projections to the caudal brain stem: a double label study using horseradish peroxidase and serotonin immunocytochemistry. *Brain Res., 239,* 258–264.

Zacks SI, Saito A (1968): Uptake of exogenous peroxidase by coated vesicles in mouse neuromuscular junctions. *J. Histochem. Cytochem., 17,* 161–170.

Ziegler MG, Thomas JA, Jacobowitz DM (1976): Retrograde axonal transport of antibody to dopamine-β-hydroxylase in the spinal cord. *Brain Res., 104,* 390–395.

CHAPTER VII

The use of radioautography for investigating transmitter-specific neurons

LAURENT DESCARRIES and ALAIN BEAUDET

> '...Radioautography stands at the cross-
> roads of Biochemistry and Morphology.'
> C.P. Leblond (1965)

1. INTRODUCTION

Not so very long ago, the physicochemical and electrophysiological analysis of neural tissues and their properties and, notably, the study of neurotransmission progressed without obvious concern for the increasingly apparent complexity of neuronal networks: the coherence of the results ensured their validity and absolved the scientist from striving for precise localization. Conversely, the neuroanatomist relied on a purely structural examination of the distribution, configuration and connectivity of nerve cells to seek understanding of their functional organization. With the development of electron-microscopy, the accrued precision and completeness of morphological descriptions even led to the belief that elucidation of neural function might emerge from considering neuronal circuitry merely in terms of excitation and inhibition.

In contrast, nowadays, one can hardly investigate any aspect of higher neuronal systems without equal consideration for both their chemical and structural heterogeneity. The number of substances more or less directly implicated in neuronal communication does not cease to grow, raising fundamental problems on the significance of this diversity. Biochemical mapping goes beyond the stage of a geographic exploration, asking questions of its own and providing clues on the respective role of so many chemical messengers.

The beginning of this new era can be dated to the advent of the histofluorescence technique, which not only allowed identification of three separate populations of biogenic amine-containing neurons in mammalian central nervous system (CNS), but, by permitting visualization of transmitter content, showed a new way to bridge the gap between neuronal structure and biochemical, pharmacological and electrophysiological properties. Another consequence of this breakthrough was to emphasize the necessity of similar approaches applicable at the electron-microscopic level. These were especially wanting in the CNS, where, at variance with the situation prevailing in some invertebrates or in the peripheral nervous system (PNS), no anatomical region comprises nerve cell bodies or axon terminals exclusive to a given transmitter type.

Three methodologies have thus far been proposed to satisfy this need: cytochemistry, radioautography and immunocytochemistry. The present chapter deals with the radioautographic method pertaining to the investigation of transmitter-specific neurons. It does not delve into the technical aspects of radioautography as such, except when they differ from those in its other domains of biological application. For reasons fully explained below, only neurons capable of transmitter uptake are amenable to radioautographic identification, i.e. those utilizing the catecholamines (CA), dopamine

Handbook of Chemical Neuroanatomy. Vol. 1: Methods in Chemical Neuroanatomy.
A. Björklund and T. Hökfelt, editors.
© Elsevier Science Publishers B.V., 1983.

(DA), noradrenaline (NA) and adrenaline (A), the indolamine 5-hydroxytryptamine (serotonin: 5-HT), the amino acids γ-aminobutyric acid (GABA), glycine, glutamate and aspartate, or acetylcholine (ACh). To further delineate the subject, most examples have been chosen from light- and electron-microscopic studies in the PNS and CNS of vertebrates, notwithstanding the importance of a great number of similar contributions made in invertebrates. Finally, since several authors have already dealt with particular aspects of this topic, emphasis has been placed on a critical reassessment of currently available data, especially when these were thought to be of interest for the future development of the field. Explicit descriptions of technical procedures and useful references on some basic aspects of radioautography have been regrouped in the Appendix (Section 8).

2. PRINCIPLES UNDERLYING THE RADIOAUTOGRAPHIC DETECTION OF CHEMICALLY-DEFINED NEURONS

2.1. PRODUCTION OF THE RADIOAUTOGRAPHIC IMAGE

As implied by its name (here preferred to the more commonly used synonym autoradiography; see Leblond 1976), radioautography (radius: ray, $\alpha\upsilon\tau os$: self, $\gamma\varrho\alpha\phi\epsilon\iota\upsilon$: write) is a method of investigation based on the production of images left in a photographic emulsion by a specimen containing radioactivity. In its current applications to the study of chemically-defined neurons, it calls for the use of transmitter molecules, or precursors or analogues thereof, labeled with low energy isotopes such as carbon-14 (^{14}C) or tritium (^{3}H). For all practical purposes, it is assumed that the isotopically-labeled molecules possess identical biological properties and undergo similar metabolic fate as their non-radioactive equivalents. Isotope exchanges are considered negligible within the time-span of the radioautographic experiments.

The production of the radioautographic image is a physicochemical process which is only partly understood. In brief, the radiolabeled molecules incorporated in a biological specimen may be considered as punctate sources emitting radiations at random. When a photographic emulsion is put in contact with a tissue section containing such sources for a more or less prolonged period of exposure, the silver halide crystals act as microdetectors of radiations: the β-particles reaching the emulsion layer induce latent images, which the photographic development subsequently reveals as silver grains observable with the light- and electron-microscopes.

The efficiency and resolution of this imaging system depend on the nature of the isotope and of the histological preparations containing it, on the type of emulsion and developer used and on the distance between the sources and photographic emulsion (see references in Section 8). For light- and electron-microscopic studies, tritiated compounds, which are now labeled with relatively high specific activities, have totally replaced [^{14}C] molecules. Tritium's low energy β-particles, which travel no more than 2 μm in histological sections and 1 μm in nuclear emulsion, indeed provide better efficiency and higher resolution.

For the sake of convenience, efficiency may be viewed as the percentage of desintegrations which result in a developed silver grain ('grain yield'). With uniformly labeled [^{3}H]methyl methacrylate, the density of which approximates that of fixed biological specimens, and using a standard emulsion, efficiencies of about 16, 11 and 7% have been respectively measured from sections 0.5, 1 and 2 μm in thickness (Falk and King 1963). Differences in specimen absorption also occur between different cellular constituents such as nucleus, nucleolus and cytoplasm (Maurer and Primbsch 1964). When osmium-fixed and metal-stained biological material is used, even a thickness of 100 nm is probably too great for self-absorption to be considered negligible. In the best conditions of exposure and development, the efficiency in sections of 100 nm or less, such as routinely used for electron-microscopy, is in the order of 20-30%.

Resolution may be defined in various ways but is often measured as the distance from point or linear sources within which half of the grains are found (half radius: HR; half distance: HD). In the light-microscope, the HD for tritium is about 0.3—0.4 μm and it is little affected by factors such as section thickness and size of emulsion crystals or developed grains (Rogers 1979). At electron-microscopic level, these factors become more critical (see refs in Section 8.3, under 'Comprehensive texts' and 'Electron-micro-scopic radioautography'). HD values of 0.1—0.15 μm have been reported for linear sources of tritium in thin sections of different thicknesses and using various types of emulsion and chemical or physical developers. In practice, however, it seems that the resolution in osmium-fixed and metal-stained biological specimens is somewhat higher, with 90% of the grains falling within 0.2 μm of point sources (Caro 1962; Gupta et al. 1973; Salpeter et al. 1978; Nadler 1979). This implies that light-microscopic radioautography will readily allow to ascribe tracer molecules to single cells and to their nucleus or cytoplasm, to thick processes such as proximal dendrites or large myelinated axons and even to axon terminals except when exceedingly small. In the electron-microscope, some large organelles, such as mitrochondria and dense bodies, will also be discernible as potential sources of labeling. On the other hand, attributing radioactivity to smaller intracellular constituents such as the synaptic vesicles will require statistical analysis of silver grain distribution, as discussed in Section 4.5, under 'Assigning silver grains to cellular constituents'.

2.2. BIOLOGICAL BASES OF LABELING

The radioautographic visualization of transmitter-defined neurons relies upon the existence of specific, high-affinity membrane transport mechanisms by which these cells take up and retain the transmitter and/or precursors involved in their normal functioning. Under proper experimental conditions, advantage can be taken of these specific uptake capacities for achieving neuronal labeling after introducing the respective compounds as radioactive tracers in the cellular environment. The extent to which the resulting radioautographic labeling will directly reflect specific uptake mechanisms is mainly dependent upon the concentrations of tracers administered and the conditions of fixation and/or histological processing. The existence of the uptake processes is nevertheless the prerequisite for obtaining identifying signals, the cellular specificity of which will ultimately be established experimentally (see Section 4.5, under 'Demonstration of specificity').

Uptake of neurotransmitters

(a) Biogenic amines

The high-affinity uptake systems for the catecholamines DA, NA and A and the indolamine 5-HT have been thoroughly investigated biochemically and pharmacologically (for reviews see Ross and Renyi 1967a; Iversen 1967, 1975; Snyder et al. 1970; Paton 1976, 1980; Horn 1979; Ross 1980). Their kinetics are those of saturable carrier-mediated membrane transport processes and are adequately described by the Michaelis-Menten equations. In all in vitro nervous tissue preparations thus far examined, the apparent Km for the high-affinity uptake of one or the other biogenic amine is in the order of 10^{-7} M. In CNS tissue, the NA, DA and 5-HT transport systems differ in their affinity for various structurally related analogues (Horn et al. 1971; Horn 1973) and they can be more or less selectively and powerfully inhibited by drugs such as desipramine (Titus and Spiegel 1962), benztropine (Coyle and Snyder 1969) and fluox-etine (Fuller et al. 1974; Wong et al. 1974), respectively. In several sympathetically-innervated organs, a low-affinity membrane transport has also been decribed for A and NA, and probably accounts for the penetration of these amines into some of their target cells (for reviews, see Iversen 1967, 1975).

Both in the PNS and CNS, the high-affinity membrane systems for catecholamines appear to be exclusively neuronal (Hamberger et al. 1964; Malmfors 1965; Hamberger. 1967; Fuxe et al. 1968). In the PNS, affinities for NA and A vary from one species to another. In rat CNS, differences in DA and NA accumulation by slices and homogenates from various anatomical regions of the brain support the likelihood of distinct carrier mechanisms for dopaminergic and noradrenergic neurons (Snyder and Coyle 1969). There is good evidence that DA and NA may be interchangeably taken up by either type of catecholaminergic neurons via their specific membrane transport systems. Thus, a high-affinity uptake of NA has been described in the DA-innervated neostriatum, although its apparent Km is considerably higher than that of DA; in areas which receive a mixed DA and NA innervation (and where the Km for NA is con-siderably lower than in the striatum), DA still inhibits NA uptake competitively and with an affinity for the NA system paradoxically greater than that for NA itself (Snyder and Coyle 1969). At high concentrations of ambient catecholamines, a low-affinity transport system has been demonstrated in CNS tissue for DA but not for NA, and it may be attributed to DA uptake into non-dopaminergic neurons (Shaskan and Snyder 1970). Berger and Glowinski (1978) have indeed shown histochemically that DA but not NA may be taken up into serotoninergic nerve terminals; such fluorescent ac-cumulation of DA does not occur in the presence of fluoxetine, which selectively in-hibits 5-HT uptake, or after destruction of 5-HT fibers by 5,7-dihydroxytryptamine.

There is also strong evidence for the existence of a high-affinity transport of 5-HT into peripheral and central serotoninergic neurons (Blackburn et al. 1967; Ross and Renyi 1967b; Chase et al. 1967; Fuxe et al. 1968; Shaskan and Snyder 1970; Robinson and Gershon 1971; Gershon and Altman 1971; Kuhar et al. 1972b; Gershon et al. 1976). In tissue exposed to relatively high concentrations of [^{3}H]5-HT, a low-affinity uptake into both dopaminergic and noradrenergic neurons is also well documented. In-itially suspected from kinetic studies in hypothalamic and striatal slices (Shaskan and Snyder 1970) and in slices from animals having received intracerebral injections of 6-hydroxydopamine (Iversen 1970), this interspecific uptake has been observed by fluorescence histochemistry (Lichtensteiger et al. 1967) and cytochemical electron-microscopy (Jaim-Etcheverry and Zieher 1968, 1969) after administration of relatively large doses of 5-HT in vivo.

(b) GABA

Demonstration of a carrier-mediated transport system responsible for rapid accumulation of γ-aminobutyric acid in CNS tissue (Elliott and Van Gelder 1958; Tsukada et al. 1963; Sano and Roberts 1963; Weinstein et al. 1965; Nakamura and Nagayama 1966) gave one of the first hints of the possible role of this amino acid as a neurotransmitter (Krnjević and Schwartz 1966).

A high-affinity uptake of GABA, with an apparent Km in the micromolar range, has since been demonstrated in brain slices and synaptosomes from various regions of the CNS (Iversen and Neal 1968; Iversen and Snyder 1968). The rate of accumulation of GABA in such preparations was shown to parallel the endogenous GABA content of the corresponding brain areas (Neal and Iversen 1969). The high-affinity transport of GABA is highly selective in that it is not competed for by other amino acids or amines but only by closely related structural analogues (for reviews, see Iversen et al. 1975; Iversen 1978). However, under certain experimental conditions, an homoexchange and/or low-affinity accumulation of GABA may prevail upon its high-affinity uptake (Levi and Raiteri 1973).

The lack of reliable cytochemical techniques for the direct cellular visualization of endogenous GABA and of cytotoxic agents capable of exclusive destruction of GABA-synthesizing neurons has made it difficult to establish the link between the high-affinity transport system for GABA and its neuronal localization as transmitter substance. Furthermore, the existence of a glial, as well as neuronal uptake of GABA, has been convincingly demonstrated (Henn and Hamberger 1971; for additional references, see Section 5.2, under 'GABA'). For instance, isolated sympathetic ganglia, which do not seem to contain GABAergic neurons, have been shown to take up and release exogenous GABA (Bowery and Brown 1971). According to Schon and Kelly (1974b), the glial and neuronal uptakes of GABA can be differentiated by the use of two false transmitters, β-alanine and diamino-butyric acid (DABA), the former being selectively taken up by glia and the latter by neurons. At high concentrations, however, DABA inhibits the neuronal uptake of GABA, which would limit its usefulness (refs in Kelly and Dick 1976). Cis-3-aminocyclohexane carboxylic acid (ACHC), another GABA uptake inhibitor (Bowery et al. 1976), could in fact be a better substrate for the neuronal as opposed to glial uptake of GABA (Neal and Bowery 1977).

(c) Glycine

Both high- and low-affinity uptake systems have been demonstrated for glycine in the CNS of mammals (Neal and Pickles 1969; Neal 1971; Johnston and Iversen 1971; Logan and Snyder 1971; Arregui et al. 1972). The high-affinity system is solely detected in spinal cord and brain stem, i.e. in anatomical regions containing glycine in high concentration and where it appears to be iontophoretically active. Similarly, glycine has been shown to be taken up by a high-affinity system in the pigeon optic tectum (Henke et al. 1976), where there is considerable evidence of its transmitter role (Cuénod and Henke 1978). As in the case of GABA, all available data regarding the cellular localization of the transport system for glycine is radioautographic (refs in Section 5.2, under 'Glycine'). Correlative evidence is therefore essential for interpreting [^{3}H]glycine localization in terms of transmitter specificity (see Section 5.2, under 'Glycine').

(d) Glutamate and aspartate

Many electrophysiological studies would seem to indicate that glutamic and aspartic acids many act as neurotransmitters in vertebrate CNS (for recent reviews, see Johnson

1978; Usherwood 1978; Johnston 1979; Cotman et al. 1981). A high-affinity uptake process for L-glutamic acid has been demonstrated in slices and homogenates from various mammalian (Logan and Snyder 1972; Balcar and Johnston 1972, 1973; Snyder et al. 1973a,b) and avian (Beart 1976b; Henke et al. 1976; Cuénod and Henke 1978) brain regions. Both L- and D-aspartate are also taken up in brain slices and by the same high-affinity uptake system as L-glutamate (Balcar and Johnston 1972; Davies and Johnston 1976). However, it has not yet been possible to determine to what extent either of these amino acids are selectively taken up by neurons likely to utilize glutamate and/or aspartate as transmitters (for review, see Shank and Aprison 1979). Several lines of evidence suggest that glial cells are also capable of high-affinity uptake of glutamate (see Section 5.2, under 'Glutamate and aspartate'). Clearly, the glial uptake sites for glutamate are distinct from those for GABA, since neither amino acid interferes significantly with each other's uptake (Schon and Kelly 1974a,b).

(e) Choline and acetylcholine

Choline is taken up by most cells and its uptake has been studied biochemically in CNS slices and synaptosomes as well as in various in vitro PNS preparations (Schuberth et al. 1966; Marchbanks 1968). The uptake of choline is sodium dependent, but one of its major components appears to be mediated by a relatively low-affinity and ubiquitous transport system (Km in the order of 10^{-4} M). In addition, a high-affinity choline transport system has been described, which might specifically belong to cholinergic neurons. Indeed, in the rat CNS, Yamamura and Snyder (1973) and Guyenet et al. (1973) detected high-affinity transport of choline with a Km in the micromolar range, and this only in anatomical areas rich in endogenous ACh, such as the corpus striatum. In guinea pig ileum, high-affinity [^{3}H]choline uptake has been found solely in the portion of this organ known to receive a cholinergic innervation (Snyder et al. 1973b). Further evidence that this high-affinity system is associated with cholinergic neurons comes from the finding in both ileum and brain homogenates that [^{3}H]choline taken up at low concentration is preferentially converted into ACh. Moreover, Kuhar et al. (1973) showed that lesions of the medial septum and diagonal band of Broca sharply reduce the high-affinity uptake of [^{3}H]choline in synaptosomes from the hippocampus, in keeping with the possibility of its selective accumulation into cholinergic neurons (see also Sorimachi and Kataoka 1974).

It has been reported by Yamamura and Snyder (1973) that in rat striatal homogenates, the high-affinity transport system for choline shows considerable affinity for ACh itself. Demonstration of this ACh uptake required incubation at low concentrations in the presence of an inhibitor of acetylcholinesterase. Subcellular fractionation of cortical slices after uptake of labeled ACh indicates that a considerable proportion of the accumulated ACh is taken up into synaptosomes (Schuberth and Sundwall 1968).

Intraneuronal binding

Because uptake mechanisms ensure trans-membranous transfer of molecules against a concentration gradient they may be viewed as the *sine qua non* for selective radioautographic identification of chemically-defined neurons. However, the intraneuronal distribution of transmitters will also depend on their intracellular binding, i.e. on physicochemical liaisons between the transmitters and cellular constituents.

Such a biological process must therefore be taken into account when considering the results of radioautography in terms of transmitter metabolism, storage and axonal transport.

Present knowledge of the mechanisms by which endogenous transmitters are naturally bound into cells remains limited to the definition and properties of various intracellular compartments involved in their utilization. In this regard, the most pertinent information derives from biochemical and cytochemical studies of noradrenergic neurons in the peripheral autonomic nervous system. Similar investigations in the CNS have been hampered by its cellular heterogeneity, whereas, in the PNS, purified subcellular fractions could be obtained from adrenergic nerve terminals (Von Euler and Lishajko 1963) and cytochemical studies performed on the latter and/or their ganglionic cell bodies (see Chapter III).

Generally speaking, a distinction has to be made between vesicular and extravesicular binding. The former refers to the storage of transmitter by the so-called synaptic vesicles aggregated into the nerve endings; the latter to all other sites of transmitter localization within the neurons.

Biochemically, vesicular binding of the biogenic amines has been characterized as a 2-step process (refs in Iversen 1975; Philippu, 1976). First, a transport system located in the vesicular membrane, which apparently differs from that of the plasma membrane by showing greatest efficiency at higher concentration of the substrate (Km in the range of 10^{-4} M). Moreover, this vesicular transport process appears largely independent of temperature or of the presence of Na^+ and K^+ in the external medium and is insensitive to many inhibitors acting upon the cellular uptake. Second, a high-affinity binding of the biogenic amines, which presumably occurs inside the vesicles of adrenergic nerves. This latter process appears to be Ca^{++} and Mg^{++} dependent and probably requires ATP. Interestingly, the kinetics of amine incorporation into splenic nerve vesicles suggest that 5-HT has a greater affinity than catecholamines for the vesicular binding sites. Among the catecholamines, DA, NA and A would exhibit comparable affinities.

Increasing biochemical evidence favors the existence of an extravesicular, cytoplasmic binding of the biogenic amines, as initially postulated to account for the ubiquitous radioautographic intracellular distribution of [^{3}H]NA taken up by noradrenergic and dopaminergic nerve cell bodies in CNS (Descarries and Droz 1970a). This notion has found support in the results of many radioisotopic studies with the catecholamines. Thus, the decay of intraventricularly administered [^{3}H]NA and [^{3}H]DA in various brain regions was found compatible with the existence of different intraneuronal pools for these exogenous amines (Glowinski and Iversen 1966). Fractionation studies have revealed the presence of both a soluble and a vesicle-bound form of NA in nerve endings from rat hypothalamus (De Robertis et al. 1965) or guinea pig cerebral cortex (Nagy et al. 1977). Many results of turnover experiments (Javoy and Glowinski 1971), radioactive metabolite studies (Gropetti et al. 1977) and in vitro investigations of the mechanisms of DA-release in neostriatum (De Belleroche et al. 1976; De Belleroche and Bradford 1978) were best explained by distinguishing between several metabolic compartments in these nerve terminals. Lastly, a cytoplasmic binding of CA has been inferred from recent analysis of the subsynaptosomal distribution of DA in neostriatum and of NA in hypothalamus and cerebral cortex under the action of various drugs (Hartman and Halaris 1980). In this regard, it is also worth recalling that there is some preliminary biochemical evidence suggesting the existence of soluble proteins with high affinity for catecholamines in CNS (Inaba and Kamata 1977; and unpublished observations of Hartman and Halaris, 1980) perhaps analogous to the 5-HT binding protein(s) demonstrated in both CNS and PNS 5-HT neurons (Tamir and Huang 1974; Jonakait et al. 1977; Rotman 1978; Tamir and Gershon 1979). In addition, cytochemical data pertaining to the intraneuronal localization of biogenic amines further support the likelihood of extravesicular binding sites playing a role in their subcellular distribution (see Chapter III).

This notion of intraneuronal binding is evidently of considerable importance also for explaining the action of certain drugs and, hence, for the assessment of their effects as observed by radioautography. Thus, the depleting actions of reserpine or similar agents on endogenous or exogenous monoamines are best accounted for by some interference with the vesicular and extravesicular binding processes. Similarly, it has been shown that substances acting as false adrenergic transmitters and which may serve to label monoaminergic neurons have the ability to replace endogenous biogenic amines in their vesicular or extravesicular stores. An eventual participation of extravesicular binding sites in the anterograde and/or retrograde axonal transport of transmitter amines is also most likely.

3. INFORMATIVE VALUE OF THE RADIOAUTOGRAPHIC APPROACH

As stated above, radioautography can be used both for identifying transmitter-specified cells and for studying transmitter metabolism. Neuronal identification will permit characterization of topographic, cytologic and ultrastructural features. Localizing the transmitters and/or their byproducts will yield information on dynamic aspects of their cellular utilization.

3.1. MORPHOLOGICAL CHARACTERIZATION OF CHEMICALLY-DEFINED NEURONS

From the strict point of view of their morphological organization, radioautographically-labeled neurons may be studied in much the same way as those identified by other cytological methods applicable at light- and electron-microscopic levels. Generally speaking, nerve cell populations and their constitutive units can be examined in terms of their distribution, composition and structural characteristics. Qualitative and quantitative data may be sought. At the light-microscopic level, nerve cell bodies and axon terminals may be mapped and their numbers estimated (Figs 1—11). At the electron-microscopic level, the nerve cell bodies and their proximal processes can be described as to size, shape, branching patterns and preferential location of relationships with other histological constituents (Figs 14, 15 and 19). Axon terminals (or varicosities) and intervaricose axonal segments can be similarly analyzed (Figs 12, 13, 16–18), and the content of identified somata, dendrites, axons and varicosities thus scrutinized for distinctive features. Furthermore, attention can be paid to terminals as afferents (Fig. 15) and to various other patterns of interconnectivity between labeled profiles themselves (Fig. 14) or the latter and terminals as afferents unidentified (Figs 12—18) or otherwise identified elements (Fig. 19). The essential merit of radioautography is to yield this information about neurons whose transmitter-identity is known, so that its real advantages and limitations are best appreciated by comparison with those of other methods available to the same ends.

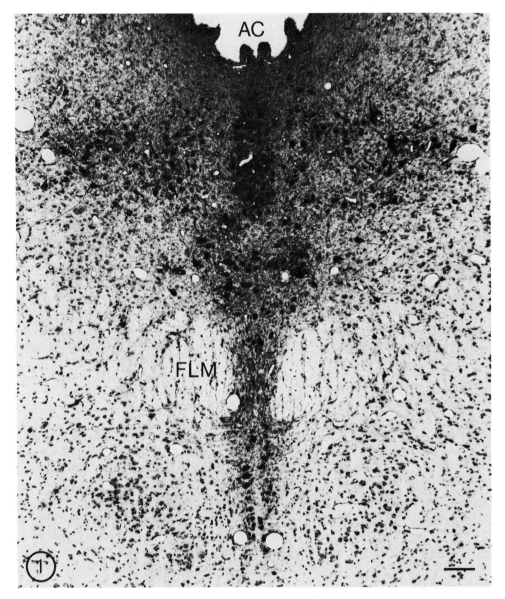

Fig. 1. Light-microscopic radioautograph across the nucleus raphe dorsalis of an adult rat injected with 300 μCi of [^{3}H]5-HT in the lateral ventricle. The tracer was infused for 2 h at a molarity of 10^{-5} M. Monoamine oxidase was inhibited. At this level, corresponding approximately to the stereotaxic plane A- 770 μm of König and Klippel's atlas (1963), 5-HT nerve cell bodies appear strongly labeled. They assume a typical distribution into two medial and one bilateral subgroups. In addition to the reactive cells laden with densely packed silver grains, there are numerous 'unlabeled' neurons which exhibit the same weak and diffuse reactivity as the whole area penetrated by the tracer. AC = aqueductus cerebri; FLM = fasciculus longitudinalis medialis. Tissue fixed by perfusion with 3.5% glutaraldehyde in phosphate buffer and embedded in paraffin. Five μm-thick section poststained with thionine and cresyl violet. Exposure time, 15 days. X 80. Calibration bar, 100 μm.

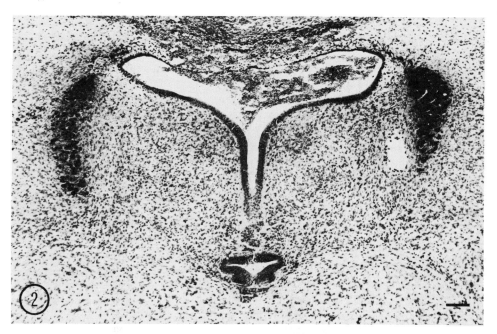

Fig. 2. Labeling of the locus ceruleus in a newborn rat pretreated with both an inhibitor of monoamine oxidase and of catechol-O-methyl transferase and injected intravenously with [³H]NA (100 μCi), 3 h earlier. All noradrenergic nerve cell bodies show equally strong reactivity, forming a compact group on either side of the fourth ventricle. Under these conditions, labeled neurons are also found in the other CA cell groups of the brain stem and in the external granular layer of the olfactory bulb. Histological and radioautographic processing as in Figure 1. X 65. Calibration bar, 100 μm. (Reproduced from Dupin et al. 1976.)

Topographic distribution

When seeking information on the topographic distribution of transmitter-defined nerve cell bodies and/or terminal arborizations, radioautography may first seem to offer little advantages over techniques such as histofluorescence or immunohistochemistry, which reveal endogenous transmitter or biosynthetic enzyme contents. Indeed, in vivo radioautographic labeling is generally limited by the restricted penetration of transmitter molecules in brain tissue (because of the necessity to bypass the blood-brain barrier) and can only be used, for mapping purposes, in periventricular or superficial regions of the brain (see Section 4.2). The in vitro approach (see Section 4.1.) will allow for more extensive surveys but requires the preparation of fresh brain slices which for all practical purposes restricts the examination to certain brain regions. Yet, radioautography remains the method of choice when quantitation is contemplated, i.e. for determining the number of chemically-defined nerve cell bodies and/or axon terminals within a given brain region (see Section 4.5, under 'Achieving integral labeling' and Section 5.1). The sensitivity of the radioautographic approach can also be an asset for identifying neurons in which the levels of transmitters and/or their synthetic enzymes appear to be too low for histofluorescence or immunohistochemical visualization. Such is apparently the case with some monoaminergic neurons during early stages of their ontogenesis, at a time when the development of their uptake properties may precede that of a full enzymatic activity or endogenous content in neurotransmitter (e.g. Verney et al. 1982). Even in adult CNS, some DA cells in retina and olfactory bulb

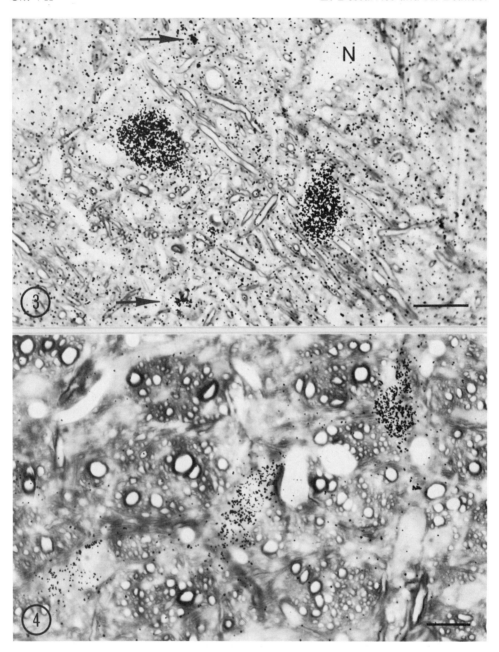

Fig. 3. Labeling by local uptake of 2 dopaminergic neurons of the zona compacta of substantia nigra, in an adult rat pretreated with a monoamine oxidase inhibitor and injected intraventricularly with 500 µCi of [³H]NA (Descarries and Droz 1968a). Note that the radioautographic reaction involves both nucleus and perikaryon. This intense and selective labeling is in contrast with the relatively weak, diffuse scattering of isolated silver grains in surrounding tissue. A neighboring nerve cell body is thus unlabeled (N). Some small and dense accumulations of silver grains (arrows) probably correspond to reactive dendrites. Tissue fixed by perfusion with glutaraldehyde followed by immersion in the same fixative and postfixation in osmium tetroxide. Two µm-thick Epon section poststained with toluidine blue. Exposure time, 7 days. X 750. Calibration bar, 20 µm.

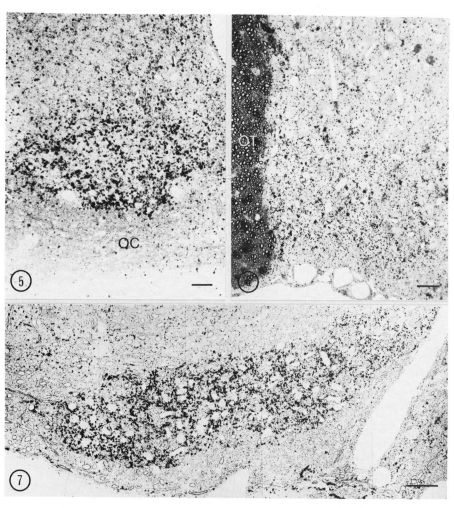

Figs. 5-7. Light-microscopic distribution of labeled monoamine axonal varicosities in various regions of the rat brain. Tissue fixed by standard glutaraldehyde perfusion followed by immersion in osmium tetroxide. One µm-thick Epon sections, poststained with toluidine blue. Exposure times, 15 days. Calibration bars, 50 µm.

Fig. 5. Suprachiasmatic nucleus after intraventricular administration of 10^{-4} M [^{3}H]5-HT in the presence of a 10-fold higher concentration of non-radioactive NA. Monoamine oxidase inhibited. 5-HT axonal varicosities having taken up and retained the tracer in high concentration are detected in the form of small and dense aggregates of silver grains and predominate in the ventral half of the nucleus. Labeled varicosities belonging to the supraependymal 5-HT plexus are also visible along the wall of the third ventricle (upper right). OC = optic chiasma. X 280. (Contributed by O. Bosler.)

Fig. 4. [^{3}H]NA-labeling by retrograde axonal transport of 3 nerve cell bodies in the medulla oblongata of an adult rat. These cells belong to Group A-3 according to the nomenclature of Dahlström and Fuxe (1964). The tracer (50 µCi) was injected stereotaxically immediately above the ipsilateral substantia nigra, about 8 mm away, 6 h earlier. Monoamine oxidase was inhibited. Note the sparing of the nucleus in the lower left neuron and the almost total absence of scattered grains in the neuropil. Fixation was carried out by double, rapid perfusion, in succession, of 3.5% glutaraldehyde and 0.5% osmium tetroxide in phosphate buffer, followed by immersion in 2% osmium tetroxide for postfixation. Large, 5 µm-thick Epon section, unstained. Exposure time, 30 days. X 420. Calibration bar, 20 µm.

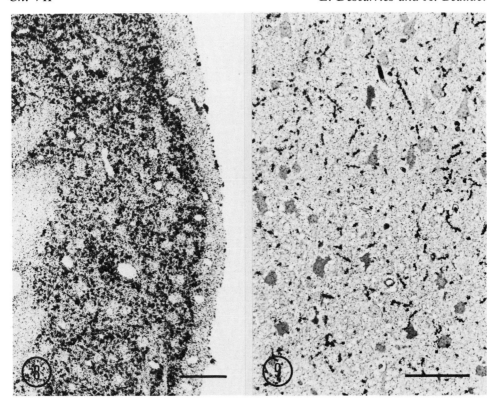

Fig. 8. Light-microscopic radioautograph from the paraventricular neostriatum of a rat injected for 3 h with 5×10^{-4} M [^{3}H]DA and 10^{-3} M non-radioactive 5-HT in the adjacent lateral cerebral ventricle (Descarries et al. 1980). The tissue was rapidly fixed and postfixed by vascular perfusion in succession of 3.5% glutaraldehyde and 0.5% osmium tetroxide solutions. This mode of fixation was essential for detecting DA axon terminals in the expected form of small and dense aggregates of silver grains. There was no such labeling in control experiments after previous destruction of the nigrostriatal dopaminergic system with 6-hydroxydopamine. One μm-thick Epon section, poststained with toluidine blue. Exposure time, 15 days. X 250. Calibration bar, 50 μm.

Fig. 9. Light-microscopic radioautograph showing dopaminergic axon terminals labeled with [^{3}H]DA in adult rat supragenual cortex. Slices were cut with a vibrating microtome and preincubated for 15 min at room temperature in the presence of a monoamine oxidase inhibitor and desipramine. [^{3}H]DA incubation also lasted 15 min, at a final concentration of 10^{-6} M. Primary fixation was carried out in 3.5% glutaraldehyde for 20—30 min and followed by exposure to osmic vapors at room temperature for 1 h prior to dehydration and resin-embedding. One μm-thick Araldite-Epon section poststained with toluidine blue. X 350. Calibration bar, 50 μm. (Reproduced from Nguyen-Legros et al. 1981.)

Fig. 6. Supraoptic nucleus after intraventricular administration of 10^{-4} M [^{3}H]NA in the presence of a 10-fold higher concentration of non-radioactive 5-HT. Monoamine oxidase inhibited. Labeled axonal varicosities are mostly observed in the ventral portion of the nucleus, which is also known to contain the greatest number of dopamine-β-hydroxylase immunoreactive terminals (Swanson and Hartman 1975; Swanson et al. 1981). OT = optic tract. X 315. (Contributed by O. Bosler.)

Fig. 7. [^{3}H]5-HT labeling in the dorsal accessory olive of a rat subjected to intraventricular injection of the neurotoxic drug 5,6-dihydroxytryptamine (75 μg in 20 μl of saline), 6 months earlier (conditions otherwise similar to those of Fig. 5). This treatment results in a severe initial loss of 5-HT terminals (90% destruction at 5 days) followed by regrowth reaching normal density after 2 months and leading to an 'hyperinnervation' with a number of 5-HT terminals almost three times greater than in controls after 6 months. Note that the zone of hyperinnervation is sharply demarcated from the surrounding reticular formation. Exposure time, 30 days. X 175. (Reproduced from Wiklund et al. 1981.)

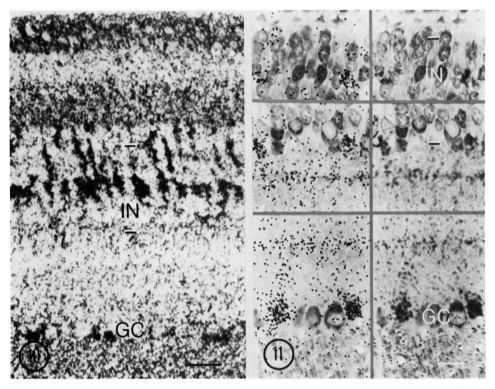

Fig. 10. Light-microscopic radioautograph from the postero-superior quadrant of the pigeon retina, 6 h after intravitreal injection of 500 μCi of [³H]D-aspartate (Beaudet et al. 1981). Note the intense and selective reactivity of Müller cells and thin processes in the inner nuclear layer (IN), and the strong accumulations of radioactive label within small cell bodies scattered in the ganglion cell layer (GC). Cell bodies of similar size and shape were found to be retrogradely labeled in this same layer following application of [³H]D-aspartate in the optic tectum, indicating that they were those of ganglion cells, rather than glial or displaced amacrine cells. Primary fixation with 5% glutaraldehyde. One μm-thick, Epon section, poststained with toluidine blue. Exposure time, 1 week. X 500. Calibration bar, 20 μm.

Fig. 11. Photomontage from a 1.5 μm-thick Epon-embedded section exemplifying the radioautographic distribution of [³H]choline uptake in the chicken retina. The tissue was incubated with 5 × 10⁻⁶ M [³H]choline for 15 min and then freeze-dried. Dry emulsion film was used for radioautography. The montage extends from the outer plexiform layer to the optic nerve fibers. Focus is on the section on the right and on the grains on the left. Selective cell body labeling is detected in both the inner nuclear (IN) and ganglion cell (GC) layers. From their position, the labeled cells in the inner nuclear layer could be amacrine and/or inner bipolar cells. Those in the ganglion cell layer are probably displaced amacrine rather than ganglion cells, as suggested by their location at the margin of the inner plexiform layer and the presence of a dense band compatible with terminal labeling in Layer 4 of the inner plexiform layer. Toluidine blue stain. Calibration bar, 10 μm. X 750. (Reproduced from Baughman and Bader 1977.)

Figs. 12 and 13. Electron-microscopic detection, in 2 consecutive thin sections, of a noradrenergic axon terminal of rat periaqueductal gray labeled by intraventricular injection of [³H]NA (Descarries and Droz 1970a). Monoamine oxidase was inhibited. The reactive bouton contains a mixed population of vesicles and makes synaptic contact with a small dendrite. Fixation as in Figure 3. Microdol-X development. Exposure time, 1 month. X 15,000. Calibration bar, 1 μm.

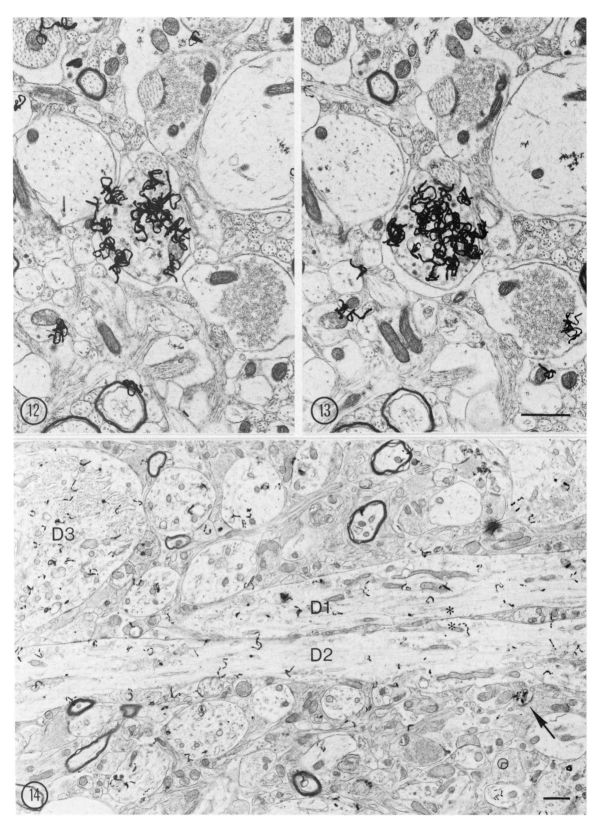

(Ehinger and Falck 1971; Halasz et al. 1977, 1978) and 5-HT neurons in hypothalamus (Beaudet and Descarries, 1979) were readily demonstrated after uptake of [³H]DA and [³H]5-HT, respectively, but required loading with exogenous transmitters or related compounds to be identified by fluorescence and/or immunohistochemistry (Fuxe and Ungerstedt 1968; Frankfurt et al. 1982).

The foregoing considerations also pertain to the usefulness of radioautography for mapping transmitter-specific neuronal projections. Admittedly, the examination of neuronal pathways labeled by local uptake of transmitter (e.g. Parent et al. 1981) will always be limited by tracer diffusion and, further, by the myelin ensheathing of some axons which also reduces their accessibility; moreover, the paucity of storage organelles along the axonal paths or intervaricose segments does not favor their labeling. However, a solution to these problems may reside in the use of the anterograde or the retrograde axonal transport of transmitters to label specific projection pathways (see Chapter VIII). While this approach remains largely to be developed for examining preterminal, branching and terminal patterns, it could yield unprecedented information on the fine structural features and intimate relationships of chemically-defined neurons when applied at the electron-microscopic level (see also Section 6).

Fig. 14. Two longitudinally (D_1, D_2) and one transversally (D_3) cut dendrites labeled in rat raphe dorsalis following prolonged intraventricular infusion of [³H]5-HT (Descarries et al. 1982). Monoamine oxidase was inhibited. All 3 dendrites exhibit the usual longitudinally oriented microtubules and neurofilaments as well as a prominent endoplasmic reticulum. The 2 central processes (D_1 and D_2) come in close apposition for a short distance (asterisks), but do not show vesicular aggregates or membrane differentiations suggestive of dendritic storage and/or release. The lower dendrite (D_2) bears a small, narrow-necked spine (arrow), overlaid by a grain cluster and receiving an unlabeled synaptic terminal. Note that this dendritic labeling is much lighter than that of the terminals illustrated above. This is partly due to the fact that perikarya and dendrites accumulate exogenous biogenic amines in much lower concentration than axon terminals, but also to the use of a physical developer, paraphenylenediamine, which is less sensitive than Microdol-X (utilized above) but has the advantage of producing smaller silver grains and thus allow for better examination of underlying structures. Exposure time, 1 month. X 8000. Calibration bar, 1 μm.

Figs 15-17. Electron-microscopic demonstration of axon terminals labeled with [³H]catecholamines in different regions of adult rat brain. Paraphenylenediamine development. Exposure times, 3 months. Calibration bars, 1 μm.

Fig. 15. [³H]DA-labeled axonal varicosities in axosomatic contact (arrows) with a nerve cell body in the nucleus lateralis septi. This innervation pattern corresponds to the pericellular arrangements of DA varicosities demonstrated by fluorescence histochemistry (Lindvall 1975). Many other terminals, unlabeled (*), are also in synaptic contact with the same nerve cell body. Of these, some are possibly serotoninergic (see Parent et al. 1981; Köhler and Steinbusch 1981). Rapid, double glutaraldehyde and osmium perfusion as in Figure 8. X 10,000.

Fig. 16. Accumulation of [³H]NA in a damaged axon of substantia grisea periventricularis, 7 days after a pretreatment with intraventricular 6-hydroxydopamine known to result in the eventual disappearance of all NA nerve cell bodies in the locus ceruleus (Descarries and Saucier 1972). This dilated profile is filled with vesicular organelles, many of which exhibit a dense core. It is partly engulfed by an adjacent microglial cell. Standard fixation. X 16,000.

Fig. 17. Axon terminal labeled with [³H]A in the nucleus arcuatus hypothalami (Bosler and Descarries 1983). This reactive varicosity is part of a tetrad synapsing on a central dendrite. The small and clear round synaptic vesicles present in all these terminals appear indistinguishable. Fixation by rapid, double-perfusion of glutaraldehyde and osmium tetroxide followed by further osmication of tissue slices. X 18,500.

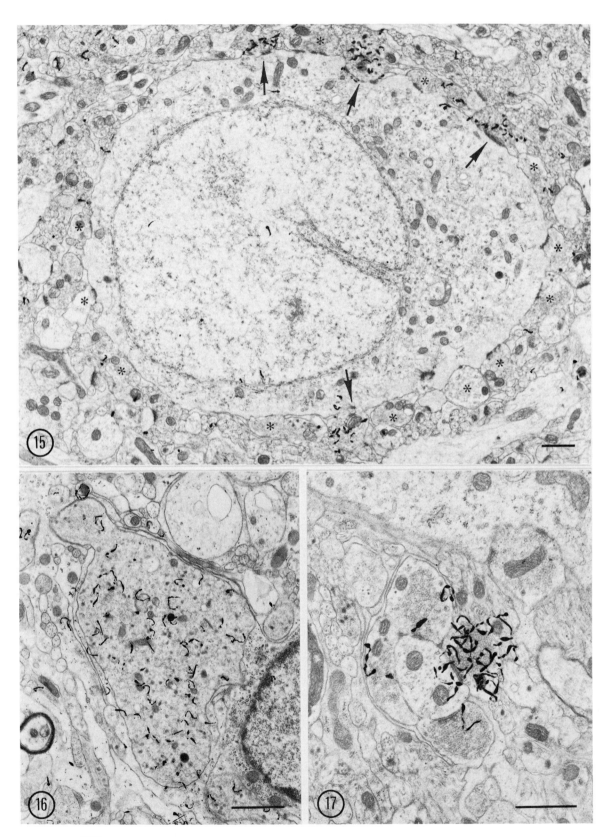

302

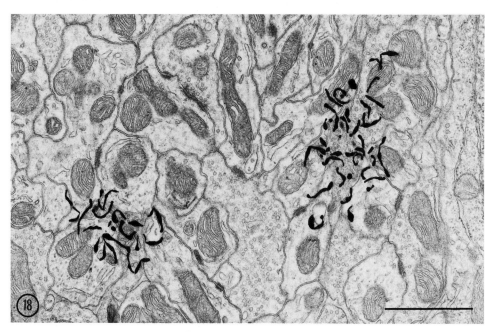

Fig. 18. Electron-microscopic radioautograph from the granular layer of rat cerebellar cortex (posterior vermis) superfused for 3 h with 10^{-4} M [^{3}H]5-HT and 10^{-3} M non-radioactive NA. Monoamine oxidase was inhibited. Two intensely labeled 5-HT varicosities are detected in the vicinity of a glomerular island. Such varicosities exhibit a denser axoplasmic matrix and smaller vesicular organelles than the surrounding unlabeled terminals. Also in contrast to other terminals, they very rarely show membrane specializations suggestive of synaptic contact. Standard perfusion fixation with 1% glutaraldehyde and 1% paraformaldehyde. Paraphenylenediamine development. Exposure time, 8 months. X 24,000. Calibration bar, 1 μm. (In collaboration with C. Sotelo.)

Cytologic features

Radioautography appears all the more suited for achieving ultrastructural characterization of transmitter-specific neurons in that it is not only compatible with conditions of tissue fixation generally superior to those of cyto- or immunocytochemistry but can also provide for the detection of every element of a type under consideration (see Section 4.5, under 'Achieving integral labeling').

Such global radioautographic visualization of cellular profiles belonging to a given category of chemically-defined neurons in turn implies that reliable topometric data may be obtained from their various parts and concerning their internal constituents. In particular, accurate measurement of the size of axon terminals will permit extrapolation of their actual number and incidence in different anatomical areas, and these estimates of innervation density give added significance to biochemical, pharmacological or electrophysiological data (e.g. Lapierre et al. 1973; Beaudet and Descarries 1976). From concomitant determinations of endogenous transmitter levels, true intraneuronal concentrations will then be measurable, and this under various experimental conditions. Lastly, the occurrence of various intraneuronal organelles and/or of special relationships with other cellular elements will be amenable to quantifications, as exemplified by the demonstration of the presence of large granular vesicles in every serotoninergic or noradrenergic axon terminal of rat cerebral cortex or of the low fre-

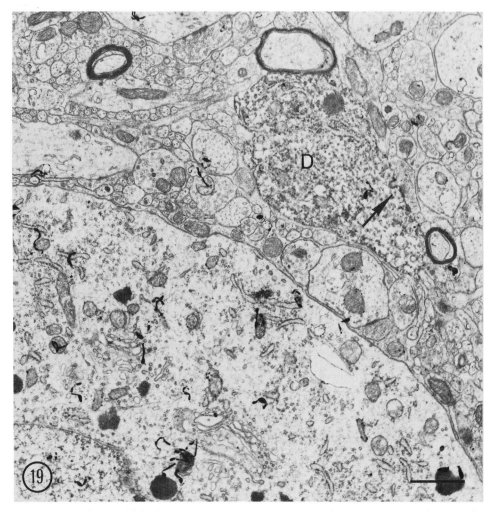

Fig. 19. Combined radioautographic and immunocytochemical identification of serotoninergic and catecholaminergic neurons in the nucleus raphe dorsalis of adult rat. The soma of a serotonin neuron (lower left) is radioautographically labeled by intraventricular injection of [³H]5-HT. The adjacent tyrosine-hydroxylase immunoreactive dendrite (presumably dopaminergic), is stained by the peroxidase-anti-peroxidase method of Sternberger. Note the indentation at the level where the immunostained dendrite receives an unlabeled synaptic terminal (arrow). Perfusion fixation with 0.5% glutaraldehyde and 4% paraformaldehyde followed by immunocytochemical processing and postfixation in osmium tetroxide. Paraphenylenediamine development. Exposure time, 7 months. X 15,000. Calibration bar, 1 μm. (Beaudet, Pickel, Joh and Cuénod, unpublished.)

quency of synaptic membrane differentiations established by such terminals in this and other parts of the rat brain (Descarries et al. 1975, 1977).

3.2. CELLULAR LOCALIZATION OF NEUROTRANSMITTERS

Another aspect of the information derived from radioautography pertains to the metabolism of transmitters. At the cellular level, identification of metabolic compartments and the extent to which they may totally or partially correspond to neurons, glia and/or target cells is indeed an essential element in the definition of transmitters. A second level of information concerns the intracellular pools implicated in transmitter turnover, i.e. synthesis, transport, degradation, binding, storage, release and/or reuptake. At both levels of investigation, a fundamental limitation of radioautography will be that silver grains revealing the presence of radioactivity tell nothing about the chemical nature of the labeled molecules. Therefore, radioautographic results will always have to be correlated with biochemical determinations to identify the labels and measure their proportion representing transmitter itself and/or byproducts, sometimes with the adjunct of pharmacological treatments aimed at preventing metabolic degradation (see Section 4.5, under 'Nature of molecules detected'). As will also be shown below, the use of precursors may be complicated by vagaries such as nonspecific incorporation, insufficient conversion to induce detectable reactions and/or artefactual retention by fixatives, explaining why radioautography presently finds little application in the study of transmitter synthesis. Nevertheless, within the constraints imposed by fixation and the resolution of the technique, visualizing the fate of transmitter molecules at different time intervals after their penetration or formation into cells may offer unique advantages such as measuring transmitter turnover in situ or localizing metabolites at their sites of formation (e.g. Descarries and Droz 1970a). After local uptake, it has not yet been possible to examine transmitter localizations imputable to physiological release. However, in this regard, changes induced by experimental manipulations (lesions, pharmacological treatments, stimulation) might eventually yield precise information by comparison with localization observed under control conditions.

4. METHODOLOGY

4.1. IN VITRO EXPERIMENTATION

Chemically-defined neurons or parts thereof may be radioautographically labeled in various isolated nervous tissue preparations (anatomical structures, slices, synaptosomes, homogenates, cultures) incubated in vitro. This approach has the main advantage of allowing for the administration of low and precise concentrations of tracer, under experimental conditions similar to those used in biochemical and/or pharmacological kinetic studies. It also permits comparisons between specimens incubated in parallel, which proves particularly useful for the assessment of drug effects. Problems with the penetration of labels may be encountered when incubating whole organs, dissected anatomical structures or even relatively thick tissue slices (see discussion in Iversen and Schon 1973). In contrast, all parts of thinner slices, homogenates, synaptosomal preparations or cultures are readily accessible to tracers. The main inconvenience of in vitro experimentation, except in the case of cultures, is that the preservation of morphology is rather poor. With tissue slices, isolated retina and PNS or CNS organs (e.g. vas deferens, spinal cord segments, pineal gland and median eminence), the integrity of cellular interrelationships is generally respected, but the cellular and subcellular structure, especially in CNS, always shows marked alterations in the form of pronounced glial and extracellular swelling and damage to neuronal perikarya and axon terminals. In homogenates and synaptosomal preparations, only fragments of glial and nerve cells are present. Synaptosomal labeling has often been used as an index of the number of terminals containing a given transmitter in different regions of the brain (see Section 5). Such results, however, must be interpreted with extreme caution since: (1) identification of synaptosomes as opposed to other cellular processes may be difficult, and (2) the proportion of synaptosomes over the total number of terminals probably varies from one region to another due to differences in size, shape and cellular relationships of terminals.

Numerous studies have demonstrated the feasibility of labeling transmitter uptake sites in vitro, as already done in various regions of CNS with most transmitters: noradrenaline (Lenn 1967), serotonin (Kuhar and Aghajanian 1973; Calas et al. 1974; Ségu and Calas 1978; Azmitia and Marovitz 1980), GABA (Iversen and Bloom 1972), glutamate (Storm-Mathisen and Iversen 1979), glycine (Hökfelt and Ljungdahl 1971; Iversen and Bloom 1972; Matus and Dennison 1971), and with [3H]choline (Baughman and Bader 1977). (Additional references will be found in Section 5.) In vitro incubation has also permitted light-microscopic identification and mapping of axon terminals which were otherwise difficult to demonstrate either because their specific labeling required special pharmacological treatments and/or because they were investigated in regions of the brain hardly accessible in vivo (e.g. Nguyen-Legros et al. 1981; Azmitia and Marovitz 1980). The in vitro approach appears particularly useful for studying transmitter specific neurons in the PNS, retina and tissue cultures (see Section 5).

4.2. IN VIVO LABELING OF PNS AND CNS NEURONS

In vivo labeling respects the anatomical, histological and cytological integrity of PNS or CNS tissue and is therefore preferable a priori for studying both the properties and morphological features of chemically-defined neurons. It must tackle, however, with the existence of the blood-brain barrier, which prevents entry of circulating biogenic amines or amino acid transmitters into adult mammalian CNS except at the level of specialized neurohemal regions. Some precursors do traverse the blood-brain barrier to a certain extent (e.g. DOPA or 5-hydroxytryptophan), but their utilization faces problems of specificity (see Section 4.5, under 'Demonstration of specificity'). For studies in the PNS, of some circumventricular organs or of immature CNS before the barrier becomes fully impermeable, tracers may be administered by the intravenous or intraperitoneal routes. The systemic approach requires the injection of large doses and has been used mainly for labeling NA and 5-HT neurons in the autonomic nervous system (see Section 5.1) or catecholaminergic neurons in the newborn rat brain (Dupin et al. 1976). In adult rats, pretreatment with an α-blocker has been proposed to prevent respiratory and cardiovascular complications at the time of [3H]NA injections (Lichtensteiger and Langemann 1966). Such experiments have shown that uptake of monoamines from the circulation is almost instantaneous. To our knowledge, successful labeling of cholinergic peripheral neurons after systemic administration of [3H]choline or [3H]ACh has never been reported.

It is for studies in the CNS that the greatest variety of approaches may be considered in terms of tracer selection, doses, routes and schedules of administration and pharmacological pretreatment(s).

Choice of tracer

All non-peptidic transmitter candidates are currently available in tritiated form.

However, as already mentioned, the various compounds toward which uptake processes have been demonstrated include not only the transmitters themselves, but also precursors, analogues or false transmitters which, because of metabolic properties and/or uptake selectivity, will sometimes be preferred for optimal radioautographic labeling. Thus, in the case of catecholaminergic neurons, interesting results might be expected from further studies with [^{3}H]α-methyl-norepinephrine (Descarries and Droz 1969), which is not degraded by monoamine oxidase once taken up intraneuronally, or with [^{3}H]6-hydroxydopamine, which has been shown to selectively accumulate in catecholaminergic neurons of both the CNS (Schubert et al. 1973) and PNS (Ljungdahl et al. 1971) thereby exerting its selective cytolytic effects (Thoenen and Tranzer 1968).

Similarly, labeling of GABA neurons may be achieved using ACHC (Neal et al. 1979), the GABA uptake inhibitor which appears more selective toward neurons than glia (Bowery et al. 1976). Cellular accumulations of [^{3}H]muscimol, a GABA antagonist, have also been reported in neurons of rat cerebellum (Chan-Palay 1978c), hippocampus (Chan-Palay 1978d) and spinal cord cultures (Chan-Palay et al. 1978), cat lateral geniculate nucleus (Sterling and Davis 1980) and frog and goldfish retina (Yazulla and Brecha 1980). Uptake of [^{3}H]muscimol has indeed been documented biochemically, in rat brain slices (Johnston et al. 1978). However, it does not seem to be confined, at least in the retina, to GABAergic neurons (Yazulla and Brecha 1980).

For investigating alleged glutamate and/or aspartate neurons, [^{3}H]D-aspartate, which is selectively taken up by the same high-affinity system as its L-stereoisomer and L-glutamate (see Section 2.2, under 'Uptake of neurotransmitters') may be chosen in view of its resistance to metabolic degradation.

Preparation of solutions

Radiochemical purity of tracer solutions must be verified, especially in the case of labile molecules such as DA, for example. Intracerebral administration generally requires that the labeled compounds, which are commercially available in non-physiological vehicles, be first evaporated dry under vacuum or under a gentle stream of nitrogen and extemporaneously redissolved in an appropriate volume of physiological saline or artificial cerebrospinal fluid. If the vehicle solution contains a non-volatile acid and there is a risk of denaturation of the labeled molecules at low pH, it may be buffered prior to evaporation. If the compound to be administered is likely to oxidise rapidly, ascorbic acid may be added to the final solution.

Routes of intracerebral administration

Various routes are available for intracerebral administration in vivo depending on the region to be investigated. Intraventricular injections were first recommended by Milhaud and Glowinski (1962) as a means to bypass the blood-brain barrier. Since the total volume of intraventricular fluid is about 150 μl in the rat, microliter amounts of tracer solution must be administered in order to avoid intraventricular overpressure. Tracers can also be introduced into the cerebrospinal fluid via the atlanta-occipital cistern, and ventriculo-cisternal or -spinal perfusions may be carried out after ventricular cannulation and cisternal or lumbar puncture, respectively, to deliver volumes in the milliliter range and thus lower tracer concentration. For studies of superficial brain structures, topical applications may be performed, the labeled solutions being directly deposited upon an exposed area of cerebral or cerebellar cortex or of the spinal cord, for example. Subarachnoid injections have also been utilized. After either ventricular, cisternal or topical administration, the observable penetration of tracers in CNS parenchyma is rather restricted, varying from 100—1200 μm according to the type, dose, specific activity and concentration of tracer used, and to the rate and duration of administration (e.g. Clark et al. 1968; Beaudet and Descarries 1976). Anatomical regions remote from both the ventricular cavities and brain surface can only be reached through intraparenchymatous microinjections. Such injections are the rule in axonal transport studies, even though positive results have also been reported after topical applications of very long duration upon wide expanses of cerebral or cerebellar cortex (Beaudet, unpublished) or optic tectum (Beaudet et al. 1981). Because of the relatively high concentrations of tracer required for intracerebral administration, the specificity of radioautographic reactions obtained under these conditions must always be rigorously assessed (see Section 4.5, under 'Demonstration of specificity').

Dose and schedule of administration

The doses of tracer have to be determined experimentally so as to provide reactions of sufficient intensity within manageable periods of radioautographic exposure. The molarity of solutions administered should ideally remain as close as possible to the Km values of the uptake systems of the neurons to be investigated. However, because of the available specific activities of radiochemicals and the small volumes which must be utilized, higher concentrations often prove necessary to ensure that sufficient quantities of radioactivity are delivered. In adopting a compromise, dilution into the cerebrospinal fluid and/or parenchyma should be taken into account.

The rate and duration of tracer administration will also influence the radioautographic labeling. In the case of lateroventricular injections, rapid delivery (e.g. 5—10 min) of a relatively large volume of solution (e.g. 50—200 μl) seems to favor intraventricular spreading and results in a more equal side-to-side labeling than slower infusions and/or smaller volumes (Descarries and Droz 1970a).

Various survival times must always be tested. With [³H]NA, for instance, a period of survival of a few hours after the end of tracer administration increases the 'signal-to-noise' ratio, i.e. selective neuronal vs ubiquitous labeling (Descarries and Droz 1970a,b). With [³H]5-HT, on the contrary, intense localized reactions have been obtained by lengthening the duration of tracer administration and carrying out tissue fixation immediately thereafter (Descarries et al. 1975). Another reason for trying various durations of tracer administration and/or periods of survival is that certain neurons may show more rapid transmitter turnover than others and hence be actually identifiable after short but not long, survival times (e.g. Bosler and Descarries 1983). In the case of [³H]GABA, short survival times apparently favor neuronal over glial accumulation, facilitating the selective identification of GABAergic neurons (Kelly and Dick 1976; see also Belin et al. 1979). Evidently, in axonal transport experiments, determining the periods of survival will be a crucial aspect of the experimentation.

Pharmacological pretreatments

Whereas certain drug effects may be revealed by radioautography, others are in fact utilized for achieving significant labeling of transmitter-specific neurons. This is particularly true in the case of biogenic amine neurons, the identification and investigation of which is greatly facilitated by pretreatment with a monoamine oxidase inhibitor in both the PNS and CNS (see Section 5.1). Blocking oxidative deamination, the main pathway for intraneuronal degradation of CA and 5-HT, has two major advantages: first, by preventing the formation of labeled metabolites intraneuronally, it ensures the persistence of strong accumulations of [^{3}H]biogenic amines into the cell bodies and axon terminals in which they have been taken up; second, since O-methylated metabolites are formed only extraneuronally and are not accumulated in nerve cells, it allows the inference that all intraneuronal accumulations of radioactivity detected after uptake of [^{3}H]CA or [^{3}H]5-HT are indeed due to the transmitters themselves rather than to labeled metabolites. Inhibition of monoamine oxidase is also required for the detection of neuronal sites labeled by anterograde or retrograde axonal transport of biogenic amines, since this process often requires survival times much longer than the biological half-life of these tracers. The best monoamine oxidase inhibitors to use are obviously those which do not interfere with uptake processes, such as β-phenyl isopropylhydrazine or pargyline. These are usually administered at least 1 h before the tracers. Inhibition of the extraneuronal O-methylation of catecholamines by substances such as pyrogallol and tropolone has not been systematically utilized for improving the labeling of catecholaminergic neurons. In fact, it appears to make little difference in the intensity of reactions observed in CNS after [^{3}H]DA or [^{3}H]NA administration, except in newborn rat where the tracer is injected intravenously and the availability of [^{3}H]NA for uptake into brain appears to be considerably increased by blockage of peripheral organ O-methylation (Dupin et al. 1976).

Amino oxyacetic acid (AOAA), which prevents intraneuronal GABA breakdown by GABA transaminase, has been recommended for studying [^{3}H]GABA uptake sites (see Iversen and Schon 1973); however, it does not appear particularly useful for achieving selective radioautographic demonstration of GABA neurons, since it also slows down the glial degradation of this amino acid.

4.3. HISTOLOGICAL PROCESSING

Rationale of chemical fixation

Whereas light-microscopic radioautography can be performed on frozen or freeze-dried tissue sections (e.g. Masuoka et al. 1971; Hökfelt and Ljungdahl 1971a,b, 1972b; Baughman and Bader 1977; Bagnoli et al. 1981), chemical fixation is really a must for electron-microscopic radioautography (see Section 4.2, under 'Electron-microscopic radioautography'). Even for light-microscopic studies, chemical fixation should be preferred whenever possible (i.e. when compatible with in situ retention of tracer molecules), in order to maintain the tissue in the best possible state of cytological and ultrastructural integrity. In some cases, the fixative may even serve as a rinsing medium capable of extracting 'undesirable' molecules such as labeled precursors and/or metabolites (see Descarries and Dupin 1974).

The physiochemical reactions leading to the retention of transmitters by the major fixatives are not fully understood. It is well established that, in test tube experiments, DA, NA, A and 5-HT react to form insoluble precipitates with strong metallic oxidants such as osmium tetroxide and potassium permanganate (Van Orden et al. 1966; Hökfelt and Jonsson 1968). DA, NA and 5-HT, but not A, are also precipitated in test tubes by glutaraldehyde (Wood and Barrnett 1964; Coupland et al. 1964; Coupland and Hopwood 1966) but not by formaldehyde fixatives (Hopsu and Makinnen 1966). The reaction with glutaraldehyde appears to leave intact the reducing power of the biogenic amines and is therefore compatible with their subsequent oxidation by postfix-atives (Bloom 1970; see also Hökfelt and Ljungdahl 1972a).

It is not known to what extent the radicals involved in cross-linkage and precipitation of biogenic amines in test tubes are in fact free and available for such reactions to occur in tissue. Besides, there are paradoxes in the observed retention of biogenic amines after in vitro or in vivo tissue labeling. For example, primary fixation with potassium permanganate, which demonstrates electron-dense cores in synaptic vesicles of peripheral and some central monoaminergic nerve terminals (Richardson 1966; Hökfelt and Jonsson 1968), is notoriously inefficient for the radioautographic detection of ex-ogenous [^{3}H]DA or [^{3}H]NA accumulated in catecholaminergic neurons (Descarries and Droz 1968; Taxi 1969). Conventional fixation with glutaraldehyde, which readily and efficiently retains [^{3}H]DA, [^{3}H]NA, [^{3}H]A or [^{3}H]5-HT taken up in axon ter-minals of the peripheral autonomic nervous system, does not succeed in doing so after [^{3}H]DA or [^{3}H]A uptake by catecholaminergic axon terminals of the CNS (see Section 4.3, under 'Special fixation procedures'; and Section 5.1, under 'Catecholamine neurons'). Those observations have led to the notion that, in vivo, fixatives might in fact react with macromolecular complexes in which the various biogenic amines are more or less tightly bound rather than directly with the biogenic amines themselves (Descarries and Droz 1970a). Upon disruption of this binding by fixation, some amines could be displaced to some extent from their 'natural' locations prior to precipitation and/or cross-linkage in new 'artefactual' sites and/or be washed out from tissue. Amino acid transmitters will also be retained in tissue by glutaraldehyde, presumably through cross-linking of their amino groups by the dialdehyde (Peters and Ashley 1967; Bergeron and Droz 1968). The usefulness of glutaraldehyde fixation for retaining ex-ogenous GABA was first recognized by Orkand and Kravitz (1971) in their study of the localization of [^{3}H]GABA at crustacean nerve muscle junctions. In model test tube ex-periments, they showed that [^{3}H]GABA could be covalently attached to proteins such as bovine serum albumin by glutaraldehyde exposure. A similar conclusion was reach-ed for glycine by Price et al. (1976), who demonstrated that this amino acid was TCA soluble and hence free in fresh tissue but largely precipitated with proteins by TCA after glutaraldehyde fixation. As already mentioned, it is the absence of such 'binding' by fixative which in the case of choline or ACh prevents their radioautographic visualization in fixed tissue.

Choice of a fixative

The choice of the primary fixative appears determinant for the eventual retention of labeled molecules. In the case of catecholamines, this stands out from the work of Devine and Laverty (1968), who demonstrated that after peripheral tissue incubation with [^{3}H]NA and immersion fixation into various solutions, the bulk of lost radioac-tivity was recovered into the primary fixative. From a comparison between osmium tetroxide, aldehydes and potassium permanganate, these authors concluded that aldehyde fixation with glutaraldehyde or a mixture of glutaraldehyde-formaldehyde was the most suitable for radioautographic studies on catecholamines. The same is true in CNS, where glutaraldehyde fixation has proven necessary for preserving exogenous catecholamines in tissue (Descarries and Droz 1970a).

Radiochemical determinations have been performed to assess quantitatively the ability of fixatives to retain exogenous biogenic amines incorporated in PNS or CNS tissue. Thus, in various peripheral organs incubated in vitro with [^{3}H]NA and fixed by immersion in a mixture of 2% glutaraldehyde and 2% formaldehyde in phosphate buffer, Devine and Laverty (1968) reported a retention of 40-60% of the radioactivity. In newborn rat brain, immersion of slices in 3.5% glutaraldehyde fixative resulted in 56% retention at a time when 70% of total brain [^{3}H] corresponded to [^{3}H]NA itself (Descarries and Dupin 1974). This proportion fell to 30% when 59% of the tracer was in the form of labeled metabolites. Since some metabolites such as [^{3}H]normetanephrine are known to be cross-linked by glutaraldehyde fixation, these experiments suggested that at least 75% of [^{3}H]NA was retained by glutaraldehyde fixation. The use of glutaraldehyde also appears to favor the retention of [^{3}H]5-HT in both peripheral organs and in the CNS. Gershon and Ross (1966) demonstrated the advantage of using glutaraldehyde over formalin for retaining [^{3}H]5-HT into various organs of mice injected with [^{3}H]5-HTP. Using hypertonic diluent buffer solutions and osmium postfixation, they found that 92.5% of the radioactivity could be kept in tissue. In the CNS, Descarries et al. (1975) reported that 80% of the radioactivity was retained in cerebral cortex superfused with [^{3}H]5-HT and fixed with 3.5% glutaraldehyde at a time when 59% of the tracer was in the form of [^{3}H]5-HT itself.

In the case of GABA, it has been shown by Iversen and Bloom (1972) that 65% of the total radioactivity incorporated in brain slices and homogenates was retained by immersion fixation in 5% glutaraldehyde. Schon and Iversen (1972) reported a proportion of 50% following in vivo perfusion with the same fixative. After [^{3}H]GABA injection in rat olfactory bulb, Halasz et al. (1979) compared the amount of radioactivity present in the whole bulb after a vascular rinse with tyrode solution or a rinse followed by fixation with glutaraldehyde at high concentration. They found that 46% of the radioactivity was retained by fixation at a time when 67% of the total radioactivity represented [^{3}H]GABA itself. In spinal cord perfused with a mixture of 4% paraformaldehyde and 0.5% glutaraldehyde, Ribeiro-Da-Silva and Coimbra (1980) reported a retention of 29%.

With [^{3}H]glycine, Iversen and Bloom (1972) measured a retention of 87% of the radioactivity in spinal cord homogenates fixed by immersion in 5% glutaraldehyde. For glutamate, 50% of the total radioactivity was retained in slices of rat hippocampal formation fixed in 5% glutaraldehyde solution at a time when 85% was known to correspond to this amino acids (Storm-Mathisen and Iversen 1979). With synaptosomal preparations, fixation of suspensions resulted in better retention than pellet fixation and yielded values in the order of 40% (Beart 1976a).

There is of course a great deal of qualitative evidence based on radioautography itself regarding the ability of fixatives to retain transmitters in situ. In this respect, it is of interest that the cellular localizations observed after fixation have sometimes been compared to those in frozen unfixed specimens by means of 'dry' radioautographic techniques. This has been done with the biogenic amines [^{3}H]NA and [^{3}H]5-HT in both the PNS and CNS (see refs in Section 5.1), and also with [^{3}H]GABA and [^{3}H]glycine in the cerebellum and spinal cord (Hökfelt and Ljungdahl 1970, 1971a).

Special fixation procedures

The radioautographic labeling of central DA nerve terminals with either [^{3}H]DA or [^{3}H]NA poses a particular problem. Conventional CNS perfusion with glutaraldehyde followed by immersion of tissue slices in glutaraldehyde solution prior to postfixation with osmium tetroxide has long given deceptive results in rat neostriatum, the region richest in DA nerve ending. The initial studies of Reivich and Glowinski (1967), Aghajanian and Bloom (1967b), Lenn (1967) and Fuxe et al. (1968) after intraventricular administration of [³H]NA, clearly indicated a preferential retention of the radioactivity in the paraventricular caudate-putamen ipsilateral to the ventricle injected. However, neither of these studies, nor those of Descarries and Droz (1968a, 1970a,b) showed clear-cut accumulations of radioactivity into DA nerve endings. Subsequently, observations on the localization of [³H]DOPA, [³H]DA or [³H]NA in rat and duck median eminence (refs in Section 5.1, under 'Catecholamine neurons') have suggested that axon terminals clearly labeled in this region were those of noradrenergic rather than dopaminergic neurons. The clearest negative observations regarding the detection of DA terminals were those of Calas et al. (1976), who found only a diffuse labeling in cat caudate nucleus superfused in vivo with [³H]DA or [³H]NA. In a later study, Arluison et al. (1978) had to resort to a statistical analysis of silver grain distribution to try and identify those axon terminals which should have taken up [³H]DA in high concentration after its administration directly into brain. The most likely explanation for these results was that the tracer had been displaced and subsequently redistributed in tissue at the time of fixation, perhaps due to weak in vivo binding of [³H]DA or [³H]NA into DA nerve terminals (see Descarries et al. 1980).

In any event, two fixation procedures were recently developed to circumvent this methodological problem (see also Section 5.1, under 'Catecholamine neurons'). Descarries et al. (1980, 1981b) found that vascular perfusion of an osmium tetroxide solution immediately after brief perfusion of the primary glutaraldehyde fixative (see Section 8.2.1) led to clear-cut detection of [³H]DA or [³H]NA accumulations over a great number of axon terminals of the neostriatum (Fig. 8). They demonstrated the dopaminergic nature of these labeled endings by showing their absence in animals whose nigro-striatal DA system had been previously destroyed by intranigral administration of 6-hydroxydopamine. Rapid perfusion in succession of both glutaraldehyde and osmium fixatives was similarly effective in maintaining [³H]A accumulated within CA neurons and some indolamine terminals of CNS (see Section 5.1, under 'Localization of [³H]adrenaline'), whereas no such accumulations could be observed following standard histological procedures (Bosler and Descarries 1982). Another satisfactory answer to the problem of detecting [³H]DA accumulations in CNS dopaminergic terminals was devised by Nguyen-Legros et al. (1983). These authors were able to visualize clear-cut reactions in specimens incubated in vitro with [³H]DA or [³H]NA, when primary fixation was carried out by brief immersion in glutaraldehyde followed by postfixation with osmic vapors instead of osmium tetroxide in solution (Fig. 9).

4.4. RADIOAUTOGRAPHIC PROCESSING

Procedures for preparing light- and electron-microscopic radioautographs from fixed nervous tissue are not different from those used with other biological specimens. The following sections deal only with some of their practicalities which the authors have found of particular value for investigating transmitter-specific neurons. Some technical details have also been included in the figure legends.

Light-microscopic radioautography

Standard protocols for the preparation of light-microscope radioautographs from frozen or paraffin- or resin-embedded specimens generally involve coating of histological sections by dipping into molten emulsion (for refs see Section 8.3). In our laboratories, 20 μm-thick frozen sections or 5 μm-thick paraffin-embedded sections are routinely used for mapping purposes. These may be cut serially from the whole brain and mounted at regular intervals for topographic studies or systematic anatomical sampling (Figs 1 and 2). Series of whole brain sections are also prepared when searching for labeled nerve cell bodies or axon terminals in axonal transport studies.

Significant benefits may be derived from using light-microscopic radioautographs processed from thick (~ 1 mm) brain slabs embedded flat in resin (see Section 8.2.2 and Fig. 4). Three to five μm-thick sections may be cut from such slices, allowing for systematic radioautographic examination of a whole rat brain in a relatively small number of sections. This sampling technique has the additional advantage of showing all possible anatomical landmarks for correlation with stereotaxic atlases prior to carving out smaller blocks for subsequent processing of high resolution radioautographs. An alternative technique offering similar advantages although lesser resolution is the cutting of alternate regular (20 μm) and thick (100—200 μm) sections of aldehyde fixed brains on a vibratome. The former can be processed for light-microscopy after defatting, and the latter postfixed by immersion and then flat-embedded in resin for electron-microscopic radioautography.

Thinner sections may be prepared from small blocks of Epon-embedded material when the best possible resolution is required at light-microscopic level (see Section 8.1.1 and Figs 3 and 5—11). A thickness of 1 μm or less ensures that all sites of tracer accumulation are actually detected and are thus amenable to quantification (see Section 4.5, under 'Achieving integral labeling').

Little use has so far been made of dry-coating techniques for the light-microscopic radioautography of transmitter-specific neurons (but see Sections 4.3, under 'Choice of a fixative', 5.1, 5.3 and Fig. 11). Such procedures should nevertheless find increasing applications for detecting water soluble molecules, such as [3H]choline or [3H]acetylcholine.

Light-microscopic radioautographs are generally developed with standard, commercially available chemical products such as Kodak Dektol or D-19 (see also Section 8.1.1). Exposure times will have to be adjusted according to the amount and localization of the radioactivity contained in the specimen. For instance, short periods of exposure (1—2 days) may provide a good signal-to-noise ratio when dealing with labeled neurons at or near sites of intracerebral injections. Conversely, durations of 6—8 weeks may be required to detect axonally-transported material. As a rule, appropriate exposures will range between 1 and 4 weeks. Longer periods should be allowed in the case of plastic-embedded as compared with frozen or paraffin-embedded sections because of greater self-absorption.

30% sodium thiosulfate is commonly used as photographic fixer. When using sections mounted on gelatinized slides, commercial fixers are preferable since they contain a hardener that will prevent softening of the gelatin support and thus improve adhesion of both sections and developed emulsion to the slides. It is also advisable to stain light-microscopic preparations after radioautographic processing, to avoid the negative chemography which may occur with certain basic dyes.

Electron-microscopic radioautography

Owing to the difficulties and limitations of cryo-ultramicrotomy and of its combination with radioautography, ultrastructural studies of transmitter-specific neurons have always been carried out on fixed nervous tissue. Techniques for the preparation of electron-microscopic radioautographs have been extensively described in several publications (for refs, see Section 8.3.3). In brief (see also Section 8.1.2), ribbons of thin (silver/gold) sections are taken from resin blocks retrimmed according to the results of previous light-microscope radioautographic examinations. These thin sections are deposited on celloidinized slides, stained with lead or doubly stained with uranyl acetate and lead, vaporized with carbon (to prevent destaining and/or negative chemography and ensure the stability of sections under the electron beam) and coated by dipping in much the same way as light-microscopic radioautographs. Exposures are invariably much longer: durations approximately 10 times those providing clear-cut signals in light-microscopic radioautographs of 1 μm-thick sections are generally needed. More or less sensitive photographic developers can be chosen. Some authors have favored the use of Phenidon (Lettré and Pawelets 1966) which allies fair sensitivity to the production of small spherical silver grains easily distinguishable from one another. For detailed scrutiny of fine structures, development with paraphenylenediamine (Caro and Van Tubergen 1962), although requiring longer duration of exposure because of low sensitivity, produces fewer, thin silver grain filaments which do not mask ultrastructural detail (compare Figs 14—19 to 12 and 13). Furthermore, the use of this developer enhances the signal-to-noise ratio, when tracer accumulations have to be detected in the presence of a fairly high amount of background radioactivity, as is often the case after intracerebral administration. When the highest possible sensitivity is desirable, as in axonal transport experiments, D-19 or Microdol-X will be utilized.

In view of the lengthy periods of exposure generally needed for electron-microscopic radioautography, it is advisable to prepare several sets of thin-sections from the same blocks and to use some as tests prior to final development. It should be emphasized that rigorous comparison of labeling intensity from one experiment to another requires simultaneous processing of electron- as well as light-microscope radioautographs. Lastly, since electron-microscopic radioautographs are particularly fragile under the electron beam, they should be collected on square meshed- rather than slit-grids for examination, even if this entails complications in the eventual recognition of labeled profiles in serial sections.

4.5. REQUIREMENTS FOR RELIABLE INTERPRETATION

In contrast to whole body or whole organ 'macroscopic' radioautography, which essentially reveals the overall density of labeling exhibited by different anatomical regions of the nervous system (e.g. Masuoka and Alcaraz 1975; Hespe et al. 1969), light- and electron-microscopic radioautography demonstrates patterns of silver grain distribution which may be ascribed to cellular constituents. The reactivity of transmitter-labeled neurons takes the form of more or less dense aggregates of silver grains superimposed over nerve cell bodies, their processes and axon terminals. In the present context, establishing the specificity of these radioautographic signals implies demonstrating the transmitter identity of their cellular sites of origin. It is only when this crucial issue is satisfactorily resolved that the information gathered on topographical and cytological features or on the intracellular localization of transmitters assumes its full significance.

Demonstration of specificity

In many radioautographic experiments, and especially those carried out in vivo, the use

314

of transmitter concentrations in the range of the Km of high-affinity uptake processes proves incompatible with the production of clear-cut radioautographic signals. Higher concentrations have to be used, which are known to trigger low-affinity uptake mechanisms in vitro. Low-affinity uptake should not often result in signals of an intensity and/or selectivity comparable to those produced by high-affinity uptake. However, the mere fact that it may be involved warrants strict specificity controls.

The first argument in favor of labeling specificity is the cellular distribution of the radioautographic signals. Selective localization, however, does not in itself constitute a proof of specificity. Indeed, selective but nonspecific labeling may be observed in neurons having taken up a transmitter different from but akin to their own. An obvious example is the reactivity of NA neurons in the peripheral autonomic system to tritiated DA or A, or that of DA or NA neurons of CNS towards one or the other of the catecholamines (see Section 5.1). Such labeling, however, is best interpreted as 'interspecific', in view of the common synthesis and uptake capacities of the neurons implicated. A similar situation is that of CA and 5-HT neurons which may at times take up each other's biogenic amine (see Section 2.2, under 'Uptake of neurotransmitters'). Thus, 5-HT axon terminals of rat neocortex have been shown to accumulate DA in vitro (Berger et al. 1978); nerve cell bodies of 5-HT neurons in the nucleus raphe dorsalis of the cat have been labeled with [^{3}H]NA after intracerebral injection (Léger et al. 1978); 5-HT axon terminals in the supraependymal plexus or subcommissural organ of the rat accumulate [^{3}H]A after intraventricular administration (Bosler and Descarries 1983). The inverse situation of PNS or CNS CA neurons labeled with [^{3}H]5-HT has also been reported, e.g. in the case of perivascular nerve endings around cerebral arteries (Chan-Palay 1976a), DA nerve cell bodies in the hypothalamus (Chan-Palay 1977b; Beaudet and Descarries 1979), and NA nerve cell bodies in cat locus ceruleus (Léger et al. 1978).

In this context, it is understandable that establishing the transmitter-identity of CNS neurons labeled in radioautographs will call for every possible correlation with the data from other complementary methods. Obviously, demonstration of specificity will be made much easier in the case of transmitter-defined systems already visualized by histofluorescence and/or immunocytochemistry, which will allow for comparisons between patterns of nerve cell bodies and/or axon terminal distributions. Even then, seemingly 'nonspecific' radioautographic labeling patterns may yet involve so-called specific high-affinity uptake mechanisms. Thus, after intraventricular administration of [^{3}H]GABA in the rat, strong reactivity of the supraependymal 5-HT plexus has been reported by Belin et al. (1980), which was abolished by a GABA high-affinity uptake inhibitor but not by concomitant administration of a 10-fold higher concentration of non-radioactive 5-HT. A possible interpretation for this type of result is the coexistence of two transmitters and of their respective uptake and binding mechanisms in the same neurons, as is apparently the case for some nerve cell bodies in nucleus raphe dorsalis which take [^{3}H]GABA and exhibit both 5-HT and GAD-like immunoreactivity (Gamrani et al. 1979; Belin et al. 1979, 1983; Nanopoulos et al. 1981, 1982).

On the other hand, other neurons appear to selectively accumulate substances which they do not use as transmitters but which could be normally released as such in their immediate environment and for which they are likely to possess receptors. This might explain the labeling of non-GABAergic neurons reported after administration of [^{3}H]muscimol (Yazulla and Brecha 1980) or that of non-catecholaminergic nerve cell bodies in the paraventricular nucleus of the thalamus, an area richly innervated by PNMT-immunoreactive terminals (Hökfelt et al. 1973, 1974), which follows intraventricular injection of [^{3}H]adrenaline (Bosler and Descarries 1983).

These examples stress the importance of using more than topographic correlations as specificity controls. Additional evidence may be gathered from correlative biochemical experiments involving, for instance, measurements of endogenous transmitter levels and/or of biosynthetic enzymes activity; pharmacological experiments using uptake blockers or non-radioactive compounds at high concentration to compete with predictable nonspecific or 'interspecific' uptake systems; lesioning experiments involving the use of cytotoxic drugs or electrocoagulation for destroying, more or less selectively, a given transmitter-identified system and thus verifying the disappearance of all observed reactions attributed to the corresponding tracer (see examples in Section 5). In this regard, 6-hydroxydopamine lesioning of the CA neurons, with or without concomitant treatment with desipramine to protect the NA system, has proven particularly useful for demonstrating the specificity of reactions observed after intracerebral administration of [^{3}H]DA (Descarries et al. 1980, 1981b), [^{3}H]NA (Descarries and Lapierre 1973a,b), [^{3}H]A (Bosler and Descarries 1983) or [^{3}H]5-HT (Descarries et al. 1975). Similarly, cytotoxic dihydroxytryptamines, with or without desipramine cotreatment (Baraban and Aghajanian 1981; Wiklund et al. 1981), or else electrolytic destruction of the midbrain raphe nuclei (Descarries et al. 1975), have been utilized to verify the specificity of reactions observed with [^{3}H]5-HT.

Obviously, the most direct demonstration of specificity will be achieved whenever it is possible to detect simultaneously a biosynthetic enzyme and/or endogenous transmitter together with accumulated tracer inside the same neurons (Chan-Palay 1979; Pickel et al. 1981). The techniques permitting such demonstrations will be all the more interesting in that they should also allow for the visualization of more than one transmitter in a given nerve cell or for the identification of two different types of transmitter-specific neurons in the same tissue sections (see Section 6).

Achieving integral labeling

Both qualitative and quantitative radioautographic analysis of chemically-defined neurons will require not only confirmation of labeling specificity, but also demonstration that all elements of the system investigated are detected in the material under consideration (see also Section 3.1). Obviously, this is indispensable for the gathering of reliable quantitative topographic or morphometric data at either the light- or electron-microscopic levels; what is less evident is that it is also necessary for qualitative analysis, and especially for the recognition of characteristic features at the electron-microscopic level. Indeed, the aspect of a given chemical type may not be very different in thin sections from that of their homologues containing other transmitters. Characterization of the shape, content and/or interrelationships of axon terminals may require extensive sampling in serial thin sections, so as to take into account variability of appearance from one thin section to another, as well as rigorous comparisons between labeled and unlabeled profiles (e.g. Descarries et al. 1975, 1977). Evidently, neither of these strategies will be applicable if many of the profiles to be characterized go unnoticed among comparable elements in their immediate vicinity and/or from one section to another. In this respect, and within the limits imposed by specificity, two kinds of experimental controls have proved particularly valuable, especially when used in combination. The first was to examine tissue prepared after the administration of widely different concentrations of tracer, the second, to use widely different periods of radioautographic exposure. When a plateau is reached in the number of labeled sites detected after decoupling the molarity of tracer administered and/or doubling the duration of radioautographic exposure, for example, it may be assumed that a vast majority if not all elements of the type to be examined have been identified.

Assigning silver grains to cellular constituents

As explained in Section 2.1, the efficiency and resolution of light- and electron-microscopic radioautography is generally sufficient to permit clear distinction between labeled and unlabeled histological elements and thus achieve their cytological identification. Most often, this will only require careful examination of the preparations and/or direct scoring of the silver grains. There are cases, however, where statistical analyses of silver grain distributions become the only means to accurately identify the real sites of labeling. This may happen even at the light-microscopic level, when small and adjacent elements are likely to be involved (e.g. thin glial ensheathings and/or axon terminals apposed to cell bodies) and to give rise to significant cross-labeling (see Storm-Mathisen and Iversen 1979). It is also the rule at the subcellular level, where organelles of small size, intermingled in the cytoplasm, need to be distinguished as eventual sources of labeling.

The principle of currently available methods of silver grain distribution analysis is to compare the actual distribution of silver grains to that which would have arisen from the very same material had it contained uniformly or randomly distributed radioactivity. Stereological techniques of silver grain sampling have been devised that take into account the isotope, section thickness, type of emulsion and developer in use for investingating various subcellular items as possible sources of labeling (for refs, see Section 8.3). Considering these single items or various combinations thereof as eventual sites of silver grain localization, the 'real' grain distribution may be compared to that of an 'hypothetical' grain distribution corresponding to a random scatter of punctual radioactive sources in the same material. When differences are detected between the two distributions, it is assumed that some sources have a higher 'specific activity' than others and a matching program is utilized to find the relative values which will result in the best fit based on a recalculation of hypothetical grain distributions. Admittedly, this technique provides only a relative index of the labeling intensity of the subcellular sources (e.g. Descarries et al. 1982). It should nevertheless become increasingly useful for comparing the intracellular distributions of different transmitters within given cell types.

Nature of molecules detected

Determining the nature of tracer molecules giving rise to the different labeling patterns observed in radioautographs is essential for gathering information on the cellular utilization of transmitters. In CNS tissue, intraneuronal accumulations are generally detected over a weak ubiquitous reactivity in background, which reflects tracer diffusion from nearby sites of administration, transmitter release after local uptake, formation of extraneuronal metabolites and/or displacement and relocation of accumulated molecules at the time of fixation. For the purpose of distinguishing between these various factors, radiochemical determinations can be carried out on unfixed tissue and/or subcellular fractions and correlated with measurements of radioactivity retained after fixation. Evaluation of the amounts of radioactivity retained after fixation according to the proportion of transmitter or of metabolites present in tissue (see Section 4.3, under 'Choice of a fixative') gives some indication of their eventual participation in the observed reactions. However, such measurements do not discriminate between intraneuronally accumulated and more diffusely located molecules. This will require control radioautographic experiments with analogues taken up intraneuronally but not metabolized or, on the contrary, with the labeled metabolites themselves (see examples in Section 5). Treatments with specific uptake inhibitors or depleting drugs will exclude the remote possibility of artefactual intraneuronal accumulations. After administration of precursors, control experiments with specific blockers of transmitter uptake or biosynthesis will allow to distinguish between intraneuronal accumulation of the precursors themselves rather than of their end-product. It is only in axonal transport experiments that exclusive localization to nerve cell bodies or axon terminals will permit direct biochemical identification after in vivo labeling (e.g. Font et al. 1982).

Significant versus artefactual intraneuronal localizations

The fact remains that intraneuronal distribution of accumulated transmitter molecules can only be analyzed in fixed tissue and that the eventuality of an intracellular localization which may thus be purely artificial can never be totally excluded. Little can be done to go beyond this interpretative limit except perhaps to compare intraneuronal distributions between neurons known to make use of the transmitter in question and others of the same region into which it has presumably penetrated by diffusion only. If this comparison shows important preferences in relative affinity of the tracer for some organelles of the neurons using the transmitter, these can be safely assumed to intervene in its utilization. On the contrary, organelles found to have comparable affinities, whether the cells normally use the transmitter or not, are likely to represent artefactual sites of localization (e.g. Descarries et al. 1982).

5. CONTRIBUTIONS OF THE RADIOAUTOGRAPHIC APPROACH

5.1. MONOAMINE NEURONS

Owing to the early recognition of their reuptake and storage capacities, monoamine-containing neurons were the first to be visualized by radioautography in both the PNS and CNS. In fact, the pioneering investigations of Samorajski and Marks (1962; see also Marks et al. 1962) and Wolfe et al. (1962) after systemic administration of [^{3}H]NA, and those of Aghajanian and Bloom after cerebroventricular injection of ([^{3}H]NA (1966, 1967a) or of [^{3}H]5-HT (1967b), were primarily intended at demonstrating such properties at the cellular level (see also Reivich and Glowinski 1967 and Lenn 1967). It was immediately realized, however, that the radioautographic detection of neuronal sites of labeled exogenous amine accumulation, which allowed their electron- as well as light-microscopic examination, might yield unprecedented information on the distribution, morphological features and cytofunctional properties of monoaminergic neurons.

Comparison of radioautographic labeling patterns with the results of fluorescence histochemistry was soon to confirm the validity of the radioautographic approach. Thus, by combining these two techniques, Gillespie and Kirpekar (1966) found that [^{3}H]NA was accumulated in adrenergic nerve terminals of the cat spleen. Masuoka and Placidi (1968; see also 1970; and Masuoka et al. 1971) and Hökfelt and Ljungdahl (1971b; see also 1972a) demonstrated an identical localization of [^{3}H]NA and of endogenous fluorescent NA to the same postganglionic nerves in heart and iris tissues. In CNS, similar findings were reported by Fuxe et al. (1968) on NA- and 5-HT-containing nerve cell bodies and axons terminals which were respectively labeled after intraventricular injections of [^{3}H]NA and [^{3}H]5-HT in various regions of the brain in normal or reserpine-nialamide pretreated rats. While subsequent radioautographic data obtained on fixed tissue eventually revealed interesting exceptions to this rule (see Section 3.1, under 'Topographic distribution', and Section 5.1, under 'Serotonin neurons'), it generally withstood the test of time and even gained further support from the correlations which could later be made with the detailed topographic data of immunohistochemistry.

Catecholamine neurons

(a) Studies in the peripheral nervous system

CA neurons of the PNS were mostly investigated at electron-microscopic level and after systemic administration of [^{3}H]NA. The initial report of Wolfe et al. (1962) revealing tracer accumulation into sympathetic axons of rat pineal gland exhibiting granular synaptic vesicles was rapidly followed by more extensive studies on this and other sympathetically innervated organs. Thus, Taxi and Droz (1966a) confirmed the localization of [^{3}H]NA to nerve fibers containing small dense-core vesicles in the pineal gland (see also Budd and Salpeter 1969), demonstrated similar labeling in the vas deferens (Taxi and Droz 1966b), and described nerve terminals which selectively concentrated [^{3}H]NA but failed to exhibit small dense-core vesicles in the intestinal submucosa and in the Auerbach's and Meissner's plexuses, at least in osmium- or glutaraldehyde and osmium-fixed tissue (Taxi and Droz 1966b). Comparable labeling patterns were reported by the same authors after administration of [^{3}H]DA, [^{3}H]A or the false transmitter [^{3}H]metaraminol (Taxi and Droz 1967; see also 1969; and Taxi 1969), but not after injection of the O-methylated metabolite of catecholamines [^{3}H]normetanephrine (Taxi and Droz 1969). These finding documented the avidity of peripheral noradrenergic neurons for molecules akin to their endogenous transmitter, and indicated that a major extraneuronal metabolite of NA did not significantly participate in their radioautographic labeling. Another important contribution of Taxi and Droz was to demonstrate effects of drugs on the storage of [^{3}H]NA. Thus, after reserpine treatment, they found that disappearance of the electron-density of small synaptic vesicles in axon terminals of the vas deferens was associated with their failure to accumulate [^{3}H]NA (Taxi and Droz 1969; see also Taxi 1969). Furthermore, in keeping with prior observations by Descarries and Droz (1968a,b) in the CNS, they showed that pretreatment of the animals with an inhibitor of monoamine oxidase resulted not only in an increased intensity of the [^{3}H]NA labeling of postganglionic adrenergic terminals, but also in a strong and ubiquitous reactivity of their parent nerve cell bodies, as exemplified in the superior cervical ganglion (Taxi and Droz 1969; see also Taxi 1976). Interestingly, Taxi (1973) later reported that, in non-pretreated rats, the same nerve cell bodies would exhibit radioautographic labeling restricted to clusters of small granular vesicles occupying a subsurface position in both the perikaryon and proximal dendrites.

Another group of electron-microscopic investigations dealt with perivascular nerve endings labeled with [^{3}H]NA in various peripheral organs such as rat intestine and mesentary (Devine 1967; Devine and Simpson 1968) and the pancreas of the cat (Lever et al. 1968). In this latter location and in the nictitating membrane muscle of the cat, Graham et al. (1968) and Esterhuizen et al. (1968) succeeded in combining radio-autography with acetylcholinesterase histochemistry on the same tissue sections to find a lack of acetylcholinesterase activity in the fibers labeled with [³H]NA.

Later radioautographic reports on noradrenergic neurons of the PNS were essentially concerned with the problem of the axonal migration of catecholamines. Following a brief description by Geffen et al. (1971) of intra-axonal labeling in the dilated proximal portions of constricted splenic nerves after [³H]NA injections in the celiac ganglion of cat, Sotelo and Taxi (1973; see also Taxi and Sotelo 1972, 1973; and Sotelo 1975) carried out more extensive investigations on ligated rat sciatic nerve after intravenous administration of [³H]NA. Both sets of experiments infirmed an earlier hypothesis according to which axonally transported NA should have been sequestered in small vesicles preformed in the nerve cell bodies.

(b) Studies in the central nervous system

Although seminal, the initial electron-microscopic results obtained on CNS tissue after cerebroventricular or in vitro administration of [³H]NA were far from conclusive in terms of selective and meaningful identification of presumptive CA neurons. Little radioactivity was present in tissue and no silver grain aggregates indicative of preferential cellular accumulation could be demonstrated. The results therefore required statistical analysis, which was all the more difficult since silver grains corresponding to [³H]NA itself could hardly be differentiated from those arising from labeled metabolites.

In this regard, a major breakthrough was the systematic recourse to pretreatment with a monoamine oxidase inhibitor (Descarries and Droz 1968a,b), which not only increased the intensity of the observed radioautographic signals but also allowed some definition of the nature of the radioactivity giving them rise. Thus, nerve cell bodies and their proximal dendrites (Fig. 3) as well as axonal varicosities ('terminals'), i.e. small axonal enlargements filled with vesicular organelles (Figs 12, 13 and 15—18), could be unequivocally demonstrated to be the exclusive sites of strong silver grain accumulations often detectable in consecutive histological or thin section (Figs 12 and 13). Moreover, in view of complementary experiments indicating that there was no uptake of [³H]normetanephrine under these very same conditions, the inference could be drawn that intraneuronal accumulations detected after [³H]NA administration were indeed representative of this amine itself rather than its labeled metabolites (Descarries and Droz 1970a).

Catecholamine nerve cell bodies

It is in the locus ceruleus and in the substantia nigra, respectively, that CA nerve cell bodies were first labeled after intraventricular injection of [³H]NA in the rat (Descarries and Droz 1968a, 1970a,b; see also Bloom 1970 and Fig. 3). In the absence of monoamine oxidase inhibition, the half-life of the tracer within these cell bodies was estimated to be approximately 1 h, i.e. 4 times shorter than in labeled axon terminals (Descarries and Droz 1970a). With or without monoamine oxidase inhibition, the accumulated silver grains overlaid the nucleus as well as perikaryon and proximal dendrites, seemingly distributed at random between the various cytoplasmic organelles. Consequently, it was suggested that, inside CA neurons, exogenous NA could be bound in the form of (a) macromolecular (protein) complex(es) and not only packaged in vesicular organelles. In subsequent investigations, more attention was paid to eventual cytological characteristics of the DA neurons of rat substantia nigra identified after administration of [³H]DA or [³H]NA. Paradoxically, the reactions always appeared stronger after [³H]NA than [³H]DA administration (Parizek et al. 1971). Despite careful ultrastructural examination, however, Sotelo (1971) and Sotelo and Riche (1974) did not detect morphological attributes which might be considered typical of these DA neurons. Sotelo (1971) also showed the presence of nerve cell bodies labeled with [³H]NA in the area postrema of the rat, whereas Ehinger and Falck (1971) and Kramer et al. (1971) demonstrated [³H]DA-accumulating cells (presumably interplexiform DA neurons) in the rabbit and the cat retina. In subsequent studies, other central DA nerve cell bodies were identified with [³H]DA or [³H]NA, notably in the periventricular arcuate nucleus complex of the hypothalamus (Scott et al. 1976; see also Bosler and Calas 1982) and the glomerular layer of the olfactory bulb (Halasz et al. 1978; Priestly et al. 1979) in the rat. Just as the NA neurons of the locus ceruleus (Descarries and Havrankova 1970), the DA cells in the hypothalamus could also be labeled after cerebroventricular administration of [³H]L-DOPA (Scott et al. 1978a,b). In fact, it now appears probable that all DA and NA nerve cell bodies in the CNS are amenable to radioautographic visualization after administration of tritiated DA, NA or L-DOPA provided that they are accessible to these tracers. In this respect, Nowaczyk et al. (1978) pointed out that the use of the intraventricular and intracisternal routes of injection results in a differential labeling of the various CA nerve cell body groups, best accounted for by the dynamics of cerebrospinal fluid circulation.

Noradrenaline axon terminals

From the start, the selective radioautographic demonstration of central NA axon terminals (Figs 6, 12, 13 and 16) was facilitated by the fact that standard fixation techniques appeared incompatible with the detection of DA nerve endings (see Section 4.3, under 'Special fixation procedures'). This was already apparent in early radioautographic investigations of the neostriatum, where only diffuse albeit preferential regional labeling had been found after intraventricular injection of [³H]NA or [³H]DA (Aghajanian and Bloom 1966; Lenn 1967; Fuxe et al. 1968). In view of various observations suggesting that the binding of endogenous or exogenous NA and DA is relatively weak within dopaminergic nerve endings (see refs in Descarries et al. 1980, 1981b), this result appeared indicative of displacement and washout of [³H]NA or [³H]DA from their dopaminergic sites of uptake in the course of standard tissue fixation, as further suggested by negative findings on cat caudate nucleus superfused in vivo with either [³H]DA or [³H]NA (Calas et al. 1976). In several early studies with [³H]NA, strong evidence could also be gathered from pharmacological and lesioning experiments to rule out the eventuality that other cell types and particularly 5-HT neurons might take up exogenous CA in sufficient amount to induce signals as strong and selective as those which arose from NA varicosities (e.g. Descarries and Lapierre 1973a,b).

In this context, it is somewhat unfortunate that NA innervations were not characterized in a greater number of CNS regions. Chronologically, results were obtained only on nucleus paraventricularis hypothalami (Aghajanian and Bloom 1967b; see also Alonso 1981); substantia grisea periventricularis and the area of the locus ceruleus (Descarries and Droz 1968a,b, 1970a,b); cerebellum (Bloom et al. 1971); area postrema (Sotelo 1971); median eminence (Cuello and Iversen 1973; Scott et al. 1976; Calas 1977); cerebral cortex (Descarries and Lapierre 1973a,b; Nelson et al. 1973;

Descarries 1975; Descarries et al. 1977; Beaudet and Descarries 1978) and nucleus raphe dorsalis (Baraban and Aghajanian 1981), always in the rat. NA terminals of the median eminence were also examined in the duck by Calas (Calas 1972, 1973, 1975, 1977; Calas and Bosc 1976). It is beyond the scope of this review to summarize the cytological information gathered in these investigations (see Volume II). It should be pointed out, however, that the frontoparietal neocortex of adult rat remains the only CNS region where every effort was made to achieve not only specific but also global identification of the NA axon terminals, and where their structural features could therefore be extensively analyzed in serial thin sections (Descarries et al. 1977; also see Beaudet and Descarries 1978).

Dopamine axon terminals

The fact that radioautographic visualization of DA nerve endings remained so long problematic (see Section 4.3, under 'Special fixation procedures') probably accounts for the almost total lack of knowledge concerning their fine structural features in most regions of the CNS (see also Bosler 1980; Bosler and Calas 1982). Cuello and Iversen (1973) and Chetverukhin et al. (1979) were the only ones to claim radioautographic identification of DA axon terminals in the CNS using conventional techniques of tissue fixation. They detected [^{3}H]DA labeled varicosities in the external part of the rat median eminence, i.e. a region otherwise known to receive dense dopaminergic but only weak noradrenergic innervation. Similarly, Bosler and Calas (1982) have recently described localized tracer accumulations of [^{3}H]DA in the intermediate and neural lobes of the pituitary, where they are unlikely to represent noradrenergic varicosities only. These findings could imply that among the various dopaminergic subsystems, tubero-infundibular and hypophyseal neurons are endowed with special binding properties toward their transmitter. Paradoxically, it has also been reported that the uptake capacity of these subclasses of DA neurons is weaker than that of DA terminals in other parts of CNS (Demarest and Moore 1979).

In any event, it is the rapid double perfusion with both a primary glutaraldehyde fixative and an osmium tetroxide postfixative, proposed by Descarries et al. (1980, 1981b), which has made it possible to achieve the first indisputable radioautographic identification of dopaminergic axonal varicosities in mammalian CNS (Fig. 8). Clearcut labeling of these nerve endings was observed in the neostriatum after intraventricular injection of [^{3}H]DA or [^{3}H]NA, and the proof of their dopaminergic identity was provided by demonstrating their total absence in animals previously subjected to selective 6-hydroxydopamine lesioning of the nigrostriatal system. Preliminary examination of other brain regions already suggests that this technique will also yield results on other DA innervations and facilitate the detection of [^{3}H]DA or [^{3}H]NA in the tubero-infundibular DA system (Bosler and Descarries, unpublished). Admittedly, the fact that DA and NA elements are simultaneously visualized in the doubly-perfused specimens raises problems of its own in terms of distinguishing between these two types of catecholaminergic neurons. However, comparison of results obtained with and without this type of tissue processing and/or before and after lesioning of the ascending noradrenergic systems, should help to resolve this issue.

Another interesting approach for the study of DA nerve terminals has been the rapid fixation of tissue slices with glutaraldehyde followed by their postfixation with osmic acid vapors (Nguyen-Legros et al. 1979, 1981; Fig. 9). This has enabled these authors to visualize specifically-labeled dopaminergic nerve endings in several regions of the rat brain (frontal and supragenual cortex, neostriatum, septum) after in vitro incubation with [³H]DA or [³H]NA in the presence of desipramine. This procedure appears particularly suitable for the acquisition of quantitative topographic information, which would hardly be obtainable after intraventricular, topical or local administration of [³H]DA or [³H]NA in vivo.

(c) Localization of [³H]adrenaline

Until recently, radioautographic studies aimed at the identification of NA and/or DA neurons did not take into account the possibility that presumed adrenergic neurons of the CNS be labeled interspecifically by [³H]NA or [³H]DA and therefore simultaneously detected. Nor had it been investigated whether [³H]A would in fact be taken up and retained in presumed adrenergic or other monoaminergic neurons of the CNS. In tissue fixed with standard perfusion technique after intraventricular administration of [³H]A, no selective neuronal accumulations showed up in rat CNS (Bosler and Descarries 1983). In contrast, when both glutaraldehyde fixation and osmium postfixation were carried out by rapid perfusion in sequence, reactive nerve cell bodies and axon terminals with a distribution corresponding to that of DA and/or NA elements were visualized in several paraventricular and paracisternal regions of the brain (Fig. 17). In addition, nerve cell bodies of unknown chemical identity in n. paraventricular thalami and serotoninergic axon terminals of the supraependymal plexus and of the subcommissural organ were found to accumulate [³H]A (Bosler and Descarries 1982). Whether or not true adrenergic neurons were actually labeled could not be determined in these experiments, since NA and/or DA-containing elements are also known to be present in all CNS regions where PNMT-immunoreactive nerve cell bodies or axon terminals have thus far been visualized (Hökfelt et al. 1973, 1974).

(d) Newborn rat

There has been only one published report (Dupin et al. 1976) of attempts to label monoaminergic neurons in vivo at early stages of CNS development, even if it has long been known that in the rat, for example, the blood brain barrier remains relatively permeable to circulating biogenic amines untill about one week after birth. This study demonstrated the feasibility of achieving a radioautographic identification of CA nerve cell bodies (Fig. 2) and NA axonal varicosities in several regions of the newborn rat brain following intravenous administration of [³H]NA in animals pretreated with both a monoamine oxidase and a catechol-O-methyltransferase inhibitors. Further experimentation along those lines might help to resolve outstanding issues such as the type of interneuronal relationships established by growing NA and DA axons, and thus shed some light into their role during development.

(e) Tissue cultures

Early radioautographic studies with labeled monoamines in cultures were performed on organ cultures of chick sympathetic ganglia and demonstrated specific accumulation of [³H]DA and [³H]NA by nerve cell bodies and processes in their outgrowth (Burdman 1968). Uptake of [³H]NA was later described in axonal sprouts of superior cervical ganglia (Silberstein et al. 1972). Subsequent investigations were carried out on CNS explants of the medulla oblongata and pons from fetal and newborn rats (Hösli et al. 1975). Strong accumulation of [³H]NA was mainly observed in nerve fibers of

323

the outgrowth zone and a small proportion of their parent nerve cell bodies. In cerebellar cultures, uptake of [³H]NA was shown to be restricted to nerve fibers (Hösli and Hösli 1976a). Radioautography has more recently been used to identify neurons grown in monolayer or suspension cultures from dissociated fetal brain tissue (Di Porzio et al. 1980). Accumulation of [³H]DA or [³H]NA into nerve cell bodies and their fibers was examined in the presence of inhibitors of uptake by noradrenergic or dopaminergic neurons, to provide evidence on their respective identity. Further studies of the factors governing the morphological and biochemical development of these nerve cells should eventually benefit from the ability of radioautography to yield quantifiable cytological data and electron-microscopic results.

Serotonin neurons

(a) Studies with [³H]5-hydroxytryptophan

Most radioautographic investigations of mammalian 5-HT neurons were performed following in vivo administration of [³H]serotonin. A few studies, however, have relied on the utilization of the 5-HT precursor 5-hydroxytryptophan for achieving selective labeling of serotoninergic neurons. Thus, in rat CNS, a subpopulation of presumptive serotonin-containing raphe neurons was detected in light-microscope radioautographs following systemic administration of [³H]5-HTP, but only in animals pretreated with para-chlorophenylalanine, a blocker of 5-HT synthesis (Petitjean et al. 1981). In the pineal gland of the rat, [³H]5-hydroxytryptophan was shown to be taken up by pinealocytes and sympathetic nerve terminals (Taxi and Droz 1966b; Bak et al. 1970), both known to contain endogenous 5-HT (Bertler et al. 1964; Jaim-Etcheverry and Zieher 1968; Tilders et al. 1974). Similarly, [³H]5-hydroxytryptophan was found to be accumulated by the serotonin-containing rudimentary photoreceptors of the pineal gland in the parakeet (Collin et al. 1975, 1976; Juillard and Collin 1976), duck (Collin et al. 1976) and lizard (Meiniel et al. 1977). In the PNS, Gershon and Ross (1966) reported labeling of nerve cell bodies in the superior cervical ganglion and of axon terminals in the myenteric plexus, following intraperitoneal injection of [³H]5-hydroxytryptophan. Interestingly, small cells in the superior cervical ganglion have been shown to be serotonin-positive by histofluorescence (Eränkö and Härkönen 1965) and more recently by immunocytochemistry (Verhofstad et al. 1981), whereas the existence of intrinsic 5-HT neurons within the enteric nervous system is now well documented (see below). On the other hand, Taxi and Droz (1966a) have reported terminal labeling in the vas deferens after systemic injection of [³H]5-hydroxytryptophan: it remains to be determined whether these sympathetic nerve fibers, as in the pineal, also metabolize and store endogenous 5-HT.

(b) Studies with [³H]5-HT in the peripheral nervous system

As stated by Gershon (1981), 'the idea that serotonin is a neurotransmitter of peripheral as well as central neurons has evolved relatively recently'. Nevertheless, converging lines of evidence have now convincingly established the existence of intrinsic serotonin neurons in the gastrointestinal tract. These neurons have been studied in several species and in both developing and adult animals by light- and electron-microscopic radioautography, following incubation of gut tissue with [³H]5-HT in the presence of an excess of non-radioactive NA (for refs, see Gershon 1981). Interestingly, the perikaria of these enteric 5-HT neurons could loose their 5-HT uptake properties during development, having only been visualized by radioautography during embryologic stages (Gershon 1981). This might also explain why labeled nerve cell bodies had not been detected in the gut following intraperitoneal administration of [³H]5-HTP in adult rats (Taxi and Droz 1966a; Gershon and Ross 1966). In contrast, enteric 5-HT axons remain amenable to radioautographic visualization in the adult, where they are found in both submucosal and myenteric plexuses.

Radioautographic evidence for the existence of serotonin-accumulating neurons in rat spinal ganglia (Calas et al. 1981) and cat nodose ganglion (Gaudin-Chazal et al. 1978; Ségu et al. 1981) has recently emerged from in vitro studies using incubation at low concentrations of [³H]5-HT. Further experimentation will be needed to determine whether these peripheral neurons also contain endogenous 5-HT.

(c) Studies with [³H]5-HT in the central nervous system

Aghajanian et al. (1966; see also Aghajanian and Bloom 1967a) were the first to achieve radioautographic localization of [³H]5-HT uptake sites in the CNS. They did so at both the light- and electron-microscopic levels, following intraventricular injection of the tritiated indolamine. Fuxe et al. (1968), in their elegant study combining histofluorescence and light-microscopic radioautography, soon confirmed that the uptake of intraventricularly administered 5-HT was largery confined to neuronal elements containing endogenous 5-HT. The development of improved labeling techniques involving prolonged topical application or intraventricular infusion of higher concentrations of [³H]5-HT in animals pretreated with a monoamine oxidase inhibitor (Calas et al. 1974; Descarries et al. 1975; Chan-Palay 1975) later generated a wealth of information concerning the fine structure, regional distribution and topographical organization of 5-HT-containing-neurons in many parts of the neuraxis (see below). While longlasting perfusions favored intraparenchymal diffusion of the tracer, the combined use of relatively high molarities of the indolamine and non-radioactive NA (Descarries et al. 1975), prevented interspecific labeling of catecholaminergic elements (Shaskan and Snyder 1970; Iversen 1970; see also Section 4.5, under 'Demonstration of specificity'). Nevertheless, in vivo labeling studies remained hampered by limited penetration of [³H]5-HT in brain tissue, explaining why incubations of brain slices using low concentrations of [³H]5-HT in vitro were occasionally preferred for light-microscope topographic investigations (Calas 1974; Ségu and Calas 1978; Azmitia and Marovitz 1980; Azmitia 1981; Calas et al. 1981; Ségu et al. 1981), particularly when these were aimed at obtaining quantitative results (Ségu and Calas 1978; Azmitia 1981).

5-HT nerve cell bodies

Light-microscopic data on the radioautographic distribution of [³H]5-HT-labeled nerve cell bodies in mammalian CNS (Chan-Palay 1977b; Léger et al. 1979; Parent et al. 1981; see Fig. 1) are essentially in accordance with those of fluorescence histochemistry or immunohistochemistry, with two exceptions. (1) A small group of hypothalamic nerve cell bodies, which normally escapes detection in the fluorescent microscope but will appear in rats pretreated with intraventricular 5-HT (Fuxe and Ungerstedt 1968), exhibits a strong and selective labeling after intraventricular injection of [³H]5-HT (Descarries and Beaudet 1978; Beaudet and Descarries 1979). These neurons, located in the ventral portion of the dorsomedial nucleus, were recently visualized by immunocytochemistry (using an anti-serotonin antibody) in animals pretreated with L-tryptophan and a monoamine oxidase inhibitor (Frankfurt et al. 1981; Steinbusch and Nieuwenhuys 1982) and are thus likely to synthesize endogenous 5-HT. (2) Several additional groups of [³H]5-HT-labeled nerve cell bodies have been reported in rat hypothalamus by Chan-Palay (1977b) following intraventricular infusion of the indolamine in the presence of non-radioactive NA. These latter findings remain to be confirmed, however, and current immunocytochemical evidence does not support the view that such cells would contain endogenous 5-HT.

Applying Abercrombie's (1946) principles to the analysis of light-microscope radioautographs, Beaudet and Descarries (1979) and Descarries et al. (1982) quantified the number of [³H]5-HT-accumulating nerve cell bodies in nucleus dorsomedialis hypothalami and raphe dorsalis, respectively. The figures obtained (2000 in hypothalamus and 11,500 in raphe dorsalis) remained unchanged after increasing the molarity of the tracer and/or the duration of radioautographic exposure, thereby confirming that optimal labeling had been achieved and that the data provided an accurate estimate of the number of 5-HT nerve cell bodies in these brain areas.

High-resolution radioautographic studies have allowed ultrastructural characterization of [³H]5-HT-labeled nerve cell bodies in several brain regions, including nucleus raphe dorsalis (Bloom et al. 1972; Chan-Palay 1976b, 1977a; Gamrani and Calas 1980; Descarries et al. 1982; Fig. 14), paragigantocellularis lateralis (Chan-Palay 1978a) and dorsomedialis hypothalami (Descarries and Beaudet 1978; Beaudet and Descarries 1979; for review, see Beaudet and Descarries 1981). Some of these investigations have dealt more particularly with the intraperikaryal distribution of [³H]5-HT, either directly taken up (Chan-Palay 1976b, 1978a; Gamrani and Calas 1980) or retrogradely transported (Araneda et al. 1980) within raphe neurons. These studies were essentially qualitative and based on direct scoring analyses, implying that only organelles overlaid by clusters of silver grains or labeled with an unexpectedly high frequency with regards to their size and/or incidence could be reliably considered as potential radioactive sources. To assess quantitatively the relative affinity for exogenous 5-HT of the different subcellular organelles in neurons of raphe dorsalis, Descarries et al. (1982) recently used the statistical method of silver grain distribution analysis devised by Blacket and Parry (1973, 1977), which, as explained above (see Section 4.5, under 'Assigning silver grains to cellular constituents') allows to compensate for the limited resolution of the radioautographic technique. Moreover, these authors compared the sequestration of [³H]5-HT in 'labeled' (i.e. 5-HT containing) versus 'unlabeled' (i.e. non-serotoninergic) neurons, to try and differentiate between biologically significant and presumably artefactual (i.e. due to aldehyde-fixation) labeling (see Section 4.5, under 'Significant versus artefactual intraneuronal localizations'). In the former, but not the latter cells, they thus demonstrated a relatively high affinity of 5-HT for dense bodies. The only other organelles showing higher labeling indices in the labeled than in the unlabeled neurons were mitochondria and the cytoplasmic membrane.

5-HT axon terminals

As recalled above, 5-HT does not cross the blood-brain barrier and most radioautographic investigations of central 5-HT neurons have relied on intraventricular injections of the tritiated amine. This probably explains why the 5-HT innervations of various circumventricular organs and of paraventricular structures were the most thoroughly investigated. Thus, the supra- and subependymal plexuses, first described in histofluorescence by Lorez and Richards (1973) and Richards et al. (1973), were examined by light- and electron-microscope radioautography in the rat or the monkey and this by a number of investigators (Alonso et al. 1974; Chan-Palay 1976a; Palay and Chan-Palay 1976; Richards 1977; Calas et al. 1978; De La Manche et al. 1981). Similarly, the distribution and fine structure of 5-HT axon terminals were studied by radioautography in most circumventricular organs, including the subcommissural and the subfornical organs (Bouchaud and Arluison 1977; Calas et al. 1978; Bouchaud 1979; Møllgård and Wiklund 1979), the organum vasculosum laminae terminalis (Bosler 1977, 1978; Calas et al.1978) and the median eminence (Calas 1972, 1973, 1975, 1977; Calas et al. 1974). Other brain areas where 5-HT nerve terminals were investigated after intraventricular injection include the neostriatum (Arluison and De La Manche 1980; Arluison 1981), the hypothalamus (Beaudet and Descarries 1979; Descarries and Beaudet 1978; Bessone 1979; see Fig. 5), the substantia nigra (Parizek et al. 1971), the cerebellar cortex and its deep nuclei (Bloom et al. 1972, Chan-Palay 1975, 1976b, 1977a; Palay and Chan-Palay 1976; Bloom and Costa 1978), the locus ceruleus (Descarries and Léger 1978; Léger and Descarries 1978), the dorsal accessory olive (Wiklund et al. 1981), and the facial (Aghajanian and McCall 1980), paratrigeminal (Chan-Palay 1978b), and paragigantocellular (Chan-Palay 1978a) nuclei. In addition, two systematic radioautographic mapping studies have described the light-microscopic distribution of [^{3}H]5-HT varicosities (and nerve cell bodies) labeled after prolonged intraventricular infusion of [^{3}H]5-HT in the rat (Chan-Palay 1977b; Parent et al. 1981).

Other approaches have been used to achieve in vivo labeling of 5-HT nerve terminals in the CNS. Thus, intraparenchymatous injections of [^{3}H]5-HT were used to visualize 5-HT elements in rat olfactory bulb (Halasz et al. 1977, 1978) and cat brain stem (Léger et al. 1978). Prolonged topical applications of [^{3}H]5-HT allowed specific identification of 5-HT varicosities in rat cerebral and cerebellar cortices (Descarries et al. 1975; Sotelo and Beaudet 1979; Beaudet and Sotelo 1981; Fig. 18), as well as in the cat caudate nucleus (Calas et al. 1978) and substantia gelatinosa (Ruda and Gobel 1980).

An initial attempt at quantifying the density of 5-HT innervation in rat CNS was that of Kuhar and Aghajanian (1973), who estimated the proportion of synaptosomes labeled with [^{3}H]5-HT in whole forebrain nuclei-free homogenates. Beaudet and Descarries (1976) were however the first to analyze quantitatively the repartition and number of 5-HT varicosities in a given brain region. They did so in rat cerebral cortex, following prolonged topical application of [^{3}H]5-HT. Control experiments were performed to demonstrate that most if not all 5-HT terminals were actually labeled in the area under scrutiny, and counts were obtained from light-microscope radioautographs of 1 μm-thick sections, to ensure that all labeled terminals present within the sections would be recorded. Volumetric extrapolations were derived by applying mathematical calculations devised by Lapierre et al. (1973) in their earlier quantitative study of the cortical NA innervation. By a similar approach, using either in vivo (topical application, intraventricular infusion) or in vitro (brain slices incubation) administration of [^{3}H]5-HT, quantitative data on the density of 5-HT innervation have also been obtained in the locus ceruleus (Léger and Descarries 1978), dorsal accessory olive (Wiklund et al. 1981), cerebellar cortex (Beaudet and Sotelo 1981) and suprachiasmatic nucleus (Bessone 1979) of the rat, and in the spinal grey (Ségu and Calas 1978) of the cat (for values, see Table I in Beaudet and Descarries 1981). Finally, Azmitia and Marovitz (1980; see also Azmitia 1981) assessed semi-quantitatively the distribution of 5-HT axons labeled in mouse, rat and monkey hippocampal slices incubated in the presence of [^{3}H]5-HT. In several of these studies, estimates of the intravaricose concentration of endogenous 5-HT could be extrapolated (using complementary biochemical data),

327

which yielded remarkably consistent values and confirmed the validity of the radioautographic approach for gathering quantitative information on innervation density.

Quantitative analyses were also carried out at the electron-microscopic level, mostly to assess the proportion of 5-HT varicosities exhibiting a given ultrastructural feature. Such studies, which again required that all 5-HT terminals be labeled in the area examined, allowed to demonstrate that, in the cerebral cortex, all 5-HT varicosities contain large dense-core vesicles (Descarries et al. 1975). More importantly, it was also established for the cortex and then in other parts of the CNS, that 5-HT varicosities often lack the junctional membrane differentiations which normally characterize chemically-transmitting synapses (for review see Beaudet and Descarries 1978, 1981). Such a conclusion could be reached either following topometric analysis of serial high-resolution radioautographs (Descarries et al. 1975), or by applying probability formulas to the processing of information gathered in randomly chosen, but systematically screened thin sections (Beaudet and Sotelo 1981; Wiklund et al. 1981).

Lastly, it should be recalled that the fate of certain 5-HT innervations has also been studied by light- and/or electron-microscopic radioautography in several pathological conditions including thiamine deficiency (Chan-Palay 1977b), cerebellar cortical agranularity (Sotelo and Beaudet 1979; Beaudet and Sotelo 1981), and following selective lesioning by 5,6-dihydroxytryptamine (Wiklund et al. 1981; see Fig. 7).

(d) Retina

Indolamine-accumulating amacrine cells have been described in the retina of a number of mammalian and non-mammalian species, using fluorescence histochemistry (for review, see Ehinger and Floren 1980). These 5-HT-accumulating cells have also been visualized by radioautography in the rabbit (Ehinger and Floren 1978) and bovine (Osborne 1980) retina. Under normal conditions, however, (i.e. without loading with exogenous 5-HT or one of its analogues), such cells are not detected by histofluorescence, even in animals pretreated with L-tryptophan and a monoamine oxidase inhibitor. For this reason, it is still unclear whether they contain only low levels of endogenous 5-HT or utilize a closely related substance as neurotransmitter.

(e) Tissue cultures

Radioautographic studies have demonstrated that, in cultures of rat brain stem, [³H]5-HT is taken up by a relatively small number of neurons, but not by glial cells. Accumulations of [³H]5-HT were also observed at the growing tips of labeled nerve fibers (Hösli et al. 1975; Hösli and Hösli 1978).

Serotonin-containing neurons have also been visualized radioautographically in the myenteric plexus grown in organotypic tissue cultures (Dreyfuss et al. 1977a,b). It was thus demonstrated that entire 5-HT neurons will develop in the cultures even if a seemingly aneural gut is removed from the chick (Gershon et al. 1980) or mouse (Rothman et al. 1979) embryos.

5.2. AMINO ACID NEURONS

Radioautographic uptake studies were until recently the only reliable approach for visualizing neurons believed to utilize amino acids as neurotransmitters. Since this approach is indirect, however, demonstration of uptake specificity had first to rely on comparisons with the regional distribution of endogenous amino acids or between labeling patterns observed using different tritiated putative transmitters. In this context, the purification of the enzyme glutamic acid decarboxylase (Wu et al. 1973) followed by the production of an antibody allowing its immunocytochemical detection (Saito et al. 1974) represented a major breakthrough in the investigation of 'amino acidergic' neurons. Thus, many of the radioautographic results obtained after [³H]GABA administration can now be correlated with those of GAD immunocytochemistry. The complementarity of the two methods has been particularly well established in a recent study by Neale et al. (1981), who demonstrated the coexistence of GAD immunoreactivity and high-affinity [³H]GABA uptake in neurons from dissociated cell cultures of the cerebral cortex. Unfortunately, immunocytochemical methods are not yet available for the detection of neurons using amino acids other than GABA, so that in many instances it remains to be formally demonstrated that their uptake capacity demonstrated by radioautography is indeed representative of their transmitter identity (see Section 2.2, under 'Uptake of neurotransmitters'). Immunocytochemical tools are clearly at hand, however, and the production of antibodies raised against aspartate aminotransferase or glutaminase (Altschuler et al. 1981), or against glutamate itself (Storm-Mathisen et al. 1982) for immunocytochemical detection of presumptive glutamate and/or aspartate neurons may be quoted as examples of promising developments.

A major problem in investigating amino acidergic neurons by radioautography is the fact that all putative amino acid transmitters are also significantly taken up by glia (see Section 2.2, under 'Uptake of neurotransmitters'). This glial uptake seriously complicates the recognition of the labeled neuronal elements, particularly at the light-microscopic level, and has thus hampered topographical distribution studies of amino acid accumulating neurons. At the electron-microscopic level, glial versus neuronal cell body labeling can be readily differentiated, but the distinction becomes arduous within terminal fields, where radioautographic signals cross-fired from glial leaflets may be mistakenly ascribed to neighbouring nerve terminals. Analysis of the data will thus often have to rely on quantitation of silver grains, particularly in the absence of clear-cut accumulations of radioactivity within nerve terminals (see Kelly and Weitsch-Dick 1978; Storm-Mathisen and Iversen 1979).

Several methods have been proposed (i.e. short injections, use of tritiated analogues, etc., see Section 4.2) to improve the selectivity of labeling of amino acidergic neurons. One of the most promising approaches could again be the use of retrograde and/or anterograde transport of the putative transmitters themselves (see Section VI; and Cuénod, Chapter VIII), which should not only allow for the tracing of these transmitter-specific pathways, but also for their light- and particularly their electron-microscopic identification in improved conditions of radioautographic visualization (Streit et al. 1980).

GABA

(a) Neuronal uptake of GABA in the central nervous system

Initial attempts at localizing GABA uptake sites by radioautography relied on intraventricular (Clark et al. 1968) or systemic administration (Hespe et al. 1969) of [¹⁴C]GABA, but showed only a diffuse distribution of the label in periventricular zones and extracerebral organs, respectively. Hökfelt and Ljungdahl (1970) were the first to detect cellular accumulations of [³H]GABA in the CNS, using light-microscopic radioautography after incubation of slices from rat cerebellar cortex; however, they could not ascertain whether this labeling affected neurons, glial cells or both (see also discussion in Hökfelt and Ljungdahl 1971b). Ehinger (1970) then reported neuronal labeling after incubation of rabbit retina in the presence of [³H]GABA, and Bloom and Iversen (1971; see also Iversen and Bloom 1972) concluded from an electron-microscope radioautographic study that the bulk of [³H]GABA incorporated into slices or homogenates from various regions of the rat brain and from the spinal cord was localized in nerve terminals.

Nerve cell bodies

The use of in vivo administration of [³H]GABA, which favors better tissue preservation than in vitro incubations, was soon to allow examination of GABA-accumulating neurons in many parts of the CNS. Thus, preferentially labeled stellate (Hökfelt and Ljungdahl 1972b; Schon and Iversen 1972; see also Iversen and Schon 1973), basket and Gogli cells (Hökfelt and Ljungdahl 1972b) were recognized in light- and electron-microscopic radioautographs of rat cerebellar cortex following intra-cerebral (Hökfelt and Ljungdahl 1972b) or intraventricular (Schon and Iversen 1972) injections of [³H]GABA or [³H]DABA. The same classes of interneurons were labeled in tissue cultures (Sotelo et al. 1972; Lasher 1974; Hösli and Hösli 1976; for review see, Sotelo 1975; Privat 1976) or intraocular transplants of rat cerebellum exposed to [³H]GABA (Ljungdahl et al. 1973). Purkinje cells, which have long been considered on biochemical, physiological and immunocytochemical grounds the most likely GABAergic candidates in the cerebellum were unequivocally labeled in cerebellar tissue cultures but, surprisingly, not in adult cerebellum, irrespective of the mode of [³H]GABA administration. To explain this discrepancy, Ljungdahl et al. (1973) hypothesized that the Purkinje cell glial enwrapping, which is absent in tissue cultures and incomplete in intraocular transplants, could constitute a barrier preventing the uptake of [³H]GABA by mature Purkinje cells. In this context, it is noteworthy that Hösli and Hösli (1978a), studying the cellular localization of [³H]GABA taken up in cultures of dorsal root ganglia, demonstrated that dorsal root ganglia neurons took up [³H]GABA when deprived of glial ensheathing but not when surrounded by satellite glial cells. In keeping with these observations, Rustioni and Cuénod (1981; see also Cuénod, Chapter VIII) have recently reported retrograde perikaryal labeling of dorsal root ganglia following intraspinal injections of [³H]GABA. Yet, similar injections in rat Deiter's nucleus failed to induce retrograde labeling of Purkinje cells (Cuénod et al.1982; see also Cuénod, Chapter VIII) while injections of [³H]GABA in the substantia nigra resulted in a clear-cut retrograde labeling of nerve cell bodies in the caudate nucleus (Streit et al. 1979; Streit 1980). Moreover, degeneration of Purkinje nerve terminals in Deiter's nucleus led to a significant decrease in GAD activity but did not affect the high affinity uptake of GABA (Storm-Mathisen 1975). Thus, the possibility that Purkinje cells loose their GABA uptake mechanisms when reaching maturity should be envisaged.

[³H]GABA-labeled nerve cell bodies have also been visualized in rat spinal cord, using both light- and electron-microscopic radioautography. These small neurons were found in laminae I—III and VI—VIII (Ljungdahl and Hökfelt 1973b) or in lamina I and in the transition zone between laminae I and II (Ribeiro-Da-Silva and Coimbra 1980), following intraspinal injections or subarachnoid instillations of [³H]GABA, respectively. At least some of these GABA-accumulating nerve cell bodies must correspond to interneurons, since they are also observed in tissue culture experiments (see below).

Despite the relatively poor penetration of [³H]GABA in brain parenchyma, intraventricular injections or combined intraventricular/intracisternal injections (Iversen and Schon 1973) have allowed the radioautographic detection of presumptive GABA neurons in several periventricular zones of the rat brain, including nucleus raphe dorsalis and periaqueductal grey (Belin et al. 1979; Gamrani et al. 1980), medio-basal hypothalamus (Makara et al. 1975) and caudate nucleus (Iversen and Schon 1973). The GABA-accumulating neurons detected in the caudate might correspond to interneurons or to some of the long projecting GABA neurons retrogradely labeled by Streit (1980; see also Streit et al. 1979) following injection of [³H]GABA into the substantia nigra.

The use of intraparenchymatous injections of [³H]GABA has also allowed radioautographic visualization of presumptive GABAergic nerve cell bodies in areas distant from the ventricular cavities, namely in rat olfactory bulb (Halasz et al. 1979), rat and monkey dentate nucleus (Chan-Palay 1977; Tolbert and Bantley 1980), cat lateral geniculate nucleus (Sterling and Davis 1980), pigeon optic tectum (Hunt and Kunzle 1976; Streit et al. 1978), and rat cerebral cortex (Hökfelt and Ljungdahl 1972b; Chrownwall and Wolff 1978, 1980). Similarly, labeled neurons have been observed in rat cerebral cortex after incubation of slices (Hökfelt and Ljungdahl 1971b) or cortical superfusions (Chrownwall and Wolff 1980). Lastly, labeled nerve cell bodies have been visualized by light-microscopic radioautography in the stratum pyramidale of rat hippocampal formation, again after incubation of brain slices in the presence of [³H]GABA (Hökfelt and Ljungdahl 1971b).

Axon terminals

All brain regions exhibiting [³H]GABA-accumulating nerve cell bodies have also been shown to contain labeled nerve terminals in keeping with the view that most GABAergic neurons are small interneurons. Presumptive GABAergic axon terminals were thus identified in light- and/or electron-microscopic radioautographs from the cerebellum (Hökfelt and Ljungdahl 1972b; Wilkin et al. 1974; Kelly et al. 1975), spinal cord (Ljungdahl and Hökfelt 1973b; Ribeiro-Da-Silva and Coimbra 1980), periaqueductal grey and nucleus raphe dorsalis (Belin et al. 1979), hypothalamus (Makara et al. 1975; Iversen and Schon 1973), caudate nucleus (Iversen and Schon 1973; Hattori et al. 1973), olfactory bulb (Halasz et al. 1979), lateral geniculate nucleus (Sterling and Davis 1980), hippocampal formation (Hökfelt and Ljungdahl 1971b; Storm-Mathisen 1978b), and cerebral cortex (Bloom and Iversen 1971; Iversen and Bloom 1972). Labeled axon terminals were also visualized in several other brain areas, namely the locus ceruleus (Schon and Iversen 1972; Iversen and Schon 1973), the substantia nigra (Schon and Iversen 1973; Hattori et al. 1973), the habenular nucleus (Iversen and Schon 1973), the median eminence (Tappaz et al. 1980), and the subcommissural organ (Gamrani et al 1981). In rat olfactory bulb (Halasz et al. 1979) and the pigeon optic tectum (Streit et al. 1978), presynaptic dendrites have also been reported to accumulate [³H]GABA. The main results of the above studies have been reviewed elsewhere (Hökfelt and Ljungdahl 1975; Iversen et al. 1975; Iversen 1978). It should also be added here that Belin et al. (1980) recently described selective and apparently specific accumulation of intracisternally administered [³H]GABA in both serotonin and non-serotonin containing fibers of the supra- and subependymal plexuses of the rat brain. These latter findings have been complemented by the results of a double immunocytochemical labeling study (Nanopoulos et al. 1981) demonstrating the existence, within the nucleus raphe dorsalis, of nerve cell bodies showing both serotonin and GAD-like immunoreactivity. It thus appears that some serotonin neurons of the rat brain may contain GAD and take up [³H]GABA by a high-affinity uptake process.

Several investigations have attemped to estimate the proportion of [³H]GABA-accumulating nerve terminals in various regions of the rat brain. These quantitative analyses were performed on electron-microscopic radioautographs from homogenates of cerebral cortex, cerebellum, spinal cord, striatum, hippocampus, hypothalamus and brain stem (Bloom and Iversen 1971; Iversen and Bloom 1972) or slices of cerebral cortex, cerebellum, striatum, globus pallidus and substantia nigra (Iversen and Schon 1973; Hattori et al. 1973; Iversen et al. 1975) incubated with [³H]GABA. Percentage of labeled axon terminals were also obtained for the locus ceruleus, hypothalamus and striatum, following intraventricular injection of the tritiated amino acid (Iversen and Schon 1973; Iversen et al. 1975). Quantitation within a given brain area using two or more different approaches often yielded remarkably similar results. Thus, for example, the proportion of [³H]GABA-accumulating terminals in rat striatum was evaluated at 34.2% in homogenates (Iversen and Bloom 1972), 33% in slices (Hattori et al. 1973) and 27% after in vivo administration of the tracer (Iversen and Schon 1973; Iversen et al. 1975).

(b) Retina

[³H]GABA has been shown by radioautography to be accumulated in amacrine cells and structures of the inner plexiform layer in rabbit, guinea pig and cat retina (Ehinger 1970; Ehinger and Falck 1971; Bauer and Ehinger 1974; Brandon et al. 1979; Pourcho 1980; Wu et al. 1981), and in both horizontal and amacrine cells in frog, goldfish, pigeon and chicken (Lam and Steinman 1971; Marshall and Voaden 1974; Voaden et al. 1974a; Neal et al. 1979; Wu et al. 1981). In the rat, however, [³H]GABA appears mainly accumulated in Müller (glial) cells (Neal and Iversen 1972; Marshall and Voaden 1974b). It has been suggested that such discrepancies may result not only from species differences, but also from the mode of tracer administration, in vivo intraocular injections or long incubation times favoring neuronal over glial accumulation.

(c) Tissue cultures

As mentioned above, radioautographic studies have demonstrated that several classes of interneurons as well as Purkinje cells and glial cells take up [³H]GABA in cerebellar tissue cultures (Sotelo et al. 1972; Lasher 1974; Hösli and Hösli 1976a; Currie and Dutton 1980). In cultures of human, rat and chick spinal cord, [³H]GABA has been shown to be taken up by many small neurons, as well as by glial cells (Hösli et al. 1972, 1975; Hökfelt and Ljungdahl 1975; Farb et al. 1979). Accumulation of [³H]GABA (or [³H]muscimol; White et al. 1980) within nerve cell bodies and their processes has also been observed in cultures of mice hippocampus (Walker and Peacock 1982) and rat brain stem (Hösli and Hösli 1978b), olfactory bulb (Currie and Dutton 1980), cerebral cortex (White et al. 1980), and dorsal root ganglia (Hösli and Hösli 1978a). Some authors have used high-resolution radioautography to characterize mature and developing presumptive GABAergic synapses in cultures of postnatal rat cerebellum (Sotelo et al. 1972; Burry and Lasher 1975).

Glycine

(a) Neuronal uptake of glycine in the central nervous system

In contrast to GABA, glycine is biosynthetically involved in general cellular metabolism, including protein synthesis. Accordingly, glycine is taken up in brain tissue by both a low- and high-affinity membrane transport system, the former presumably subserving its metabolic and the latter its transmitter function (see Section 2.2, under 'Uptake of neurotransmitters'). Glycine's low-affinity uptake is ubiquitous, and as such complicates the radioautographic detection of putative glycinergic neurons by giving rise to high background levels against which selective signals can only be unequivocally ascertained through quantitative analysis (Price et al. 1976; Ribeiro-Da-Silva and Coimbra 1980; Wilkin et al. 1981).

Presumptive glycinergic nerve terminals were first visualized by high-resolution radioautography in slices of rat spinal cord incubated with [^{3}H]glycine (Hökfelt and Ljungdahl 1971a; Matus and Dennison 1971). Double-labeling experiments on whole spinal cord homogenates indicated that [^{3}H]glycine-accumulating nerve terminals were distinct from those taking up [^{3}H]GABA (Iversen and Bloom 1972). [^{3}H]glycine-labeled boutons characteristically exhibited 'flat' synaptic vesicles (Matus and Dennison 1971, 1972; Ljungdahl and Hökfelt 1973a,b). This finding, together with physiological data regarding the intraneuronal origin of inhibitory synapses in the spinal cord and the correlation between interneurons loss and decrease in endogenous glycine in the ventral horn, prompted the suggestion that these presumptive glycinergic terminals might arise from inhibitory interneurons (Matus and Dennison 1972). In agreement with this interpretation, small, intensely labeled nerve cell bodies were detected in both ventral and dorsal horns of rat and cat spinal cord following in vivo injections of [^{3}H]glycine into the spinal cord itself (Ljungdahl and Hökfelt 1973a,b; Price et al. 1976), the central canal (Dennison et al. 1976), or the subarachnoid space (Ribeiro-Da-Silva and Coimbra 1980). Similarly, both nerve cell bodies and axon terminals were found to selectively accumulate [^{3}H]glycine in tissue cultures of human and rat spinal cord (Hösli et al. 1972; Ljungdahl and Hökfelt 1973; Hösli and Hösli 1978).

Quantitative estimates of the number of axon terminals radioautographically labeled in rat spinal cord homogenates (Iversen and Bloom 1972) or in tissue slices (Hökfelt and Ljungdahl 1975) incubated with [^{3}H]glycine both yielded values in the order of 25%. A significantly higher percentage (40%) was found to be labeled in the ventral horn proper, following intraspinal injection of the tracer (Price et al. 1976).

The possibility that some of the nerve terminals associated with cerebellar glomeruli might selectively accumulate [^{3}H]glycine has been envisaged on the basis of biochemical (Wilkin et al. 1979) as well as light- (Hökfelt and Ljungdahl 1972) and electron- (Kelly and Dick 1976) microscope radioautographic studies after in vitro or in vivo administration of [^{3}H]glycine, respectively. Recently, Wilkin et al. (1981), using high-resolution radioautography on fragments of cerebellar glomeruli or slices of rat cerebellum, were able to demonstrate that a subpopulation of Golgi neurons, distinct from those accumulating [^{3}H]GABA, selectively accumulates [^{3}H]glycine by a high-affinity uptake process. In this context, it is likely that the few neurons which have been shown to take up [^{3}H]glycine in dissociated (Lasher 1974) or organotypic (Hösli and Hösli 1978) cultures of rat cerebellum also correspond to Golgi cells. It is also of interest that retrogradely labeled putative glycinergic nerve cell bodies have been visualized by light- (Hunt et al. 1977) and electron- (Streit et al. 1980) microscopic radioautography in the pigeon subtectal nucleus isthmi, pars parvocellularis, following injection of [³H]glycine at the level of their terminal field within the optic tectum (see also Chapter VIII).

(b) Retina

Radioautographic studies on the retina of a number of species, including human, rat, cat, rabbit, pigeon, chicken and frog, have consistently shown a selective accumulation of [³H]glycine by cells in the position of amacrine interneurons (Ehinger and Falck 1971; Ehinger 1972b; Bruun and Ehinger 1974; Voaden et al. 1974; Marshall and Voaden 1974; Pourcho 1980; Lam and Hollyfield 1980). In the rabbit retina (Ehinger and Falck 1971; Bruun and Ehinger 1972) and in light adapted frog retinas (Voaden et al. 1974), [³H]glycine was also found to be taken up by a subpopulation of ganglion cells.

Glutamate and aspartate

(a) Neuronal uptake of glutamate and aspartate in the central nervous system

Glutamate and aspartate are taken up in brain slices by what appears to be a common high-affinity uptake system (see Section 2.2, under 'Uptake of neurotransmitters'). This implies, a priori, that the use of neither of these excitatory amino acids will allow a radioautographic distinction between neurons allegedly utilizing glutamate, aspartate, or both as neurotransmitters. Moreover, glutamate and aspartate, like glycine, are involved in general cellular metabolism and, as such, are ubiquitously taken up in brain tissue by a low-affinity uptake mechanism, which complicates the radioautographic detection of their selective, high-affinity uptake sites. As mentioned earlier (Section 4.2, under 'Choice of tracer'), this problem can be alleviated by using D-aspartate, a metabolically stable compound which is taken up by the same high-affinity system as its L-stereoisomer and L-glutamate. Still, like other transmitter amino acids, D-aspartate is accumulated by both neurons and glial cells, implying that accurate radioautographic assessment of its neuronal uptake sites at the electron-microscopic level may require, as that of glutamate (Storm-Mathisen and Iversen 1979), detailed statistical analysis. In fact, early radioautographic investigations following in vitro or in vivo administration of [³H]glutamate first led to the conclusion that the amino acid was mainly taken up in glia (Hökfelt and Ljungdahl 1972a; Schon and Kelly 1974; McLennan 1976). Yet Beart (1976a,b), using radioautography on homogenates of rat cerebral cortex and pigeon optic tectum incubated with [³H]glutamate, was able to demonstrate preferential uptake of the amino acid by the synaptosomal fraction and to evaluate at 14-15% and 10-30% the proportion of labeled synaptosomes in cerebral cortex and optic tectum, respectively.

The hippocampal formation was the first structure in which topographical identification of putative glutamate and/or aspartate neurons was to be radioautographically achieved, its low content in glial elements presumably serving to unmask neuronal uptake (Storm-Mathisen and Iversen 1979). Combining lesion experiments with surface radioautography of hippocampal slices incubated with [³H]L-glutamate, L-aspartate or D-aspartate, Storm-Mathisen and coworkers were thus able to demonstrate, at the light-microscopic level, a lamination of glutamate/aspartate high-affinity uptake sites compatible with a preferential labeling of the terminal fields of the three main excitatory neuronal projections in the hippocampal formation: the perforant path, the mossy fibers and the pyramidal cell axons (Storm-Mathisen 1977, 1978a,b). These results were confirmed by a quantitative high-resolution radioautographic study, which showed preferential accumulation of [³H]glutamate within axon terminals arising from the same three fiber systems (Storm-Mathisen and Iversen 1979). The absence of radioautographic labeling in the soma and large dendrites of the parent neurons (i.e. granular and pyramidal cells) was interpreted as resulting from their relatively poor preservation in incubated tissue slices. Indeed, perikaryal labeling of CA 3/4 pyramidal cells, although curiously not of granule cells, was recently observed in the hippocampus of rat, mouse and hamster, following intraventricular injection of [³H]D-aspartate (Storm-Mathisen 1981; Storm-Mathisen and Wold 1981).

The topographical distribution of [³H]glutamate/aspartate uptake sites has now been assessed by light-microscopic radioautography in several other brains regions including the septum, striatum and neocortex of the rat (Taxt and Storm-Mathisen 1979; Storm-Mathisen and Wold 1981), and in the barrel subfield of the somatosensory cortex of the mouse (Soreide and Fonnum 1980). [³H]glutamate-accumulating nerve terminals have also been identified by electron-microscopic radioautography in the cat oculomotor nucleus (Denêmes and Raymond 1982).

A new and potentially powerful approach to the problem of selectively identifying putative glutamate and/or aspartate neurons by radioautography has stemmed from the work of Streit (1980), who observed retrograde nerve cell body labeling in rat neocortex following injection of [³H]D-aspartate into the neostriatum. Both retrograde and anterograde transport of [³H]D-aspartate were subsequently demonstrated in two other probable glutamate and/or aspartate pathways: the pigeon retino-tectal system (Cuénod et al. 1980; Beaudet et al. 1981) and the monkey cortico-geniculate projection (Baughman and Gilbert 1980, 1981). Finally, retrograde labeling with [³H]D-aspartate was recently demonstrated in rat primary sensory neurons (Cuénod et al. 1982), spinal interneurons and cortico-dorsal nuclei path (Rustioni and Cuénod 1982) and cerebellar climbing fibers (Wiklund et al. 1982).

(b) Retina

As in the CNS, the first glutamate/aspartate uptake sites to be radioautographically recognized in the retina were glial in nature (Ehinger and Falk 1971; Ehinger 1972a; Bruun and Ehinger 1974; Neal 1976; White and Neal 1976). Selective radioautographic labeling of photoreceptor inner segments and of a small population of ganglion cells has since been reported in the rabbit, guinea pig and pigeon retinas, following in vitro (Ehinger 1981) or in vivo (Ehinger 1981; Beaudet et al. 1981; see Fig. 10) administration of [³H]D-aspartate. In the pigeon retina, both anterograde and retrograde labeling experiments confirmed that most of the labeled perikarya detected in the ganglion cell layer after intraocular injection of [³H]D-aspartate indeed corresponded to ganglion cells, rather than to glial or displaced amacrine cells (Beaudet et al. 1981). Preferential labeling of horizontal cells (Ehinger 1977) and amacrine cells (Redburn 1981) was also observed in the rabbit retina, following incubation with [³H]L-glutamate.

(c) Tissue cultures

Radioautographic studies on the cellular localization of [³H]L-glutamate and [³H]L-aspartate uptake in cultures of human and rat spinal cord and brain stem have shown that both amino acids were accumulated by a relatively large number of neurons and by almost all glial cells (Hösli and Hösli 1976b, 1978b). In contrast, in cultures of dissociated cerebellum, [^{3}H]glutamate appeared to be exclusively accumulated by glial elements (Hökfelt and Ljungdahl 1972; Lasher 1974). Finally, high-affinity uptake of [^{3}H]glutamate was found to occur in approximately 30% of the neurons present in monolayer cultures from embryonic retina (Hyndman and Adler 1982).

5.3. CHOLINERGIC NEURONS

The radioautographic visualization of cholinergic neurons has thus far exclusively relied upon the cellular detection of [^{3}H]choline high-affinity uptake sites (see Section 2.2, under 'Uptake of neurotransmitters'). For this purpose, 'dry' radioautographic techniques applied on unfixed, frozen or freeze-dried tissue were a logical choice since choline and ACh are both water-soluble molecules that will not be retained in tissue in the course of standard histological and/or dipping procedures. This type of approach has allowed Baughman and Bader (1977), in an elegant investigation combining biochemistry and radioautography, to localize [^{3}H]choline high-affinity uptake sites in the chicken retina (Fig. 11). The label was shown to be concentrated in certain cell bodies of the inner nuclear and ganglion cell layers and in two bands in the inner plexiform layer, suggesting the involvement of amacrine and inner bipolar cells. More recently, Ruch et al. (1982) have reported marked accumulations of radioactivity within the motor end-plates of stimulated mouse phrenic nerve-hemidiaphragm preparations incubated with [^{3}H]choline and radioautographed by apposition to emulsion-coated coverslips. Using the same 'coverslip technique' developed by Young and Kuhar (1979) for receptor binding studies, Bagnoli et al. (1981) were able to demonstrate selective retrograde labeling of presumptive cholinergic nerve cell bodies in rat septal nucleus and nucleus of the diagonal band and in pigeon nucleus dorsolateralis anterior thalami, following injection of [^{3}H]choline in their territories of projection, i.e. the hippocampal formation in the rat and the visual wulst in the pigeon. Similarly, injections of [^{3}H]choline into rat spinal cord were recently found to induce selective retrograde labeling of rubrospinal, vestibulospinal and part of reticulospinal pathways, thereby suggesting that these might be cholinergic (Paré et al. 1982). Interestingly, the latter authors were able to detect similar labeling in tissue fixed by rapid perfusion of an aldehyde solution containing a high concentration of magnesium.

In view of the difficulties involved in the detection of diffusible substances by electron-microscopic radioautography, there has been no attempt at localizing [^{3}H]choline high-affinity uptake sites at the ultrastructural level. Yet, two independent light-microscopic investigations have raised the possibility that these might be amenable to radioautographic visualization after conventional fixation procedures, provided that sufficient amounts of [^{3}H]choline are incorporated into phospholipids. Barald and Berg (1979a,b) were thus able to identify cells that displayed high-affinity choline uptake mechanisms in dissociated cell cultures of chick spinal cord, ciliary ganglia and rat superior cervical ganglia. Similarly, Woodward and Lindstrom (1977) reported selective radioautographic labeling of motoneurons following injection of [^{3}H]choline in cat spinal cord. It nevertheless appears likely that in the near future the use of tritiated antibodies raised against choline acetyltransferase (Park et al. 1982; Ross et al. 1983) will provide a more specific approach for the radioautographic identification of cholinergic neurons at both the light- and electron-microscopic levels.

6. STATE OF THE ART AND ANTICIPATED DEVELOPMENTS

This retrospective look at the contributions of radioautography calls for several concluding remarks. The first is that a great deal of information is still to be gained from the radioautographic examination of transmitter-specific neurons. Initially utilized to answer a few precise questions, this experimental approach, like many others, has progressively enlarged its scope and has become a method of choice not only for identifying and/or characterizing chemically-defined neurons, but also for studying cytofunctional properties related to transmitter utilization. Yet, it is clear that with none of the transmitters thus far recognized has radioautography been exploited to the full extent of its possibilities particularly for investigating cellular and subcellular correlates of transmitter biosynthesis, metabolism and release or the effects of drugs on these processes.

In the case of monoamine neurons, we have seen that the recent development of radioautographic procedures for visualizing labeled dopaminergic elements at the light- and electron-microscopic levels appears extremely promising in terms of analyzing their regional distribution, fine structure and intracellular relationships. One might believe that more complete data are already at hand on noradrenergic neurons. Here again, however, a critical appraisal of the literature reveals much ignorance, in most brain regions, of the fine structural feature of noradrenergic nerve cell bodies, axonal projections and their terminal arborizations. As regards presumptive adrenergic neurons, these have not even yet been formally identified radioautographically in any part of the CNS. Serotoninergic neurons are probably the ones which have been the most thoroughly investigated. Qualitative as well as quantitative data on both the distribution and ultrastructure of 5-HT nerve cell bodies and axon terminals have thus been gathered in several parts of the neuraxis. These results will now need to be completed, enlarged to other species than the rat and further analyzed in correlation with the data on other chemically-defined neuronal systems.

The radioautographic visualization of the neuronal uptake of [^{3}H]GABA has greatly contributed to establish the transmitter role of this amino acid in the CNS and to demonstrate its prevalence in many anatomical regions. The difficulties involved in identifying presumptive glycinergic and particularly glutamate and aspartate neurons by either light- and/or electron-microscopic radioautography have been commented upon. The same can be said about cholinergic neurons, for which immunocytochemical studies, although in their preliminary stage, appear not only as an alternative but as a unique mean to achieve specific ultrastructural identification (Park et al. 1982; Ross et al. 1983).

Little use has thus far been made of radioautography for visualizing transmitter-specific neuronal systems during normal and abnormal development and/or for studying their adaptive properties following mechanical or chemical injury, X-irradiation or grafting. In this respect, it appears reasonable to believe that the systems best defined in the normal adult animal will provide the most suitable models.

Emphasis has been placed on the methodological and interpretational problems associated with radioautographic labeling achieved by local uptake after intracerebral administration of transmitters. In this context, the recent utilization of radioautography after specific retrograde and/or anterograde transport of transmitters constitutes a major breakthrough. The first attempt at exploiting axonal transport properties for the radioautographic demonstration of chemically-defined neurons of the CNS was that of McGeer et al. 1975. Unfortunately, this experiment was carried out on the nigrostriatal DA system and it is now clear that the procedures of tissue fixation available at the time were inappropriate to maintain in situ [³H]DA or [³H]NA conveyed intra-axonally into dopaminergic terminals. Recent results obtained with the same system, but after rapid, double-perfusion of glutaraldehyde and osmium tetroxide fixatives, suggest that such anterograde axonal labeling could be sufficiently intense not only to delineate the nigrostriatal system at the light-microscopic level, but also to allow electron-microscopic identification of neostriatal DA terminals (Descarries et al. unpublished). Furthermore, [³H]DA and [³H]NA and/or their byproducts may be transported retrogradely into CA nerve cell bodies located at considerable distance from terminal uptake sites (Hunt et al. 1977; Léger et al. 1977; Streit et al. 1979; Streit 1980; see also Fig. 4), which offers an additional means to achieve their electron-microscopic characterization. Indeed, the same approach has already allowed ultrastructural identification of serotonin nerve cell bodies retrogradely labeled after injection of [³H]serotonin in rat olfactory bulb (Araneda et al. 1980) and that of presumptive glycinergic nerve cell bodies in the pigeon nucleus isthmi, pars parvocellularis, after application of [³H]glycine at their site of termination in the optic tectum (Streit et al. 1980). Similar ultrastructural studies in other neuronal systems in which selective anterograde and/or retrograde transmitter axonal transport has been demonstrated (see Chapter VIII) are likely to yield results in the near future.

New perspectives are also being opened-up by the combination of radioautography with other techniques for light- and electron-microscopic identification of chemically-defined neurons and notably immunocytochemistry. In recent years, a number of double-labeling techniques have been proposed (see Chapter VI). Most of these, however, are not applicable at the electron-microscopic level (e.g. histo- or immunofluorescence and retrograde labeling with horseradish peroxidase or fluorescent dyes). Others, suitable for electron-microscopic studies, provide only indirect information on the nature of transmitters (e.g. combination of radioautography or immunocytochemistry with lesion techniques or peroxidase tract tracing). While radioautography and immunocytochemistry have already been combined for simultaneous light-microscopic visualization of different transmitters in the same cells (Chan-Palay 1979) or detection of two types of transmitter-specific neurons (Beaudet et al. 1980; Pickel et al. 1980), their conjunction appears of even greater interest at the electron-microscopic level (see Fig. 19), where it may not only help to establish the specificity of radioautographic reactions (Pickel et al. 1981), but also provide information on the colocalization of different transmitters in the same axon terminals and permit analysis of morphological interrelationships between chemically-defined neurons (Pickel et al. 1982). Moreover, combination of radioautography and immunocytochemistry should eventually allow for the simultaneous visualization of transmitter-identified neurons and of receptors to their own or other transmitters. Thus, Möhler et al. (1981) have recently reported concomitant detection of GABA terminals, immunostained with an anti-GAD antibody, and of benzodiazepine receptors radioautographically demonstrated by photoaffinity labeling (on the use of radioautography for localizing receptors, see Chapter IX).

The increasingly rapid advances and diversified applications of radioautography have somehow preceded the consolidation of much basic knowledge essential for the comprehension of the results it was yielding. It can only be hoped that this rapid evolution does not leave behind too many unexplored avenues which might have led to a better understanding of the reality it was meant to explore.

7. ACKNOWLEDGEMENTS

The authors thank MM Daniel Cyr and Charles Hodge for expert photographic work. They are also grateful to Ms Marie Hélène Lévy, Elizabeth Mullin, Claire Goguen and Maud Lerebours and to Mr Kenneth C. Watkins for clerical help in preparing the manuscript. Most of the personal studies referred to in the text were supported by the Medical Research Council of Canada, of which Dr Alain Beaudet is currently a Scholar.

8. APPENDIX (with the collaboration of K.C. Watkins and S. Garcia)*

8.1. A PROTOCOL FOR HIGH-RESOLUTION RADIOAUTOGRAPHY

The following 2-step technique to prepare epoxy resin-embedded material for light- and electron-microscopic radioautography is mainly derived from the work of Lacassagne et al. (5), Bélanger and Leblond (6), Kopriwa and Leblond (9), Caro and Van Tubergen (17), Granboulan (21) and Salpeter and Bachmann (22). It has already been described in some details by Larra and Droz (23), Descarries (25) and Chan-Palay (26). In the first step, light-microscopic radioautographs are processed from relatively thick (1-5 μm) sections of blocks or slices of tissue. This allows extensive sampling and initial survey of entire biological specimens for purposes of detecting labeled histological constituents and assessing their regional distribution and reactivity in various experimental conditions. In the second step, electron-microscopic radioautographs are obtained from thin sections of smaller areas trimmed from the same blocks or slices, thereby ensuring exact knowledge of the anatomical location and representativity of labeled cellular elements when characterizing their fine structural features and analyzing the intracellular disposition of tracers.

8.1.1. Light-microscopic radioautography (see Section 4.4)

(a) Cleaning glass slides

Soak in chromic sulfuric acid solution	10 min
Wash in running tap water	10 min
Rinse in distilled water	3×5 min
Dry in dust-free atmosphere and store in aluminium foil-wrapped packets	

(b) Preparing semi-thin sections for light-microscopic radioautography

One μm-thick sections from small blocks of epoxy-embedded material are usually processed since they provide for excellent resolution and optimal detection of tritiated compounds. The same procedure also applies to larger sections prepared as described in Section 8.2.2.

> For each block, deposit 3-5 sections on clean slides at approximately one third the distance from one of their extremities.
> Using a diamond scribe, engrave the block number at the opposite end, on the side of the slide bearing the sections.
> Section-bearing slides are conveniently stored in light-proof plastic boxes without liners. By convention, they are always stacked in the same manner (e.g. specimen number on the right,

---

*In this section, the numbers in brackets refer to the references listed under the subtitle 'Selected readings on basic and technical aspects of radioautography' (Section 8.3).

sections facing the front of boxes). Affixing an embossed label on the front and lower part of the boxes will permit their correct orientation (and that of the slides) in the darkroom.

Prepare a minimum of 3 slides for each block, and add several spares to each series to be used as tests for exposure-times, staining, etc. Two series plus a few test slides will usually be coated together. The third is saved as a substitute in case of technical failure or future needs.

Before coating, place slides in 60°C oven for a minimum of 24 h to ensure permanent adherence of sections to glass and prevent slippage or wrinkling during subsequent processing.

(c) Coating with emulsion

Much of this protocol also applies to electron-microscope radioautographs (Section 8.1.2.e). For light-microscopy, Ilford K-5 or Kodak NTB-2 emulsions are commonly used (K-5 emulsion is relatively unstable and should always be tested when older than 3 months from its manufacturing date).

Assemble the following material in a photographic darkroom equipped with a safelight (15 watt light bulb behind a Wratten No. 2 red filter):
  Water bath providing a constant temperature of 40°C
  Thermometer
  Filter paper
  4 porcelain spoons or glass stirring rods
  5 unused clean slides
  Section-bearing slides in their respective boxes
  Plexiglass racks with slots allowing 80° angulation of slides
  Black plastic electrical tape
  Scissors
  Emulsion flask
  Dipping container: Jolly tube (oval section) for up to 20 slides or Borel tube (round section) for up to 40 slides, bearing black marks at 3 and 6 cm from their base.
Fill dipping container with distilled water up to the 3 cm mark and immerse in the water bath at 40°C.
Under safelight illumination, ladle emulsion into the dipping container until the water level reaches the 6 cm mark (providing a 1:1 dilution).
Switch off safelight and return emulsion flask to refrigerator.
At 20-min intervals, re-enter the darkroom to stir the melting emulsion with a clean porcelain spoon, agitating gently enough to avoid air bubbles.
After the third stirring, begin coating under safelight illumination. First, dip 4-5 clean unused slides to remove air bubbles or dust particles from the melted emulsion. These coated slides may be brought against the safelight to verify the homogeneity of the emulsion coat.
Holding section-bearing slides by their numbered end, lower each one to the bottom of the emulsion container and remove slowly and uniformly (in 1-2 sec) touching the slide edge to the rim of the container to steady the movement.
Briefly stand each slide on filter paper to drain excess emulsion.
Line up the coated slides sequentially on drying racks, labeled end up, facing forward and angled backward. Keep each series on a different rack for subsequent identification.
Note the position of racks and their respective series of slides, switch off safelight and take out empty slide boxes upon leaving the darkroom.
Let coated slides dry for a minimum of 3-4 h.
Just before returning to darkroom, place in each slide box a small packet (~20 g) of phosphorous pentoxide or Drierite wrapped in facial tissue and partially enveloped in aluminium foil. Secure this packet between the labeled end of the box and a clean unused slide. In the darkroom, store each series of dry, coated slides in their respective boxes keeping the same orientation as before.
Seal boxes with light-tight, black plastic electrical tape.

(d) Exposure

Duration of exposure may vary from a few days to several months depending on the conditions and purposes of the experiments. The boxes may be kept at room temperature, preferably in a dry enclosure, and should stand vertically on their labeled end.

(e) Development of light-microscope radioautographs

For optimal results the D-19 developer and sodium thiosulfate fixer should be freshly prepared.

To make 250 ml of D-19, dissolve in distilled water, in the given order: 0.5 g Metol, 2.25 g Quinol (hydroquinone), 18 g sodium sulfite, 12 g sodium carbonate and 1 g potassium bromide.

To prepare 250 ml of fixer, dissolve 75 g of sodium thiosulfate in distilled water.

Development is carried out at 18°C, according to the following schedule:

Immersion in full strength D-19 developer	4 min
Rinse in distilled water	10 sec
Immersion in fixer	5-10 min
Wash in distilled water	3×5 min

After the third wash, the slides are usually put for 1-3 min in distilled water warmed to 40°C to clean them of emulsion debris.

All solutions should be replaced after processing a maximum of 50 slides/250 ml.

Developed slides are left to dry on racks in dust-free atmosphere.

(f) Poststaining with toluidine blue

Stock solution: 1% toluidine blue in 1% sodium tetraborate.

Filter stock solution and dilute 1:10 with 70% ethanol.

Place slides on a hot plate (50-60°C) and stain for 45-60 sec with a sufficient amount of dilute solution to cover the whole slide.

Rinse and differentiate with 70% ethanol, wipe-off excess alcohol and evaporate any residue by heat.

Clear the sections with a drop of xylene and mount the coverslip with Permount or Eukitt.

8.1.2. Electron-microscopic radioautography (see Section 4.4)

(a) Preparation of celloidin-coated slides

Prepare a 2% solution of celloidin (Parlodion) in amyl acetate, allowing 24 h to dissolve (will keep for at least 1 month in a closely stoppered container).

Using a diamond scribe, engrave slides with 2 small markings, 5 mm from their lateral edges and 25 mm from one end. Then, clean the slides as described earlier (Section 8.1.1).

Mark the outside of a Borel tube 5 cm from its internal base and fill it to the mark with filtered celloidin solution.

Working in a dust-free area, dip the scribed end of each slide, drain briefly, and allow to dry at an angle of 30° with the scribed surface facing downward.

After thorough drying (2-3 h), re-dip the lower end of each slide to a depth of 0.5-1 cm and dry as before. This will reinforce the film at the re-dipped end and avoid premature stripping-off.

Celloidin-coated slides may be stored for months.

(b) Transferring thin sections to celloidin-coated slides

Remove ribbons of silver-gold sections from the cutting trough with a 3-4 mm diameter wire loop. To avoid breaking the ribbons, approach them from below.

Lower the loop containing the sections opposite the markings on the slide.

Draw-off the cutting solution by touching the lower edge of the ring with a small piece of filter paper, thereby depositing the floating sections onto the celloidin. Deposition of sections may be facilitated by putting a small drop of cutting solution on the slide prior to placement of sections. During the whole operation, care should be taken not to tear the fragile film.

Inscribe the block number at the uncoated end of the slide.

At least 3 slides (each bearing 2 ribbons of sections) should be prepared from every block. A few extras may be useful for exposure tests. Some sections should also be picked up on grids to test staining.

Section-bearing slides are stored in dust-free boxes, orientated as previously indicated.

(c) Staining with lead citrate

The following procedure is recommended whether or not the tissue has been block-stained with uranyl acetate.

Prepare a stock solution of Reynold's lead citrate solution by dissolving separately 2.66 g lead nitrate and 2.52 g sodium citrate, each in 30 ml of distilled water; mix the 2 solutions together and stir for 30 min. Add 16 ml of fresh 1 N NaOH and bring the volume to 100 ml with distilled water.

Depending on the intensity of staining required, use solution as such or diluted 1:1 with 0.01 N NaOH.

Stain for 2-4 min in Jolly tubes filled to a height of 3 cm and changing tube every 2 slides. Wash the immersed part of slides thoroughly, with a stream of distilled water meticulously directed to avoid the upper end of the celloidin film.

Allow the slides to dry upright in racks, for a minimum of 1 h, in a dust-free atmosphere.

(d) Carbon coating

Carbon-coating is a necessity. It favors uniform layering of the emulsion, protects against negative chemography, avoids destaining during radioautographic processing and provides greater stability of the sections under the electron beam. The thickness of the carbon required should produce a faint shade of gray on paper. It can be controlled by placing in the vacuum coating unit, along with the slides, a small piece of filter paper, half of which is covered with high-vacuum grease.

(e) Coating with emulsion

Technique identical to that described in Section 8.1.1 except that Ilford L-4 emulsion is used and the dilution is 1:4 (Jolly tube bearing marks at 48 and 60 mm from bottom).

The Ilford L-4 emulsion is more stable than K-5 and may be kept for longer periods of time in the refrigerator. It may be checked for background by light-microscopic radioautography, using a 1:1 dilution and a 5-min development in D-19.

(f) Exposure

Same conditions as for light microscope radioautographs. Depending on the sensitivity of the developer, optimal exposure usually requires a period 5-15 times longer than for light-microscopic radioautography. The dessicant in slide boxes should be replaced monthly.

(g) Development of electron-microscopic radioautographs

We use one of 3 developers depending on the efficacy and/or size and shape of grains desired (see Section 4.4 and refs in Section 8.3.3.b). D-19 has the highest efficiency. It is freshly made (see above), diluted 1:5, and development for 1 min at 20°C produces thin, filamentous and highly convoluted silver grains.

Microdol-X is of intermediate efficiency. It is commercially available (Kodak), can be prepared in advance (keeps for 1 month) but must be filtered before use. A 4-min development at 18°C produce complete silver grains in the shape of moderately convoluted, comparatively thick filaments. Underdeveloped grains may sometimes be preferred and can be obtained by shortening the duration of development.

Paraphenylenediamine has a very low efficiency but gives much smaller and thinner grains. It is prepared by dissolving 270 mg of this product in 250 ml of distilled water containing 3.15 g of sodium sulfite and warmed at 50°C. Filter before use. Development should last exactly 1 min at 20°C.

> Proceed as described above (Section 8.1.1.e). Make sure to agitate gently during development and to carry out fixation and washing at the same or slightly lower temperature to prevent peeling-off of the celloidin film.
>
> For the sake of convenience, slides may be kept in the refrigerator for a few hours in the last rinsing bath.

(h) Stripping of celloidin film and placement of grids on sections

> Assemble the following material:
>> Large crystallizing dish filled to the brim with distilled water and resting in a tray lined with black paper
>> Flask of distilled water
>> Glass rod
>> Clean razor blade
>> Mounted needle
>> Fine forceps
>> Clean copper grids (we generally use 150-mesh)
>> Whatman No. 1 filter paper
>> Pencil
>> Scissors
>
> Stand all slides on a drying rack and cover with an inverted jar, together with a wet facial tissue to maintain a high level of humidity.
>
> Holding a slide by its numbered end, detach the thick edge of the celloidin film with the razor blade.
>
> With the section facing downward, scrape both lateral edges of the slide with the razor blade.
>
> With the section facing upward, bring the lower extremity of the slide to rest against the rim of the crystallizing dish and, at a sharp angle, slowly lower the slide into the water. The celloidin film should strip-off and float onto the water surface. Gentle pulling with the mounted needle may facilitate this operation.
>
> Under an illuminated magnifier, place a grid, shiny side down, over each ribbon of thin sections.
>
> Write the slide number on a piece of filter paper.
>
> Breathe on the floating film to humidify its surface and bring a piece of filter paper in full contact with it.
>
> As soon as the paper is completely wet, pull it out of the water, lifting the thinner end of the celloidin film first.
>
> Cut out excess paper around the celloidin film and place, filter paper down, in a Petri dish.

Before proceeding to the next slide, add water to the crystallizing dish and clean the surface by running the glass rod across it.

(i) Thinning the celloidin film

After drying in a 40°C oven for 1-2 h, free grids from the surrounding film by puncturing around them with a fine forceps.
Dissolving the celloidin support will greatly improve contrast in the electron-microscope. This is conveniently done in small Petri dishes, lined with filter paper, by immersing each grid for 2.5-3 min in pure amyl acetate.
Let dry for 1 h at 40°C before examination.
Electron-microscope radioautographs may be handled and stored in the same manner as regular thin sections for electron-microscopy.

8.2. SPECIAL PROCEDURES

8.2.1. Successive perfusion of aldehyde and osmium fixatives (see also Section 4.3)

The double vascular perfusion of an aldehyde and then an osmium fixative is not a new procedure per se. The novelty here is to perform it with a high flow-rate pumping device, so that the duration of the primary aldehyde fixation may be considerably shortened and this step immediately followed by rapid osmication of the entire CNS. When used for preserving [³H]catecholamines in situ (see comments and references in Sections 4.3 and 5.1), glutaraldehyde should be present in the primary fixative at a minimal concentration of 1%, whereas the concentration of the osmium tetroxide perfusate may be as low as 0.2%. Overall preservation of the morphology appears to be improved when slices of the double-fixed tissue are further osmicated by immersion in a 1-2% osmium postfixative as is usually done after aldehyde fixation in standard fixation sequences. Otherwise, the composition of both fixatives and their buffers may be varied to suit the needs of the investigation. The following technique has been devised for adult rat.

The perfusion apparatus consists of a graduated 1-liter reservoir, a controllable flow-rate roller pump (Varistaltic, Manostat) and a metal canula (14-gauge needle, curved and shortened to 15 mm, with blunted bevelled end) linked to the container with flexible tubing (Manostat, Manosil, i.d. 1/4", 1/16"-thick and i.d. 1/8", 1/32"-thick). The system is filled with filtered aldehyde fixative, care being taken to eliminate all air bubbles. The flow-rate is set to 200 ml/min at the end of the canula, the tube clamped and the canula plunged in a small beaker containing the fixative.

The perfusion takes place in a large plastic tray where the anesthetized rat is secured on a dissection board, its head maintained in extension with adhesive tape. The skin is incised on the midline from abdomen to neck and reflected over the thorax. A laparectomy is performed and the descending aorta clamped immediately above the renal arteries. With two scissor cuts, the chest wall is opened in a V and reclined. The tip of the heart is grasped with toothed forceps and the muscle itself sectioned in its lower two thirds, across both ventricles. The metal canula is inserted through the left ventricle into the origin of the aortic arch and immobilized with a special clamp machined to fit snugly around it. The tubing from the pump is unclamped and the perfusion begun usually less than 20 sec after chest opening.

600 ml of aldehyde fixative are thus perfused in 3-5 min. When the reservoir is almost empty, 500-600 ml of osmium fixative are slowly poured into it. The perfusion tray is immediately covered with a polythylene sheet and the returning liquids and the fumes aspirated into a vacuum flask connected to a water suction system. The osmium perfusion is usually terminated within 5 min, and, after thorough rinsing of the whole animal and tray, the hood is removed to begin dissection. Doubly-fixed tissue is then processed according to standard techniques, except for the modifications described below for preparing whole brain sections for microscopic radioautography.

8.2.2. Preparing epoxy resin-embedded sections of the whole rat brain for light-microscopic radioautography (see also Section 4.4)

The following technique has been devised to reconcile the advantages of a systematic light-microscope radiographic survey of the whole rat brain (such as may be carried out with serial frozen or paraffin-embedded sections) with those of high-resolution radioautography (light- and electron-microscopy on the same specimens). It was especially developed to examine tissue fixed by double-perfusion of aldehyde and osmium, but may be useful after standard fixation as well. In brief, immediately after the perfusion, the entire brain is cut into 1-mm slices which are postfixed, dehydrated, embedded in epoxy resin, sectioned and radioautographed by procedures similar to those used for small tissue blocks.

(a) Postfixation

Whether the tissue has been previously osmicated or not by perfusion (0.2-0.5% osmium tetroxide), 1 mm-thick slices should be postfixed for at least 2-3 h in 1-2% osmium tetroxide, at room temperature.

(b) Staining 'en bloc'

Semi-thin sections of tissue stained with uranyl acetate exhibit numerous α-tracts when radioautographed. This staining procedure is therefore avoided or used only on alternate slices from which small blocks will be taken for electron-microscopy.

(c) Dehydration

Slices are conveniently dehydrated at room temperature, in increasing concentrations of ethanol or methanol: 35% (3 × 5 min), 50, 70, 80, 90, 95% (10 min each), absolute (3 × 10 min). Transfer to propylene oxide for 3x10 min:

(d) Embedding

The best results have so far been obtained with Epon (50:50 mixture, according to Luft). Agitation is required during infiltration.

1:1 mixture of propylene oxide-Epon	60 min
3:1 mixture of propylene oxide-Epon	90 min
Pure Epon	overnight

Each slice is embedded individually in a small peel-away, disposable cubic mold filled with fresh Epon. The specimens are polymerized for 20-24 h at 60°C.

(e) Cutting

The block face is trimmed to a square or rectangular shape. Three to five μm-thick sections are conveniently cut on a heavy-duty sliding microtome equipped with a tungsten carbide knife for extremely hard specimens (we have used the Jung Microtome K). Wetting the block face and knife edge with 70% alcohol improves the smoothness of sectioning. The sections are picked-up with a soft brush and transferred to a bath of 70% alcohol warmed at 45°C, from which they are mounted on chrome alum-gelatin coated slides. This is done by holding the slide half immersed in the alcohol bath and bringing one edge of the section in contact with the slide. The section is then unrolled and flattened by gently lifting it out of the bath. It is immediately blotted with bibulous paper to eliminate air bubbles and left to dry on a hot plate at 60°C for 24 h.

(f) Light-microscopic radioautography

The large sections may be processed as above (Section 8.1.1) except that after development they are immediately dehydrated in increasing concentrations of alcohol (70% to absolute), cleared in xylene and mounted. No staining is required because of the osmication.

8.3. SELECTED READING ON BASIC AND TECHNICAL ASPECTS OF RADIOAUTOGRAPHY

This is a list of publications that the authors have found particularly instructive on the fundamentals of the radioautographic method and/or useful in the planning and interpretation of radioautographic experiments.

8.3.1. Comprehensive texts

1. Roth LJ, Stumpf WE (Eds) (1969): *Autoradiography of Diffusible Substances,* pp. 1–371. Academic Press, New York.
2. Cowan WM, Cuénod M (Eds) (1975): *The Use of Axonal Transport for Studies of Neuronal Connectivity,* pp. 1–365. Elsevier, Amsterdam.
3. Droz B, Bouteille M, Sandoz D (Eds) (1976): *Techniques in Radioautography. J. Microsc. Biol. Cell., 27,* 71–292.
4. Rogers AW (1979): *Techniques of Autoradiography,* 3rd ed., pp. 1–429. Elsevier, Amsterdam.

8.3.2. Light-microscopic radioautography

5. Lacassagne A, Lattes J, Lavedan J (1925): Étude expérimentale des effets biologiques du polonium introduit dans l'organisme. *J. Radiol. Electrol., 9,* 1–14.
6. Bélanger LF, Leblond CP (1946): A method for locating radioactive elements in tissue by covering histological sections with photographic emulsion. *Endocrinology, 39,* 8–13.
7. Gross J, Bogoroch R, Nadler NJ, Leblond CP (1951): The theory and methods of the radioautographic localization of radioelements in tissue. *Am. J. Roentgenol. Radium Ther., 65,* 420–458.
8. Nadler NJ (1953): The quantitative estimation of radioisotopes by radioautography. *Am. J. Roentgenol. Radium Ther., 70,* 814–823.
9. Kopriwa BM, Leblond CP (1962): Improvements in the coating technique of radioautography. *J. Histochem. Cytochem., 10,* 269–284.
10. Appleton TC (1964): Autoradiography of soluble labeled compounds. *J. R. Microsc. Soc. 83,* 277–281.

8.3.3. Electron-microscopic radioautography

(a) Resolution and assessment of silver grain distribution

11. Caro LG (1962): High-resolution radioautography. II. The problem of resolution. *J. Cell Biol., 15,* 189–199.
12. Bachmann L, Salpeter MM (1965): Autoradiography with the electron-microscope. A quantitative evaluation. *Lab. Invest., 14,* 303–315.
13. Williams MA (1969): The assessment of electron-microscope autoradiographs. In: Barer R, Cosslett VE (Eds), *Advances in Optical and Electron-Microscopy, Vol. III,* pp. 219–272. Academic Press, London.
14. Blackett NM, Parry DM (1977): A simplified method of 'hypothetical grain' analysis of electron-microscope autoradiographs. *J. Histochem. Cytochem., 25,* 206–214.

15. Salpeter MM, McHenry FA, Salpeter EE (1978): Resolution in electron-microscopic autoradiography. IV. Application to analysis of autoradiographs. *J. Cell Biol., 76,* 127–145.
16. Nadler NJ (1979): Quantitation and resolution in electron-microscopic radioautography. *J. Histochem. Cytochem., 27,* 1531–1533.

(b) Emulsions and developers

17. Caro LG, Van Tubergen RP (1962): High-resolution autoradiography. I. Methods. *J. Cell Biol., 15,* 173–188.
18. Lettré H, Paweletz N (1966): Probleme der elektromikroskopischen Autoradiographie. *Naturwissenschaften, 53,* 268–271.
19. Kopriwa BM (1967): The influence of development on the number and appearence of silver grains in electron-microscopic autoradiography. *J. Histochem. Cytochem., 15,* 501–515.
20. Kopriwa BM (1975): A comparison of various procedures for fine grain development in electron-microscopic radioautography. *Histochemistry, 44,* 201–224.

8.3.4. Detailed technical descriptions

21. Granboulan P (1965): Comparison of emulsions and techniques in electron-microscopic radioautography. In: Leblond CP, Warren KB (Eds), *The Use of Radioautography in Investigating Protein Synthesis,* pp. 43–63. Academic Press, New York.
22. Salpeter MM, Bachmann L (1965): Assessment of technical steps in electron-microscopic autoradiography. In: Leblond CP, Warren KB (Eds), *The Use of Radioautography in Investigating Protein Synthesis,* pp. 23–39. Academic Press, New York.
23. Larra F, Droz B (1970): Techniques radioautographiques et leur application à l'étude du renouvellement des constituants cellulaires. *J. Microsc. (Paris), 9,* 845–880.
24. Kopriwa BM (1973): A reliable, standardized method for ultrastructural electron-microscopic radioautography. *Histochemistry, 37,* 1–17.
25. Descarries L (1975): High-resolution radioautography of noradrenergic axon terminals in the neocortex. Appendix II: A technique for high-resolution radioautography. In: Ali MA (Ed), *Vision in Fishes,* pp. 224–232. Plenum Press, New York.
26. Chan-Palay V (1977): *Cerebellar Dentate Nucleus: Organization, Cytology and Transmitters,* pp. 507–511. Springer-Verlag, Berlin-Heidelberg-New York.
27. Beaudet A (1982): High-resolution radioautography of central 5-hydroxytryptamine (5-HT) neurons. *J. Histochem. Cytochem., 30,* 765–768.

9. REFERENCES

Abercrombie M (1946): Estimation of nuclear population from microtome sections. *Anat. Rec., 94,* 239–247.
Aghajanian GK, Bloom FE (1966): Electron-microscopic autoradiography of rat hypothalamus after intraventricular ^{3}H-norepinephrine. *Science, 153,* 308–310.
Aghajanian GK, Bloom FE (1967a): Localization of tritiated serotonin in rat brain by electron-microscopic autoradiography. *J. Pharmacol. Exp. Ther., 156,* 23–30.
Aghajanian GK, Bloom FE (1967b): Electron-microscopic localization of norepinephrine in rat brain: Effect of drugs. *J. Pharmacol. Exp. Ther., 156,* 407–416.
Aghajanian GK, McCall RB (1980): Serotonergic synaptic input to facial motoneurons: Localization by electron-microscopic autoradiography. *Neuroscience, 5,* 2155–2162.
Aghajanian GK, Bloom FE, Lovell B, Sheard M, Freedman DX (1966): The uptake of 5-hydroxytryptamine-^{3}H from the cerebral ventricles: Autoradiographic localization. *Biochem. Pharmacol., 15,* 1401–1403.
Alonso G (1981): Etudes morphologiques et functionelles des neurones neurosécrétoires hypothalamoneurohypophysaires chez le rat. Thèse de Sciences, Université des Sciences et Techniques du Languedoc, Montpellier.

Alonso G, Pons F, Cadilhac J (1974): Mise en évidence par radioautographie de terminaisons indolaminergiques dans les parois ventriculaires cérébrales chez le rat. *C. R. Séances Soc. Biol. Paris, 168,* 1021–1024.

Altschuler RA, Mosinger JL, Wenthold RJ, Hoffman DW, Parakkal M (1981): Immunocytochemical localization of aspartate aminotransferase and enkephalin immunoreactivities in the guinea pig retina. *Soc. Neurosci. Abstr., 7,* 916.

Araneda S, Gamrani H, Font C, Calas A, Pujol JF, Bobillier P (1980). Retrograde axonal transport following injection of [^{3}H]serotonin in the olfactory bulb. II. Radioautographic study. *Brain Res., 196,* 417–427.

Arluison M (1981): Les fibres nerveuses sérotonergiques du striatum chez le rat et leurs caractéristiques ultrastructurales. *J. Physiol. (Paris), 77,* 45–51.

Arluison M, De La Manche IS (1980): High resolution radioautographic study of the serotonin innervation of the rat corpus striatum after intraventricular administration of [^{3}H]5-hydroxytryptamine. *Neuroscience, 5,* 229–240.

Arluison M, Agid Y, Javoy F (1978): Dopaminergic nerve endings in the neostriatum of the rat. 2. Radioautographic study following local microinjections of tritiated dopamine. *Neuroscience, 3,* 675–683.

Arregui A, Logan WJ, Bennett JP, Snyder SH (1972): Specific glycine-accumulating synaptosomes in the spinal cord of rats. *Proc. Nat. Acad. Sci. USA, 69,* 3485–3489.

Azmitia EC (1981): The visualization and characterization of 5-HT reuptake sites in the rodent and primate hippocampus. A preliminary Study. *J. Physiol. (Paris), 77,* 175–182.

Azmitia EC, Marovitz W (1980): In vitro hippocampal uptake of tritiated serotonin (^{3}H-5HT): A morphological, biochemical, and pharmacological approach to specificity. *J. Histochem. Cytochem., 28,* 636–664.

Bagnoli P, Beaudet A, Stella M, Cuénod M (1981): Selective retrograde labeling of cholinergic neurons with [^{3}H]choline. *J. Neurosci., 7,* 691–695.

Bak IJ, Kim JH, Hassler R (1970): Electron-microscopic autoradiography for demonstration of pineal serotonin in rat. *Z. Zellforsch. Mikrosk. Anat., 105,* 167–175.

Balcar VJ, Johnston GAR (1972): The structural specificity of the high affinity uptake of L-glutamate and L-aspartate by rat brain slices. *J. Neurochem., 19,* 2657–2666.

Balcar VJ, Johnston GAR (1973): High affinity uptake of transmitters: Studies on the uptake of L-aspartate, GABA, L-glutamate and glycine in cat spinal cord. *J. Neurochem., 20,* 529–539.

Baraban JM, Aghajanian GK (1981): Noradrenergic innervation of serotonergic neurons in the dorsal raphe: Demonstration by electron-microscopic autoradiography. *Brain Res., 204,* 1–11.

Barald KF, Berg DK (1979a): Autoradiographic labeling of spinal cord neurons with high affinity choline uptake in cell culture. *Dev. Biol. Suppl., 72,* 1–14.

Barald KF, Berg DK (1979b): Ciliary ganglion neurons in cell culture: High affinity choline uptake and autoradiographic choline labeling. *Dev. Biol. Suppl., 72,* 15–23.

Bauer B, Ehinger B (1978): Retinal uptake and release of [^{3}H]DABA. *Exp. Eye Res., 26,* 275–289.

Baughman RW, Bader CR (1977): Biochemical characterization and cellular localization of the cholinergic system in the chicken retina. *Brain Res., 138,* 469–485.

Baughman RW, Gilbert CD (1980): Aspartate and glutamate as possible neurotransmitters of cells in layer 6 of the visual cortex. *Nature, 287,* 448–489.

Baughman RW, Gilbert CD (1981): Aspartate and glutamate as possible neurotransmitters in the visual cortex. *J. Neurosci., 1,* 427–439.

Beart PM (1976a): The autoradiographic localization of L-^{3}H glutamate in synaptosomal preparations. *Brain Res., 103,* 350–355.

Beart PM (1976b): An evaluation of L-glutamate as the transmitter released from optic nerve terminals of the pigeon. *Brain Res., 110,* 99–114.

Beaudet A, Descarries L (1976): Quantitative data on serotonin nerve terminals in adult rat neocortex. *Brain Res., 111,* 301–309.

Beaudet A, Descarries L (1978): The monoamine innervation of rat cerebral cortex: Synaptic and nonsynaptic axon terminals. *Neuroscience, 3,* 851–860.

Beaudet A, Descarries L (1979): Radioautographic characterization of a serotonin-accumulating nerve cell group in adult rat hypothalamus. *Brain Res., 160,* 231–243.

Beaudet A, Descarries L (1981): The fine structure of central serotonin neurons. *J. Physiol. (Paris), 77,* 193–203.

Beaudet A, Sotelo C (1981): Synaptic remodeling of serotonin axon terminals in rat agranular cerebellum. *Brain Res., 206,* 305–329.

Beaudet A, Pickel VM, Joh TH, Miller RJ, Cuénod M (1980): Simultaneous detection of serotonin and tyrosine hydroxylase or enkephalin containing neurons by combined radioautography and immunocytochemistry in the central nervous system of the rat. *Soc. Neurosci. Abstr., 6,* 353.

Beaudet A, Burkhalter A, Reubi J-C, Cuénod M (1981): Selective bidirectional transport of [³H]D-aspartate in the pigeon retino-tectal pathway. *Neuroscience, 6,* 2021–2034.

Belin MF, Aguera M, Tappaz M, McRae-Degueurce A, Bobillier P, Pujol JF (1979): GABA-accumulating neurons in the nucleus raphe dorsalis and periaqueductal gray in the rat: A biochemical and radioautographic study. *Brain Res., 170,* 279–297.

Belin MF, Gamrani H, Aguera M, Calas A, Pujol JF (1980): Selective uptake of ³H-γ-aminobutyrate by rat supra and subependymal nerve fibers. Histological and high resolution radioautographic studies. *Neuroscience, 5,* 241–254.

Belin MF, Nanopoulos D, Didier M, Aguera M, Steinbusch HWM, Verhofstad AAJ, Vincendon G, Maitre M, Pujol JF (1983): Immunohistochemical evidence for the presence of γ-aminobutyric acid and serotonin in one nerve cell. A study on the raphe nuclei of the rat using antibodies to glutamate decarboxylase and serotonin. *Brain Res.,* in press.

Berger B, Glowinski J (1978): Dopamine uptake in serotoninergic terminals in vitro. A valuable tool for the histochemical differentiation of catecholaminergic and serotoninergic terminals in rat cerebral structures. *Brain Res., 147,* 29–45.

Bergeron M, Droz B (1968): Analyse critique des conditions de fixation et de préparation des tissus pour la détection radioautographique des protéines néoformées en microscopie électronique. *J. Microsc. (Paris), 7,* 51–62.

Bertler A, Falck B, Owman C (1964): Studies on the 5-hydroxytryptamine stores in pineal gland of rat. *Acta Physiol. Scand., 63, Suppl. 239,* 1–18.

Bessone R (1979): Étude morphologique et fonctionnelle de l'innervation sérotoninergique du noyau suprachiasmatique chez le rat. Thèse Spéc. Sci. Biol., Université des Sciences et Techniques du Languedoc, Montpellier.

Blackburn KJ, French PC, Merrills RJ (1967): 5-hydroxytryptamine uptake by rat brain in vitro. *Life Sci., 6,* 1653–1663.

Blackett NM, Parry DM (1973): A new method for analyzing electron-microscope autoradiographs using hypothetical grain distributions. *J. Cell Biol., 57,* 9–15.

Blackett NM, Parry DM (1977): A simplified method of 'hypothetical grain' analysis of electron-microscope autoradiographs. *J. Histochem. Cytochem., 25,* 206–214.

Bloom FE (1970): The fine structural localization of biogenic monoamines in nervous tissue. In: Pfeiffer CC, Smythies JR (Eds), *Internat. Rev. Neurobiol., Vol. 13,* pp. 27–66. Academic Press, New York.

Bloom FE, Costa E (1971): The effects of drugs on serotoninergic nerve terminals. In: Clementi F, Ceccarelli B (Eds), *Advances in Cytopharmacology, Vol. 1,* pp. 379–395. Raven Press, New York.

Bloom FE, Iversen LL (1971): Localization of [³H]-GABA in nerve terminals of rat cerebral cortex by electron-microscopic autoradiography. *Nature, 229,* 628–630.

Bloom FE, Hoffer BJ, Siggins GR (1971): Studies on norepinephrine-containing afferents to Purkinje cells of rat cerebellum. I. Localization of the fibers and their synapses. *Brain Res., 25,* 501–521.

Bloom FE, Hoffer BJ, Siggins GR, Barker JL, Nicoll RA (1972): Effects of serotonin on cental neurons: Microiontophoretic administration. *Fed. Proc., Fed. Am. Soc. Exp., 31,* 97–106.

Bosler O (1977): The organum vasculosum laminae terminalis. A cytophysiological study in the duck Anas Platyrhynchos. *Cell. Tissue Res., 1982,* 383–399.

Bosler O (1978): Radioautographic identification of serotonin axon terminals in the rat organum vasculosum laminae terminalis. *Brain Res., 150,* 177–181.

Bosler O (1980): Radioautographie des systèmes monoaminergiques centraux. Nouvelle possibilité d'investigation des neurones dopaminergiques. *Les Entretiens du CARLA, 1,* 31–46.

Bosler O, Calas A (1982): Radioautographic investigation of monoaminergic neurons. An evaluation. *Brain Res. Bull., 9,* 151–169.

Bosler O, Descarries L (1983): Uptake and retention of ³H-adrenaline by central monoaminergic neurons: A light- and electron-microscope radioautographic study after intraventricular administration in the rat. *Neuroscience, 8,* 561–581.

Bouchaud C (1979): Evidence for a multiple innervation of subcommissural ependymocytes in the rat. *Neurosci. Lett., 12,* 253–258.

Bouchaud C, Arluison M (1977): Serotoninergic innervation of ependymal cells in the rat subcommissural organ. A fluorescence, electron-microscopic and radioautographic study. *Biol. Cell., 30,* 61–64.

Bowery NG, Brown DA (1971): Observations on ³H-γ-aminobutyric acid accumulation and efflux in isolated sympathetic ganglia. *J. Physiol. (Lond.), 218,* 32P–33P.

Bowery NG, Jones GP, Neal MJ (1976): Selective inhibition of neuronal GABA uptake by cis-1,3-aminocyclohexane carboxylic acid. *Nature, 264,* 281–282.

Brandon C, Lam DMK, Wu J-Y (1979): The γ-aminobutyric acid system in rabbit retina: Localization by immunocytochemistry and autoradiography. *Proc. Nat. Acad. Sci. USA, 76,* 3557–3561.

Bruun A, Ehinger B (1972): Uptake of the putative neurotransmitter, glycine, into the rabbit retina. *Invest. Ophtalmol., 11,* 191–198.

Bruun A, Ehinger B (1974): Uptake of certain possible neurotransmitters into retinal neurons of some mammals. *Exp. Eye Res., 19,* 435–447.

Budd GC, Salpeter MM (1969): The distribution of labeled norepinephrine within sympathetic nerve terminals studied with electron-microscope radioautography. *J. Cell Biol., 41,* 21–32.

Burdman JA (1968): Uptake of [³H]catecholamines by chick embryo sympathetic ganglia in tissue culture. *J. Neurochem., 15,* 1321–1323.

Burry RW, Lasher RS (1975): Uptake of GABA in dispersed cell cultures of postnatal rat cerebellum: An electron-microscope autoradiographic study. *Brain Res., 88,* 502–507.

Calas A (1972): Capture et rétention de monoamines dans des fibres nerveuses de l'éminence médiane. Étude in vivo chez le canard par radioautographie à haute résolution. *CR Acad. Sci. (Paris), 274,* 925–927.

Calas A (1973): L'innervation monoaminergique de l'éminence médiane. Etude radioautographique et pharmacologique chez le canard Anas Platyrhynchos. *Z. Zellforsch. Mikrosk. Anat., 138,* 503–522.

Calas A (1975): The avian median eminence as a model for diversified neuroendocrine routes. In: Knigge KM, Scott DE, Kobayashi H, Ishi S (Eds), *Brain Endocrine Interaction. II. The Ventricular System in Neuroendocrine Mechanisms,* pp. 54–69. S. Karger, Basel.

Calas A (1977): Radioautographic studies of aminergic neurons terminating in the median eminence. In: Costa E, Gessa GL (Eds), *Neostriatal Dopaminergic Neurons Advances in Biochemical Psychopharmacology, Vol. 16,* pp. 79–88. Raven Press, New York.

Calas A, Bosc S (1976): Identification de fibres noradrénergiques et sérotoninergiques dans l'Eminence Médiane: Étude radioautographique, pharmacologique et microspectrofluorimétrique. *Ann. Histochim., 21,* 77–82.

Calas A, Alonso G, Arnauld E, Vincent JD (1974): Demonstration of indolaminergic fibres in the median eminence of the duck, rat and monkey. *Nature, 250,* 242–243.

Calas A, Besson MJ, Gauchy C, Alonso G, Glowinski J, Cheramy A (1976): Radioautographic study of in vivo incorporation of ³H-monoamines in the cat caudate nucleus: Identification of serotonergic fibers. *Brain Res., 118,* 1–13.

Calas A, Bosler O, Arluison M, Bouchaud C (1978): Serotonin as a neurohormone in circumventricular organs. In: Scott DE, Kozlowski GP, Weindl A (Eds), *Brain-Endocrine Interaction. III. Neural Hormones and Reproduction,* pp. 238–250. S. Karger, Basel.

Calas A, Dupuy JJ, Gamrani H, Gonella J, Mourre C, Condamin M, Pellissier JF, Van Den Bosch P (1981): Radioautographic investigation of serotonin cells. In: Haber B, Gabay S, Issidorides MR, Alivisatos SGA (Eds), *Serotonin-Current Aspects of Neurochemistry and Function, Advances in Experimental Medicine and Biology, Vol. 133,* pp. 51–66. Plenum Press, New York, London.

Caro LG (1962): High resolution radioautography. II. The problem of resolution. *J. Cell Biol., 15,* 189–199.

Caro LG, Van Tubergen RP (1962): High resolution radioautography. I. Methods. *J. Cell Biol., 15,* 173–188.

Chan-Palay V (1975): Fine structure of labelled axons in the cerebellar cortex and nuclei of rodents and primates after intraventricular infusions with tritiated serotonin. *J. Anat. Embryol., 148,* 235–265.

Chan-Palay V (1976a): Serotonin axons in the supra- and subependymal plexuses and in the leptomeninges: Their roles in local alterations of cerebrospinal fluid and vasomotor activity. *Brain Res., 102,* 103–130.

Chan-Palay V (1976b): On the identification of CAT₂ serotonin axons in the mammalian cerebellum. The roles of large granular, small, and granular alveolate vesicles in transmitter storage discharge, and reuptake – an hypothesis. In: Eränkö O (Ed), *Sif Cells, Fogarty International Center Proceedings, No. 30,* pp. 227–249. DHEW Publication, Washington.

Chan-Palay V (1977a): *Cerebellar Dentate Nucleus. Organization, Cytology and Transmitters,* pp. 390–454. Springer-Verlag, Berlin.

Chan-Palay V (1977b): Indoleamine neurons and their processes in the normal rat brain and in chronic diet-induced thiamine deficiency demonstrated by uptake of ³H-serotonin. *J. Comp. Neurol., 176,* 467–494.

Chan-Palay V (1978a): Morphological correlates for transmitter synthesis, transport, release, uptake and catabolism: A study of serotonin neurons in the nucleus paragigantocellularis lateralis. In: Fonnum F (Ed), *Amino Acids as Chemical Transmitters,* pp. 1–30. Plenum Press, New York.

Chan-Palay V (1978b): The paratrigeminal nucleus. II. Identification and interrelations of catecholamine axons, indolamine axons, and substance P immunoreactive cells in the neuropil. *J. Neurocytol., 7,* 419–442.

Chan-Palay V (1978c): Autoradiographic localization of γ-aminobutyric acid receptors in the rat central nervous system by using [^{3}H]muscimol. *Proc. Nat. Acad. Sci. USA, 75,* 1024–1028.

Chan-Palay V (1978d): Quantitative visualization of γ-aminobutyric acid receptors in hippocampus and area dentata demonstrated by [^{3}H]muscimol autoradiography. *Proc. Nat. Acad. Sci. USA, 75,* 2516–2520.

Chan-Palay V (1979): Combined immunocytochemistry and autoradiography after in vivo injections of monoclonal antibody to substance P and ^{3}H-serotonin: Coexistence of two putative transmitters in single cells and fiber plexuses. *J. Anat. Embryol., 156,* 241–254.

Chan-Palay V, Yonezawa T, Yoshida S, Palay SL (1978): γ-Aminobutyric acid receptors visualized in spinal cord cultures by (^{3}H) muscimol autoradiography. *Proc. Nat. Acad. Sci. USA, 75,* 6281–6284.

Chase TN, Breese GR, Kopin IJ (1967): Serotonin release from brain slices by electrical stimulation. Regional differences and effect of LSD. *Science, 157,* 1461–1463.

Chetverukhin VK, Belenky MA, Polenov AL (1979): Quantitative radioautographic light and electron-microscopic analysis of the localization of monoamines in the median eminence of the rat. I. Catecholamines. *Cell Tissue Res., 203,* 469–485.

Chrownwall BM, Wolff JR (1978): Classification and location of neurons taking up [^{3}H]GABA in the visual cortex of rats. In: Fonnum F (Ed), *Amino Acids as Chemical Transmitters,* pp. 297–303. Plenum Press, New York.

Chrownwall BM, Wolff JR (1980): Prenatal and postnatal development of GABA accumulating cells in the occipital neocortex of rat. *J. Comp. Neurol., 190,* 187–208.

Clark WG, Vivonia CA, Baxter CF (1968): Accurate freehand injection into the lateral brain ventricle of the conscious mouse. *J. Appl. Physiol., 25,* 319–321.

Collin J-P, Juillard M-T, Brisson P (1975): Synthèse des indolamines dans l'organe pinéal d'oiseau: Étude radio-autographique chez la perruche (Mélopsittacus undulatus, Shaw). *CR Acad. Sci. (Paris), 280,* 93–96.

Collin J-P, Calas A, Juillard M-T (1976): The avian pineal organ. Distribution of exogenous indoleamines: A qualitative study of the rudimentary photoreceptor cells by electron-microscopic radioautography. *Exp. Brain Res., 25,* 15–33.

Cotman CW, Foster A, Lantorn T (1981): An overview of glutamate as neurotransmitter. In: Di Chiara G, Gessa GL (Eds), *Glutamate as a Neurotransmitter, Advances in Biochemical Psychopharmacology, Vol. 27,* pp. 1–27. Raven Press, New York.

Coupland RE, Hopwood D (1966): The mechanism of the differential staining reaction for adrenaline- and noradrenaline-storing granules in tissues fixed in glutaraldehyde. *J. Anat., 100,* 227–243.

Coupland RE, Pyper AS, Hopwood D (1964): A method for differentiating between noradrenaline- and adrenaline-storing cells in the light- and electron-microscope. *Nature, 201,* 1240–1242.

Coyle JT, Snyder SH (1969): Antiparkinsonian drugs: Inhibition of dopamine uptake in the corpus striatum as a possible mechanism of action. *Science, 166,* 899–901.

Cuello AC, Iversen LL (1973): Localization of tritiated dopamine in the median eminence of the rat hypothalamus by electron-microscope autoradiography. *Brain Res., 62,* 474–478.

Cuénod M, Henke H (1978): Neurotransmitters in the avian visual system. In: Fonnum F (Ed), *Amino Acids as Chemical Transmitters,* pp. 221–239. Plenum Press, New York.

Cuénod M, Beaudet A, Canzek V, Streit P, Reubi JC (1981): Glutamatergic pathways in the pigeon and the rat brain. In: Di Chiara G, Gessa GL (Eds), *Glutamate as a Neurotransmitter, Advances in Biochemical Psychopharmacology, Vol. 27,* pp. 57–68 Raven Press, New York.

Cuénod M, Bagnoli P, Beaudet A, Rustioni A, Wiklund L, Streit P (1982): Transmitter-specific retrograde labeling of neurons. In: Chan-Palay V, Palay SL (Eds), *Cytochemical Methods in Neuroanatomy,* pp. 17–44. Alan R. Liss, New York.

Currie DN, Dutton GR (1980): (^{3}H)GABA uptake as a marker for cell type in primary cultures of cerebellum and olfactory bulb. *Brain Res., 199,* 473–481.

Dahlström A, Fuxe K (1964): Evidence for the existence of monoamine-containing neurons in the central nervous system. I. Demonstration of monoamines in the cell bodies of brain stem neurons. *Acta Physiol. Scand., 62, Suppl. 232,* 1–55.

Davies LP, Johnston GAR (1976): Uptake and release of D- and L-aspartate by rat brain slices. *J. Neurochem., 26,* 1007–1014.

De Belleroche JS, Bradford HF (1978): Compartmentation of synaptosomal dopamine. In: Roberts PJ, Woodruff GN, Iversen LL (Ed), Dopamine, *Advances in Biochemical Psychopharmacology, Vol. 19,* pp. 57–73. Raven Press, New York.

De Belleroche JS, Bradford HF, Jones DA (1976): A study of the metabolism and release of dopamine and amino acids from nerve endings isolated from sheep corpus striatum. *J. Neurochem., 26,* 561–571.

351

De La Manche IS, Arluison M, Bouchaud C (1981): Experimental ultrastructure modifications of the content of serotoninergic supraependymal nerve fibers in the rat. *J. Physiol. (Paris), 77,* 225–231.

Demarest KT, Moore KE (1979): Lack of a high affinity transport system for dopamine in the median eminence and posterior pituitary. *Brain Res., 171,* 545–551.

Denêmes D, Raymond J (1982): Radioautographic identification of [³H]glutamic acid-labeled nerve endings in the cat oculomotor nucleus. *Brain Res., 231,* 433–437.

Dennison ME, Jordan CC, Webster RA (1976): Distribution and localization of tritiated amino acids by autoradiography in the cat spinal cord in vivo. *J. Physiol. (London), 258,* 55–56P.

De Robertis E, De Iraldi AP, De Lores Arnaiz GR, Zieher LM (1965): Synaptic vesicles from the rat hypothalamus. Isolation and norepinephrine content. *Life Sci., 4,* 193–201.

Désarménien M, Santangelo F, Linck G, Headly PM, Feltz P (1981): Physiological study of amino acid uptake and receptor desensitization: the GABA system in dorsal root ganglia. In: DeFeudis FV, Mandel P (Eds), *Amino Acid Neurotransmitters, Advances in Biochemical Psychopharmacology, Vol. 29,* pp. 309–319. Raven Press, New York.

Descarries L (1975): High resolution radioautography of noradrenergic axon terminals in the rat neocortex. In: Ali MA (Ed), *Vision in Fishes,* pp. 211–230. Plenum Press, New York.

Descarries L, Beaudet A (1978): The serotonin innervation of adult rat hypothalamus. In: *Biologie Cellulaire des Processus Neurosécrétoires Hypothalamiques, Colloques Int. CNRS, no. 280,* pp. 135–153. Paris.

Descarries L, Droz B (1968a): Incorporation de noradrénaline –³H (NA–³H) dans le système nerveux central du rat adulte. Étude radioautographique en microscopie électronique, *CR Acad. Sci. (Paris), 266,* 2480–2482.

Descarries L, Droz B (1968b): Electron-microscope radioautographic detection of norepinephrine –³H in the central nervous system of the rat. In: Bocciarelli DS (Ed), *Electron-Microscopy 1968, Vol. II,* pp. 527–528. Tipographia Poliglotta Vaticana, Rome.

Descarries L, Droz B (1969): Storage and renewal of tritiated norepinephrine and α-methyl-norepinephrine in catecholaminergic neurons of the central nervous system. A radioautographic study. In: Paoletti R, Fumagalli R, Galli C (Eds), *IInd Internat. Meet. Internat. Soc. Neurochem.,* p. 150. Tamburini Editore, Milan.

Descarries L, Droz B (1970a): Intraneural distribution of exogenous norepinephrine in the central nervous system of the rat. *J. Cell Biol., 44,* 385–399.

Descarries L, Droz B (1970b): Neurones catécholaminergiques du système nerveux central. Étude radioautographique. In: Benoit J, Kordon C (Eds), *Neuroendocrinologie, Coll. Nat. CNRS, Vol. 927,* pp. 49–56. Éditions du CNRS, Paris.

Descarries L, Dupin JC (1974): Retention of noradrenaline-³H in brain and preferential extraction of labeled metabolites by glutaraldehyde fixation. *Experientia, 30,* 1164–1165.

Descarries L, Havrankova J (1970): Catécholamines endogènes marquées dans le système nerveux central. Étude radioautographique après L-3,4 dihydroxyphénylalanine tritiée (DOPA-³H). *CR Acad. Sci. (Paris), 271,* 2392–2395.

Descarries L, Lapierre Y (1973a): Noradrenergic axon terminals in the cerebral cortex of rat. I. Radioautographic visualization after topical application of DL-[³H] norepinephrine. *Brain Res., 51,* 141–160.

Descarries L, Lapierre Y (1973b): Characterization of cortical noradrenergic axon terminals with high resolution radioautography. In: Usdin E, Snyder SH (Eds), *Frontiers in Catecholamine Research,* pp. 463–465. Pergamon Press, Oxford.

Descarries L, Léger L (1978): Serotonin nerve terminals in the locus coeruleus of adult rat. In: Garattini S, Pujol JF, Samanin R (Eds), *Interactions Between Putative Neurotransmitters,* pp. 355–367. Raven Press, New York.

Descarries L, Saucier G (1972): Disappearance of the locus coeruleus in the rat after intraventricular 6-hydroxydopamine. *Brain Res., 37,* 310–316.

Descarries L, Beaudet A, Watkins KC (1975): Serotonin nerve terminals in adult rat neocortex. *Brain Res., 100,* 563–588.

Descarries L, Watkins KC, Lapierre Y (1977): Noradrenergic axon terminals in the cerebral cortex of rat. III. Topometric ultrastructural analysis. *Brain Res., 133,* 197–222.

Descarries L, Bosler O, Berthelet F, Des Rosiers MH (1980): Dopaminergic nerve endings visualized by high-resolution autoradiography in adult rat neostriatum. *Nature, 284,* 620–622.

Descarries L, Berthelet F, Garcia S (1981a): Axophoresis of [³H]DA and [³H]NA by central catecholaminergic neurons: Radioautographic demonstration. *Soc. Neurosci. Abstr., 7,* 802.

Descarries L, Bosler O, Berthelet F, Des Rosiers MH (1981b): Innervation dopaminergique du néostriatum: Nouvelle possibilité d'investigation radioautographique. *J. Physiol. (Paris), 77,* 53–61.

Descarries L, Watkins KC, Garcia S, Beaudet A (1982): The serotonin neurons in nucleus raphe dorsalis of adult rat: A light- and electron-microscope radioautographic study. *J. Comp. Neurol., 207*, 239–254.

Devine CE (1967): Electron-microscope autoradiography of rat arteriolar axons after noradrenaline infusion. *Proc. Univ. Otago Med. Sch., 45*, 7–8.

Devine CE, Laverty R (1968): Fixation for electron-microscopy and the retention of ^{3}H-noradrenaline by tissues. *Experientia, 24*, 1156–1157.

Devine CE, Simpson FO (1968): Localization of tritiated norepinephrine in vascular sympathetic axons of the rat intestine and mesentery by electron-microscopic radioautography. *J. Cell Biol., 38*, 184–192.

Di Porzio U, Daguet MC, Glowinski J, Prochiantz A (1980): Effect of striatal cells on in vitro maturation of mesencephalic dopaminergic neurones grown in serum-free conditions. *Nature, 288*, 370–373.

Dreyfus CF, Sherman D, Gershon MD (1977): Uptake of serotonin by intrinsic neurons of the myentric plexus grown in organotypic tissue culture. *Brain Res., 128*, 109–123.

Dupin JC, Descarries L, De Champlain J (1976): Radioautographic visualization of central catecholaminergic neurons in newborn rat after intravenous administration of tritiated norepinephrine. *Brain Res., 102*, 588–596.

Ehinger B (1970): Autoradiographic identification of rabbit retinal neurons that take up GABA. *Experientia, 26*, 1063–1964.

Ehinger B (1972a): Cellular location of the uptake of some amino acids into the rabbit retina. *Brain Res., 46*, 297–311.

Ehinger B (1972b): Uptake of tritiated glycine into neurons of the human retina. *Experientia, 28*, 1042–1043.

Ehinger B (1977): Glial and neuronal uptake of GABA, glutamic acid, glutamine and glutathione in the rabbit retina. *Exp. Eye Res., 25*, 221–234.

Ehinger B (1981): (^{3}H)D-aspartate accumulation in the retina of pigeon guinea-pig and rabbit. *Exp. Eye Res., 33*, 381–392.

Ehinger B, Falck B (1971): Autoradiography of some suspected neurotransmitter substances: GABA, glycine, glutamic acid, histamine, dopamine, and L-DOPA. *Brain Res., 33*, 157–172.

Ehinger B, Florén I (1978): Quantitation of the uptake of indoleamines and dopamine in the rabbit retina. *Exp. Eye Res., 26*, 1–11.

Ehinger B, Florén I (1980): Retinal indoleamine accumulating neurons. *Neurochemistry, 1*, 209–229.

Elliott KAC, Van Gelder NM (1958): Occlusion and metabolism of γ-aminobutyric acid by brain tissue. *J. Neurochem., 3*, 28–40.

Eränkö O, Härkönen M (1965): Monoamine-containing small cells in the superior cervical ganglion of the rat and an organ composed of them. *Acta Physiol. Scand., 63*, 511–512.

Esterhuizen AC, Graham JDP, Lever JD, Spriggs TLB (1968): Catecholamine and acetylcholinesterase distribution in relation to noradrenaline release. An enzyme histochemical and autoradiographic study on the innervation of the cat nictitating membrane. *Br. J. Pharmacol. Chemother., 32*, 46–56.

Falk GJ, King RC (1963): Radioautographic efficiency for tritium as a function of section thickness. *Radiat. Res., 20*, 466–470.

Farb DH, Berg DK, Fischbach GD (1979): Uptake and release of [3]Hγ-aminobutyric acid by embryonic spinal cord neurons in dissociated cell culture. *J. Cell Biol., 80*, 651–661.

Fonnum F, Lund Karlsen R, Malthe-Sorenssen D, Sterri S, Walaas I (1980): High affinity transport systems and their role in transmitter action. In: Cotman CW, Poste G, Nicolson GL (Eds), *The Cell Surface and Neuronal Function*, pp. 455–504. Elsevier, Amsterdam.

Font C, Araneda S, Pujol JF, Bobillier P (1982): Biochemical and autoradiographic investigation of the retrograde axonal transport of labeled material following [3]Hnorepinephrine injection in the olfactory bulb. *Neurochem. Int., 4*, 569–575.

Frankfurt M, Lauder JM, Azmitia EC (1982): The immunocytochemical localization of serotonergic neurons in the rat hypothalamus. *Neurosci. Lett., 24*, 227–232.

Fuller RW, Perry KW, Molloy BB (1974): Effect of an uptake inhibitor on serotonin metabolism in rat brain: Studies with 3-(p-trifluoromethylphenoxy)-N-methyl-3-phenylpropylamine (Lilly 110140). *Life Sci., 15*, 1161–1171.

Fuxe K, Ungerstedt U (1968): Histochemical studies on the distribution of catecholamines and 5-hydroxytryptamine after intraventricular injections. *Histochemie, 13*, 16–28.

Fuxe K, Hökfelt T, Ritzen M, Ungerstedt U (1968): Studies on uptake of intraventricularly administered tritiated noradrenaline and 5-hydroxytryptamine with combined fluorescence and autoradiographic techniques. *Histochemie, 16*, 186–194.

Gamrani H, Calas A (1980): Cytochemical, stereological and radioautographic studies of rat raphe neurons. *Mikroskopie, 36*, 1–11.

Gamrani H, Calas A, Belin MF, Aguera M, Pujol JF (1979): High resolution radioautographic identification of ^{3}H-GABA labeled neurons in the rat nucleus raphe dorsalis. *Neurosci. Lett., 15*, 43–48.

Gamrani H, Belin MF, Aguera M, Calas A, Pujol JF (1981): Radioautographic evidence for an innervation of the subcommissural organ by GABA-containing nerve fibres. *J. Neurocytol., 10,* 411–424.

Gaudin-Chazal G, Daszuta A, Ségu L, Ternaux JP, Puizillout JJ (1978): Serotonin containing neurons in the nodose ganglia of the cat. *Waking and Sleeping, 2,* 149–151.

Geffen LB, Descarries L, Droz B (1971): Intraaxonal migration of ^{3}H-norepinephrine injected in the coeliac ganglion of cats: Radioautographic study of the proximal segment of constricted splenic nerves. *Brain Res., 35,* 315–318.

Gershon MD (1981): Properties and development of peripheral serotonergic neurons. *J. Physiol. (Paris), 77,* 257–265.

Gershon MD, Altman RF (1971): An analysis of the uptake of 5-hydroxytryptamine by the myenteric plexus of the small intestine of the guinea pig. *J. Pharmacol. Exp. Ther., 179,* 29–41.

Gershon MD, Ross LL (1966): Location of sites of 5-hydroxytryptamine storage and metabolism by radioautography. *J. Physiol. (London), 186,* 477–492.

Gershon MD, Robinson RG, Ross LL (1976): Serotonin accumulation in the guinea pig's myenteric plexus: Ion dependence, structure activity relationship and the effect of drugs. *J. Pharmacol. Exp. Ther., 198,* 548–561.

Gershon MD, Epstein ML, Hegstrand L (1980): Colonization of the chick gut by progenitors of enteric serotoninergic neurons: Distributon, differentiation, and maturation within the gut. *Dev. Biol., 77,* 41–51.

Gillespie JS, Kirkepar AM (1966): The histological localization of noradrenaline in the cat's spleen. *J. Physiol. (London), 187,* 69–79.

Glowinski J, Iversen LL (1966): Regional studies of catecholamines in the rat brain. I. The disposition of (^{3}H)-norepinephrine, (^{3}H)-dopamine and ^{3}H-dopa in various regions of the rat brain. *J. Neurochem., 13,* 655–669.

Glowinski J, Kopin IJ, Axelrod J (1965): Metabolism of ^{3}H-norepinephrine in the rat brain. *J. Neurochem., 12,* 25–30.

Graham JDP, Lever JD, Spriggs TLB (1968): An examination of adrenergic axons around pancreatic arterioles of the cat for the presence of acetylcholinesterase by high resolution radioautographic and histochemical methods. *Br. J. Pharmacol. Chemother., 33,* 15–20.

Gropetti A, Algeri S, Cattabeni F, Di Giulio AM, Galli CL, Ponzio F, Spano PF (1977): Changes in specific activity of dopamine metabolites as evidence of a multiple compartmentation of dopamine in striatal neurons. *J. Neurochem, 28,* 193–197.

Gupta BL, Moreton RB, Cooper NC (1963): Reconsideration of resolution in EM autoradiography using a biological line source. *J. Microsc., 99,* 1–25.

Guyenet P, Lefresne P, Rossier J, Beaujouan JC, Glowinski J (1973): Inhibition by hemicholinium-3 of ^{14}C-acetylcholine synthesis and ^{3}H-choline high affinity uptake in rat striatal synaptosomes. *Mol. Pharmacol., 9,* 630–639.

Halaris AE, De Met EM (1978): Active uptake of [^{3}H]5-HT by synaptic vesicles from rat brain. *J. Neurochem., 31,* 591–597.

Halasz N, Hökfelt T, Ljungdahl A, Johansson O, Goldstein M (1977): Dopamine neurons in the olfactory bulb. In: Costa E, Gessa GL (Eds), *Nonstriatal Dopaminergic Neurons, Advances in Biochemical Psychopharmacology, Vol. 16,* pp. 169–177. Raven Press, New York.

Halasz N, Ljungdahl A, Hökfelt T (1978): Transmitter histochemistry of the rat olfactory bulb. II. Fluorescence histochemical, autoradiographic and electron-microscopic localization of monoamines. *Brain Res., 154,* 253–271.

Halasz N, Ljungdahl A, Hökfelt T (1979): Transmitter histochemistry of the rat olfactory bulb. III. Autoradiographic localization of [^{3}H]GABA. *Brain Res., 167,* 221–240.

Hamberger B (1967): Reserpine-resistant uptake of catecholamines in isolated tissues of the rat. *Acta Physiol. Scand., Suppl. 295,* 1–56.

Hamberger B, Malmfors T, Norberg KA, Sachs C (1964): Uptake and accumulation of catecholamines in peripheral adrenergic neurons of reserpinized animals, studied with a histochemical method. *Biochem. Pharmacol., 13,* 841–844.

Hartman JA, Halaris AE (1980): Compartmentation of catecholamines in rat brain: Effects of agonists and antagonists. *Brain Res., 200,* 421–436.

Hattori T, McGeer PL, Fibiger HC, McGeer EG (1973): On the source of GABA-containing terminals in the substantia nigra. Electron-microscopic autoradiographic and biochemical studies. *Brain Res., 54,* 103–144.

Hendry SH, Jones EG (1981): Sizes and distributions of intrinsic neurons incorporating tritiated GABA in monkey sensory-motor cortex. *J. Neurosci., 1,* 390–408.

354

Henke H, Schenxer TM, Cuénod M (1976): Uptake of neurotransmitter candidates by pigeon optic tectum. *J. Neurochem., 26,* 125–130.

Henn FA, Hamberger A (1971): Glial cell function: Uptake of transmitter substances. *Proc. Nat. Acad. Sci. USA, 68,* 2686–2690.

Henn FA, Goldstein MN, Hamberger A (1974): Uptake of neurotransmitter candidate glutamate by glia. *Nature, 249,* 663–664.

Hespe W, Roberts E, Prins H (1969): Autoradiographic investigation of the distribution of [^{14}C]GABA in tissues of normal and aminooxyacetic acid-treated mice. *Brain Res., 14,* 663–671.

Hökfelt T (1968): In vitro studies on central and peripheral monoamine neurons at the ultrastructural level. *Z. Zellforsch. Mikrosk. Anat., 91,* 1–74.

Hökfelt T, Jonsson G (1968): Studies on reaction and binding of monoamines after fixation and processing for electron-microscopy with special reference to fixation with potassium permanganate. *Histochemie, 16,* 45–67.

Hökfelt T, Ljungdahl A (1970): Cellular localization of labeled gamma-aminobutyric acid (^{3}H-GABA) in rat cerebellar cortex: An autoradiographic study. *Brain Res., 22,* 391–396.

Hökfelt T, Ljungdahl A (1971a): Light and electron-microscopic autoradiography on spinal cord slices after incubation with labeled glycine. *Brain Res., 32,* 189–194.

Hökfelt T, Ljungdahl A (1971b): Uptake of [^{3}H]noradrenaline and [^{3}H]gamma-aminobutyric acid in isolated tissues of rat: An autoradiographic- and fluorescence-microscopic study. In: Eränkö O (Ed), *Histochemistry of Nervous Transmission, Progress in Brain Research, Vol. 34,* pp. 87–102. Elsevier, Amsterdam.

Hökfelt T, Ljungdahl A (1972a): Application of cytochemical techniques to the study of suspected transmitter substances in the nervous system. In: Costa E, Iversen LL, Paoletti R (Eds), *Studies of Neurotransmitters at the Synaptic Level, Advances in Biochemical Psychopharmacology, Vol. 6,* pp. 1–36. Raven Press, New York.

Hökfelt T, Ljungdahl A (1972b): Autoradiographic identification of cerebral and cerebellar cortical neurons accumulating labeled gamma-aminobutyric acid ([^{3}H]-GABA). *Exp. Brain Res., 14,* 354–362.

Hökfelt T, Ljungdahl A (1975): Uptake mechanisms as a basis for the histochemical identification and tracing of transmitter-specific neuron populations. In: Cowan WM, Cuénod M (Eds), *The Use of Axonal Transport for Studies of Neuronal Connectivity,* pp. 251–305. Elsevier, Amsterdam.

Hökfelt T, Fuxe K, Goldstein M, Johansson O (1973): Evidence for adrenaline neurons in the rat brain. *Acta Physiol. Scand., 89,* 286–288.

Hökfelt T, Fuxe K, Goldstein M, Johansson O (1974): Immunohistochemical evidence for the existence of adrenaline neurons in the rat brain. *Brain Res., 66,* 235–251.

Hopsu UK, Makinen EO (1966): Two methods for the demonstration of noradrenaline-containing adrenal medullary cells. *J. Histochem. Cytochem., 14,* 434–435.

Horn AS (1973): Structure-activity relations for the inhibition of catecholamine uptake into synaptosomes from noradrenaline and dopaminergic neurons in rat brain homogenates. *Br. J. Pharmacol., 47,* 332–338.

Horn AS (1979): Characteristics of dopamine uptake. In: Horn AS, Korf J, Westerink BHC (Eds), *The Neurobiology of Dopamine,* pp. 217–235. Academic Press, London.

Horn AS, Coyle JT, Snyder SH (1971): Catecholamine uptake by synaptosomes from rat brain. *Mol. Pharmacol., 7,* 66–80.

Hösli L, Hösli E (1972): Autoradiographic localization of the uptake of glycine in cultures of rat medulla oblongata. *Brain Res., 45,* 612–616.

Hösli E, Hösli L (1976a): Autoradiographic studies on the uptake of ^{3}H-noradrenaline and ^{3}H-GABA in cultured rat cerebellum. *Exp. Brain Res., 26,* 319–324.

Hösli E, Hösli L (1976b): Uptake of L-glutamate and L-aspartate in neurones and glial cells of cultured human and rat spinal cord. *Experientia, 32,* 219–222.

Hösli E, Hösli L (1978a): Autoradiographic localization of the uptake of [^{3}H]GABA and [^{3}H]L-glutamic acid in neurones and glial cells of cultured dorsal root ganglia. *Neurosci. Lett., 7,* 173–176.

Hösli L, Hösli E (1978b): Action and uptake of neurotransmitters in CNS tissue culture. *Rev. Physiol. Biochem. Pharmacol., 81,* 136–188.

Hösli E, Ljungdahl A, Hökfelt T, Hösli L (1972): Spinal cord tissue cultures – a model for autoradiographic studies on uptake of putative neurotransmitters such as glycine and GABA. *Experientia, 28,* 1342–1344.

Hösli E, Bucher UM, Hösli L (1975): Uptake of ^{3}H-noradrenaline and ^{3}H-5-hydroxytryptamine in cultured rat brainstem. *Experientia, 31,* 354–356.

Hunt SP, Künzle H (1976): Selective uptake and transport of label within three identified neuronal systems after injections of [^{3}H]GABA into the pigeon optic tectum: An autoradiographic and Golgi study. *J. Comp. Neurol., 170,* 173–190.

Hunt SP, Streit P, Künzle H, Cuénod M (1977): Characterization of the pigeon isthmo-tectal pathway by selective uptake and retrograde movement of radioactive compounds and by Golgi-like horseradish peroxidase labeling. *Brain Res., 129,* 197–212.

Hyndman AG, Adler R (1982): Analysis of glutamate uptake and monosodium glutamate toxicity in neural retina monolayer cultures. *Dev. Brain Res., 2,* 303–314.

Inaba M, Kamata K (1977): Catecholamine binding macromolecule in soluble fraction of rat brain. *Jpn. J. Pharmacol., 27,* 213–225.

Iversen LL (1967): *The Uptake and Storage of Noradrenaline in Sympathetic Nerves,* pp.1–253. Cambridge University Press, Cambridge.

Iversen LL (1970): Neuronal uptake processes for amines and amino acids. In: Costa E, Giacobini E (Eds), *Biochemistry of Simple Neuronal Models, Advances in Biochemical Psychopharmacology, Vol. 2,* pp. 109–132. Raven Press, New York.

Iversen LL (1975): Uptake processess for biogenic amines. In: Iversen LL, Iversen SD, Snyder SH (Eds), *Biochemistry of Biogenic Amines, Handbook of Psychopharmacology, Vol. 3,* pp. 381–442. Plenum Press, New York.

Iversen LL (1978): Identification of transmitter-specific neurons in CNS by autoradiographic techniques. In: Iversen LL, Iversen SD, Snyder SH (Eds), *Chemical Pathways in the Brain, Handbook of Psychopharmacology, Vol. 9,* pp. 41–68. Plenum Press, New York.

Iversen LL, Bloom FE (1972): Studies of the uptake of ^{3}H-GABA and ^{3}H-glycine in slices and homogenates of rat brain and spinal cord by electron-microscopic autoradiography. *Brain. Res., 41,* 131–143.

Iversen LL, Neal MJ (1968): The uptake of ^{3}H-GABA by slices of rat cerebral cortex. *J. Neurochem., 15,* 1141–1149.

Iversen LL, Schon F (1973): The use of autoradiographic techniques for the identification and mapping of transmitter-specific neurones in CNS. In: Mandell AJ (Ed), *New Concepts in Neurotransmitter Regulation,* pp. 153–193. Plenum Press, New York.

Iversen LL, Snyder SH (1968): Synaptosomes: Different populations storing catecholamines and gamma-aminobutyric acid in homogenates of rat brain. *Nature, 220,* 796–798.

Iversen LL, Dick F, Kelly JS, Schon F (1975): Uptake and localization of transmitter amino acids in the nervous system. In: Berl S, Clarke DD, Schneider D (Eds), *Metabolic Compartmentation and Neurotransmission,* pp. 65–89. Plenum Press, New York.

Jaim-Etcheverry G, Zieher LM (1968): Cytochemistry of 5-hydroxytryptamine at the electron-microscopic level. II. Localization in the autonomic nerves of rat pineal gland. *Z. Zellforsch. Mikrosk. Anat., 86,* 393–400.

Jaim-Etcheverry G, Zieher LM (1969): Ultrastructural cytochemistry and pharmacology of 5-hydroxytryptamine in adrenergic nerve endings. I. Localization of exogenous 5-hydroxytryptamine in the autonomic nerves of the vas deferens. *J. Pharmacol. Exp. Ther., 166,* 264–271.

Javoy F, Glowinski J (1971): Dynamic characteristics of the 'functional compartment' of dopamine in dopaminergic terminals of the rat striatum. *J. Neurochem., 18,* 1305–1311.

Johnson JL (1978): The excitant amino acids glutamic and aspartic acid as transmitter candidates in the vertebrate central nervous system. *Prog. Neurobiol., 10,* 155–202.

Johnston GAR (1979): Central nervous system receptors for glutamic acid. In: Filer LJ, Garattini S, Kare MR, Reynolds WA, Wurtman RJ (Eds), *Glutamic Acid, Advances in Biochemistry and Physiology,* pp. 177–185. Raven Press, New York.

Johnston GAR, Iversen LL (1971): Glycine uptake in rat central nervous system slices and homogenates: Evidence for different uptake systems in spinal cord and cerebral cortex. *J. Neurochem., 18,* 1951–1961.

Johnston GAR, Kennedy SME, Lodge D (1978): Muscimol uptake, release and binding in rat brain slices. *J. Neurochem., 31,* 1519–1523.

Jonakait JM, Tamir H, Rapport MM, Gershon MD (1977): Detection of a soluble serotonin-binding protein in the mammalian myenteric plexus and other peripheral sites of serotonin storage. *J. Neurochem., 28,* 277–284.

Juillard M-T, Collin J-P (1976): L'organe pinéal aviare: Étude ultracytochimique et pharmacologique d'un 'pool' granulaire de 5-Hydroxytryptamine chez la perruche (Melopstittacus undulatus, Shaw). *J. Microsc. Biol. Cell., 26,* 133–138.

Kelly JS, Dick F (1976): Differential labeling of glial cells and GABA-inhibitory interneurons and nerve terminals following the micro-injection of ^{3}H-β-alanine, ^{3}H-DABA and ^{3}H-GABA into single folia of the cerebellum. In: *The Synapse, Cold-Spring Harbor Symposia on Quantitative Biology, Vol. XL,* pp. 93–106. Cold Spring Harbor Laboratory.

Kelly JS, Weitsch-Dick F (1978): A critical evaluation of the use of autoradiography as a tool in the localization of amino-acids in the mammalian CNS. In: Fonnum F (Ed), *Amino Acids as Chemical Transmitters*, pp. 103–121. Plenum Press, New York.

Kelly JS, Dick F, Schon F (1975): The autoradiographic localization of the GABA-releasing nerve terminals in cerebellar glomeruli. *Brain Res., 85,* 255–259.

Köhler C, Steinbusch HMW (1981): Distribution and origin of serotonin fibers in the septal area. A combined immunohistochemical and fluorescent retrograde tracing study in the rat. *Neurosci. Lett., Suppl. 7,* S398.

König JFR, Klippel RA (1963): *The Rat Brain, A Stereotaxic Atlas,* William and Wilkins Co., Baltimore.

Kramer SG, Potts AM, Mangnall Y (1971): Dopamine: A retinal neurotransmitter. II. Autoradiographic localization of ^{3}H-dopamine in the retina. *Invest. Ophthal., 10,* 617–624.

Krnjević K, Schwartz S (1966): Is γ-aminobutyric acid an inhibitory transmitter. *Nature, 211,* 1372–1374.

Kuhar MJ, Aghajanian GK (1973): Selective accumulation of ^{3}H-serotonin by nerve terminals of raphe neurones: An autoradiographic study. *Nature, 241,* 187–189.

Kuhar MJ, Aghajanian GK, Roth RH (1972a): Tryptophan hydroxylase activity and synaptosomal uptake of serotonin in discrete brain regions after midbrain raphe lesions: Correlations with serotonin levels and histochemical fluorescence. *Brain Res., 44,* 165–176.

Kuhar MJ, Roth RH, Aghajanian GK (1972b): Synaptosomes from forebrains of rats with midbrain raphe lesions: Selective reduction of serotonin uptake. *J. Pharmacol. Exp. Ther., 181,* 36–45.

Kuhar MJ, Sethy VH, Roth RH, Aghajanian GK (1973): Choline: Selective accumulation by central cholinergic neurones. *J. Neurochem., 20,* 581–593.

Lam DMK, Hollyfield JG (1980): Localization of putative amino acid neurotransmitters in the human retina. *Exp. Eye Res., 31,* 729–732.

Lam DMK, Steinman L (1971): The uptake of (γ-^{3}H)aminobutyric acid in the goldfish retina. *Proc. Nat. Acad. Sci. USA, 68,* 2777–2781.

Lapierre Y, Beaudet A, Demianczuk N, Descarries L (1973): Noradrenergic axon terminals in the cerebral cortex of rat. II. Quantitative data revealed by light and electron-microscope radioautography of the frontal cortex. *Brain Res., 63,* 175–182.

Lasher RS (1974): The uptake of [^{3}H]GABA and differentiation of stellate neurons in cultures of dissociated postnatal rat cerebellum. *Brain Res., 69,* 235–254.

Leblond CP (1965): What radioautography has added to protein lore. In: Leblond CP, Warren KB (Eds), *The Use of Radioautography in Investigating Protein Synthesis,* pp. 321–339. Academic Press, New York.

Leblond CP (1976): Interpretations in radioautography. In: Droz B, Bouteille M, Sandoz D (Eds), *Techniques in Radioautography, J. Microsc. Biol. Cell., 27,* 73–79.

Léger L, Descarries L (1978): Serotonin nerve terminals in the locus coeruleus of adult rat: A radioautographic study. *Brain Res., 145,* 1–13.

Léger L, Pujol JF, Bobillier P, Jouvet M (1977): Transport axoplasmique de la sérotonine par voie rétrograde dans les neurones monoaminergiques centraux. *CR Acad. Sci. (Paris), 205,* 1179–1182.

Léger L, Mouren-Mathieu AM, Descarries L (1978): Identification radioautographique de neurones monoaminergiques centraux par microinstallation locale de sérotonine ou de noradrénaline tritiées chez le chat. *CR Acad. Sci. (Paris), 286,* 1523–1526.

Léger L, Wiklund L, Descarries L, Persson M (1979): Description of an indolaminergic cell component in the cat locus coeruleus: A fluorescence histochemical and radioautographic study. *Brain Res., 168,* 43–56.

Léger L, McRae-DeGueurce A, Pujol JF (1980): Origine de l'innervation sérotoninergique du locus coeruleus chez le rat. *CR Acad. Sci. (Paris), 290,* 807–810.

Lenn NJ (1967): Localization of uptake of tritiated norepinephrine by rat brain in vivo and using electron-microscopic radioautography. *Amer. J. Anat., 120,* 377–390.

Lettré H, Pawelets N (1966): Probleme der elektromikroskopischen Autoradiographie. *Naturwissenschaften, 53,* 268–271.

Lever JD, Spriggs TLB, Graham JDP (1968): A formol-fluorescence, fine-structural and autoradiographic study of the adrenergic innervation of the vascular tree in the intact and sympathectomized pancreas of the cat. *J. Anat., 103,* 15–34.

Levi G, Raiteri M (1973): Detectability of high and low affinity uptake systems for GABA and glutamate in rat brain slices and synaptosomes. *Life Sci., 12,* 81–88.

Lichtensteiger W, Langemann H (1966): Uptake of exogenous catecholamines by monoamine-containing neurons of the central nervous system: Uptake of catecholamines by arcuato-infundibular neurons. *J. Pharmacol. Exp. Ther., 151,* 400–408.

Lichtensteiger W, Mutzner U, Langemann H (1967): Uptake of 5-hydroxytryptamine and 5-hydroxytryptophan by neurons of the central nervous system normally containing catecholamines. *J. Neurochem., 14,* 489–497.

Lindvall O (1975): Mesencephalic dopaminergic afferents to the lateral septal nucleus of the rat. *Brain Res.*, *87*, 89–95.

Ljungdahl A, Hökfelt T (1973a): Accumulation of ^{3}H-glycine in interneurons of the cat spinal cord. *Histochem.*, *33*, 277–280.

Ljungdahl A, Hökfelt T (1973b): Autoradiographic uptake patterns of [^{3}H]GABA and [^{3}H]glycine in central nervous tissues with special reference to the cat spinal cord. *Brain Res.*, *62*, 587–595.

Ljungdahl A, Hökfelt T, Jonsson G, Sachs C (1971): Autoradiographic demonstration of uptake and accumulation of ^{3}H-6-hydroxydopamine in adrenergic nerves. *Experientia*, *27*, 297–299.

Ljungdahl A, Seiger A, Hökfelt T, Olsson L (1973): ^{3}H-GABA uptake in growing cerebellar tissue: Autoradiography of intraocular transplants. *Brain Res.*, *61*, 379–384.

Logan WJ, Snyder SH (1971): Unique high affinity uptake systems for glycine, glutamic and aspartic acids in central nervous tissue of the rat. *Nature*, *234*, 297–299.

Logan WJ, Snyder SH (1972): High affinity uptake systems for glycine, glutamic and aspartic acids in synaptosomes of rat central nervous tissue. *Brain Res.*, *42*, 413–431.

Lorez HP, Richards JG (1973): Distribution of indolealkylamine nerve terminals in the ventricles of rat brain. *Z. Zellforsch. Mikrosk. Anat.*, *144*, 511–522.

Majocha RE, Pearse RN, Baldessarini RJ, Delong GR, Walton KG (1981): The noradrenergic system in cultured aggregates of fetal rat brain cells: Morphology of the aggregates and pharmacological indices of noradrenergic neurons. *Brain Res.*, *230*, 235–252.

Makara GB, Rappay G, Stark E (1975): Autoradiographic localization of ^{3}H-Gamma-aminobutyric acid in the medial hypothalamus. *Exp. Brain Res.*, *22*, 449–455.

Makara GB, Gyévai A, Rappay G (1976): ^{3}H-GABA uptake and acetylcholinesterase activity in dissociate cell cultures of the medial hypothalamus. *Acta Biol. Acad. Sci. Hung.*, *27*, 191–197.

Malmfors T (1965): Studies on adrenergic nerves. *Acta Physiol. Scand.*, *62, Suppl. 248*, 1–93.

Marc RE, Lam DMK (1981a): Uptake of aspartic and glumatic acid by photoreceptors in goldfish retina. *Proc. Nat. Acad. Sci. USA*, *78*, 7185–7189.

Marc RE, Lam DW (1981b): Glycinergic pathways in the goldfish retina. *J. Neurosci.*, *1*, 152–165.

Marchbanks RM (1968): The uptake of ^{14}C-choline into synaptosomes in vitro. *Biochem. J.*, *110*, 533–541.

Marks BH, Samorajski T, Webster EJ (1962): Radioautographic localization of norepinephrine-H^3 in the tissues of mice. *J. Pharmac. Exp. Ther.*, *138*, 376–381.

Marshall J, Voaden M (1974a): An autoradiographic study of the cells accumulating [^{3}H]γ-aminobutyric acid in the isolated retinas of pigeons and chickens. *Invest. Ophthal.*, *13*, 602–607.

Marshall J, Voaden M (1974b): An investigation of the cells incorporating [^{3}H]GABA and [^{3}H]-glycine in the isolated retina of the rat. *Exp. Eye Res.*, *18*, 367–370.

Masuoka DT, Alcaraz AF (1975): An autoradiographic method of mapping the distribution and density of monoamine neurons in mouse brain. *Eur. J. Pharmacol.*, *33*, 125–130.

Masuoka DT, Placidi G-F (1968): A combined procedure for the histochemical fluorescence demonstration of monoamines and microautoradiography of water-soluble drugs. *J. Histochem. Cytochem.*, *16*, 659–662.

Masuoka DT, Placidi G-F (1970): Uptake of ^{3}H-norepinephrine by fluorescent nerves of the heart. *J. Histochem.*, *18*, 660–666.

Masuoka DT, Placidi G-F, Gosling JA (1971): Histochemical fluorescence-microscopy and microautoradiography techniques combined for localization studies. In: Eränkö O (Ed), *Histochemistry of Nervous Transmission, Progress in Brain Research, Vol. 34*, pp. 77–86. Elsevier, Amsterdam.

Matus AI, Dennison ME (1971): Autoradiographic localisation of tritiated glycine at 'flat-vesicle' synapses in spinal cord. *Brain Res.*, *32*, 195–197.

Matus AI, Dennison ME (1972): An autoradiographic study of uptake of exogenous glycine by vertebrate spinal cord slices in vitro. *J. Neurocytol.*, *1*, 27–34.

Maurer W, Primbsch E (1964): Grösse der beta-Selfabsorption bei der ^{3}H-Autoradiographie. *Exp. Cell Res.*, *33*, 8–18.

McGeer PL, Hattori T, McGeer EG (1975a): Chemical and autoradiographic analysis of γ-Aminobutyric acid transport in Purkinje cells of the cerebellum. *Exp. Neurol.*, *47*, 26–41.

McGeer EG, Hattori T, McGeer PL (1975b): Electron-microscopic localization of labeled norepinephrine transported in nigro-striatal neurons. *Brain Res.*, *86*, 478–482.

McLennan H (1976): The autoradiographic localization of L-[^{3}H]glutamate in rat brain tissue. *Brain Res.*, *115*, 139–144.

Meiniel A, Collin J-P, Calas A (1977): Incorporation du 5-hydroxytryptophane (5-HTP) dans l'organe pinéal du Lacertilien Lacerta vivipara (L): Étude par radioautographie à haute résolution. *CR Acad. Sci. (Paris)*, *274*, 2897–2900.

Milhaud G, Glowinski J (1962): Métabolisme de la dopamine-^{14}C dans le cerveau du rat. Etude du mode d'administration. *CR Acad. Sci. (Paris), 255,* 203–205.

Möhler H, Wu J-Y, Richards JG (1981): Benzodiazepine receptors: Autoradiographical and immunocytochemical evidence for their localization in regions of gabaergic synaptic contacts. In: Costa E, Di Chiara G, Gessa GL (Eds), *GABA and Benzodiazepine Receptors, Advances in Biochemical Psychopharmacology, Vol. 26,* pp. 139–146. Raven Press, New York.

Møllgård K, Wiklund L (1979): Serotoninergic synapses on ependymal and hypendymal cells of the rat subcommissural organ. *J. Neurocytol., 8,* 445–467.

Nadler NJ (1979): Quantitation and resolution in electron-microscope radioautography. *J. Histochem. Cytochem., 27,* 1531–1533.

Nagy A, Varady G, Joo F, Rakonczay Z, Pilc A (1977): Separation of acetylcholine and catecholamine containing synaptic vesicles from brain cortex. *J. Neurochem., 29,* 449–459.

Nakamura R, Nagayama M (1966): Amino acid transport by slices from various regions of the brain. *J. Neurochem., 13,* 305–313.

Nanopoulos D, Maitre M, Belin MF, Aguera M, Pujol JF, Gamrani H, Calas A (1981): Autoradiographic and immunocytochemical evidence for the existence of GABAergic neurons in the nucleus raphe dorsalis - possible existence of neurons containing 5-HT and glutamate decarboxylase. In: DeFeudis FV, Mandel P (Eds), *Amino Acid Neurotransmitters, Advances in Biochemical Psychopharmacology, Vol. 29,* pp. 519–525. Raven Press, New York.

Nanopoulos D, Belin MF, Maitre M, Vincendon G, Pujol JF (1982): Immunocytochemical evidence for the existence of GABAergic neurons in the nucleus raphe dorsalis. Possible existence of neurons containing serotonin and GABA. *Brain Res., 232,* 375–389.

Neal MJ (1971): The uptake of [^{14}C]glycine by slices of mammalian spinal cord. *J. Physiol. (Lond.), 215,* 103–117.

Neal MJ (1976): Amino acid transmitter substances in the vertebrate retina. *Gen. Pharmacol., 7,* 321–332.

Neal MJ, Bowery NG (1977): Cis-3-aminohexanecarboxylic acid: A substrate for the neuronal GABA transport system. *Brain Res., 138,* 169–174.

Neal MJ, Iversen LL (1969): Subcellular distribution of endogenous and ^{3}H-γ-aminobutyric acid in rat cerebral cortex. *J. Neurochem., 16,* 1245–1252.

Neal MJ, Iversen LL (1972): Autoradiographic localization of ^{3}H-GABA in rat retina. *Nature, 235,* 217–218.

Neal MJ, Pickles HG (1969): Uptake of [^{14}C]glycine by spinal cord. *Nature, 222,* 679–680.

Neal MJ, Cunningham JR, Marshall J (1979): The uptake and radioautographical localization in the frog retina of [^{3}H](γ)aminocyclohexane carboxylic acid, a selective inhibitor of neuronal GABA transport. *Brain Res., 176,* 285–296.

Neale EA, Oertel WH, Bowers LM (1981): Co-existence of GAD immunoreactivity and high affinity ^{3}H-GABA uptake in neurons in dissociated cell cultures of cerebral cortex. *Soc. Neurosci. Abstr., 7,* 916.

Nelson CN, Hoffer BJ, Chu N-S, Bloom FE (1973): Cytochemical and pharmacological studies on polysensory neurons in the primate frontal cortex. *Brain Res., 62,* 115–133.

Nguyen-Legros J, Berger B, Alvarez C (1979): Identification radioautographique des axones dopaminergiques dans le SNC du rat. Marquage in vitro par la dopamine et la noradrénaline tritiées. *CR Acad. Sci. (Paris), 289,* 1311–1314.

Nguyen-Legros J, Berger B, Alvarez C (1981): High resolution radioautography of central dopaminergic fibers labelled in vitro with ^{3}H-dopamine or ^{3}H-norepinephrine. *Brain Res., 213,* 265–276.

Nowaczyk T, Pujol JF, Valatx JL, Bobillier P (1978): Differential radioautographic visualization of central catecholaminergic neurons following intracisternal or intraventricular injection of tritiated norepinephrine. *Brain Res., 152,* 567–572.

Orkand P, Kravitz A (1971): Localization of the sites of γ-aminobutyric acid (GABA) uptake in lobsters nerve muscle preparations. *J. Cell Biol., 49,* 75–89.

Osborne NN (1980): In vitro experimentation on the metabolism, uptake and release of 5-hydroxytryptamine in bovine retina. *Brain Res., 184,* 283–297.

Palay SL, Chan-Palay V (1976): A guide to the synaptic analysis of the neuropil. In: *The Synapse, Cold Spring Harbor Symposia on Quantitative Biology, Vol. XL.* pp. 1–16. Cold Spring Harbor Laboratory.

Paré MF, Jones BE, Beaudet A (1982): Application of a selective retrograde labeling technique to the identification of acetylcholine subcorticospinal neurons. *Soc. Neurosci. Abstr., 8,* 517.

Parent A, Descarries L, Beaudet A (1981): Organization of ascending serotonin systems in the adult rat brain. A radioautographic study after intraventricular administration of [^{3}H]5-hydroxytryptamine. *Neuroscience, 6,* 115–138.

Parizek J, Hassler R, Bak IJ (1971): Light- and electron-microscopic autoradiography of substantia nigra of rat after intraventricular administration of tritium labelled norepinephrine, dopamine, serotonin and the precursors. *Z. Zellforsch. Mikrosk. Anat., 115,* 137–148.

Park DH, Ross ME, Pickel VM, Reis DJ, Joh TH (1982): Antibodies to rat choline acetyltransferase for immunochemistry and immunocytochemistry. *Neurosci. Lett., 34,* 129–135.

Paton DM (1976): Characteristics of uptake of noradrenaline by adrenergic neurons. In: Paton DM (Ed), *The Mechanism of Neuronal and Extraneuronal Transport of Catecholamines,* pp. 49–66. Raven Press, New York.

Paton DM (1980): Neuronal transport of noradrenaline and dopamine. *Pharmacology., 21,* 85–92.

Peters T, Ashley CA (1967): An artefact in radioautography due to binding of free amino acids to tissue by fixatives. *J. Cell Biol., 33,* 53–60.

Petitjean F, Touret M, Buda C, Janin M, Salvert D, Jouvet M, Bobillier P (1981): Monoamines et sommeil: Identification de neurones contenant des indolamines dans une situation pharmacologique particulière (PCPA, 5-HTP), en relation avec le sommeil. *J. Physiol. (Paris), 77,* 237–240.

Philippu A (1976): Transport in intraneuronal storage vesicles. In: Paton DM (Ed), *The Mechanism of Neuronal and Extraneuronal Transport of Catecholamines,* pp. 215–246. Raven Press, New York.

Pickel VM, Beaudet A, Beckley S, Joh TH, Reis DJ, Cuénod M (1980): Combined immunocytochemical and radioautographic study of dopaminergic terminals in the neotriatum. *Soc. Neurosci. Abstr., 6,* 352.

Pickel VM, Beaudet A, Joh TH, Reis DJ, Cuénod M (1981): Combined immunocytochemical and radioautographic study of dopaminergic terminals in the neostriatum. In: Usdin E, Weiner N, Youdin MBH (Eds), *Function and Regulation of Monoamine Enzymes: Basic and Clinical Aspects,* pp. 353–360. MacMillan, London.

Pickel VM, Chan J, Joh TH, Beaudet A (1982): Serotonergic terminals in the nucleus tractus solitarius: Ultrastructure and synaptic associations with catecholaminergic neurons. *Soc. Neurosci. Abstr., 8,* 122.

Pourcho RG (1980): Uptake of [³H]glycine and [³H]GABA by amacrine cells in the cat retina. *Brain Res., 198,* 333–346.

Price DL, Stocks A, Griffin JW, Young A, Peck K (1976): Glycine-specific synapses in rat spinal cord. *J. Cell Biol., 68,* 389–395.

Priestly JV, Kelly JS, Cuello AC (1979): Uptake of [³H] dopamine in periglomerular cells of the rat olfactory bulb: An autoradiographic study. *Brain Res., 165,* 149–155.

Privat A (1976): High resolution radioautographic localization of GABA. A critical study. *J. Microsc. Biol. Cell., 27,* 253–256.

Redburn DA (1981): GABA and glutamate as retina neurotransmitters in rabbit retina. In: Di Chiara G, Gessa GL (Eds), *Glutamate as a Neurotransmitter, Advances in Biochemical Psychopharmacology,* Vol. 27, pp. 79–89. Raven Press, New York.

Reivich M, Glowinski J (1967): An autoradiographic study of the distribution of C¹⁴-norepinephrine in the brain of the rat. *Brain, 40,* 633–646.

Ribeiro-Da-Silva A, Coimbra A (1980): Neuronal uptake of [³H]GABA and [³H]Glycine in laminae I-III (Substantia gelatinosa rolandi) of the rat spinal cord. An autoradiographic study. *Brain Res., 188,* 449–464.

Richards JG (1977): Autoradiographic evidence for the selective accumulation of [³H]5-HT by supraependymal nerve terminals. *Brain Res., 134,* 151–157.

Richards JG, Lorez HP, Tranzer JP (1973): Indolealkylamine nerve terminals in cerebral ventricles: Identification by electron-microscopy and fluorescence histochemistry. *Brain Res., 57,* 277–288.

Richardson KC (1966): Electron-microscopic identification of autonomic nerve endings. *Nature, 210,* 756.

Robinson RG, Gershon MD (1971): Synthesis and uptake of 5-hydroxytryptamine by the myenteric plexus in the guinea pig ileum: A histochemical study. *J. Pharmacol. Exp. Ther., 179,* 311–324.

Rogers AW (1979): *Techniques of Autoradiography,* 3rd ed., pp. 61–110. Elsevier, Amsterdam.

Ross SB (1980): Neuronal transport of 5-hydroxytryptamine. *Pharmacology, 21,* 123–131.

Ross SB, Renyi AL (1967a): Inhibition of the uptake of tritiated catecholamines by antidepressant and related agents. *Eur. J. Pharmacol., 2,* 181–186.

Ross SR, Renyi AL (1967b): Accumulation of tritiated 5-hydroxytryptamine in brain slices. *Life Sci., 6,* 1407–1415.

Ross ME, Park DH, Teitelman G, Pickel VM, Reis DJ, Joh TH (1983): Immunohistochemical localization of choline acetyltransferase using a monoclonal antibody: A radioautographic method. *J. Neurosci.,* in press.

Rothman RP, Dreyfus CF, Gershon MD (1979): Differentiation of enteric neurons from unrecognizable precursors within the microenvironment of cultured fetal mouse gut. *Soc. Neurosci. Abstr., 5,* 176.

Rotman A (1978): Partial purification of serotonin binding protein by affinity chromatography. *Brain Res., 146,* 141–144.

Ruch GA, Koelle GB, Sanville UJ (1982): Autoradiographic demonstration of the sodium-dependent high-affinity choline uptake system. *Proc. Nat. Acad. Sci. USA, 79,* 2714–2716.

Ruda MA, Gobel S (1980): Ultrastructural characterization of axonal endings in the substantia gelatinosa which take up [³H]serotonin. *Brain Res., 184,* 57–83.

Rustioni A, Cuénod M (1981): Selective retrograde labeling of central and spinal ganglion neurons after injections of D-aspartate and GABA in the spinal cord and cuneate nucleus of the rat. *Soc. Neurosci. Abstr., 7,* 322.

Rustioni A, Cuénod M (1982): Selective retrograde transport of D-aspartate in spinal interneurons and cortical neurons of rats. *Brain Res., 236,* 143–155.

Saito K, Barber R, Wu J-Y, Matsuda T, Roberts E, Vaughn JE (1974): Immunohistochemical localization of glutamic acid decarboxylase in rat cerebellum. *Proc. Nat. Acad. Sci. USA, 71,* 269–273.

Salpeter MM, McHenry FA, Salpeter EE (1978): Resolution in electron-microscope autoradiography. IV. Application to analysis of autoradiographs. *J. Cell Biol., 76,* 127–145.

Samorajski T, Marks BH (1962): Localization of tritiated norepinephrine in mouse brain. *J. Histochem. Cytochem., 10,* 392–399.

Sano K, Roberts E (1963): Binding of γ-aminobutyric acid by mouse brain preparations. *Biochem. Pharmacol., 12,* 489–502.

Schon F, Iversen LL (1972): Selective accumulation of ³H-GABA by stellate cells in rat cerebellar cortex in vivo. *Brain Res., 42,* 503–507.

Schon F, Iversen LL (1974): The use of autoradiographic techniques for the identification and mapping of transmitter-specific neurones in the brain. *Life Sci., 15,* 157–175.

Schon F, Kelly JS (1974a): Autoradiographic localisation of [³H]GABA and [³H]-glutamate over satellite glial cells. *Brain Res., 66,* 275–288.

Schon F, Kelly JS (1974b): The characterization of ³H-GABA uptake into the satellite glial cells of rat sensory ganglia. *Brain Res., 66,* 289–300.

Schubert P, Kreutzberg GW, Reinhold K, Herz A (1973): Selective uptake of ³H-6-hydroxydopamine by neurones of the central nervous system. *Exp. Brain Res., 17,* 539–548.

Schuberth J. Sundwall A (1968): Differences in the subcellular localization of choline, acetylcholine and atropine taken up by mouse brain slices in vitro. *Acta Physiol. Scand., 72,* 65–71.

Schuberth J, Sundwall A, Sorbo B, Lindell JA (1966): Uptake of choline by mouse brain slices. *J. Neurochem., 13,* 347–352.

Scott DE, Sladek JR, Knigge KM, Krobisch-Dudley G, Kent DL, Sladek CD (1976): Localization of dopamine in the endocrine hypothalamus of the rat. *Cell Tissue Res., 166,* 461–473.

Scott DE, McNeill TH, Krobisch-Dudley G (1978a): Fine structural localization of radiolabelled L-Dopa in the mammalian hypothalamus. In: Scott DE, Kozlowski GP, Weindl A (Eds), *Brain Endocrine Interaction. III. Neural Hormones and Reproduction,* pp. 228–237. S. Karger, Basel.

Scott DE, Scott PM, Krobisch-Dudley G (1978b): Ultrastructural localization of radiolabelled L-Dopa in the endocrine hypothalamus of the rat. *Cell Tissue Res., 195,* 29–43.

Ségu L, Calas A (1978): The topographical distribution of serotoninergic terminals in the spinal cord of the cat: Quantitative radioautographic studies. *Brain Res., 153,* 449–464.

Ségu L, Gaudin-Chazal G, Seyfritz N, Puizillout JJ (1981): A serotoninergic system in the nodose ganglia of the cat: Radioautographic studies. *J. Physiol. (Paris), 77,* 187–189.

Shank RP, Aprison MH (1979): Biochemical aspects of the neurotransmitter function of glutamate. In: Filer LJ, Garatini S, Kare MR, Reynolds WA, Wurtman RJ (Eds), *Glutamic Acid, Advances in Biochemistry and Physiology,* pp. 139–150. Raven Press, New York.

Shaskan EG, Snyder SH (1970): Kinetics of serotonin accumulation into slices from rat brain: Relationship to catecholamine uptake. *J. Pharmacol. Exp. Ther., 175,* 404–418.

Silberstein SD, Johnson DG, Hanbauer I, Bloom FE, Kopin IJ (1972): Axonal sprouts and [³H]norepinephrine uptake by superior cervical ganglia in organ culture. *Proc. Nat. Acad. Sci. USA, 69,* 1450–1454.

Snyder SH, Coyle JT (1969): Regional differences in ³H-norepinephrine and ³H-dopamine uptake into rat brain homogenates. *J. Pharmacol. Exp. Ther., 165,* 78–86.

Snyder SH, Kuhar MJ, Green AI, Coyle JT, Shaskan EG (1970): Uptake and subcellular localization of neurotransmitters in the brain. *Int. Rev. Neurobiol., 13,* 127–158.

Snyder SH, Logan WJ, Bennett JP, Arregui A (1973a): Amino acids as central nervous transmitters: Biochemical studies. *Neurosci. Res., 5,* 131–157.

Snyder SH, Yamamura HI, Pert CB, Logan WJ, Bennett JP (1973b): Neuronal uptake of neurotransmitters and their precursors in studies with 'transmitter' amino acids and choline. In: Mandell AJ (Ed), *New Concepts in Neurotransmitter Regulation,* pp. 195–238. Plenum Press, New York.

Soreide AJ, Fonnum F (1980): High affinity uptake of D-aspartate in the barrel subfield of the mouse somatic sensory cortex. *Brain Res., 201,* 427–430.

Sorimachi M, Kataoka K (1974): Choline uptake by nerve terminals: A sensitive and a specific marker of cholinergic innervation. *Brain Res., 72,* 350–353.

Sotelo C (1971): The fine structural localization of norepinephrine-^{3}H in the substantia nigra and area postrema of the rat. An autoradiographic study. *J. Ultrastruct. Res., 36,* 824–841.

Sotelo C (1975): Radioautography as a tool for the study of putative neurotransmitters in the nervous system. In: Stockinger L (Ed), *Principles of Neurotransmission, J. Neural Transm. Suppl. 12,* pp. 75–95. Springer-Verlag, Wien.

Sotelo C, Beaudet A (1979): Influence of experimentally induced agranularity on the synaptogenesis of serotonin nerve terminals in rat cerebellar cortex. *Proc. R. Soc. Lond., Ser. B., 206,* 133–138.

Sotelo C, Riche D (1974): Ultrastructural identification of nigral dopaminergic cells in the rat. *Excerpta Med. Int. Congr. Ser., 359,* 425–433.

Sotelo C, Taxi J (1973): On the axonal migration of catecholamines in constricted sciatic nerve of the rat. A radioautographic study. *Z. Zellforsch. Mikrosk. Anat., 138,* 345–370.

Sotelo C, Privat A, Drian MJ (1972): Localization of ^{3}H-GABA in tissue culture of rat cerebellum using electron-microscopy radioautography. *Brain Res., 45,* 302–308.

Steinbusch HWM, Nieuwenhuys R (1982): The raphe nuclei of the rat brainstem: A cytoarchitectonic and immunohistochemical study. In: *Serotoninergic Neurons in the Central Nervous System of the Rat,* pp. 165–278. Thesis, Nijmegen.

Sterling P, Davis TL (1980): Neurons in cat lateral geniculate nucleus that concentrate exogenous [^{3}H]-γ-aminobutyric acid (GABA). *J. Comp. Neurol., 192,* 737–749.

Storm-Mathisen J (1975): High affinity uptake of GABA in presumed GABAergic nerve endings in rat brain. *Brain Res., 84,* 409–427.

Storm-Mathisen J (1977): Glutamic acid and excitatory nerve endings: Reduction of glutamic acid uptake after axotomy. *Brain Res., 120,* 379–386.

Storm-Mathisen J (1978a): Localization of putative transmitters in the hippocampal formation with a note on the connections to septum and hypothalamus. In: *Functions of the Septo-Hippocampal System, Ciba Foundation Symposium, Vol. 58 (new series),* pp. 49–86. Elsevier/Excerpta Medica/North Holland, Amsterdam.

Storm-Mathisen J (1978b): Localization of transmitter amino acids: Application to hippocampus and septum. In: Fonnum F (Ed), *Amino Acids as Chemical Transmitters,* pp. 155–171. Plenum Press, New York.

Storm-Mathisen J (1981): Glutamate in hippocampal pathways. In: Di Chiara G, Gessa GL (Eds), *Glutamate as a Neurotransmitter, Advances in Biochemical Psychopharmacology, Vol. 27,* pp. 43–55. Raven Press, New York.

Storm-Mathisen J, Iversen LL (1979): Uptake of [^{3}H]glutamic acid in excitatory nerve endings: Light- and electron-microscopic observations in the hippocampal formation of the rat. *Neuroscience, 4,* 1237–1253.

Storm-Mathisen J, Wold JE (1981): In vivo high-affinity and axonal transport of D-(2,3-^{3}H)aspartate in excitatory neurons. *Brain Res., 230,* 427–433.

Storm-Mathisen J, Leknes A, Bore AB (1982): Immunohistochemical visualization of glutamate in excitatory boutons. *Neuroscience, 7,* S-203.

Streit P (1980): Selective retrograde labeling indicating the transmitter of neuronal pathways. *J. Comp. Neurol., 191,* 429–463.

Streit P, Knecht E, Reubi JC, Hunt SP, Cuénod M (1978): GABA-specific presynaptic dendrites in pigeon optic tectum: A high resolution autoradiographic study. *Brain Res., 149,* 204–210.

Streit P, Knecht E, Cuénod M (1979): Transmitter-specific retrograde labeling in the striato-nigral and raphe-nigral pathways. *Science, 205,* 306–308.

Streit P, Knecht E, Cuénod M (1980): Transmitter-related retrograde labeling in the pigeon optic lobe: A high resolution autoradiographic study. *Brain Res., 187,* 59–67.

Swanson LW, Hartman BK (1975): The central adrenergic system: An immunofluorescence study of the location of cell bodies and their efferent connections in the rat utilizing dopamine-β-hydroxylase as a marker. *J. Comp. Neurol., 163,* 467–505.

Swanson LW, Sawchenko PE, Bérod A, Hartman BK, Helle KB, Van Orden DE (1981): An immunohistochemical study of the organization of catecholaminergic cells and terminals fields in the paraventricular and supraoptic nuclei of the hypothalamus. *J. Comp. Neurol., 196,* 271–285.

Tamir H, Gershon MD (1979): Storage of serotonin and serotonin binding protein in synaptic vesicles. *J. Neurochem., 33,* 35–44.

362

Tamir H, Huang YL (1974): Binding of serotonin to soluble binding protein from synaptosomes. *Life Sci.,* *14,* 83–93.

Tappaz M, Aguera M, Belin MF, Pujol JF (1980): Autoradiography of GABA in the rat hypothalamic median eminence. *Brain Res., 186,* 379–391.

Taxi J (1969): Morphological and cytochemical studies on the synapses in the autonomic nervous system. In: Akert K, Waser PG (Eds), *Mechanisms of Synaptic Transmission, Progress in Brain Res., Vol. 31,* pp. 5–20. Elsevier, Amsterdam.

Taxi J (1973): Observations complémentaires sur l'ultrastructure des ganglions sympathiques des mammifères (en particulier les connexions intercellulaires). *Trab. Inst. Cajal Invest. Biol., 65,* 9–40.

Taxi J (1976): General principles of neurotransmitter detection. Problems and application to catecholamines. *J. Microsc. Biol. Cell., 27,* 243–248.

Taxi J, Droz B (1966a): Étude de l'incorporation de noradrénaline-^{3}H (NA-^{3}H) et de 5-hydroxy-tryptophane-^{3}H (5-HTP-^{3}H) dans l'épiphyse et le ganglion cervical supérieur. *CR Acad. Sci. (Paris), 263,* 1326–1329.

Taxi J, Droz B (1966b): Étude de l'incorporation de noradrénaline-^{3}H (NA-^{3}H) et de 5-hydroxy-tryptophane-^{3}H (5-HTP-^{3}H) dans les fibres nerveuses du canal déférent et de l'intestin. *CR Acad. Sci. (Paris), 263,* 1237–1240.

Taxi J, Droz B (1967): Localisation d'amines biogènes dans le système neurovégétatif périphérique. (Etude radioautographique en microscopie électronique après injection de noradrénaline-^{3}H et de 5-hydroxytryptophane-^{3}H). In: Stutinsky F (Ed), *Neurosecretion, IV International Symposium on Neurosecretion,* pp. 191–202. Springer-Verlag, Berlin.

Taxi J, Droz B (1969): Radioautographic study of the accumulation of some biogenic amines in the autonomic nervous system. In: Barondes SH (Ed), *Cellular Dynamics of the Neuron, Symp. Internat. Soc. Cell Biol., Vol. 8,* pp. 175–190. Academic Press, New York.

Taxi J, Sotelo C (1972): Le problème de la migration des catécholamines dans les neurones sympathiques. *Rev. Neurol., 127,* 23–36.

Taxi J, Sotelo C (1973): Cytological aspects of the axonal migration of catecholamines and of their storage material. *Brain Res., 62,* 431–437.

Taxt T, Storm-Mathisen J (1979): Tentative localization of glutamergic and aspartergic nerve endings in brain. *J. Physiol. (Paris), 75,* 677–684.

Thoenen H, Tranzer J-P (1968): Chemical sympathectomy by selective destruction of adrenergic nerve endings with 6-hydroxydopamine. *Naunyn-Schmiedebergs Arch. Pharmak. Exp. Pathol, 261,* 271–288.

Tilders FJH, Ploem JS, Smelik PG (1974): Quantitative microfluorimetric studies on formaldehyde-induced fluorescence of 5-hydroxytryptamine in the pineal gland of the rat. *J. Histochem. Cytochem., 22,* 967–975.

Titus EO, Spiegel HE (1962): Effects of desmethylimipramine (DMI) on uptake of norepinephrine-7-H^3-NE in heart. *Fed. Proc., Fed. Am. Soc. Exp. Biol., 21,* 179.

Tolbert DL, Bantli H (1980): Uptake and transport of ^{3}H-GABA (gamma-aminobutyric acid) injected into the cat dentate nucleus. *Exp. Neurol., 70,* 525–538.

Tsukada Y, Nagata Y, Hirano S, Matsutani T (1963): Active transport of amino acid into cerebral cortex slices. *J. Neurochem., 10,* 241–256.

Usherwood PNR (1978): Amino acids as neurotransmitters. *Adv. Comp. Physiol. Biochem., 7,* 227–309.

Van Orden LS, Bloom FE, Barrnett RJ, Giarman NJ (1966): Histochemical and functional relationships of catecholamines in adrenergic nerve endings. I. Participation of granular vesicles. *J. Pharmacol. Exp. Ther., 154,* 185–199.

Verhofstad AAJ, Steinbusch HWM, Penke B, Varga J, Joosten HWV (1981): Serotonin-immunoreactive cells in the superior cervical ganglion of the rat. Evidence for the existence of separate serotonin- and catecholamine-containing small ganglion cells. *Brain Res., 212,* 39–49.

Verney C, Berger B, Adrien J, Vigny A, Gay M (1982): Development of the dopaminergic innervation of the rat cerebral cortex. A light-microscopic immunocytochemical study using anti-tyrosine hydroxylase antibodies. *Dev. Brain Res., 5,* 41–52.

Voaden MJ, Marshall J, Murani M (1974): The uptake of [^{3}H]γ-aminobutyric acid and [^{3}H]-glycine by the isolated retina of the frog. *Brain Res., 67,* 115–132.

Von Euler US, Lishajko F (1963): Catecholamine release and uptake in isolated adrenergic nerve granules. *Acta Physiol. Scand., 57,* 468–480.

Walker CR, Peacock JH (1982): Development of GABAergic function of dissociated hippocampal cultures from fetal mice. *Dev. Brain Res., 2,* 541–555.

Weinstein H, Varon S, Muhlemann DR, Roberts E (1965): A carrier-mediated transfer model for the accumulation of ^{14}C-γ-aminobutyric acid by subcellular particles. *Biochem. Pharmacol., 14,* 273–288.

Wenthold RJ, Haser WG, Altschuler RA, Harmison GG, Neises GR, Fex J (1981): Immunocytochemical localization of aspartate amino-transferase and glutaminase in the auditory nerve. *Soc. Neurosci. Abst.*, *7*, 916.

White TD (1976): Evidence that the rapid binding of newly accumulated noradrenaline within synaptosomes involves synaptic vesicles. *Brain Res.*, *108*, 87–96.

White RD, Neal MJ (1976): The uptake of L-glutamate by the retina. *Brain Res.*, *111*, 79–93.

White WF, Snodgrass SR, Dichter M (1980): Identification of GABA neurons in rat cortical cultures by GABA uptake autoradiography. *Brain Res.*, *190*, 139–152.

Wiklund L, Descarries L, Møllgård K (1981): Serotoninergic axon terminals in the rat dorsal accessory olive: Normal ultrastructure and light-microscopic demonstration of regeneration after 5,6-dihydroxytryptamine lesioning. *J. Neurocytol.*, *10*, 1009–1027.

Wiklund L, Toggenburger G, Cuénod M (1982): Aspartate: Possible neurotransmitter in cerebellar climbing fibers. *Science*, *216*, 78–80.

Wilkin G, Wilson JE, Balazs R, Schon F, Kelly JS (1974): A comparison of GABA uptake into the excitatory and inhibitory nerve terminals of the isolated cerebellar glomerulus. *Nature*, *252*, 397–399.

Wilkin GP, Csillag A, Balazs R, Kingsbury AE, Wilson JE, Johnson AL (1981): Localization of high affinity [³H]glycine transport sites in the cerebellar cortex. *Brain Res.*, *216*, 11–33.

Wolfe DE, Potter LT, Richardson KC, Axelrod J (1962): Localizing tritiated norepinephrine in sympathetic axons by electron-microscopic radioautography. *Science*, *138*, 440–442.

Wong DT, Horng JS, Bymaster FP, Hauser KL, Molloy BB (1974): A selective inhibitor of serotonin uptake: Lilly 110140 3-(p-trifluoromethylphenoxy)-N-methyl-3-phenylpropylamine. *Life Sci.*, *15*, 471–479.

Wood JG, Barrnett RJ (1964): Histochemical demonstration of norepinephrine at a fine structural level. *J. Histochem. Cytochem.*, *12*, 197–209.

Woodward WR, Lindström SH (1977): A potential screening technique for neurotransmitters in the CNS: Model studies in the cat spinal cord. *Brain Res.*, *137*, 37–52.

Wu J-Y, Matsuda T, Roberts E (1973): Purification and characterization of glutamate decarboxylase from the mouse brain. *J. Biol. Chem.*, *248*, 3029–3034.

Wu J-Y, Brandon C, Su YYT, Lam DMK (1981): Immunocytochemical and autoradiographic localization of GABA system in the vertebrate retina. *Mol. Cell. Biochem.*, *39*, 229–238.

Yamamura HI, Snyder SH (1973): High affinity transport of choline into synaptosomes of rat brain. *J. Neurochem.*, *21*, 1355–1374.

Yazulla S, Brecha N (1980): Binding and uptake of the GABA analogue, ³H-muscimol, in the retinas of goldfish and chicken. *Invest. Ophtalmol. Vis. Sci.*, *19*, 1415–1426.

Young III WS, Kuhar MJ (1979): A new method for receptor autoradiography: [³H]Opioid receptors in rat brain. *Brain Res.*, *179*, 255–270.

Young JAC, Brown DA, Kelly JS, Schon F (1973): Autoradiographic localization of sites of ³H-γ-aminobutyric acid accumulation in peripheral autonomic ganglia. *Brain Res.*, *63*, 479–486.

CHAPTER VIII

Neuronal tracing using retrograde migration of labeled transmitter-related compounds*

M. CUÉNOD and P. STREIT

1. INTRODUCTION

The need for chemical neuroanatomy, in both basic neurobiology and its clinical applications, has long been recognized: fluorescence histochemistry has allowed the visualization of aminergic pathways and immunohistochemistry has been essential for defining neurons chemically, when the transmitter or one of its specific enzymes can be used to produce antibodies. The last approach has been used successfully for the neuropeptides and for markers such as glutamic acid decarboxylase in GABA neurons or cholineacetyltransferase in cholinergic ones. However, immunohistochemistry alone does not allow to trace a given pathway and at the same time to define its transmitter characteristics, unless it is combined with a nonselective tracer. The method presented here could prove to be both reliable and simple for delineating pathways according to their transmitter, particularly those using amino acids and acetylcholine.

The principle on which this approach relies is that some transmitters or related molecules, after having been selectively taken up by the nerve terminals in which they are normally utilized, migrate retrogradely (possibly in a modified form) toward the perikaryon where they are accumulated (Fig. 1). This basic assumption rests on 2 cellular properties of the neuron: (1) the selective uptake of transmitters or their metabolites in the terminal, which has been documented for amino acids, choline and the biogenic amines (Snyder et al. 1973; Hökfelt and Ljungdahl 1975; Iversen et al. 1975); and (2) the retrograde, somatopetal intra-axonal migration of material from the terminal to the cell body, a phenomenon that has been established for various endogenous or exogenous compounds, but not as yet for transmitter-like molecules (for review see, Grafstein and Forman 1980; Weiss 1982).

Experimentally, after administration of a radioactive marker such as a transmitter, or in certain cases its precursor, in a restricted area of the central nervous system, only the neurons with an affinity uptake mechanism selective for that given marker would be retrogradely labeled and autoradiograms would reveal silver grains almost exclusively confined to their cell bodies of origin and their axons leading to the injected zone. This contrasts with nonselective retrograde markers such as horseradish peroxidase (HRP) or wheat germ agglutinin (WGA), which label non-differentially all neurons with terminals exposed to them. In the striatum for example, while a WGA injection

*This study was supported by Grants 3.636.75, 3.505.79 and 3.506.79 of the Swiss National Science Foundation and the Dr Eric Slack-Gyr-Foundation.

Handbook of Chemical Neuroanatomy. Vol. 1: Methods in Chemical Neuroanatomy.
A. Björklund and T. Hökfelt, editors.

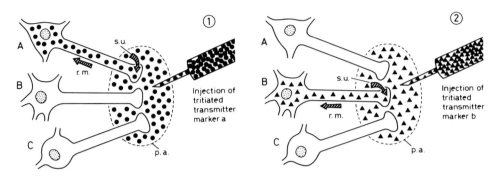

Fig. 1. Schematic representation of the method's principle. In situation 1 the tritiated transmitter marker 'a' is injected into the projection area (p.a.) of pathways 'A'-'C'. There is a specific uptake (s.u.) system for this transmitter marker only in pathway 'A' which uses this or a related molecule as transmitter. The marker (possibly in a modified form) reaches the perikarya of pathway 'A' after intra-axonal retrograde migration (r.m.). The radioactivity accumulated in these perikarya is located by means of autoradiography. No retrograde labeling is found in pathways 'B' and 'C'. In situation 2 transmitter marker 'b', which is identical with or related to the transmitter used in pathway 'B', is applied in the same terminal area. Selective retrograde labeling is found in pathway 'B'.

leads to the labeling of all its inputs, specific markers label only selected pathways: [³H]dopamine delineating the nigrostriatal neurons, [³H]serotonin the raphe-striatal ones, and D-[³H]aspartate the cortico- and thalamo-striatal ones (Streit et al. 1979b; Streit 1980a,b).

We shall restrict ourselves here only to an outline of the method, since a detailed description has been included in the Appendix. The concentrated radioactive compound is drawn into a glass micropipette which, guided by a micromanipulator, is introduced into the appropriate brain area of an anesthetized animal, either under visual control or according to stereotactic coordinates. The injection is made using a temperature controlled expansion device, which allows the delivery of 30–60 nl containing 15–30 µCi over a period of 10–20 min. After a survival time of a few hours to a few days, in most cases the anesthetized animal is perfused with glutaraldehyde and the brain sections prepared for light-microscopic autoradiography by conventional techniques, using an exposure time of 3–6 weeks. In cases where the molecules are not fixed by glutaraldehyde, such as choline or one of its metabolites, an autoradiographic procedure for diffusible substances like the dry-mount technique has to be applied in order to preserve the localization of the tracer (Bagnoli et al. 1981).

The initial experiments leading us to the concept of transmitter-related selective retrograde tracing were carried out by Hunt in our laboratory in 1975 (Hunt et al. 1975, 1976, 1977). After injection of [³H]glycine, [³H]serine and [³H]alanine into the pigeon optic tectum, he observed an accumulation of silver grains over the perikarya in the nucleus isthmi pars parvocellularis (Ipc) which has a reciprocal connection with the tectum (Fig. 2). This observation was best explained by assuming a selective uptake and retrograde migration of the radioactivity. Since the available evidence strongly suggests that Ipc-tectal neurons use glycine as transmitter (see below), the hypothesis of a selective transmitter-related retrograde labeling of neurons was proposed. In 1977, Leger et al. reported labeled perikarya in the nucleus raphe dorsalis after [³H]serotonin injections in the rat striatum, a finding which was also consistent with the idea of transmitter-specific retrograde tracing of serotonergic neurons.

The hypothesis proposed has been tested in various pathways where transmitters have been established or suggested on the basis of neurochemical, physiological, pharmacological or histochemical evidence. Selective labeling was successfully obtained with the amino acids glycine (gly), γ-aminobutyric acid (GABA), D-aspartate (D-asp) and possibly proline (pro), with choline, and with the amines dopamine (DA) and serotonin (5-HT). These experiments, performed partly in our laboratory and partly in others, will be reviewed in the main part of the chapter and are summarized in Table 1. As will be discussed in detail at the end, the results are to a large extent compatible with the proposal that transmitter-specific retrograde labeling takes place in pathways known — according to other methods — to use the tested transmitter, whereas it does not occur in pathways that do not. However, in some cases, there is a discrepancy between the results obtained with the technique proposed here and those from other, better established methodologies. This leads to what may be termed 'false-positive' and 'false-negative' results, whereby it often remains open if the cause of the discrepancy, the 'fault', lies in the specific retrograde labeling or in the other available evidence. At any rate, it should be clear that the method suggested here is by no means fully established as yet and that its limitations have to be defined and if possible explained.

2. GLYCINE

The *Ipc-tectal neurons in the pigeon* have been well characterized morphologically by both anterograde and retrograde labeling (see, Cuénod and Streit 1979). The cell bodies and dendrites are located in the nucleus Ipc and the axons project topographically, at distances of 3–4 mm, to Layers 2 to 7 of the optic tectum. There is good evidence that glycine, a well established inhibitory transmitter in the vertebrate spinal cord (Aprison and Nadi 1978), could be a transmitter also in the pigeon optic tectum (Barth and Felix 1974; Zukin et al. 1975; Henke et al. 1976a; Henke and Cuénod 1978; Le Fort et al. 1978; Cuénod et al. 1982). In particular, both exogenously (Reubi and Cuénod 1976) and endogenously (Wolfensberger et al. 1981) released glycine could be collected with a push-pull cannula from the tectum during electrical stimulation of Ipc.

[3H]Glycine, injected into the superficial layers of the lateral optic tectum or applied to its surface led to perikaryal labeling of a small group of neurons arranged as a column within the Ipc as shown by Hunt et al. (1977) and Streit et al. (1980) (Fig. 2). At the electron-microscopic level, the silver grains lay predominantly over elements intrinsic to Ipc, namely dendrites, perikarya and initial axon segments, whereas presynaptic terminals remained practically free of label (Streit et al. 1980). This pattern is best explained by assuming an intra-axonal retrograde migration of a radioactive compound, after the same molecule or its precursor has been taken up in the zone of termination of the isthmo-tectal neurons. Extracellular diffusion of the tritiated glycine followed by uptake in Ipc would have resulted in a considerably more diffuse distribution of labeled neurons, rather than in the observed columnar pattern. Diffusion can further be excluded because an injection of [3H]glycine into the depth of the optic tectum, below the main layers of the Ipc-tectal termination, leads to a much less pronounced perikaryal labeling, even though the focus from which the tracer spreads is closer to the Ipc (Hunt et al. 1977). In contrast, neurons projecting also to the optic tectum and originating in nuclei other than Ipc were not covered by silver grains. Selective labeling of Ipc neurons was also observed after injections of [3H]serine and [3H]α-alanine in the lateral tectum, while [3H]GABA injections in the rostral tectum led to perikaryal labeling in the anterior part of the Ipc. In the glycine experiments, retrograde labeling

TABLE 1. *Summary of studies on retrograde transport of transmitter-related compounds in the CNS of rat, cat or pigeon*

	Injection or superfusion (S)	Perikaryal labeling		Transmitter status	Species (rat, pigeon)	References
Gly	Tectum (lat)	Ipc	+	+	P	Hunt et al. (1977)
						Streit et al. (1980)
GABA	Tectum (ant)	Tectum	+	?	P	Streit et al. (1980)
	Pretectum	Tectum	+	?	P	Hunt and Künzle (1976)
	Substantia nigra	Striatum	+	+ +	R	Streit (1980)
	Deiters' n.	Purkinje	−	+ +	R	Wiklund et al. (1982)
	DCN	Interneurons	−	?	R	Rustioni and Cuénod (1982)
	Dorsal horn	Interneurons	−	?	R	Rustioni and Cuénod (1982)
	Pallidum	Subthalamic n.	+	?	C	Nauta and Cuénod (1982)
Proline	Spinal cord	Cortex, n. Ruber	+	?	Monkey	Künzle (1976)
	Retina	Mes. tegm.	+	?	Lamprey	Repérant et al. (1980)
	Sup. Colliculus	Cortex	+	?	C	LeVay and Sherk (1981)
D-asp	Tectum (+S)	Retina	+	+ + asp/glu	P	Beaudet et al. (1981)
	DCN, dorsal horn	Prim. afferents	+	(+)	R	Rustioni et al. (1982)
	Cerebellum (+S)	Inferior olive	+	+ + asp/(glu)	R	Wiklund et al. (1982)
		Granule cell	−	+ + glu	R	Wiklund et al. (1982)
	Striatum	Thalamus	+	?	R	Streit (1980)
	Striatum	Cortex (V)	+	+ + glu/asp	R	Streit (1980)
	Claustrum (visual)	Cortex (VI)	+	?	C	LeVay and Sherk (1981)
	Substantia nigra	Cortex (V)	+	+ glu/asp	R	Streit (1980)
	LGN	V. Cortex (VI)	+	+ glu/asp	C/R	Baughman and Gilbert (1981)
	Thalamus: VB	S.M. Cortex (VI)	+	+ glu/asp	R/C	Rustioni et al. (1982)
	S. Colliculus	Cortex	−	+ glu/asp	C/R	Baughman and Gilbert (1981)
	DCN	Cortex	+	+ glu/asp	R	Rustioni and Cuénod (1982)
	Dorsal horn	Cortex	(+)	+ glu/asp	R	Rustioni and Cuénod (1982)
	Pontine n.	Cortex (V)	+	+	R	Wiklund and Perschak (unpubl.)
	Raphe magnus	PAG	+	?	R	Persson and Wiklund (unpubl.)
	Vestibular complex	N.Edinger-Westphal	+	?	R	Wiklund et al. (unpubl.)
	Inf. Colliculus	N. sagulum	+	?	R	Wiklund et al. (unpubl.)

	Injection or superfusion (S)	Perikaryal labeling	Transmitter status	Species (rat, pigeon)	References
Choline (ACh)	Hippocampus	Medial septum	+	++	R	Bagnoli et al. (1981)
	Wulst	Thalamus (DLAmc)	+	++	P	Bagnoli et al. (1981)
	Cortex	N. basalis magnocellularis Meynert	+	++	R	Wiklund (unpubl.)
	Intralam. thal.	Parabrachial complex	+	+	R	Wiklund (unpubl.)
DA	Striatum	S.N., A8, A10	+	++	R	Streit (1980)
		Dorsal raphe	(+)	-?	R	Streit (1980)
Serotonin	Striatum	Dorsal raphe	+	++	R	Leger et al. (1977), Streit (1980)
		S.N., A8, A10	(+)	-	R	Leger et al. (1977), Streit (1980)
		Cortex, Thalamus	(+)	-	R	Streit (1980)
	Substantia nigra	Dorsal raphe	+	++	R	Streit (1980)
	Cortex (S)	Dorsal raphe	+	++	R	Beaudet et al. (1981)
	Cerebellum	Raphe	+	++	R	Yamamoto et al. (1980)
		Inf.ol., LC, Vest.n., ret. Lat., pont.n.	+	-	R	Yamamoto et al. (1980)
	Olfactory bulb	Raphe	+	++	R	Araneda et al. (1980)

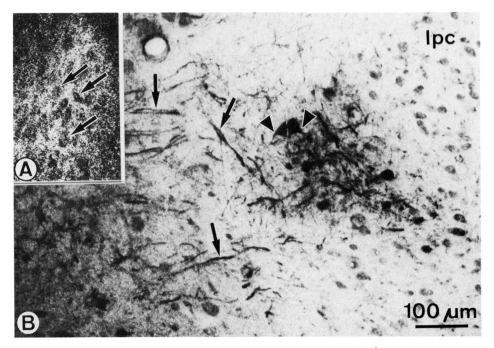

Fig. 2.(A) Bright-field autoradiograph of the Ipc nucleus following injection of [³H]glycine (50 μCi in 0.2 μl during 10 min) into the pigeon lateral optic tectum. Some heavily labeled perikarya are situated in a limited field of labeled neuropil. Note fibrous processes (arrow-heads) arising from perikarya and labeled fibers (arrows) in the space between tectum and Ipc. (5% glutaraldehyde perfusion 20 min after injection, 50 μm slice, cresylecht-violet staining.) (From Cuénod and Streit 1979.) (B) Dark-field autoradiograph showing mainly neuropil labeling in Ipc after tectal injection of [³H]proline. Note the low density of silver grains over perikarya (arrows); 24-h survival. Same magnification as in A. (From Hunt et al. 1977.)

was observed after survival times as short as 20 min, indicating a speed of migration in the order of 150–250 mm/day, which is well compatible with that of retrograde axonal transport (Streit et al. 1980). Under these conditions, a high density of silver grains was detected over the structures mentioned above when glutaraldehyde was used as fixative while only faint labeling was observed after formaldehyde perfusion. This suggests that most of the radioactivity reaching Ipc neurons is in a soluble form (Cuénod and Streit 1979; Streit et al. 1980). After survival times of 24 h, more radioactivity seems to be incorporated in macromolecules which are fixed by formaldehyde (Hunt et al. 1977).

Thus, a part of the isthmo-tectal pathway seems to release glycine upon stimulation and is retrogradely labeled selectively after application of [³H]glycine to the terminals.

3. GABA

GABA is one of the best established amino acid inhibitory transmitters in the vertebrate central nervous system (Curtis and Johnston 1974). Patterns of selective retrograde labeling were observed following intracerebral injections of [³H]GABA in the pigeon optic tectum, in the rat substantia nigra, dorsal column nuclei (DCN) and dorsal horn of the spinal cord and in the cat pallidal complex.

In the *pigeon optic tectum*, two types of extrinsic neurons have been retrogradely labeled with [³H]GABA (reviewed in (Cuénod and Streit 1979; Henke 1983): One belongs to the isthmo-tectal pathway — already described above in relation to glycine — but in the rostral aspect of the tectum as observed by Hunt et al. (1977). The other, described by Hunt and Künzle (1976), has cell bodies in Layer 10 of the tectum, radial processes in Layer 7, and axons projecting through Layer 1 to the pretectum and the ventral thalamus. Both show an affinity for tritiated GABA which labels them retrogradely, but no other evidence is available to support the notion that they are using GABA as transmitter.

In mammals, GABA is well established as transmitter in a population of striatal neurons projecting to the *substantia nigra* (Kim et al. 1971; Precht and Yoshida 1971; Fonnum et al. 1974; Kataoka et al. 1974; Jessell et al. 1978; Nagy et al. 1978). Six hours after [³H]GABA injection in the rat substantia nigra, Streit et al. (1979a) and Streit (1980a) observed labeled fibers leading to the caudoputamen, where medium-sized neuronal perikarya were overlaid with silver grains (Fig. 3). Perikaryal labeling was not observed in projections to the substantia nigra involving other transmitters such as the ones originating in the cerebral cortex or nucleus raphe dorsalis. These observations are consistent with the suggestion that striatonigral neurons containing GABA were

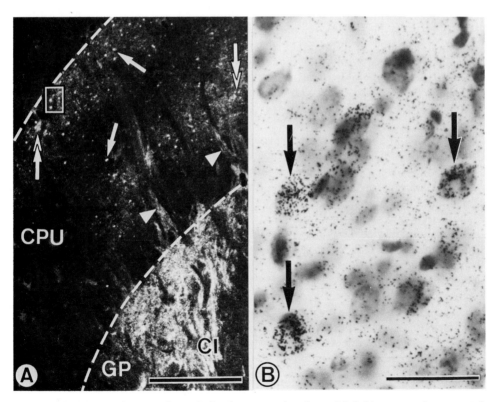

Fig. 3. Light-microscopic autoradiograph showing neuronal perikarya labeled by retrograde transport (arrows) 6 h after injection of [³H]GABA (15 µCi in 0.05 µl) in substantia nigra of the rat. (A) Labeling of perikarya and small fiber bundles (arrow-heads) in the caudoputamen (CPU). Many strongly labeled fibers can be seen in capsula interna (CI). GP = globus pallidus. Dark field illumination; bar: 500 µm. (B) Enlargement of rectangle in A. Bright field illumination; cresylecht-violet staining; bar: 50 µm. (From Streit et al. 1979.) (Copyright 1982 by the American Association for the Advancement of Science.)

retrogradely labeled in a selective way, although the involvement of neurons using substance P as mediator cannot be readily excluded. Substance P immunoreactive neurons, however, have been observed in more rostral portions of the caudoputamen than the ones labeled after intra-nigral injection of [³H]GABA (Brownstein et al. 1977; Jessell et al. 1978). Similar injections of tritiated precursors of GABA, like L-glutamate or L-glutamine, were ineffective in labeling retrogradely striatal neurons and/or their fibers (Streit et al. 1979a; Streit 1980a).

Recently, Somogyi et al. (1981) described selective labeling of superficial interneurons following [³H]GABA injections into the deep layers of the Rhesus monkey visual cortex, an observation which they interpreted in terms of retrograde migration of labeled material.

Retrograde labeling was observed in the subthalamic nucleus and in the putamen by Nauta and Cuénod (1982) following injections of [³H]GABA into the cat *pallidal complex*, while no other afferent neurons were covered with silver grains. Application of D-[³H]aspartate or [³H]serotonin to the pallidal complex did not lead to perikaryal labeling in the subthalamic nucleus. These observations show that the subthalamo-pallidal projection is selectively labeled by [³H]GABA and indicate that these neurons use GABA as transmitter, a suggestion supported by recent electrophysiological results (Perkins and Stone 1981; Rouzaire-Dubois et al. 1983).

After [³H]GABA injections in the *dorsal column nuclei* (DCN) of the rat, Rustioni and Cuénod (1982) did not observe perikaryal labeling either outside the injection site in the spinal segments, or at the brain stem or cortical levels. Similarly, injections administered in the *dorsal horn* of the rat cervical spinal cord, did not give rise to central perikaryal labeling imputable to retrograde translocation of the radioactivity (Rustioni and Cuénod 1982). Thus, long axon CNS neurons containing GABA do not project to the DCN or the cervical cord or, if they exist, they do not show an affinity for exogenous GABA.

Injections of [³H]GABA in Deiters' nucleus or deep cerebellar nuclei failed to label retrogradely *Purkinje cells* in the cerebellar cortex (Wiklund, Künzle and Cuénod, 1983). This negative result comes as a surprise in view of the strong evidence that GABA is a transmitter of these cells (Obata et al. 1967; Obata and Takeda 1969; McLaughlin et al. 1974; Storm-Mathisen 1976; Ribak et al. 1978). However, degeneration of Purkinje nerve terminals in Deiters' nucleus, which leads to a significant decrease in glutamic acid decarboxylase (GAD) activity, does not affect the high-affinity uptake of GABA (Storm-Mathisen 1975, 1976). This suggests that Purkinje cells lack the high-affinity uptake mechanism for GABA at their terminals, a property also apparently shared by their perikarya and dendrites since these are not labeled following a [³H]GABA injection within the cerebellar cortex (Hökfelt and Ljungdahl 1975). The lack of an uptake mechanism would explain the absence of retrograde labeling of Purkinje neurons after [³H]GABA injection into Deiters' nucleus, since the uptake of transmitter substances by the nerve terminals appears to represent a crucial step for the initiation of their retrograde migration (see discussion below).

4. D-ASPARTATE

The amino acids L-glutamate (glu) and L-aspartate (asp) have been proposed as excitatory transmitters in the vertebrate central nervous system on the basis of physiological, biochemical and pharmacological evidence (for review see, Curtis and

Johnston 1974; Johnson 1978; Cotman et al. 1981). The nerve terminals of such excitatory pathways are often characterized by a mechanism of high-affinity uptake for these two amino acids. However, as long as tritiated L-glu or L-asp were tested for their ability to retrogradely label selective neurons, the attempts remained unsuccessful, presumably because the role of these amino acids in the general metabolism precludes their migration. D-Asp, which is not metabolized, acts as a false transmitter and is taken up by the same high-affinity mechanisms as the L-forms of asp and glu at least in the cerebral cortex (Balcar and Johnston 1972; Davies and Johnston 1976; Takagaki 1977; Storm-Mathisen and Woxen Opsahl 1978; Storm-Mathisen 1979). Selective retrograde labeling of cortical pyramidal neurons was first observed following D-[^{3}H]-asp injection into the rat striatum (Streit and Cuénod 1979; Streit 1980a), delineating a pathway well known for its use of glu and/or asp as transmitter (Spencer 1976; Divac et al. 1977; Kim et al. 1977; McGeer et al. 1977; Reubi and Cuénod 1979; Reubi et al. 1980). D-[^{3}H]glu, tested by Baughman and Gilbert (1981) in the cat cortico-geniculate pathway, gave the same, although weaker labeling pattern as [^{3}H]D-asp. It should be pointed out that it is not easy to distinguish, at the moment, between glu and asp with respect to their transmitter role in specific neurons (however, see below). Therefore, they will be treated here as a unit, although this is most probably an oversimplification; indeed, in the goldfish retina, a differential uptake of aspartic and glutamic acid by photoreceptors has been reported by Marc and Lam (1981).

4.1. RETINO-TECTAL NEURONS IN THE PIGEON

Many lines of evidence point to a transmitter role of glu and asp in the retino-tectal neurons of the pigeon (Henke et al. 1976b; Cuénod and Henke 1978; Cuénod and Streit 1979; Canzek et al. 1981; Henke 1981; Fonnum and Henke 1982). Following D-[^{3}H]asp application to the zone of termination of the optic nerve fibers in the optic lobe, either by intratectal injection or by tectal superfusion (concentration: 10^{-5} M), Beaudet et al. (1981) and Cuénod et al. (1981) could trace labeled axons through Layer 1 down to the optic tract, within the optic nerve and in the fiber layer of the contralateral retina; some ganglion cells were covered with silver grains in a zone topographically related to the site of D-asp application to the tectum (Fig. 4). In this zone, the labeled ganglion cells were small (6–7 μm in diameter), rounded, and intermingled with numerous unlabeled cell bodies of similar size and shape. This pattern contrasts with that observed after comparable tectal injections of HRP, where virtually all ganglion cells showed the enzyme reaction (Burkhalter et al., in preparation). The differential labeling suggests that D-[^{3}H]asp migrates selectively within a subpopulation of retinal ganglion cells. It should also be noted that intravitreal injections of D-[^{3}H]asp led to the labeling of a small percentage of perikarya in the ganglion cell layer heterogeneously distributed throughout the retina (Beaudet et al. 1981; Ehinger 1981). These cells were especially numerous in the postero-superior quadrant (Beaudet et al. 1981) which is known to project to the ventro-caudal aspect of the tectum (McGill et al. 1966). From the retina, anterograde filling of the axons could be detected, tracing the pathway to the contralateral tectum (mainly in Layers 1–3 and 5), as well as to some, but not all mesencephalic primary visual relay nuclei. Thus, in the pigeon retino-tectal neurons, in which stimulation induces a liberation of endogenous glu and asp (Canzek et al. 1981), D-[^{3}H]asp appears to label, both retrogradely and anterogradely, a selected subpopulation of neurons.

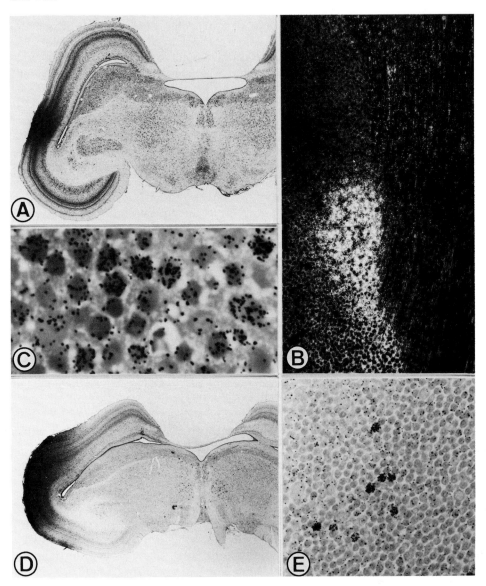

Fig. 4. (A-C) Light-microscopic autoradiographs of the left optic tectum (A) and contralateral retina (B, C) from the same pigeon, 6 h after intratectal injection of D-[^{3}H]aspartate (25 μCi in 0.05 μl). (A) Coronal section through the optic tectum at the level of the injection site. The latter stands out as a patch of dense and diffuse radioautographic labeling, spreading across 2 mm^2 over the lateral aspect of the tectum and involving all layers. Exposure 2 weeks. $\times$5. (B) One μm-thick, Epon-embedded, tangential section through the foveal region of the contralateral retina under dark-field illumination. The left half of the micrograph runs through the ganglion cell layer and the right half through the fiber layer. Note the clustering of the labeled cells at the level of the fovea and, on the right hand side, the discrete retrograde labeling of their efferent axons. $\times$100. (C) The same section, illustrated at higher power and under bright-field illumination. Ganglion cell layer. Small round, retrogradely labeled cells are visible amidst unlabeled perikarya of similar size and shape. Note the variability in the intensity of labeling. Exposure 6 weeks. $\times$600. (D,E) Light-microscopic radioautographs of the left optic tectum (D) and the contralateral retina (E) from a pigeon submitted to a 4-h tectal superfusion with 10^{-5} M D-[^{3}H]aspartate. (D) Coronal section through the optic tectum illustrating the extent of tracer penetration. An intense and ubiquitous diffuse reaction, corresponding to D-[^{3}H]aspartate retained in tissue in the course of glutaraldehyde fixation, pervades the external aspect of the

4.2. SPINAL PRIMARY AFFERENTS

It has been suggested, on the basis of biochemical and physiological evidence, that glutamate might play a role in the primary afferents to the spinal cord (Curtis and Johnston 1974; Johnson 1978). After D-[^{3}H]asp injection, either in the dorsal horn at the cervical level or in the cuneate nucleus, Rustioni et al. (in preparation) observed retrograde labeling of the afferent neurons in the corresponding spinal ganglia (Fig. 5). The labeled cells were large and amounted to about 5% of the neuronal population in the ganglion. While it is not possible to decide whether the same neurons are labeled after spinal and cuneate injection, it appears that a subpopulation of primary afferents, particularly large-sized ones, have an affinity for D-asp and are likely candidates as users of acidic amino acid transmitters.

4.3. OLFACTORY AFFERENTS

Fischer et al. (1982c) observed perikaryal labeling in the nucleus of the olfactory tract, mainly ipsilaterally, following D-[^{3}H]asp injections in the rat basolateral amygdala.

Thus, in three sensory systems, the pigeon optic nerve and the rat spinal primary afferents as well as the olfactory system, D-[^{3}H]asp labels retrogradely a small subpopulation of their cell bodies of origin.

4.4. CEREBELLAR AFFERENT SYSTEMS

The numerous granule cells, which give rise to parallel fibers, have been proposed to

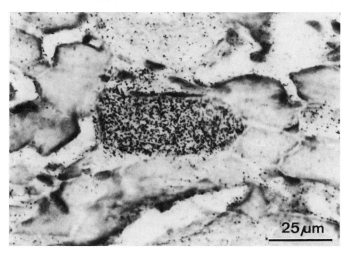

Fig. 5. Autoradiographic labeling in a part of the rat dorsal root ganglion C8 24 h after injection of 0.05 μl D-[^{3}H]aspartate (spec. act. 16.8 Ci/mmol) at cervical levels. Example of one of the relatively few heavily labeled perikarya. (From Rustioni, unpublished.)

tectum, spreading across all layers. A preferential labeling of the fiber layer (Layer I) is clearly distinguishable along the ventral border. Exposure 2 weeks. $\times$5. (E) Five μm thick, paraffin-embedded, tangential section through the ganglion cell layer of the contralateral retina. Retrogradely labeled cells, similar in size and shape to those depicted in (C) and to their unlabeled congeners, dot the red field area (temporo-superior quadrant). Exposure time 3 months. $\times$400. (From Beaudet et al. 1981.)

use glu as transmitter (Young et al. 1974; Hudson et al. 1976; Sandoval and Cotman 1978; Hackett et al. 1979; Rhode et al. 1979). Furthermore, after destruction of the olivo-cerebellar climbing fiber system, decreased contents of asp (Nadi et al. 1977; Rea et al. 1980) and reduced in vitro release of endogenous asp (Toggenburger et al. 1983) in the cerebellum suggest that climbing fibers may use this excitatory amino acid. After injections of D-[^{3}H]asp into various parts of the cerebellar vermis, hemispheres and deep nuclei, retrograde labeling of the *olivocerebellar climbing fiber pathway* was observed by Wiklund et al. (1982) (Fig. 6). Corroborative results were obtained after prolonged vermal superfusions with D-[^{3}H]asp at concentrations in the range of K_m for high-affinity uptake (10^{-5} and 10^{-4} M; see, Davies and Johnston 1976). The climbing fibers were strongly labeled along their entire trajectory through the cerebellum and brain stem. In addition, labeling of presumed climbing fiber collaterals in the deep nuclei and distant parts of the cerebellar cortex suggested anterograde migration of tracer from branching points of the axon. Furthermore, the density of labeled cell bodies was such that all olivary neurons were likely to have the capacity for uptake and transport of D-[^{3}H]asp retrogradely.

Most *parallel fibers* and *granule cells* exposed to high levels of D-[^{3}H]asp at the site of injection or superfusion appeared unlabeled by the tracer (Wiklund et al. 1982). This

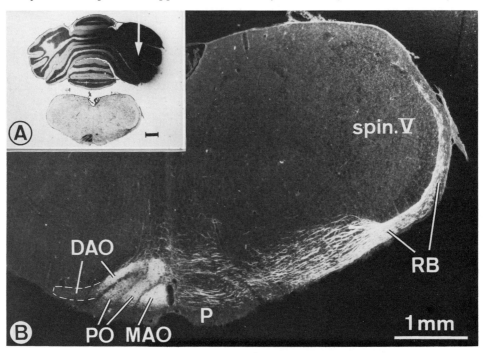

Fig. 6. (A) Bright-field micrograph of rat cerebellum and medulla oblongata 24 h after an injection of D-[^{3}H] aspartate (25 µCi in 0.05 µl) involving crus II and lobulus paramedianus (arrow). The retrograde labeling in the inferior olive can easily be distinguished at this low magnification (bar: 1 mm). (B) Dark-field micrograph of the same section. Retrogradely labeled nerve fibers are seen in the restiform body (RB), and traversing the ventral medulla oblongata from their origin in the contralateral inferior olive. At this rostral level of the inferior olive, strongly labeled perikarya are present in the medial accessory (MAO), principal, (PO) and medial part of the dorsal accessory (DAO) nucleus. The lateral part of the dorsal accessory nucleus (outlined), which projects to the vermis of lobuli I-VI, is not labeled. P = pyramid; spin. V = spinal trigeminal nucleus. (From Wiklund et al. 1982.) (Copyright 1982 by the American Association for the Advancement of Science.)

result was surprising since these cerebellar interneurons are believed to use glu as transmitter. Small groups of well-labeled granule cells and corresponding parallel fibers were, however, regularly observed. These seemed to appear consistently in a transverse plane along the axis of the folium and to be transected by the pipette penetration. It is therefore likely that the labeled granule cells correspond to neurons subjected to mechanical injury. These observations invite the speculation that intact granule cells fail to become labeled because they lack the necessary uptake mechanisms (Sandoval and Cotman 1978; Gordon et al. 1980), but injured granule cells, whose 'barrier' may have been opened, demonstrate the capacity to accumulate and retain the tracer. The effect of the lesion did not appear indiscriminately, because Purkinje's cells and inhibitory interneurons, although also likely to be subject to fortuitous injury, did not appear labeled by D-[^{3}H]asp. Tentatively, the observations point to the possibility that the transmitter-selective labeling involves several processes, which may include uptake at the membrane level as well as intracellular capacity to retain the exogenous tracer. No *mossy fiber* afferents from the brain stem (for review see, Gould 1980) or spinal cord (Matsushita et al. 1979) were labeled by D-[^{3}H]asp.

4.5. BRAIN STEM

D-[^{3}H]asp injection into the nucleus raphe magnus of the rat resulted in retrograde labeling of the neurons in the mesencephalic periventricular gray (Persson, Wiklund and Cuénod, in preparation), suggesting that this connection, postulated to play a role in the inhibitory nociceptive control, may utilize an excitatory amino acid as transmitter. Neurons within the Edinger-Westphal nucleus were labeled after D-[^{3}H]asp injections in the rat vestibular complex (Wiklund, Perschak, Büttner-Ennever and Cuénod, in preparation). Finally, retrogradely labeled cell bodies were observed in the nucleus sagulum after injections of D-[^{3}H]asp involving the inferior colliculus (Wiklund, unpublished observations).

4.6. CORTICOFUGAL SYSTEMS

There is accumulating evidence suggesting that many cortico-cortical and corticofugal neurons use glu/asp as transmitter. The commissural, striatal, nigral, thalamic, tectal, pontine, cuneate and spinal projections of the neocortex, among others, also appear to utilize, at least in part, these transmitters according to neurochemical, physiological and pharmacological data (see, Stone 1976; Fonnum et al. 1981; Thangnipon and Storm-Mathisen 1981; Young et al. 1981). Application of D-[^{3}H]asp to the zone of termination of many of these corticofugal projections has led to their selective retrograde labeling, i.e. without simultaneous labeling of most other pathways.

Injection of D-[^{3}H]asp was first attempted in the rat *caudoputamen* by Streit and Cuénod (1979) and Streit (1980a). Within 6 h it led to retrograde perikaryal and dendritic labeling of medium-sized pyramidal neurons in Layer V, mainly within the ipsilateral frontal cortex (Streit 1980a) (Fig. 7). This observation correlates well with the convincing evidence in favor of glu and asp as transmitters in the corticostriatal neurons (Spencer 1976; Divac et al. 1977; Kim et al. 1977; McGeer et al. 1977; Reubi and Cuénod 1979; Reubi et al. 1980). Furthermore, cell bodies were labeled in the central medial, central lateral and parafascicular thalamic nuclei (Streit 1980a). Finally, no perikaryal labeling was detected in the pars compacta of the substantia nigra, in the dopaminergic cell groups A10 and A8, in the dorsal raphe nucleus or in the n. locus ceruleus.

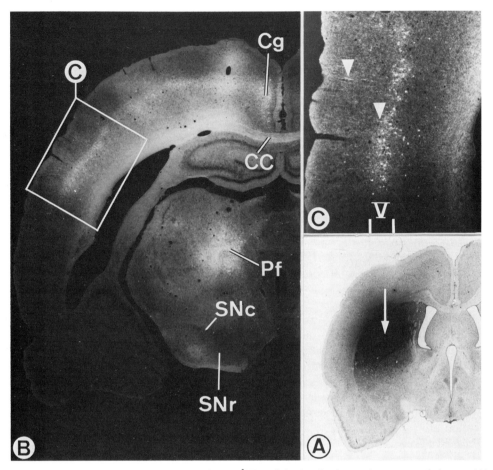

Fig. 7. Cortical cell's retrograde labeling after D-[³H]asp injection in the caudoputamen of the rat. (A) Autoradiogram at the injection site (arrow) 6 h after [³H]D-aspartate application (14 μCi in 0.05 μl). Bright-field illumination. ×5. (B) Same case as in A. Perikaryal labeling patterns (dark-field illumination) in Layer V of the dorsolateral cortex, in cingulate cortex (Cg), and in parafascicular nucleus (Pf). Rather heavy background labeling over deeper layers of the dorsal cortex. Note absence of perikaryal labeling in the region of substantia nigra; only weak neuropil labeling in lateral part of pars reticulat (SNr). SNc = substantia nigra pars compacta. Frame C indicates area shown in (C). ×8.5. (C) Detail indicated in (B). Perikaryal labeling in Layer V of lateral cortex. Some perikarya in Layer VI are labeled too. Arrow-heads point to accumulations of silver grains shaped like apical dendrites. ×21.5. (From Streit 1980.)

Recently, after injections in the rat basolateral amygdala, Storm-Mathisen and his collaborators reported perikaryal labeling in the lateral entorhinal cortex and in the hippocampus (CAl) as well as in the nucleus of the lateral olfactory tract and the interanteromedial and paraventricular nuclei of the thalamus (Fischer et al. 1982c).

Injections of D-[³H]asp in the *substantia nigra* gave rise to perikaryal labeling over scattered pyramidal neurons in Layer V of the cerebral cortex, in the n. accumbens septi, in the rostral caudoputamen and in the hypothalamus. A few cells were labeled in the dorsal raphe nucleus but none in the n. locus ceruleus (Steit 1980a).

Baughman and Gilbert (1980, 1981) injected D-[³H]asp or D-[³H]glu in the cat *lateral geniculate nucleus* (LGN) and observed, in the topographically appropriate cortical region, many labeled pyramidal cells in Layer VI as well as a diffuse band of label in Layer IV (Fig. 8). They interpreted this pattern as being compatible with a retrograde

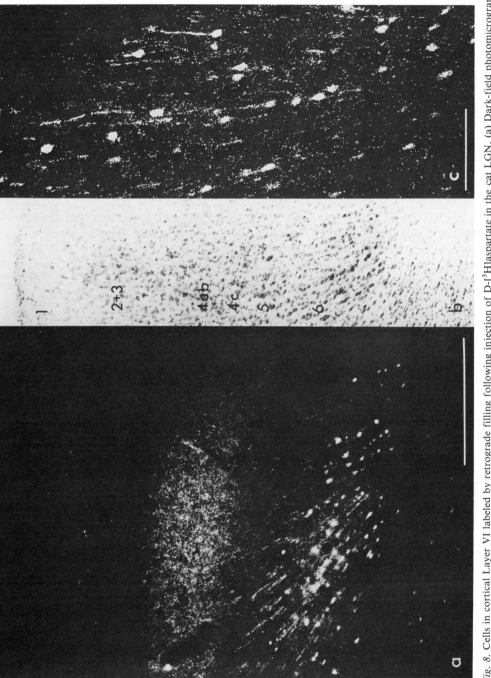

Fig. 8. Cells in cortical Layer VI labeled by retrograde filling following injection of D-[³H]aspartate in the cat LGN. (a) Dark-field photomicrograph showing labeled cells in Layer VI and a band of diffuse label in Layer IV. Bar = 500 μm. (b) Bright-field photomicrograph of the right side of field shown in (a), indicating positions of layers. (c) Higher-power dark-field photomicrograph of labeled Layer VI cells, indicating pyramidal morphology. Bar = 100 μm. (From Baughman and Gilbert 1981.)

labeling of the cortico-thalamic Layer VI pyramidal cells with a filling of their collateral ramification in Layers IV and VI (Gilbert and Wiesel 1979). These observations were confirmed by LeVay and Sherk (1981a), who also reported labeling of Layer VI neurons in the visual cortex following D-[³H]asp injections in the claustrum. The cortico-claustrum cell population is distinct from and smaller than the cortico-geniculate cell population; in addition it does not send collaterals to Layer IV. In contrast, injection of D-[³H]asp or D-[³H]glu in the dorsal layers of the *superior colliculus*, the site of projection of cortical Layer V cells, induced no labeling at all in the visual cortex.

Selective retrograde labeling of the cortico-pontine projection has been observed by Wiklund et al. (in preparation): Cortical neurons in Layer V are covered with silver grains after D-[³H]asp injections in the pontine nuclei.

Similarly, after D-[³H]asp injections in the ventrobasal complex of the thalamus of rats and cats, Rustioni et al. (1982) observed an intense autoradiographic labeling of Layer VI cortical neurons in the area projecting to the injected target, while the major source of ascending projections to the ventro-basal complex, the dorsal column and trigeminal nuclei, remained unlabeled. Furthermore, following D-[³H]asp injections in the cuneate nucleus of the *dorsal column nuclei*, Rustioni and Cuénod (1982) observed labeling over fibers in the pyramidal tract, internal capsule and over Layer V pyramidal cells in the area of the forelimb representation within the sensorimotor cortex (Fig. 9). This is in keeping with both physiological (Stone 1976) and neurochemical (Young et al. 1981) data which suggest that glu and asp play a role in the cortical fibers ter-

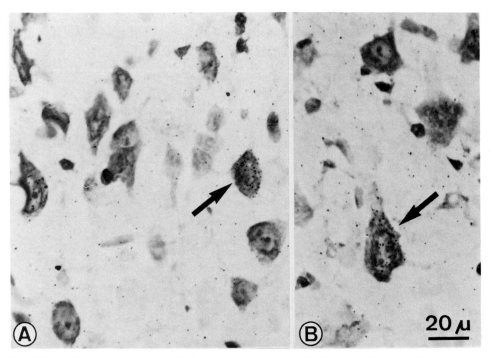

Fig. 9. Layer V pyramidal neurons in the sensorimotor cortex labeled by autoradiographic silver grains (arrows) after contralateral injection of 0.05 μl of D-[³H]aspartate in the cuneate rat nucleus; 24 h survival time. Note the fairly uniform perikaryal size of labeled elements and the absence of labeling in smaller cortical neurons. Same magnification in A and B; bright-field illumination. (From Rustioni and Cuénod 1982.)

minating in the DCN. In contrast, none of the perikarya from the spinal cord and brain stem known to project to DCN appeared labeled.

Besides the primary afferents mentioned above, a fraction of the perikarya in the substantia gelatinosa and a sparser population of larger neurons in Laminae IV to VI were labeled over a distance of a few segments above and below the D-[³H]asp injection site in the dorsal horn of the cervical *spinal cord* as reported by Rustioni and Cuénod (1982). These interneurons might correspond to the neurons which degenerate in the cat lumbar cord following temporary occlusion of the thoracic aorta, a lesion accompanied by a decrease of asp but not glu (Davidoff et al. 1967). Silver grains, though not observed over brain stem neuronal perikarya, are seen overlaying pyramidal tract fibers on the side contralateral to the injection. These fibers presumably arise from within the cerebral cortex, but labeled pyramidal neurons were not observed at any of the survival times allowed (6–72 h) (Rustioni and Cuénod 1982). Thus, these results indicate that in the somatosensory system, corticofugal neurons projecting to the afferent relay nuclei, at the diencephalic, bulbar and, most likely, spinal levels, possess a selective affinity for D-asp suggestive of a possible transmitter role of asp or glu.

Cortico-cortical labeling following D-[³H]asp injections has been observed in the rat frontal (Streit 1980a) and sensorimotor (Fischer et al. 1982b) cortex and in the cat visual cortex (Baugman and Gilbert 1981). Within a few millimeters surrounding the site of application, labeled neurons were observed in Layers III to VI after frontal injections and in Layers VI after visual cortex injections. In the homologous area of the contralateral cortex, Layer V neurons were reported to be labeled after both frontal and sensorimotor cortex injections. Commissural interhippocampal (CA3) were also labeled with D-[³H]asp (Fischer et al. 1982a). Köhler (personal communication), after D-[³H]asp injections into the septal part of the hippocampus, observed a selective retrograde labeling of perikarya in Layer II of the dorsal part of the ipsilateral entorhinal cortex and of cells in the contralateral hippocampus while the other hippocampal inputs remained free of label. This is consistent with the biochemical evidence suggesting excitatory amino acids as transmitter in these two afferent pathways.

4.7. CONCLUSION

Summing up these results, it should be stressed that the retrograde labeling obtained with D-[³H]asp is highly selective, as only a few of the many inputs to the injected zones are detected in autoradiographs. This has been seen (a) in a relatively small fraction of neurons in three sensory afferent systems, visual and spinal olfactory, (b) in the olivary-climbing fibers of the cerebellum, and (c) in various corticofugal neurons projecting to the striatum, the substantia nigra, the lateral geniculate body, the ventrobasal thalamic complex, the claustrum, the dorsal column nuclei and most likely the spinal cord. In most of these pathways, neurochemical, physiological and/or pharmacological evidence is available suggesting that L-asp is involved in their synaptic transmission, in conjunction with L-glu.

5. PROLINE

There are some indications that proline might be an inhibitory transmitter (for review see, Felix and Künzle 1974; 1976): high-affinity uptake has been observed for proline in synaptosomes (Bennett et al. 1974; Balcar et al. 1976; Henke et al. 1976b). At the site of [³H]proline injection, selective autoradiographic localization has been described in the lateral reticular nucleus (Künzle and Cuénod 1973), the cerebellum (Felix and Künzle 1974), the dorsal column nuclei (Berkley 1975; Berkley et al. 1977; Molinari and Berkley 1981), and the inferior olive (Groenewegen and Voogd 1977). Iontophoretic application of L-proline induces inhibition of neuronal discharge in the vertebrate brain (Curtis and Johnston 1974; Felix and Künzle 1974) and has both agonistic and antagonistic effects on glu induced excitation in hippocampal slices (Van Harreveld and Strumwasser 1981).

Künzle (1977) was the first to report retrogradely labeled cell bodies in the cortex and nucleus ruber of the monkey following [³H]proline injections in the spinal cord. More recently, Repérant et al. (1980) described the retrograde labeling of a retinopetal pathway in the lamprey following intraocular injection of [³H]proline. Finally, LeVay and Sherk (1981b) reported selective retrograde labeling of Layer V neurons of the cat visual cortex following [³H]proline injections in the pulvinar, superior colliculus and pons. Thus, proline, which is an inhibitory transmitter candidate, might be retrogradely transported in a selective manner, although no evidence is available yet that the pathways retrogradely labeled after [³H]proline application are indeed prolinergic. Molinari and Berkley (1981) have argued that in the DCN, the available evidence does not favor a transmitter role of proline.

6. CHOLINERGIC SYSTEMS

Cholinergic neurons and terminals pick up choline by a high-affinity transport mechanism (Yamamura and Snyder 1973; Whittaker and Dowdall 1975; Dowdall et al. 1976; Baughman and Bader 1977; Jope 1979). Therefore, Bagnoli et al. (1981) tested whether [³H]choline could be used to trace retrogradely cholinergic neurons in a selective way. Following intracerebral injection of [³H]choline, the autoradiographic distribution of the radioactivity follows two distinct patterns: (1) a diffuse, neuropil labeling present in all structures known to receive a projection from the injected area; this can be detected with conventional autoradiographic techniques and most likely corresponds to nonselective anterograde migration of nondiffusible molecules, probably lipids (Droz et al. 1978, 1979); (2) grain accumulations in the form of small circular foci centered over cell bodies, with a halo of decreasing grain density expanding beyond the limits of the perikarya (Fig. 10). These foci could be observed only in dry-mounted material (Young and Kuhar 1979; see Appendix for technical details) and were present exclusively over neuronal populations known to send a cholinergic projection to the injected area. The radioactivity is likely to be present in choline, acetylcholine or phosphorylcholine (Baughman and Bader 1977).

6.1. SEPTO-HIPPOCAMPAL NEURONS

The cholinergic input to the hippocampus originates in the medial septal nucleus (MS) and in the nucleus of the diagonal band (DB) and reaches its target via the fimbria. Lesion of this pathway led to a drastic decrease in hippocampal choline acetyltransferase (CAT) activity, acetylcholine (ACh) levels and turnover, while septal stimulation is followed by an increase in ACh hippocampal release and turnover. Other inputs to the hippocampus are considered to use glu, asp, serotonin and catecholamines as transmitters (for review see, Storm-Mathisen 1977; Fonnum et al. 1979).

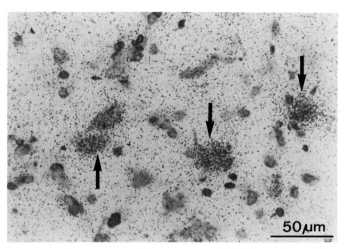

Fig. 10. Retrograde labeling of neurons (arrows) in the parabrachialis complex after [³H]choline injection (25 μCi in 0.05 μl; spec. act. 77 Ci/mmol) in the ipsilateral caudal thalamus of the rat. Autoradiography according to the dry-mount technique. (Wiklund, unpublished.)

After [³H]choline injections in the rat hippocampus, diffuse, most likely anterograde, labeling is observed in the contralateral hippocampus, in the ipsilateral entorhinal cortex, and in the lateral septum. Perikaryal foci of silver grains are present in the ipsilateral medial septal nucleus and nucleus of the diagonal band, suggesting a retrograde labeling of this cholinergic pathway. No focal labeling can be detected in the contralateral hippocampus, in the entorhinal area, in the locus ceruleus or in the raphe nuclei (Bagnoli et al. 1981).

6.2. OTHER SYSTEMS

In the pigeon, lesion of the visual thalamic relay induces a 40% decrease in CAT activity in the visual projection to the hyperstriatum (visual Wulst) (Vischer et al. 1980, 1982; Csoknay et al. in preparation), suggesting that the thalamo-Wulst projection contains cholinergic neurons. [³H]Choline injections into the Wulst led to a retrograde labeling of nerve cell bodies in the n. dorsolateralis anterior thalami, pars magnocellularis (Bagnoli et al. 1981) and not in other neurons projecting to the Wulst, either from the thalamus or the mid-brain (Bagnoli et al. 1981; Bagnoli and Burkhalter 1982). Here also, diffuse anterograde labeling is present in the target zones of Wulst efferent fibers.

More recently, Wiklund et al. (unpublished) injected [³H]choline in the rat *neocortex* and observed retrograde labeling of neurons in the nucleus basalis magnocellularis Meynert consistent with its being source of cholinergic innervation to the neocortex (Divac 1975; Lewis and Shute 1978; Lehman et al. 1980; Wenk et al. 1980; Johnston et al. 1981; Kimura et al. 1981), while thalamic and brain stem afferents remained unlabeled. Injections involving the *intralaminar nuclei of the thalamus* led to retrograde labeling of the perikarya in the parabrachial complex of the brain stem (Wiklund et al., unpublished), (Fig. 10) which is well established as the source of cholinergic innervation (Lewis and Shute 1978; Saper and Loewy 1980; Kimura et al. 1981).

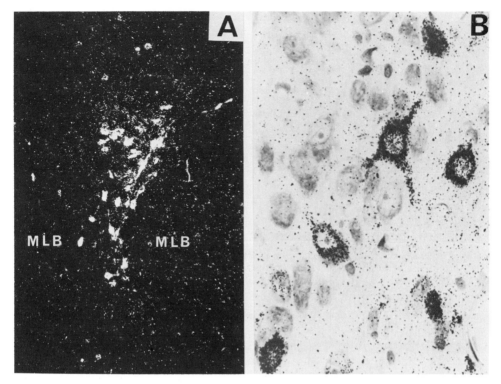

Fig. 11. Light-microscopic radioautographs 24 h after a unilateral injection of [^{3}H]5-HT (100 μCi) in the rat olfactory bulb. Exposure time: 1 month. (A) Ipsilateral labeled cell bodies in the raphe dorsalis nucleus. MLB = medial longitudinal bundle. ×80. (B) Retrogradely labeled cell bodies in the raphe dorsalis nucleus. Note the positive labeling of dendrites. ×440. (From Araneda et al. 1980b.)

7. BIOGENIC AMINES: DOPAMINE AND SEROTONIN

The systems using biogenic amines as transmitter in the central nervous system have been extensively investigated and their distribution is well established, owing to the excellent histochemical methods available to outline them. Thus, it was attractive to test the hypothesis of transmitter specific retrograde tracing on serotonergic and catecholaminergic pathways.

7.1. DOPAMINERGIC PROJECTIONS

[^{3}H]Dopamine injections in the rat caudoputamen led to intense perikaryal labeling throughout the zona compacta of the ipsilateral substantia nigra, in the ipsilateral groups A10 and A8 and to weak labeling in the dorsal raphe nucleus. Labeled perikarya were never detected either in the cerebral cortex or in the thalamus. Striatal injection of tritiated tyrosine, the amino acid precursor for dopamine, was ineffective in distant labeling of perikarya in any brain region (Streit 1980a). Dopamine injections in the rat substantia nigra resulted in perikaryal labeling in the ipsilateral locus ceruleus, and to a lesser extent the dorsal raphe nucleus, while the caudoputamen was free of perikaryal labeling (Streit 1980a). Thus, dopamine appears to label retrogradely the well established dopaminergic pathways originating in the substantia nigra, or in groups A8 and A10 and projecting to the caudoputamen (reviewed in Lindvall and Björklund 1978; Moore and Bloom 1978); however, it also labels cells in the dorsal raphe nucleus. This could be related to a crossed specificity of the uptake mechanism between dopamine and serotonin, leading to 'false' labeling of a serotonergic raphe projection with [³H]dopamine. Alternatively, as a population of dopaminergic neurons has been demonstrated in the raphe nucleus and since dopaminergic neurons have been shown by Steinbusch et al. (1981) and Steinbusch and Nieuwenhuys (1982) to project to the neostriatum, it is also possible that this retrograde labeling with [³H]dopamine indeed reveals a dopaminergic pathway. A similar interpretation has recently been proposed by Descarries et al. (1981). Clearly, noradrenergic neurons of the nucleus locus ceruleus were cross-labeled by [³H]dopamine injections (Streit 1980a).

7.2. SEROTONINERGIC PROJECTIONS

Leger et al. (1977) were the first to report retrograde perikaryal labeling in the nucleus raphe dorsalis after an injection of [³H]serotonin into the rat *caudoputamen*. They also showed that cell bodies in the substantia nigra and in groups A10 and A8 were labeled as well. These observations were confirmed by Streit et al. (1979a, 1980a) and Beaudet et al. (in preparation), who also found retrogradely labeled cells in the cortex and in the thalamus, in the absence of pretreatment with a monoaminoxidase inhibitor. Striatal injection of tritiated tryptophan, the amino acid precursor for serotonin, was ineffective in distant labeling of perikarya, even in the nucleus raphe dorsalis (Streit 1980a).

[³H]Serotonin injections into the rat *substantia nigra* led to perikaryal labeling in the ipsilateral nucleus raphe dorsalis and occasionally in the cortex but not in the caudoputamen (Streit 1980a).

Superfusion of rat *cerebral cortex* with 10^{-4} M [³H]serotonin, which leads locally to an intense labeling of axonal varicosities, induced retrograde perikaryal labeling in the nucleus raphe dorsalis, raphe medialis and locus ceruleus (Beaudet et al. in preparation).

Araneda et al. (1980a,b) demonstrated, by both biochemical and autoradiographic techniques, retrograde labeling in the dorsal raphe nucleus after [³H]serotonin injections in the *olfactory bulb* in rats pretreated with a monoaminoxidase inhibitor (Fig. 11). 30–50% of the radioactivity was recovered in the form of serotonin, and the migration took place at the rates of 48 and 16 mm/day. When injected in the olfactory bulb, [³H]norepinephrine was ineffective in labeling raphe neurons.

Yamamoto et al. (1980) injected [³H]serotonin into the rat *cerebellum* and observed not only a perikaryal labeling of the raphe nuclei but also of many other non-serotoninergic brain stem nuclei known to project to the cerebellum, such as the inferior olive, the vestibular nuclei, parvocellular pontine nuclei, subtrigeminal part of the nucleus reticularis lateralis, nucleus prepositus hypoglossi and locus ceruleus.

Thus, after injecting [³H]serotonin one may encounter two problems: not only does it seem to crosslabel catecholamine neurons, as might be expected from the established crossed specificity of their uptake mechanisms (Shaskan and Snyder 1970; Berger and Glowinski 1978), but it also appears to become, under some circumstances, an almost nonspecific marker which labels all the inputs to the injected area, just as horseradish peroxidase or wheat germ agglutinin would do. Nonspecific labeling with serotonin injections has been observed also after striatal injections in the absence of pargyline (Streit 1980a), after cerebellar injection (Yamamoto et al. 1980), and after striatal injections associated with 'cold' noradrenaline or with the uptake blocker citalopram (Beaudet et al., in preparation). Furthermore, following injection of [³H]serotonin in the tongue, intense perikaryal labeling was observed within the ipsilateral nucleus of the 12th nerve, indicating the labeling of a known cholinergic neuron (Beaudet et al., in preparation). General retrograde labeling of afferents was also found after [³H]serotonin injection into the pigeon optic tectum (Streit, unpublished observations).

It is possible that the effective concentration of serotonin in situ is critical for the specific labeling. Araneda et al. (1981) have indeed observed that above a certain serotonin concentration, the retrograde labeling becomes nonspecific.

8. ASSESSMENT AND LIMITATIONS OF THE METHOD

Selective, transmitter-specific retrograde neuronal labeling has been presented for the amino acids glycine, GABA and D-aspartate (as a marker for L-asp/L-glu neurons), for choline (as a marker of cholinergic neurons) and for the biogenic amines dopamine, noradrenaline and serotonin. Successful results have been obtained in the pigeon, the rat and the cat.

The data reviewed above fall into four classes based on the correlation between the results obtained with this new method and those available from established biochemical, histochemical, physiological and pharmacological methodologies. The first two classes are double-positive (A) and double-negative (B), the last two offer a more challenging view and can be considered as the 'false-negative' (C) and the 'false-positive' (D). (A) First, there are pathways for which a given transmitter candidate is relatively well established and which are retrogradely labeled after application of the appropriate marker. To this class belong, among others, the glycinergic isthmo-tectal neurons, the GABAergic striatonigral neurons, the 'aspartatergic' retino-tectal neurons, spinal primary afferents, olivo-climbing fibers of the cerebellum as well as the cortico-fugal neurons to the striatum, the substantia nigra, the lateral geniculate nucleus, the ventro-basal thalamus, pontine nuclei, the dorsal column nuclei and the spinal cord, the cholinergic septo-hippocampal and thalamo-Wulst neurons, the dopaminergic nigrostriatal neurons and the serotonergic efferents of the raphe nucleus to the nigra, striatum, cortex and olfactory bulb.

(B) A second class pertains to the neurons for which no evidence is available to date indicating that they use a given transmitter, and which correspondingly are not retrogradely labeled after application of the appropriate marker. It would be impossible to list all examples in this class, but throughout this review a bulk of evidence has been offered for the high selectivity of retrograde labeling: as an example, one should be reminded that the majority of inputs to the cerebellum, DCN and dorsal horn of the spinal cord were not labeled with injection of [³H]D-asp, or that most afferents to the hippocampus were not labeled with [³H]choline. The body of evidence supplied by Classes A and B supports the hypothesis of transmitter-selective retrograde labeling.

(C) The third class is made up of those with 'false-negative' results, namely cases in which a transmitter marker fails to label a group of neurons believed to release the corresponding transmitter: the failure to label GABAergic Purkinje neurons after [³H]GABA injections into Deiters' nucleus is the prototype of this category. Also, the absence of interneurons labeled by GABA in the neighborhood of the DCN or the spinal dorsal horn is puzzling. Finally, the absence of labeling of the cerebellar granule cells and that in the cortico-collicular projection after D-[³H]asp injection could possibly fall into the 'false-negative' category. These data do not support the hypothesis proposed here and alternative explanations will be sought. In the case of Purkinje's cells, it is possible, as discussed above, that they are lacking in the GABA specific high-affinity uptake — a mechanism believed to be essential to selective retrograde labeling. The GABAergic interneurons in the dorsal horn or the DCN might not exist, or might possess axons so short that the perikarya are lost in the high density of grains at the site of injection. It should also be pointed out that in all experiments with [³H]GABA in the spinal cord or DCN, 6–72 h elapsed between injection and sacrifice, a period probably too long for visualizing local perikaryal uptake (Kelly and Dick 1976). The status of acidic excitatory amino acids is not yet as established as that of the other transmitters discussed here, and, therefore, some revision of the basic concepts about their mechanisms of action might be needed in the future. At any rate, these 'false-negative' results do not really warrant a rejection of the hypothesis, but point out the limitation of the method, especially in relation to the importance of selective uptake mechanisms. At any rate, the absence of labeling cannot be taken as evidence that a transmitter is not being used.

Furthermore, since an active uptake mechanism seems to play a crucial role it is not surprising that to date there are no studies demonstrating the type of retrograde labeling discussed here in transmitter systems for which no uptake has been found. This is the case for the neuropeptide substance P in its intact form (Iversen et al. 1976; Segawa et al. 1976, 1978). Recently, however, evidence has been obtained for a high- and low-affinity uptake of substance P carboxy-terminal hepta-peptide (5–11) (Nakata et al. 1981). This cleavage product (Kato et al. 1980b) as well as the responsible endopeptidase have also been detected in brain material (Blumberg et al. 1980; Kato et al. 1980a). Uptake of certain peptide breakdown products may allow to test the present hypothesis even in pathways using neuropeptides as transmitters. It should therefore be possible to cover the last group of transmitters remaining to be addressed.

(D) The fourth class consists of those with 'false positive' results, that is to say cases in which the application of a tritiated marker leads to retrograde perikaryal labeling of neurons for which the corresponding transmitter has not been suspected on the basis of other experimental approaches. This situation has presented among the biogenic amines, which usually crosslabel each other, and also with serotonin, which, under some circumstances, becomes a universal retrograde marker. In the case of the amines, one is most likely dealing with a problem of crossed sensitivity of the uptake mechanism. As far as serotonin is concerned, it might turn out, as discussed above, that its concentration at the relevant sites is highly critical so that various levels of sensitivity might be present, the most sensitive uptake being restricted to serotonergic neurons and the next one includes the catecholamines, while high concentrations affect all neurons, a phenomenon which nevertheless might be of physiological significance.

Finally, there is still much data, made up of positive and negative retrograde perikaryal labeling, which cannot be correlated with information derived from other methods. Their value as convincing proof will depend on the reliability of the method developed and they can only be used at present as suggestive evidence to promote further research.

9. CONCLUSION

In conclusion, the evidence which favors selective retrograde labeling of pathways has been reviewed for amino acids, choline and biogenic amines. In many cases this selectivity has shown to be specific for the transmitter used. Positive results have been recorded in neurons using glycine, GABA, aspartate and/or glutamate, acetylcholine, dopamine and serotonin as transmitters. 'False-negative' observations were made in some pathways using GABA or asp/glu, while 'false-positive' ones occurred with dopamine and, in particular, with serotonin, which seems, under some conditions, to become a universal marker. The phenomenon seems to depend upon an uptake mechanism in the nerve terminal. It is indeed present in many cases following superfusion at concentrations in the range of high-affinity uptake (Beaudet et al. 1981; Wiklund et al. 1982; Beaudet et al., in preparation) and could be blocked by high-affinity uptake antagonists in the case of serotonin (Araneda et al. 1980a; Beaudet et al., in preparation). It is also dependent upon a retrograde transport sensitive to tubulin-binding agents (Araneda et al. 1980a; Beaudet et al., in preparation). The selectivity could rest on the uptake, and possibly also on the retrograde transport. Considering the limited amount of data available so far, as well as the limitations and pitfalls discussed, the proposed hypothesis of a transmitter-specific retrograde labeling cannot be considered as definitively established. However, in view of the predictive value of the results obtained, further investigation of this phenomenon with emphasis on its mechanisms and its possible biological significance is certainly justified.

10. APPENDIX

(Prepared by Leif Wiklund, Department of Histology, University of Lund, Sweden)

10.1. TECHNIQUE FOR TRANSMITTER-RELATED RETROGRADE LABELING OF AMINO ACID AND MONOAMINE TRANSMITTERS

1. *Stereotaxic microinjection* of tracer in aqueous solution (from Amersham)

[³H]D-aspartate	10–30 Ci/mmol
[³H]GABA	50–70 Ci/mmol
[³H]glycine	10–30 Ci/mmol
[³H]serotonin	10–20 Ci/mmol
[³H]dopamine	5–15 Ci/mmol

These tracers are supplied in a dilute aqueous or ethanol solution (1 mCi/ml). They are therefore evaporated under a stream of N_2, and redissolved to desired concentration. For injection, we routinely dissolve 1 mCi of the tracer in 2 μl aq.dest., and of this solution 30–60 nl is injected slowly over 10 min through a glass micropipette (40 μm in diameter broken or beveled). (The concentration of the injected tracer under these conditions is in the order of 10^{-2} M.)

2. *Survival* 6, 12, 24 h (for long connections, up to 48 h).

3. *Perfusion-fixation*
   (a) rinse out blood; 50–100 ml 5% Rheomacrodex;
   (b) 3.5–5% glutaraldehyde in 0.2 M phosphate buffer, 1000 ml
       (Glutaraldehyde, and not formaldehyde, is necessary as fixative, since the retrogradely transported molecules are not incorporated in macromolecules);
   (c) the dissected brains are routinely left in the same fixative overnight in order to ensure thorough fixation (4°C).

4. *Tissue processing and sectioning*
The brains can either be sectioned on a freezing microtome 30 μm (10 μm), or paraffin-embedded and -sectioned.

   A.   For sectioning on freezing microtome:
      (a)   The fixed brain is transferred to 30% sucrose in 0.2 M phosphate buffer (4°C); overnight or until the brain sinks.
      (b)   Sectioning on freezing microtome (10–30 μm).
      (c)   Wash the sections in 3 changes of aq.dest. (to ensure washing out of excess fixative and salts).
      (d)   Mounting on gelatine-chromalum subbed slides.
      (e)   Adherence of mounted sections ensured by drying overnight at 40°C.
      (f)   De-fatting of mounted sections in xylene, and pass through falling series of alcohols to aq.dest. Dry sections overnight. (The sections are thereafter ready for dipping in photographic emulsion.)

   B.   For paraffin-embedding and -sectioning
      (a)   Dehydration of tissue:

Ethanol 70%	1 bath	90 min	
Ethanol 80%	1 bath	90 min	
Ethanol 95%	2 baths	2 min each	
Ethanol 100%	2 baths	2 min each	
Amyl acetate	3 baths	2 min each	

Note: amyl acetate is used in place of xylene in order to keep the glutaraldehyde fixed tissue soft enough for sectioning.
      (b)   Embedding in paraffin.
      (c)   Sectioning (e.g. 10 μm). Sections stretched on water and mounted on gelatinized slides.
      (d)   Dry-mounted sections overnight (40°C).
      (e)   Deparaffinize through 3 baths of xylene (each 20 min), rehydrate through decreasing series of alcohol, and wash in aq-dest. Dry section-bearing slides overnight (40°C).

5. *Autoradiography*
      (a)   Section bearing slides are dipped in the dark in liquid emulsion (e.g. Kodak NTB-2, diluted 1:1 with aq.dest., melted at 43°C).
      (b)   After air-drying, the emulsion-coated slides are stored for exposure in light-proof slideboxes in the presence of a desiccating agent (e.g. silica gel). Exposure time: 3 and 6 weeks.
      (c)   Photographic development:
            90 sec in Dektol (Kodak; diluted 1:2 with aq.dest.) at 18°C;
            30 sec rinse in water;
            8–10 min fixation in sodiumthiosulfate (75 g in 250 ml aq.dest.);
            3×5 min rinse in aq.dest.

6. *Cresylviolet staining*, and coverslipping.

7. *Microscopy* in bright- and darkfield.

10.2. TECHNIQUE FOR SELECTIVE RETROGRADE LABELING OF CHOLINERGIC SYSTEMS

1. *Stereotaxic microinjection*
[^{3}H]Choline (60–85 Ci/mmol, Amersham); 30–50 nl containing 15–25 μCi (equivalent to ca. 0.7×10^{-2} M).

389

2. *Survival* 6–12 h (longer not yet tested).

3. *Sacrifice*: dissected fresh brain tissue is rapidly frozen, e.g. using 2-methylbutane cooled to −40° by crushed dry ice.

4. *Cryostat sectioning*
   15–20 μm sections are thaw-mounted onto gelatinized slides, and rapidly dried on a hotplate (+60°C).

5. *Autoradiography* for diffusable substances following the method of Young and Kuhar (1979).

   (a) Acid-washed coverslips (25 × 77 mm No. O; thin and flexible) are dipped in the dark to ca. half their length in NTB-2 emulsion (diluted 1:1 with aq.dest.) at 43°C.

DIPPING OF COVERSLIPS (IN DARK)

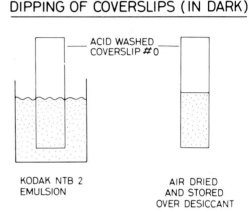

Dry the dipped coverslips in the air for (4h - overnight).

   (b) Glue the coverslips onto the section-bearing slides in the dark. The coverslip should protrude a little below the edge of the microscope slide. (We recommend: Loctite IS495 superfast cyanoacrylate adhesive.)

   (c) After the glue sets, a square of teflon is put on top of the coverslip, and the assembly held together with a clip.

ASSEMBLY PROCEDURE (IN DARK)

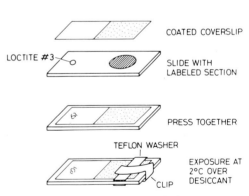

   (d) Exposure in light-safe slide boxes for 3 and 6 weeks, in presence of desiccant.

   (e) For development, the clips and teflon squares are removed in the dark, the coverslip carefully bent away from the section, and a spacer in the form of a thin plastic rod inserted.

   (f) Development: 90 sec, Dektol, 18°C, by immersing the section-bearing half of the assembly.

DEVELOPMENT (IN DARK)

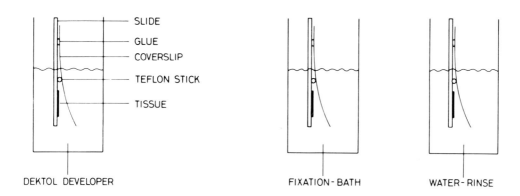

Rinse: 30 sec in aq.dest.
Fixation: 10 min in sodiumthiosulfate
Rinse: 3 × 5 min in aq.dest. at 4°C.

(Note: It is important to agitate the assemblies during development and fixation.)

FIXATION AND STAINING

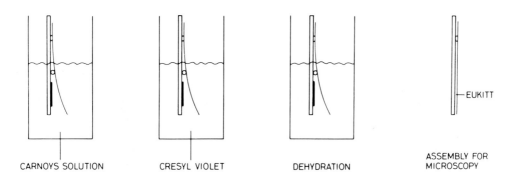

(g) Fixation of tissue in Carnoy's solution (60 ml ethanol abs., 30 ml chloroform and 10 ml acetic) by immersion of the section-bearing half of the assembly.

(Note: Carnoy's solution may dissolve the glue.)

(h) Stain in cresylviolet, followed by:
3 × absolute alcohol, agitate
3 × xylene; leave the assemblies in the last bath of xylene until
mounting with suitable medium (e.g. Eukitt or Permount)
place a weight on the coverslip until the mounting mediums solidifies in order to bring the silver grains in close apposition to the underlying tissue section.

6. *Microscopy* in bright- and darkfield.

11. ACKNOWLEDGEMENTS

The authors wish to thank Drs P. Bagnoli, A. Beaudet, H.J.W. Nauta, A. Rustioni and L. Wiklund for their invaluable contributions throughout these studies. We also thank Mrs M. Jäckli and E. Schneider and Mr J. Künzli for their secretarial, graphic and photographic help.

This chapter is an adapted version of the symposium report 'Transmitter-specific retrograde labeling of neurons' by Cuénod, Bagnoli, Beaudet, Rustioni, Wiklund and Streit in *'Cytochemical Methods in Neuroanatomy'*, S.L. Palay and V. Chan-Palay (Eds.), Alan R. Liss, 1982.

12. REFERENCES

Aprison, MH, Nadi NS (1978): Glycine: Inhibition from the sacrum to the medulla. In; Fonnum F (Ed) *Amino Acids as Chemical Transmitters*, pp. 531–570. Plenum Press, New York.

Araneda S, Bobillier P, Buda M, Pujol J-F (1980a): Retrograde axonal transport following injection of [³H]serotonin in the olfactory bulb. I. Biochemical study. *Brain Res., 196*, 405–415.

Araneda S, Gamrani H, Font C, Calas A, Pujol J-F, Bobillier P (1980b): Retrograde axonal transport following injection of [³H]serotonin into the olfactory bulb. II. Radioautographic study. *Brain Res., 196*, 417–427.

Araneda S, Font C, Pujol J-F, Bobillier P (1981): Is the retrograde axonal transport of ³H-5-HT a specific process of serotoninergic neurons? *J. Physiol. (Paris) 77*, 233–235.

Balcar VJ, Johnston GAR (1972): The structural specificity of the high-affinity uptake of L-glutamate and L-aspartate by rat brain slices. *J. Neurochem., 19*, 2657–2666.

Balcar VJ, Johnston GAR, Stephanson AL (1976): Transport of L-proline by rat brain slices. *Brain Res., 102*, 143–151.

Bagnoli P, Burkhalter A (1983): Organization of the afferent projections to pigeon visual Wulst: A retrograde transport study. *Comp. Neurol., 214*, 103–113.

Bagnoli P, Beaudet A, Stella M, Cuénod M (1981): Selective retrograde labeling of cholinergic neurons with [³H]choline. *J. Neurosci., 1*, 691–695.

Barth R, Felix D (1974): Influence of GABA and glycine and their antagonists on inhibitory mechanisms of pigeon's optic tectum. *Brain Res., 80*, 532–537.

Baughman RW, Bader CR (1977): Biochemical characterization of the cholinergic system in the chicken retina. *Brain Res., 138*, 469–485.

Baughman RW, Gilbert CD (1980): Aspartate and glutamate as possible neurotransmitters of cells in Layer VI of the visual cortex. *Nature, 287*, 848–849.

Baughman RW, Gilbert CD (1981): Aspartate and glutamate as possible neurotransmitters in the visual cortex. *J. Neurosc., 1*, 427–439.

Beaudet A, Burkhalter A, Reubi JC, Cuénod M (1981): Selective bidirectional transport of [³H]D-aspartate in the pigeon retinotectal pathway. *Neuroscience, 6*, 2021–2034.

Bennett JP, Mulder AH, Snyder SH (1974): Neurochemical correlates of synaptically active amino acids. *Life Sci., 15*, 1045–1056.

Berger B, Glowinski J (1978): Dopamine uptake in serotoninergic terminals in vitro: A valuable tool for the histochemical differentiation of catecholaminergic and serotoninergic terminals in rat cerebral structures. *Brain Res., 147*, 29–45.

Berkley KJ (1975): Different targets of different neurons in nucleus gracilis of the cat. *J. Comp. Neurol., 163*, 285–304.

Berkley KJ, Graham J, Jones EG (1977): Differential incorporation of tritiated proline and leucine by neurons of the dorsal column nuclei in the cat. *Brain Res., 132*, 485–505.

Blumberg S, Teichberg VI, Charli JL, Hersh LB, McKelly JF (1980): Cleavage of substance P to an N-terminal tetrapeptide and a C-terminal heptapeptide by a post-proline cleaving enzyme from bovine brain. *Brain Res., 192*, 477–486.

Brownstein MJ, Mroz EA, Tappaz ML, Leeman SE (1977): On the origin of substance P and glutamic acid decarboxylase (GAD) in the substantia nigra. *Brain Res., 135*, 315–324.

Burkhalter A, Wang SJ, Streit P (1983): Distribution and classification of retinal ganglion cells after horseradish peroxidase injections in the dorsolateral thalamus and the optic textum of the pigeon. In preparation.

Canzek V, Wolfensberger M, Amsler U, Cuénod M (1981): In vivo release of glutamate and aspartate following optic nerve stimulation as determined by mass fragmentographic technique. *Nature, 293*, 572–574.

Cotman CW, Foster A, Lanthorn T (1981): An overview of glutamate as a neurotransmitter. In: Di Chiara G, Gessa GL (Eds), *Glutamate as a Neurotransmitter*, pp. 1–27. Raven Press, New York.

Csoknay A, Vischer A, Bagnoli P, Henke H (1982): Cholinergic and GABAergic innervation in the pigeon visual Wulst: Effect of thalamic lesions. In preparation.

Cuénod M, Henke H (1978): Neurotransmitters in the avian visual system. In: Fonnum F (Ed), *Amino Acids as Chemical Transmitters*, pp. 221–239. Plenum Press, New York.

Cuénod M, Streit P (1979): Amino acid transmitters and local circuitry in optic tectum. In: Schmitt FO, Worden FG (Eds), *The Neurosciences: Fourth Study Program*, pp. 989–1004. MIT Press, Cambridge, MA.

Cuénod M, Beaudet A, Canzek V, Streit P, Reubi JC (1981): Glutamatergic pathways in the pigeon and the rat brain. In: Di Chiara G, Gessa GL (Eds), *Glutamate as a Neurotransmitter*, pp. 57–68. Raven Press, New York.

Cuénod M, Bagnoli P, Beaudet A, Rustioni A, Wiklund L, Streit P (1982): Transmitter-specific retrograde labeling of neurons. In: Chan-Palay V, Palay SL (Eds), *Cytochemical Methods in Neuroanatomy,* pp. 17–44 Alan R. Liss Co.

Curtis DR, Johnston GAR (1974): Amino acid transmitters in the mammalian central nervous system. *Ergeb. Physiol. Biol. Chem. Exp., 69,* 97–188.

Davidoff RA, Graham Jr LT, Shank RP, Werman R, Aprison MH (1967): Changes in amino acid concentrations associated with loss of spinal interneurons. *J. Neurochem., 14,* 1025–1031.

Davies LP, Johnston GAR (1976): Uptake and release of D- and L-aspartate by rat brain slices. *J. Neurochem., 26,* 1007–1014.

Descarries L, Berthelet F, Garcia S (1981): Axophoresis of [³H]DA and [³H]NA by central catecholaminergic neurons in rat brain: Radioautographic demonstration. *Soc. Neurosci. Abstr., 7,* 802.

Divac I (1975): Magnocellular nuclei of the basal forebrain project to neocortex, brain stem and olfactory bulb: Review of some functional correlates. *Brain Res., 93,* 385–398.

Divac I, Fonnum F, Storm-Mathisen J (1977): High-affinity uptake of glutamate in terminals of corticostriatal axons. *Nature, 266,* 377–378.

Dowdall MJ, Fox G, Wachtler K, Whittaker VP, Zimmermann H (1976): Recent studies on the comparative biochemistry of the cholinergic neuron. In: *Proceedings, Cold Spring Harbor Symposia on Quantitative Biology, Vol. 40, The Synapse,* pp. 65–81. Cold Spring Harbor Laboratory, New York.

Droz B, DiGiamberardino L, Koenig HL, Boyenval J, Hassig R (1978): Axon-myelin transfer of phospholipid components in the course of their axonal transport as visualized by radioautography. *Brain Res., 155,* 347–353.

Droz B, Burnetti M, DiGiamberardino L, Koenig HL, Porcelatti G (1979): Transfer of phospholipid constituents to glia during axonal transport. *Soc. Neurosci. Symp., 4,* 344–360.

Ehinger B (1981): [³H]D-aspartate accumulation in the retina of pigeon, guinea-pig and rabbit. *Exp. Eye Res., 33,* 381–391.

Felix D, Künzle H (1974): Iontophoretic and autoradiographic studies on the role of proline in nervous transmission. *Pflügers Arch. Ges. Physiol., 350,* 135–144.

Felix D, Künzle H (1976): The role of proline in nervous transmission. In: Costa E, Giacobini E, Paoletti R (Eds), *Advances in Biochemical Psychopharmacology, Vol. 15,* pp. 165–173. Raven Press, New York.

Fischer BO, Ottersen OP, Storm-Mathisen J (1982a): Anterograde and retrograde axonal transport of D-[³H]aspartate (D-asp) in hippocampal excitatory neurons. *Neuroscience, Suppl. 7,* S68.

Fischer BO, Ottersen OP, Storm-Mathisen J (1982b): Axonal transport of D-[³H]aspartate in the claustrocortical projection. *Neuroscience, Suppl. 7,* S69.

Fischer BO, Ottersen OP, Storm-Mathisen J (1982c): Labelling of amygdalopetal and amygdalofugal projections after intra-amygdaloid injections of tritiated D-aspartate. *Neuroscience, Suppl. 7,* S69.

Fonnum F, Henke H (1982): The topographical distribution of alanine, aspartate, γ-aminobutyric acid, glutamate, glutamine and glycine in the pigeon optic tectum and the effect of retinal ablation. *J. Neurochem., 38,* 1130–1134.

Fonnum F, Grofova I, Rinvik E, Storm-Mathisen J, Walberg F (1974): Origin and distribution of glutamate decarboxylase in substantia nigra of the cat. *Brain Res., 71,* 77–92.

Fonnum F, Lund Karlsen R, Malthe-Sørensen D, Skrede KK, Walaas I (1979): Localization of neurotransmitters, particularly glutamate, in hippocampus, septum, nucleus accumbens and superior colliculus. In: Cuénod M, Kreutzberg G, Bloom F (Eds), *Development and Chemical Specificity of Neurons, Progress in Brain Research,* pp. 167–191. Elsevier, Amsterdam.

Fonnum F, Søreide A, Kvale I, Walker J, Walaas I (1981): Glutamate in cortical fibers. In: Di Chiara G, Gessa GL (Eds), *Glutamate as a Neurotransmitter*, pp. 29–41. Raven Press, New York.

Gilbert CD, Wiesel TN (1979): Morphology and intracortical projections of functionally characterized neurons in the cat visual cortex. *Nature, 280,* 120–125.

Gordon RD, Wilkin GP, Gallo V, Levi G, Balazs R (1980): High-affinity transport of L-glutamate and D-aspartate into cell types of the cerebellum. *Neurosci. Lett. Suppl. 5,* 78.

Gould BB (1980): Organization of afferents from the brain stem nuclei to the cerebellar cortex on the cat. *Adv. Anat. Embryol. Cell Biol., 62,* 1–79.

Grafstein B, Forman DS (1980): Intracellular transport in neurons. *Physiol. Rev., 60,* 1167–1283.

Groenewegen JH, Voogd J (1977): The parasagittal zonation within the olivocerebellar projection. I. Climbing fiber distribution in the vermis of cat cerebellum. *J. Comp. Neurol., 174,* 417–488.

Hackett JT, Hou S-M, Cochran SL (1979): Glutamate and synaptic depolarization of Purkinje's cells evoked by parallel fibers and by climbing fibers. *Brain Res., 170,* 377–380.

Henke H (1983): The central part of the avian visual system. In: Nistico G, Bolis L (Eds) *Progress in Nonmammalian Brain Research.* CRC Press Inc., Boca Raton, USA. In press.

Henke H, Cuénod M (1978): Uptake of L-alanine, glycine and L-serine in the pigeon central nervous system. *Brain Res., 152,* 105–119.

Henke H, Schenker TM, Cuénod M (1976a): Uptake of neurotransmitter candidates by pigeon optic tectum. *J. Neurochem., 26,* 125–130.

Henke H, Schenker TM, Cuénod M (1976b): Effects of retinal ablation on uptake of glutamate, glycine, GABA, proline and choline in pigeon tectum. *J. Neurochem., 26,* 131–134.

Hökfelt T, Ljungdahl AA (1975): Uptake mechanisms as a basis for the histochemical identification and tracing of transmitter-specific neuron populations. In: Cowan WM, Cuénod M (Eds), *The Use of Axonal Transport for Studies of Neuronal Connectivity,* pp. 249–305. Elsevier, Amsterdam.

Hudson DB, Valcana T, Bean G, Timiras PS (1976): Glutamic acid: A strong candidate as neurotransmitter of the cerebellar granule cell. *Neurochem. Res., 1,* 83–92.

Hunt SP, Künzle H (1976): Selective uptake and transport of label within three identified neuronal systems after injection of [^{3}H]GABA into the pigeon optic tectum: An autoradiographic and Golgi study. *J. Comp. Neurol., 170,* 173–190.

Hunt SP, Künzle H, Cuénod M (1975): The retrograde transport of amino acids and a glycinergic system within the optic lobe. *Exp. Brain Res., S23,* 189.

Hunt SP, Henke H, Künzle H, Reubi JC, Schenker T, Streit P, Felix D, Cuénod M (1976): Biochemical neuroanatomy of the pigeon optic tectum. In: Creutzfeldt O (Ed) *Afferent and Intrinsic Organization of Laminated Structures in the Brain, Exp. Brain Res. Suppl. 1,* pp. 521–525. Springer New York.

Hunt SP, Streit P, Künzle H, Cuénod M (1977): Characterization of the pigeon isthmo-tectal pathway by selective uptake and retrograde movement of radioactive compounds and by Golgi-like HRP. *Brain Res., 129,* 197–212

Iversen LL, Dick F, Kelly JS, Schon F (1975): Uptake and localization of transmitter amino acids in the nervous system. In: Berl S, Clarke DD, Schneider D (Eds), *Metabolic Compartmentation and Neurotransmission,* pp. 65–87. Plenum Press, New York.

Iversen LL, Jessell T, Kanazawa I (1976): Release and metabolism of substance P in rat hypothalamus. *Nature, 264,* 81–83.

Jessell TM, Emson PC, Paxinos G, Cuello AC (1978): Topographic projections of substance P and GABA pathways in the striato- and pallidonigral system: A biochemical and immunohistochemical study. *Brain Res., 152,* 487–498.

Johnson JL (1978): The excitant amino acids glutamic and aspartic acid as transmitter candidates in the vertebrate central nervous system. *Prog. Neurobiol., 10,* 155–202.

Johnston MV, McKinney M, Coyle JT (1981): Neocortical cholinergic innervation: A description of extrinsic and intrinsic components in the rat. *Exp. Brain Res., 43,* 159–172.

Jope RS (1979): High-affinity choline transport and acetylCoA production in brain and their roles in the regulation of acetylcholine synthesis. *Brain Res. Rev., 1,* 313–345.

Kataoka K, Bak IJ, Hassler R, Kim JG, Wagner A (1974): L-glutamate decarboxylase and choline acetyltransferase activity in the substantia nigra and the striatum after surgical interruption of the strionigral fibres of the baboon. *Exp. Brain Res., 19,* 217–227.

Kato T, Nakano T, Kojima K, Nagatsu T, Sakakibara S (1980a): Changes in prolylendopeptidase during maturation of rat brain and hydrolysis of substance P by the purified enzyme. *J. Neurochem., 35,* 527–535.

Kato T, Okada M, Nakano T, Nagatsu T, Emura J, Sakakibara S, Iizuka Y, Tsushima S, Nakazawa N, Ogawa H (1980b): The presence of substance P carboxy-terminal heptapeptide in pig brain stem. *Proc. Jpn. Acad. B., 56,* 388–399.

Kelly JS, Dick F (1976): Differential labeling of glial cells and GABA-inhibitory interneurons and nerve terminals following the microinjection of [β-^{3}H]DABA and [^{3}H]GABA into single folia of the cerebellum.

In: *Proceedings Cold Spring Harbor Symposia on Quantitative Biology, Vol. 40,* The Synapse, pp. 93–106. Cold Spring Harbor Laboratory, New York.

Kim JS, Bak IJ, Hassler R, Okada Y (1971): Role of γ-aminobutyric acid in the extrapyramidal motor system. 2. Some evidence for the existence of a type of GABA strionigral neurons. *Exp. Brain Res., 14,* 95–104.

Kim JS, Hassler P, Haug P, Paik KS (1977): Effect of frontal cortex ablation on striatal glutamic acid level in rat. *Brain Res., 132,* 370–374.

Kimura H, McGeer PL, Peng JH, McGeer EG (1981): The central cholinergic system studied by choline acetyltransferase immunohistochemistry in the cat. *J. Comp. Neurol., 200,* 151–201.

Künzle H (1977): Evidence for selective axon-terminal uptake and retrograde transport of label in cortico- and rubrospinal systems after injection of [³H]proline. *Exp. Brain Res., 28,* 125–132.

Künzle H, Cuénod M (1973): Differential uptake of [³H]proline and [³H]leucine by neurons: Its importance for the autoradiographic tracing of pathways. *Brain Res., 62,* 213–217.

Le Fort D, Henke H, Cuénod M (1978): Glycine specific [³H]strychnine binding in the pigeon CNS. *J. Neurochem., 30,* 1287–1291.

Leger L, Pujol JF, Bobillier P, Jouvet M (1977): Transport axoplasmique de la sérotonine par voie retrograde dans les neurones monoaminergiques centraux, *CR Acad, Sci. (Paris), 285,* 1179–1182.

Lehman J, Nagy JI, Atmodja S, Fibiger HC (1980): The nucleus basalis magnocellularis: The origin of a cholinergic projection to the neocortex of rat. *Neuroscience, 5,* 1161–1174.

LeVay S, Sherk H (1981a): The visual claustrum of the cat. I. Structure and connections. *J. Neurosci., 1,* 956–980.

LeVay S, Sherk H (1981b): Retrograde transport of L-[³H]-proline by cortical Layer V pyramidal cells. *Soc. Neurosci. Abstr., 36/17,* 112.

Lewis PR, Shute CCD (1978): Cholinergic pathways in CNS. In: Iversen LL, Iversen SD, Snyder SH (Eds), *Handbook of Psychopharmacology, Vol. 9, Chemical Pathways in the Brain,* pp. 315–355. Plenum Press, New York.

Lindvall O, Björklund A (1978): Organization of catecholamine neurons in the rat central nervous system. In: Iversen LL, Iversen SD, Snyder SH (Eds), *Handbook of Psychopharmacology, Vol. 9, Chemical Pathways in the Brain,* pp. 139–231. Plenum Press, New York.

Marc RE, Lam DMK (1981): Uptake of aspartic and glutamic acid by photoreceptors in goldfish retina. *Proc. Nat. Acad. Sci. USA, 78,* 7185–7189.

Matsushita M, Hosoya Y, Ikeda M (1979): Anatomical organization of the spinocerebellar system in the cat as studied by retrograde transport of horseradish peroxidase. *J. Comp. Neurol., 184,* 81–106.

McGeer PL, McGeer EG, Scherer U, Singh K (1977): A glutamatergic corticostriatal path? *Brain Res., 128,* 369–373.

McGill JI, Powell TPS, Cowan WM (1966): The retinal representation upon the optic tectum and isthmo-optic nucleus in the pigeon, *J. Anat., 100,* 5–33.

McLaughlin BJ, Wood JG, Saito K, Barber R, Vaughn JE, Robert E, Wu J-Y (1974): The fine structural localization of glutamate decarboxylase in synaptic terminals of rodent cerebellum. *Brain Res., 76,* 377–391.

Molinari HH, Berkley KJ (1981): Differences in glial and neuronal labeling following [³H]proline or [³H]leucine injections into the dorsal column nuclei of cats. *Neuroscience, 6,* 2313–2334.

Moore RY, Bloom FE (1978): Central catecholamine neuron systems: Anatomy and physiology of the dopamine system. *Annu. Rev. Neurosci., 1,* 129–169.

Nadi NS, Kanter D, McBride WJ, Aprison MH (1977): Effects of 3-acetylpyridine on several putative neurotransmitter amino acids in the cerebellum and medulla of the rat. *J. Neurochem., 28,* 661–662.

Nagy JI, Carter DA, Fibiger HC (1978): Anterior striatal projections to the globus pallidus, entopeduncular nucleus and substantia nigra in the rat: The GABA connection. *Brain Res., 158,* 15–29.

Nakata Y, Kusaka Y, Yajima H, Segawa T (1981): Active uptake of substance P carboxy-terminal heptapeptide (5–11) into rat brain and rabbit spinal cord slices. *J. Neurochem., 37,* 1529–1534.

Nauta HJW, Cuénod M (1982): Perikaryal cell labelling in the subthalamic nucleus following the injection of [³H]GABA into the pallidal complex: An autoradiographic study in the cat. *Neuroscience, 7,* 2725–2734.

Obata K, Takeda K (1969): Release of γ-aminobutyric acid into the fourth ventricle induced by stimulation of the cats cerebellum. *J. Neurochem., 16,* 1043–1047.

Obata K, Ito M, Ochi R, Sano N (1967): Pharmacological properties of the postsynaptic inhibition by Purkinje's cell axons and the action of γ-aminobutyric acid on Deiter's neurons. *Exp. Brain Res., 4,* 43–57.

Perkins MN, Stone TW (1981): Ionotophoretic studies on pallidal neurons and the projection from the subthalamic nucleus. *Quart. J. Exp. Physiol., 66,* 225–236.

Precht W, Yoshida M (1971): Blockade of caudate-evoked inhibition of neurons in the substantia nigra by picrotoxin. *Brain Res., 32,* 229–233.

Rea MA, McBride WJ, Rohde BH (1980): Regional and synaptosomal levels of amino acid neurotransmitters in the 3-acetylpyridine deafferented rat cerebellum. *J. Neurochem., 34,* 1106–1108.

Repérant J, Vesselkin NP, Ermakova TV, Kenigfest NB, Kosareva AA (1980): Radioautographic evidence for both orthograde and retrograde axonal transport of labeled compounds after intraocular injection of [³H]proline in the lamprey (Lampetra fluviatilis). *Brain Res., 200,* 179–183.

Reubi JC, Cuénod M (1976): Release of exogenous glycine in the pigeon optic tectum during stimulation of a midbrain nucleus. *Brain Res., 112,* 347–361.

Reubi JC, Cuénod M (1979): Glutamate release in vitro from corticostriatal terminals. *Brain Res., 176,* 185–188.

Reubi JC, Toggenburger G, Cuénod M (1980): Asparagine as precursor for transmitter aspartate in corticostriatal fibres. *J. Neurochem., 35/4,* 1015–1017.

Rhode BH, Rea MA, Simon JR, McBridge WJ (1979): Effects of X-irradiation induced loss of cerebellar granule cells on the synaptosomal levels and the high-affinity uptake of amino acids. *J. Neurochem., 32,* 1431–1435.

Ribak CE, Vaughn JE, Saito K (1978): Immunocytochemical localization of glutamic acid decarboxylase in neuronal somata following colchicine inhibition of axonal transport. *Brain Res., 140,* 315–332.

Rouzaire-Dubois B, Scarnati E, Hammond C, Crossman AR, Shibazaki T (1983): Microiontophoretic studies on the nature of the neurotransmitter in the subthalamo-entopenduncular pathway of the rat. *Brain Res.,* in press.

Rustioni A, Cuénod M (1982): Selective retrograde transport of D-aspartate in spinal interneurons and cortical neurons of rats. *Brain Res., 236,* 143–155.

Rustioni A, Schmechel DE, Spreafico R, Cheema S, Cuénod M (1983): Excitatory and inhibitory amino acid putative neurotransmitters in the ventralis posterior complex: An autoradiographic and immunocytochemical study in rats and cats. In: Macchi G, Rustioni A, Spreafico R (Eds), *Somatosensory Integration in the Thalamus,* Elsevier, Amsterdam. In press.

Sandoval ME, Cotman CW (1978): Evaluation of glutamate as a neurotransmitter of cerebellar parallel fibers. *Neuroscience, 3,* 199–206.

Saper CB, Loewy AD (1980): Efferent connections of the parabrachial nucleus in the rat. *Brain Res., 197,* 291–317.

Segawa T, Nakata Y, Nakamura K, Yajima H, Kitagawa K (1976): Substance P in the central nervous system of rabbits: Uptake system differs from putative transmitters. *Jpn. J. Pharmacol., 26,* 757–760.

Segawa T, Nakata Y, Yajima H, Kitagawa K (1978): Further observation on the lack of active uptake system for substance P in the central nervous system. *Jpn. J. Pharmacol., 27,* 573–580.

Shaskan E, Snyder SH (1970): Kinetics of serotonin accumulation into slices from rat brain: Relationship to catecholamine uptake. *J. Pharmacol. Exp. Ther., 175,* 404–418.

Snyder SH, Yamamura HI, Pert CB, Logan WJ, Bennett JP (1973): Neuronal uptake of neurotransmitters and their precursors in studies with 'transmitters' amino acids and choline. In: Mandell AJ (Ed), *New Concepts in Neurotransmitter Regulation,* pp. 195–222. Plenum Press, New York.

Somogy P, Cowey A, Halasz N, Freund TF (1981): Vertical organization of neurones accumulating [³H]GABA in visual cortex of rhesus monkey. *Nature, 294,* 761–763.

Spencer HJ (1976): Antagonism of cortical excitation of striatal neurons by glutamic acid diethyl ester: Evidence for glutamic acid as an excitatory transmitter in the rat striatum. *Brain Res., 102,* 91–101.

Steinbusch HWM, Nieuwenhuys R (1982): The raphe nuclei of the rat brain stem. A cytoarchitectonic and immunohistochemical study. In: Emson P (Ed), *Chemical Neuroanatomy.* Raven Press, New York. In press.

Steinbusch HWM, Nieuwenhuys R, Verhofstad AAJ, Vanderkooy D (1981): The nucleus raphe dorsalis of the rat and its projection upon the caudato putamen. A combined cytoarchitectonic immunohistochemical and retrograde transport study. *J. Physiol. (Paris), 77,* 157–174.

Stone TW (1976): Blockade by amino acid antagonists of neuronal excitation mediated by the pyramidal tract. *J. Physiol. (London), 257,* 187–198.

Storm-Mathisen J (1975): High-affinity uptake of GABA in presumed GABAergic nerve endings in rat brain. *Brain Res., 84,* 409–427.

Storm-Mathisen J (1976): Distribution of the components of GABA system in neuronal tissue: Cerebellum and hippocampus - effects of axotomy. In: Roberts E, Chase TN, Tower DB (Eds), *GABA in Nervous System Function,* pp. 149–168. Raven Press, New York.

Storm-Mathisen J (1977): Localization of transmitter candidates in the brain: The hippocampal formation as a model. *Prog. Neurobiol., 8,* 119–181.

Storm-Mathisen J (1979): Autoradiographic and microchemical localization of high-affinity uptake of glutamate and aspartate. In: *Proceedings, Seventh Meeting of the International Society for Neurochemistry, Jerusalem,* p. 109.

Storm-Mathisen J, Woxen Opsahl H (1978): Aspartate and/or glutamate may be transmitters in hippocampal efferents to septum and hypothalamus. *Neurosci. Lett., 9,* 65–70.

Streit P (1980a): Selective retrograde labeling indicating the transmitter of neuronal pathways. *J. Comp. Neurol., 191,* 429–463.

Streit P (1980b): Retrograder axonaler Transport und neuronale Transmittorspezifität. *Bull. Schweiz. Akad. Med. Wiss., 36.* 21–51.

Streit P, Cuénod M (1979): Transmitter specificity and connectivity revealed by differential retrograde labeling of neural pathways. *Neurosci. Lett. Suppl. 3,* 340.

Streit P, Knecht E, Cuénod M (1979a): Transmitter specific retrograde labeling in the striatonigral and raphe-nigral pathways. *Science, 205,* 306–308.

Streit P, Reubi JC, Wolfensberger M, Henke H, Cuénod M (1979b): Transmitter-specific retrograde tracing of pathways? In: Cuénod M, Kreutzberg G, Bloom F (Eds), *Development and Chemical Specificity of Neurons, Progress in Brain Research,* pp. 489–496. Elsevier, Amsterdam.

Streit P, Knecht E, Cuénod M (1980): Transmitter-related retrograde labeling in the pigeon optic lobe: A high resolution autoradiographic study. *Brain Res., 187,* 59–67.

Takagaki G (1977): Properties of the accumulation of D-[^{14}C]-aspartate into rat cerebral crude synaptosomal fraction. In: Fonnum F (Ed), *Amino Acids as Chemical Transmitters,* pp. 357–361. Plenum Press, New York.

Thangnipon W, Storm-Mathisen J (1981): K$^+$-evoked CA^{2+}-dependent release of D-[^{3}H]aspartate from terminals of the cortico-pontine pathway. *Neurosci. Lett., 23,* 181–186.

Toggenburger G, Wiklund L, Henke H, Cuénod M (1983): Release of endogenous and accumlated exogenous amino acids form slices of normal and climbing fibers deprived rat cerebellar slices. *J. Neurochem.,* in press.

Van Harrenveld A, Strumwasser F (1981): Glutamate agonistic and antagonistic activity of L-proline investigated in the hippocampal slice. *Neuroscience, 6,* 2495–2503.

Vischer A, Fäh A, Burkhalter A, Henke H (1980): Kainic acid toxicity in the pigeon thalamus and consequent decrease in the hyperstriatal choline acetyltransferase and glutamic acid decarboxylase. *Experientia, 36,* 703.

Vischer A, Cuénod M, Henke H (1982): Neurotransmitter receptor ligand binding and enzyme regional distribution in the pigeon visual system. *J. Neurochem.,* in press.

Weiss D (1982): *Axoplasmic Transport.* Raven Press, New York. In press.

Wenk H, Bigl V, Meyer U (1980): Cholinergic projections from magnocellular nuclei of the basal forebrain to cortical areas in rats. *Brain Res. Rev., 2,* 295–316.

Whittaker VP, Dowdall MJ (1975): Current state of research on cholinergic synapses. In: Waser PG (Ed), *Cholinergic Mechanisms,* pp. 35–40. Raven Press, New York.

Wiklund L, Künzle H, Cuénod M (1983): Failure to demonstrate retrograde labeling of cerebellar Purkinje cells after injection of [^{3}H]GABA in Deiters' nucleus. *Neurosci. Lett.,* in press.

Wiklund L, Toggenburger G, Cuénod M (1982): Aspartate: Possible neurotransmitter in cerebellar climbing fibers. *Science, 216,* 78–79.

Wolfensberger M, Reubi JC, Canzek V, Redweik U, Curtius HCh, Cuénod M (1981): Mass fragmentographic determination of endogenous glycine and glutamic acid released in vivo from the pigeon optic tectum. Effect of electrical stimulation of a midbrain nucleus. *Brain Res., 224,* 327–336.

Yamamoto M, Chan-Palay V, Palay SL (1980): Autoradiographic experiments to examine uptake, anterograde and retrograde transport of tritiated serotonin in the mammalian brain. *Anat. Embryol., 159,* 137–149.

Yamamura HI, Snyder SH (1973): High-affinity transport of choline into synaptosomes of rat brain. *J. Neurochem. 21,* 1355–1374.

Young III WS, Kuhar MJ (1979): A new method for receptor autoradiography: [^{3}H]Opioid receptors in rat brain. *Brain Res., 179,* 255–270.

Young AB, Oster-Granite ML, Herndon RM, Snyder SH (1974): Glutamic acid: Selective depletion by viral-reduced granule cell loss in hamster cerebellum. *Brain Res., 73,* 1–13.

Young AB, Bromberg MBM, Penney Jr JB (1981): Decreased glutamate uptake in subcortical areas deafferented by sensorimotor cortical ablation in the cat. *J. Neurosci., 1,* 241–249.

Zukin SR, Young AB, Snyder SH (1975): Development of the synaptic glycine receptor in chick embryo spinal cord. *Brain Res., 83,* 525–530.

CHAPTER IX

Autoradiographic localization of drug and neurotransmitter receptors

MICHAEL J. KUHAR

1. INTRODUCTION

In recent years it has become possible to identify receptor proteins directly by biochemical binding methods using radioactive ligands (Snyder and Bennett 1976; Yamamura et al. 1978). Along with these biochemical studies, there has been a great need for and some success in developing microscopic methods for localizing receptors. The success of biochemical binding studies and the earlier development of autoradiographic techniques for localizing diffusible molecules (Stumpf and Roth 1966; Roth and Stumpf 1969) have also been very important in the evolution of light-microscopic autoradiographic studies of receptors. The rationale for localizing receptors at the microscopic level has been simple. Radioactive drugs or chemicals are placed in contact with tissues under conditions such that the drugs bind to receptors with a high degree of specificity. In biochemical studies, the bound ligand is measured by scintillation counting whereas most light-microscopic studies involve detection of ligand by autoradiography. This chapter discusses the progress in the area of the autoradiographic localization of receptors. The goal is to provide an overview of the issues, findings, limitations, advantages, expectations and to emphasize the methodology involved.

2. LIGHT-MICROSCOPIC METHODS

2.1. IN VIVO LABELING AUTORADIOGRAPHY

Since the greatest success in identifying receptors was by using biochemical in vitro techniques, it is somewhat surprising that in vivo binding techniques were the first to be applied in the autoradiographic localization of receptors. The probable reason for this is the success of various methods for localizing steroid hormone receptors following in vivo administration of radiolabeled steroid hormones (Stumpf and Roth 1966). The work in our laboratory on localizing drug and neurotransmitter receptors was initially based on these techniques (Kuhar and Yamamura 1974, 1975, 1976).

When using microscopic autoradiography methods for localizing receptors, two main methodologic factors must be taken into account. First, the receptors must be labeled with a fairly high degree of selectivity. In this case, the bulk of the autoradiogram will show the distribution of receptors rather than the distribution of nonspecifically bound drug in tissue sections. Second, autoradiographic methods

Handbook of Chemical Neuroanatomy. Vol. 1: Methods in Chemical Neuroanatomy.
A. Björklund and T. Hökfelt, editors.
© Elsevier Science Publishers B.V., 1983.

which prevent or minimize diffusion of the drug from receptor must be used. If significant diffusion of ligand from receptor occurs before or during the generation of an autoradiogram, there will be a serious loss of anatomical resolution and perhaps a misleading distortion of the autoradiogram. When one labels receptors with irreversible ligands, one need be concerned with diffusion only minimally or perhaps not at all; however, irreversible ligands exist in only a couple of cases and most receptors are studied with reversible, diffusible ligands. Hence, it was very useful to have some early work on the techniques for localizing diffusible molecules by autoradiography (Stumpf and Roth 1966; Roth and Stumpf 1969).

The term in vivo 'receptor labeling' is used to describe the procedure by which receptors are labeled in intact tissues in vivo after systemic administration of drug. When there is a ligand with a very high affinity for receptor, tracer quantities of the drug can be injected into the animal, and after a relatively short time interval, the drug is carried to the brain by the blood, diffuses into the brain and binds to the receptors. The nonreceptor bound drug is then removed from the brain and other tissues by various excretory processess. The high affinity of the drug for receptor causes a retention of the radioactive ligand on or in the vicinity of the receptor.

Some of the earliest studies of in vivo labeling of receptors involved cholinergic muscarinic receptors (Yamamura et al. 1974; Kuhar and Yamamura 1974, 1975, 1976). Later, interesting studies involved the opiate receptor (Pert et al. 1975) and the dopamine receptor (Kuhar et al. 1978; Laduron et al. 1978; Hollt and Schubert 1978). Figure 1 shows the labeling of radioactive spiperone by dopamine receptors following intraveneous administration of radioactive spiperone. Injections of tracer doses of tritiated drug into the tail veins of mice resulted in the striking regional distribution of the drug in accordance with the regional distribution of receptors. Additional studies

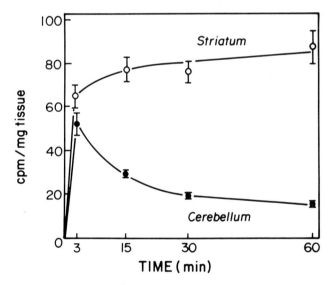

Fig. 1. Time course of ^{3}H-spiperone accumulation in the striatum and cerebellum. Animals were injected with 25 μCi of ^{3}H-spiperone. Note that the level of ^{3}H-spiperone in the striatum is maintained while that in the cerebellum declines. The striatum has very high concentrations of dopamine receptors while the cerebellum, by comparison, has negligible levels. These and other data are indicative of an in vivo labeling of dopamine and other neuroleptic-related receptors with ^{3}H-spiperone. (Reproduced from Kuhar et al. 1978).

on the subcellular localization of the binding sites, the pharmacological specificity of the binding sites and the additional regional studies of the binding sites indicated that the drug retained in the brain is mostly receptor-bound drug or drug bound to other specific neuroleptic related sites (Kuhar et al. 1978; Laduron et al. 1978). Of course, it can be seen that not all drug in the brain is bound to receptor. There is a certain amount of residual drug in the blood stream and perhaps in other compartments that is nonreceptor bound. This can be seen in the cerebellum which has a negligible quantity of dopamine receptors compared to the striatum. This relatively low quantity of radioactivity in the cerebellum reflects nonreceptor-bound drug and is fortunately small in comparison to that bound in regions such as the striatum where there are high levels of receptor.

The strategy for carrying out successful in vivo labeling experiments is as follows. First, a drug which is known to have a high degree of specificity and a very high affinity for some receptor is selected. The dissociation constant (K_d) should probably be less than one nanomolar. Small quantities of the drug should be injected (probably less than 10 μg/kg at first), and the regional distribution of drug localization as a function of time should be studied. If the regional distribution in brain is found to be uneven and parallels the known distribution of receptors, some measure of success has been achieved in obtaining in vivo labeling of receptors. A demonstration of pharmacological specificity is an extremely important factor in proving the identification of a specific receptor. In experiments involving in vivo labeling, injection of large quantites of unlabeled drugs with an affinity for the same receptor should block the binding of the tracer doses of the ligand to the site; for example, if working with opiates, opiate drugs should block the radiolabeled accumulation of radiolabeled ligand in various regions. In addition to a regional localization and pharmacological specificity, it is useful to show other factors such as saturability and binding to membranes. Examples of successful in vivo labeling experiments can be found in the literature as already mentioned (Yamamura et al. 1974; Pert et al. 1975; Kuhar et al. 1975; Laduron et al. 1978).

Once the conditions for labeling a given receptor in vivo have been identified, one can then proceed to generate autoradiograms which will provide information on the distribution of receptor binding sites at the microscopic level. As mentioned above, one must generate autoradiograms by methods that minimize diffusion of drug from binding sites. We and others have utilized thaw-mounting or dry-mounting of cryostat cut sections to emulsion-coated slide in the dark (Stumpf and Roth 1966; Kuhar 1978). Dry-mounting has the advantage that diffusion is less of a problem, but it has the disadvantage of being considerably more laborious. When cutting the sections for mounting, one of course must take the usual care that the tissue is frozen so as to minimize ice crystal formation as well as diffusion. In order to prevent diffusion, the animals are not perfused by aldehyde fixatives after receptor labeling as this frequently washes out the receptor bound drug from the brain. Hence, animals are sacrificed and fresh-frozen unfixed tissues with receptors labeled with radioactive ligands are frozen directly onto microtome chucks. 4–10 μm sections of these frozen tissue blocks can then be picked up on emulsion-coated slides for the generation of autoradiograms (Kuhar 1978). These sections are stored dry, and an important feature of this overall procedure is that the mounted tissue sections or the brain from which they are derived are not subject to fixatives or other aqueous environments where the ligand could diffuse away from the receptors. Only after the autoradiograms are formed can one treat the tissue and the slides in such a way that the ligand might be lost (Stumpf and Roth 1966; Kuhar 1978). While care must obviously be taken in these studies, several publications indicate that this approach can be used successfully (Kuhar et al. 1974, Pert et al. 1975; Kuhar et al. 1978).

In the autoradiograms, investigators find a distribution of autoradiographic grains that is expected; for example, since synapses occur in between cell bodies, or in the neuropil, it is to be expected that the bulk of receptors are found in the neuropil. In autoradiographic studies, it has indeed been found that the bulk of receptor-bound ligand occurs in the neuropil. In in vivo labeling experiments where the tissue sections and emulsion-coated surface of the slide are immediately apposed and attached, one

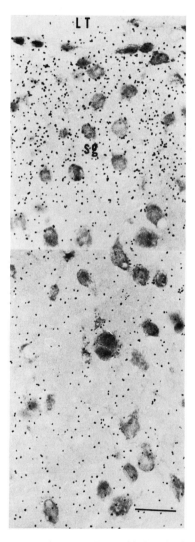

Fig. 2. The autoradiographic localization of opiate receptors in the rat spinal cord. This is a brightfield micrograph showing regions of the dorsal horn. Note the high concentrations of autoradiographic grains (hence, opiate receptors) over the substantia gelatinosa (sg) while there is a much lower level over Lissauer's tract (LT) and an intermediate level over Lamina IV. (Reproduced from Atweh and Kuhar 1977a).

TABLE 1. *Advantages of in vitro labeling autoradiography over in vivo labeling autoradiography*

1. Control of metabolism
2. Circumvention of the blood-brain barrier
3. Controlled binding milieu
   (a) good specific-to-nonspecific binding ratios
   (b) testing of ionic and other chemical influences (e.g. nucleotides, various displacers)
4. Enhanced sensitivity (nanogram size regions studied quantitatively)
5. Different radiolabeled ligands or conditions in consecutive sections
6. Relative low cost (versus in vivo labeling autoradiography)
7. Use of human postmortem tissue

can view the distribution of receptors and the fixed and stained tissues simultaneously (Fig. 2).

While in vivo labeling autoradiography has been successful and important in the field, it has serious limitations. It seems that a very important factor in these experiments is the availability of a ligand with a very high affinity for the receptor. Also, one cannot control the binding conditions so as to increase specificity. Also, it can be somewhat expensive in that an entire animal must be loaded with radioactive ligand whereas only small portions of the brain are actually used to obtain information. Because of this, it is clear that labeling of individual tissue sections in vitro would have many advantages and eliminate many of the problems associated with in vivo labeling.

2.2. IN VITRO LABELING AUTORADIOGRAPHY

In in vitro labeling procedures, slide-mounted tissue sections are incubated with radioactive ligands so that receptors are labeled under very controlled conditions (Young and Kuhar 1979a). Following the labeling, the sections can be rinsed to remove as much as possible of the nonreceptor-bound drug. Autoradiograms can then be produced in various ways which will be described (see Appendix). The advantages of in vitro labeling over in vivo labeling are listed in Table 1.

A significant advantage of the in vitro labeling procedures is that one can carry out the labeling and then remove the sections from the slide and count the radioactivity in the sections by liquid scintillation counting. Hence, extensive preliminary studies to define the optimal conditions for labeling receptors can be carried out. Once the receptors have been labeled with a high degree of specificity, the localization of these binding sites can be carried out. The procedure developed by Young and Kuhar for localizing receptors by in vitro labeling is shown in Figure 3 and discussed in the Appendix. After labeling the receptors in vitro, the tissue sections with labeled receptors are apposed to emulsion-coated coverslips. After a suitable exposure, where the patterns of radioactivity in the tissues are recorded in the emulsion, the emulsion is developed, the tissue fixed and the coverslips reapposed to the tissues which have been stained. Under these conditions, it is possible to identify the distribution of receptor sites in the tissues.

It was clear in early experiments that receptor binding to slide-mounted tissue sec-

Fig. 3. The procedure of in vitro labeling autoradiography. Frame 1 shows the preparation of subbed microscope slides. Frame 2 shows the acid washing of the No. 0 coverslips. Frame 3 shows the in vitro labeling of thaw-mounted tissue sections on slides and the subsequent rinsing to obtain high ratios of specific-to-nonspecific receptor bindings. Frame 4 shows the assembly of emulsion-coated coverslips with receptor labeled tissue to produce autoradiograms. Frame 5 shows the temporary separation of coverslip from tissue and the development of the emulsion. Frame 6 shows the fixing and staining of the tissue and the reapposition of the coverslip and slide for microscopy. (Reproduced from Young and Kuhar 1979a).

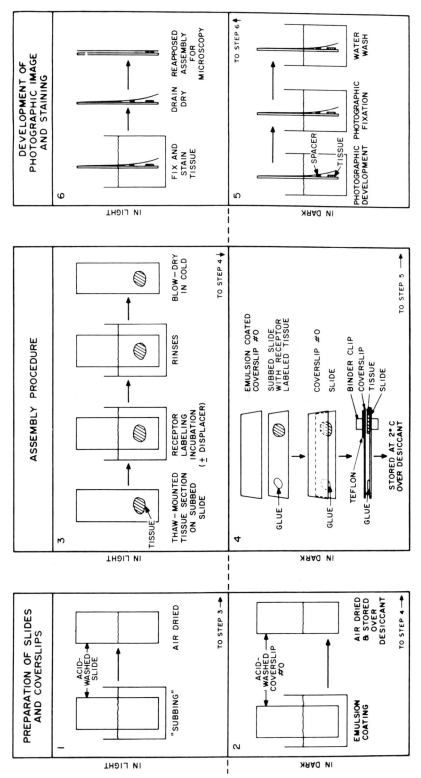

tions could be carried out in much the same way as with homogenates of tissue in biochemical experiments (Young and Kuhar 1978). The earliest attempts at producing autoradiograms involved dipping of labeled, slide-mounted tissue sections into molten nuclear emulsion (Young and Kuhar 1978); however, diffusion of ligand into the molten emulsion as well as adverse problems with the tissues pretty much eliminates this as a useful approach. Some investigators claim that fixing the tissue prior to dipping (Herkenham and Pert 1980) or placing of barriers over the tissues before dipping (Itoga et al. 1981) provides workable techniques. While it appears that these approaches show promise, they must be undertaken with care; for example, recent experiments have shown that fixation of tissue before dipping still results in a very large loss of label from the tissue during dehydration procedures indicating additional opportunity for diffusion of ligand (Kuhar, unpublished).

While the coverslip method is somewhat laborious, it has provided excellent results; for example, GABA receptors have been localized to the granule cell layer in the rat cerebellum (Fig. 4). Darkfield microscopy has often been used to examine the autoradiographic grain distribution in these experiments.

Another interesting way to generate an autoradiogram after in vitro labeling of receptors in slide-mounted tissue sections is to use tritium-sensitive sheet film. By these procedures labeled, slide-mounted tissue sections are arranged in cassettes, in rows, and large films that are sensitive to tritium, such as LKB Ultrofilm, are then apposed to the tissue sections. While the autoradiograms produced in these cases are useful and identical to those produced by other methods (Fig. 5), there is a considerable loss of resolution because the grain size in the film tends to be much larger than that in the nuclear emulsions. Thus, the autoradiograms are usually viewed at a lower microscopic power; however, the advantages of using the tritiated sheet film are great especially in that one can utilize densitometric procedures and computerized procedures in analyzing the autoradiogram (Palacios et al. 1981b; Unnerstall et al. 1982).

The success of in vitro labeling procedures is evident by the many receptors which have been explored using this approach (Table 2).

2.3. QUANTITATION OF AUTORADIOGRAPHS

A main advantage of biochemical studies of receptors is that they are not only rapid but also quantitative. It is often necessary to quantitate autoradiographs. It is clear from the numerous experiments over the past years that autoradiography in general is quantitative. Many methods have been used and these include: grain counting, photometry, densitometry and still others (Rogers 1973).

When attempting to quantitate autoradiograms, it is necessary that autoradiographic standards be utilized. The use of standards allows one to directly translate grain densities into molar quantities of the ligand bound. In these calculations, it is necessary to know the quantity of radioactivity in the standards and the specific activity of the ligand used. Also, a reasonable standard would probably consist of the same material as the sample. Thus, Unnerstall et al. (1981) have devised autoradiographic standards made by mixing tritiated compounds with brain paste. The brain paste was useful because it has the same cutting, mounting and absorptive characteristics as the brain sections used in receptor autoradiographic studies. Autoradiographs of these standards are shown in Figure 6. A relationship between grain density and exposure time is shown in Figure 7. In these studies, grain densities were measured by direct visual counting with an eyepiece with a superimposed grid for measuring areas.

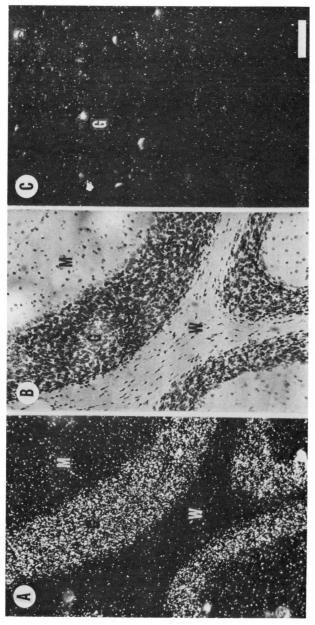

Fig. 4. Autoradiographic localization of high affinity GABA receptors in the rat cerebellum. The darkfield micrograph in *A* was taken from the tissue shown in the brightfield micrograph in *B*. An adjacent section incubated with 0.2 mM unlabeled GABA was used to produce a blank as shown in *C*. The radioactive ligand used to label the high affinity GABA receptors was ^{3}H-muscimol. A high receptor density in the molecular layer (M). Background levels were found in the white matter (W). Bar = 100 μm (Reproduced from Palacios et al. 1980b).

When one uses tritium-sensitive sheet film (^{3}H-Ultrofilm), the grain density can be measured on the film by microdensitometry; for example, optical densities can be determined utilizing a Gamma Scientific DR-2H microdensitometer system at 100 μm resolution, and the relationship between OD and concentration of radioactivity for various exposure times can be determined (Unnerstall et al. 1982). By this approach, curves relating optical density to exposure can be drawn (Fig. 8). These curves can be used to translate optical density to radioactive levels.

One of the most interesting uses of the sheet film is in computerized densitometry. Equipment that can accept the film and analyze the density on the sheet film is available. When the densitometer is coupled to an appropriate display, the autoradiogram can be reconstructed quantitatively. This entire procedure can take a matter of minutes (Fig. 9); this is an incredibly small fraction of the time that it would take to quantitate this much information by visual grain counting. It is also possible to use color coded computerized reconstructions to greatly facilitate the quantitation visually (Palacios et al., 1981).

While it is clear that in vitro labeling autoradiography is very useful, it has its limitations (Table 3). One of the most significant of these is the lack of ultrastructural resolution.

3. ULTRASTRUCTURAL LOCALIZATION OF RECEPTORS

While the light-microscopic localization of receptors is a well studied topic, considerably less work has been done in the electron-microscopic localization of receptors. A barrier against advances in this area is the lack of resolution of electron-microscopic

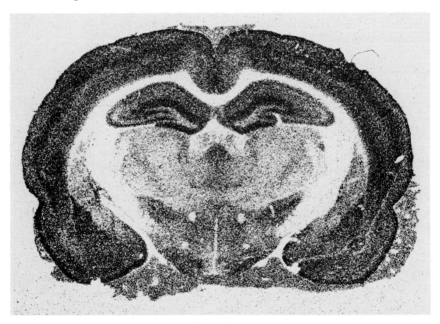

Fig. 5. Autoradiographic localization of benzodiazepine receptors in a coronal section of rat brain using tritium-sensitive sheet film. This is an excellent reproduction of earlier results using emulsion-coated coverslips. This is a brightfield micrograph taken directly from the sheet film using a 1 × objective and Leitz orthoplan microscope. (Reproduced from Palacios et al. 1981b).

TABLE 2. *Receptor localization in the literature*[a]

Receptor	Reference
Muscarinic cholinergic	Kuhar and Yamamura 1974, 1975, 1976
	Wamsley et al. 1981
	Rotter et al. 1979a,b
Nicotinic cholinergic	Hunt and Schmidt 1978
	Lentz and Chester 1977
	Segal et al. 1978
	Arimatsu et al. 1978
Dopamine	
*(actually receptors labeled	[*]Hollt and Schubert 1978
by neuroleptics)	[*]Kuhar et al. 1978
	Murrin and Kuhar 1979
	[*]Goldsmith et al. 1979
	Palacios et al. 1981a
Opiate	Pert et al. 1975
*(mu vs delta)	Atweh et al. 1977a,b,c
	Herkenham and Pert 1980
	[*]Goodman et al. 1980
	Person et al. 1980
	Young and Kuhar 1979a
GABA (high affinity)	Palacios et al. 1980b
	Palacios et al. 1981
Benzodiazepines	Young and Kuhar 1980b
*(receptor subtypes)	[*]Young et al. 1981
	Mohler et al. 1980
Neurotensin	Young and Kuhar 1981
Serotonin	Young and Kuhar 1980c
	Meibach 1980
α-Adrenergic	Young and Kuhar 1980a
β-Adrenergic	Palacios and Kuhar 1980
Glycine	Zarbin and Kuhar 1981
Histamine (H1)	Palacios et al. 1980a

[a]The tabulation is not intended to be complete, but rather an extensive introduction to the literature. Another useful tabulation, including nonneurotransmitter receptors is found in Barnard 1979.

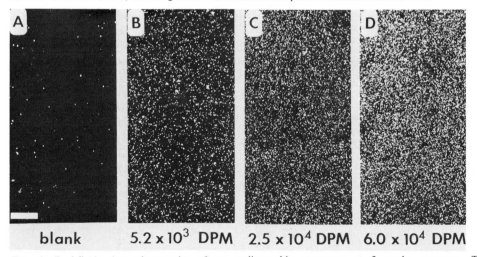

Fig. 6. Darkfield photomicrographs of autoradiographic standards at 2 weeks exposure. The autoradiographic grains appear as white dots in these and subsequent figures, whereas the tissue is not visible. DPMs refer to the concentration of radioactivity per milligram of tissue dry weight for each source as determined by scintillation spectrometry. Bar = 100 μm. (Reproduced from Unnerstall et al. 1981.)

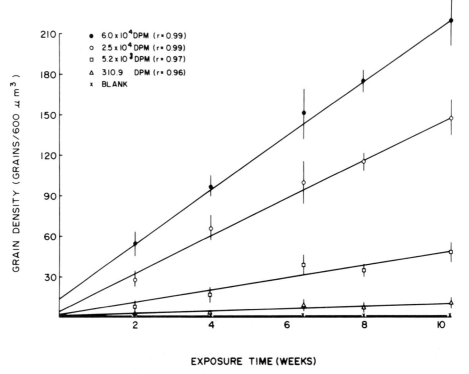

Fig. 7. Relationship between grain density and exposure time in the standardized sources of varying specific activities. DPMs refer to the concentration of radioactivity per milligram of tissue in each source. Grain density increased linearly with time and was proportional to the specific radioactivity in the standards. In autoradiographic experiments, equivalent standards can be exposed simultaneously with the tissue being studied. In all instances, grain densities should be within the range of the standards. (Reproduced from Unnerstall et al. 1981.)

(EM) autoradiography. Since most methods for labeling of receptors involve radioactive ligands, autoradiography again is the method of choice; however, there are great limits in the resolution of electron-microscopic autoradiography and one cannot localize the receptor to specific membranes by this approach (Salpeter et al. 1969). It is clear that one can use EM autoradiography to show that receptors are associated with synapses or synaptic boutons. Other approaches, possibly immunocytochemical ones (Lentz and Chester 1977; Goldsmith 1979), will be more feasible once antibodies to receptors are available. It seems that the development of electron-microscopic methods for localizing receptors with sufficient resolution should be given high priority.

4. SOME USES OF RECEPTOR LOCALIZATION STUDIES

While the uses of receptor localization studies may be obvious to some and while we have already discussed much of this, it seems worthwhile to summarize these. One might ask that since receptors can be measured biochemically, why should one do so by autoradiography. Receptor autoradiography has two great advantages: One is increased anatomical resolution; since one is looking at receptor densities at the microscopic level, such densities can be measured in small areas. Another important advantage is

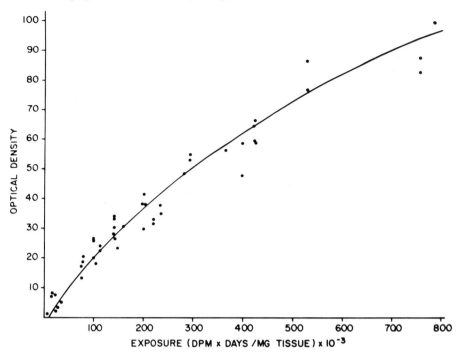

Fig. 8. Response curve (optical density as a function of exposure) of ^{3}H-Ultrofilm to varying concentrations of tritium in tissue sections exposed under conditions identical to those used for quantitative autoradiography of neurotransmitter receptors. Each point represents the mean of 6–10 densitometry readings using the Gamma Scientific DR-2H system from autoradiograms generated from tissue sections containing 10 different concentrations of radioactivity (9.45×10^{-2} to 1.22×10^6 DPM/mg tissue dry weight) exposed for 6 different lengths of time (1–6 weeks). Optical density values greater than 100 are not shown in this graph. (Reproduced from Unnerstall et al. 1982.)

sensitivity. Since the receptors are being measured in small areas and in very small pieces of tissue, one has a great sensitivity of measurement for receptors. The light-microscopic autoradiographic studies can be 4-5 orders of magnitude greater in sensitivity than biochemical assays. This great sensitivity of measurement and this great anatomic resolution have been important, for example, in experiments examining the axonal flow of receptors (Young et al. 1980).

In studies of the brain, which is a tissue of great intrinsic organization, the distribution of receptors is of interest in itself. When one produces maps of receptor distributions in the brain, it is a unique view of the structure and biochemical organization of the brain.

Probably an important use of receptor maps is that they complement other maps of the distribution of neurotransmitters or related enzymes; for example, fluorescence histochemistry has been used to produce maps of the catecholamines. Immunocytochemistry has been used to produce maps of catecholamine synthesizing enzymes. The maps of catecholamine receptors can be used in conjunction with these other histochemical maps to provide a more complete view of adrenergic neurotransmission in the brain.

The maps of receptor distribution are also useful to pharmacologists. It has always been known that centrally acting drugs have a variety of effects; for example, opiate drugs are analgesic, produce euphoria, sedation, cause respiratory depression, 'pin-

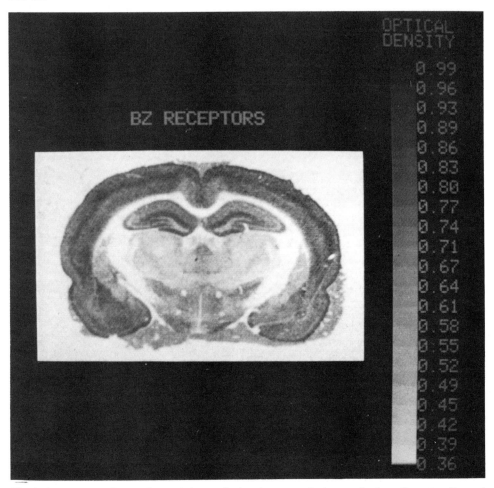

Fig. 9. A reconstructed monochromatic image displayed on an cathode ray tube from the autoradiograph shown in Figure 5. (Reproduced from Palacios et al. 1981.)

point' pupils as well as an alteration in visceral reflexes. Regional distribution and related physiologic studies have provided evidence that this diversity of drug action is due to the localization of receptors in different neuronal circuits within the brain (Atweh and Kuhar 1977a,b,c.). Thus, receptor maps provide remarkable insights to drug action, and this has been shown in many cases.

Another potential use of receptor maps is that they are a guide to regions of the brain

TABLE 3. *Limitations of in vitro labeling autoradiography*

1. Diffusion of ligand from receptor after incubation[*]
2. Lack of ultrastructural resolution
3. Morphological defects[*]
    freezing induced
    incubation and photographic development induced
4. Freezing may destroy receptors[*]
5. Low affinity sites (K_d probably greater than 10^{-8} M) not localized

[*]These do not appear to be signficant limitations, at least in our studies.

410

rich in receptors. This can be useful when one has a need to test the effects of drugs on neurons; for example, the locus ceruleus has a very high density of opiate and α_2-adrenergic receptors. Thus, it makes good sense to select these cell bodies when examining the effects of these drugs on electrical activity. This, of course, has been done (Aghajanian 1978). Receptor maps can also be useful guides to those planning behavioral studies with direct injections of drugs into brain.

5. CONCLUSION

It is possible to develop autoradiographic techniques for localizing drug and neurotransmitter receptors in brain. Since most ligands available for labeling receptors are reversible, techniques must be utilized which prevent or minimize diffusion of drug from binding site. One can label receptors by in vivo administration or by the more versatile approach of in vitro labeling. These methods for receptor mapping have many important uses such as being valuable complements to other histochemical methods and for providing another view of brain organization. They can also be used to provide valuable new hypotheses about how drugs produce various effects. The autoradiographic methods are quantitative and one can measure receptor densities in small tissue areas. The successful use of computers to quantitatively map receptor densities provides a highly rapid and reliable way to produce receptor maps. An important frontier is the development of electron-microscopic methods with enough resolution to localize receptors to distinct membranes.

6. APPENDIX

DESCRIPTION OF IN VITRO LABELING AUTORADIOGRAPHIC PROCEDURES

The method involves labeling tissue sections mounted on slides and attaching flexible, emulsion-coated coverslips to these slides for autoradiography. The overall procedure is shown schematically in Figure 3. Many useful variations are possible. The following procedure is the one used in our laboratory and contains relevant basic information.

Tissue preparation

Male, 180–225 g, Sprague-Dawley rats (Madison, WI) are often used and are sacrificed by decapitation; however, any species may be used, including human postmortem tissue. In an attempt to improve the tissue morphology, pentobarbital anesthetized rats may be perfused with 100–200 ml of low concentrations of formaldehyde (1 ml concentrated reagent per 1 of phosphate-buffered saline; Fisher, Fairlawn, NJ). The effects of fixatives are not significant if the concentration is low (Young and Kuhar 1979). However, this must be monitored carefully, and the amount of fixative used can vary depending on the ligand studied. Perfusion can even be omitted without any problems. The brains are then rapidly removed and 1–3 mm slices of appropriate regions are frozen onto microtome chucks and stored in liquid nitrogen if not used immediately.

In vitro tissue section labeling

The tissues can be cut on a Harris cryostat microtome (Harris Manufacturing Co., N. Billerica, MA) or a similar instrument, thaw-mounted onto subbed (0.5 g/100 ml gelatin and 50 mg/100 ml chromium potassium sulfate) slides and stored for 7–14 days at −20°C to permit adhesion of the tissues to the slides. In general, we use 6–14 μm thick sections.

The slides with tissue sections are brought to room temperature individually immediately before incubation. Preincubations, incubations and washes are performed in 5 and 8 slot Coplin jars containing 25 and 50 ml of solution, respectively. Tris-HCl (170 mH, pH 7.4–7.7) is often the buffer used depending on the binding optimum of the receptor under investigation. However, the choice of buffer can be quite important depending on the ligand used. Some receptors or ligands require the presence of certain ions, metabolic inhibitors or enzyme inhibitors. The concentration of the buffers represents an osmolality of 320 mOsm. Occasionally, preincubation was necessary to at least partially remove a competing endogenous ligand from the tissue (Palacios et al. 1980).

Initially, ice-water temperatures were chosen for biochemical studies to minimize any possibility of metabolism or degradation of receptor or ligand; however, if satisfactory specific to nonspecific ratios were not obtained or binding equilibrium was reached only after several hours, we then employed higher incubation temperatures (e.g. 20°C). The time of incubation selected for routine studies was the time at which equilibrium was reached. Nonspecific binding was obtained by adding 1000-fold excess (i.e. 1000 × K_d concentration) of a related compound. Of course, it is better not to use the same compound that is being studied so that isotopic dilution and displacement of nonspecific binding are not concerns.

The purpose of the washing is to reduce nonspecific binding to a greater degree than specific binding. The washing times are determined empirically and vary for each receptor. It was generally found that two short washes were better than one longer one. Occasionally, the specific binding had a short half-time of dissociation (e.g. ^{3}H-flunitrazepam), and only one short wash was used to avoid excessive loss of specific binding. All washes are carried out at ice-water temperatures to retard dissociation of specific binding. The nonspecific binding, because of its low affinity, generally dissociated quite rapidly even at this temperature.

As mentioned in the text, an important aspect of in vitro autoradiography is the ability to extensively characterize the receptor biochemically before beginning the autoradiographic study. For the biochemical studies, the tissues can be wiped off the slides with Whatman GF/B filters, placed in scintillation jars with 15 ml of 947 scintillation fluid, kept overnight at 4°C, and counted. These biochemical studies allow one to ascertain that ligand binding on the slide-mounted tissue sections has the expected properties and to identify potential binding artifacts. The kinetics of the binding is of great importance. The association and dissociation rates as well as the dissociation constant (K_d) should be determined. The number of receptors in the tissue (B_{max}) can also be determined.

Of no less importance is the chemical specificity of the binding. The receptor should show the appropriate stereospecificity, and only pharmacologically related compounds should displace the tritiated ligand (and they should show appropriate K_i's). Ion and nucleotide effects are important to check as well. Another important consideration is regional binding specificity. If the cerebellum, for example, contained few receptors in homogenate studies, it should show few in the mounted section binding also. Finally, thin-layer chromatography or other procedures can be used to assure that no degradation of the ligand is occurring.

Autoradiography

Once biochemical studies on the mounted tissue sections indicate that receptor binding is occurring under the selected conditions, one can proceed to autoradiographic studies. Instead of wiping off the sections for biochemical assay, washing and drying of the slides can be completed. The labeled sections on the slides were dipped very briefly (approximately 2 sec) into distilled H_2O

and then placed on a cold plate where cool, dry air was blown over the sections to dry them. The water dip hastens the drying procedure by removing some of the salts as well as preventing salt artifacts in the emulsion.

The apposition technique of Roth et al. (1974) was adapted for all autoradiographic studies. Acid-washed coverslips (25 × 77 mm, Corning No. 0, Corning , NY) were dipped into Kodak NTB-3 emulsion (Rochester, NY), diluted 1:1 with water, dried for 3 h and stored with dessicant in black, light-tight boxes for 24 h to 7 days. The background was higher if older coverslips were used. The use of Kodak NTB2, Ilford L4 (Ilford, England) and other nuclear emulsions is also possible.

The emulsion-coated coverslips were attached to the slides with the tissue sections in the presence of a Whatman No. 2 safelight. This was accomplished by placing a drop of glue (Super Glue No. 3, Loctite Corp., Cleveland, OH) on the end of the slide away from the tissue section. After the glue set (25 sec), squares of teflon (1/8'' thick) were put on top of the coverslips and the assemblies were held together with No. 20 binding clips. The assemblies were placed in a slide box containing dessicant and wrapped with a light opaque tape. The box itself was stored in a Tupperware bread box (Dart Industries; Orlando, FL) with more dessicant at 2–4°C for varying exposure times. As a rule of thumb, we allowed 6–8 weeks of exposure for 1500 d.p.m./mg tissue and extrapolated from that value for other cases (see Unnerstall et al. 1982). The production of spurious grains (positive chemography) should be assessed in all experiments. Negative chemography can be assessed by using emulsion-coated coverslips which have been exposed to light briefly.

After exposure, the binding clips were removed and the coverslips gently bent away from the tissue sections with a round spacer. The emulsion was developed in Dektol (Kodak; 1:1 with water) for 2 min, fixed in Kodak Liquid Hardener (1:13 with water) for 15 sec, fixed in Kodak Rapid Fix for 3 min and rinsed in distilled water for 20 min. Different development times were also examined. The tissues were then fixed in Carnoy's solution and stained with pyronin Y. The tissue sections were dried for several hours at 40°C and then the spacers were removed and the coverslips reapposed with Permount (Fisher, Fair Lawn, NJ).

When the Ilford L4 emulsion was used, a different development system was adopted. Stock D170 (25 g Na_2SO_3 and 1 g KBr/200 ml distilled water) was diluted 4:1 with water and 0.45 g of 2,4-diaminophenol dihydrochloride was added. The autoradiograms (2:1 and 1:1 coatings of emulsions) were then developed in this solution for 7 min at 18°C. This was followed by a quick water rinse, 24% sodium thiosulfate for 5 min, a second water rinse and then 2 min in water. The assemblies were processed routinely after this point.

Instead of using the emulsion-coated coverslips for apposition to produce autoradiograms, a tritium-sensitive film (^{3}H-Ultrofilm; LKB Industries) can be used. This has several advantages (Palacios et al. 1981b). When using the film, the slide-mounted tissue sections are placed in GAF cassettes in rows and are held in place with strips of 2-sided adhesive tape. Sheets of the film are placed on top of the tissue sections to produce autoradiograms. The film is developed for 5 min at 22°C in Kodak D19 developer. After an acid-water rinse, the film is fixed in Kodak Rapidfix for 5 min, washed in distilled water and dried. Standards can be used with both the coverslips and the film so that optical densities or grain densities can be converted to moles of ligand bound (Unnerstall et al. 1981, 1982).

Several different microscopes were used to evaluate the autoradiograms. We used a Zeiss Standard microscope (Carl Zeiss, FRG) with an oil immersion 40 × or 100 × objective in conjunction with a calibrated eye-piece grid for counting grains. A Leitz Ortholux microscope equipped with a Hinsch-Goldman box (Bunton Instrument Co., Inc., Rockville, MD) or an Olympus Stereoscope with a JM brightfield/darkfield illuminator (Olympus Optical Co., Ltd., New York, NY) was used to obtain lower-power darkfield micrographs.

Other papers that include important technical information are Young and Kuhar 1979a, 1981; Kuhar 1978; Palacios et al. 1980, 1981b; Unnerstall et al. 1982, and Stumpf and Roth 1966. Also, see individual papers dealing with specific ligands (Table 2).

7. REFERENCES

Aghajanian GK (1978): Tolerance of locus coeruleus neurones to morphine and suppression of withdrawal response by clonidine. *Nature, 276,* 186–188.

Arimatsu Y, Seto A, Amano T (1978): Localization of alphabungarotoxin binding sites in mouse brain by light- and electron-microscopic autoradiography. *Brain Res., 147,* 165–169.

Atweh SF, Kuhar MJ (1977a): Autoradiographic localization of opiate receptors in rat brain. I. Spinal cord and lower medulla. *Brain Res., 124,* 53–68.

Atweh SF, Kuhar MJ (1977b): Autoradiographic localization of opiate receptors in rat brain. II. The brainstem. *Brain Res., 129,* 1–12.

Atweh SF, Kuhar MJ (1977c): Autoradiographic localization of opiate receptors in rat brain. III. The telencephalon. *Brain Res., 134,* 393–405.

Barnard EA (1979): Visualization and counting of receptors at the light- and electron-microscope levels. In: O'Brien RD (Ed), *The Receptors, Vol. 1, General Principles and Procedures,* pp. 247–310. Plenum Press, New York.

Goldsmith PC, Cronin MJ, Weiner RI (1979): Dopamine receptor sites in the anterior pituitary. *J. Histochem. Cytochem., 27,* 1205–1207.

Goodman RR, Snyder SH, Kuhar MJ, Young III WS (1980): Differentiation of delta and mu opiate receptor localizations by light-microscopic autoradiography. *Proc. Nat. Acad. Sci. USA, 77,* 6239–6243.

Herkenham M, Pert DB (1980): In vitro autoradiography of opiate receptors in rat brain suggest loci of 'opiatergic' pathways. *Proc. Nat. Acad. Sci. USA, 77,* 5532–5536.

Hollt V, Schubert P (1978): Demonstration of neuroleptic sites in mouse brain by autoradiography. *Brain Res., 151,* 149–153.

Hunt SP, Schmidt J (1978): The electron-microscopic autoradiographic localization of alpha-bungarotoxin binding sites within the central nervous system of the rat. *Brain Res., 142,* 152–159.

Itoga E, Kito S, Kishida T (1981): Morphological studies on neurotransmitter receptors in brain. In: Yamamura S (Ed), *Taniguchi Symposium on Receptors,* John Wiley and Sons, Inc. In press.

Kuhar MJ (1978): Histochemical localization of neurotransmitter receptors. In: Yamamura HI, Enna SJ, Kuhar MJ (Eds), pp. 113–126. Raven Press, New York.

Kuhar MJ, Yamamura HI (1974): Light-microscopic autoradiographic localization of cholinergic muscarinic sites in rat brain. *Proc. Soc. Neurosci., 4,* 29.

Kuhar MJ, Yamamura HI (1975): Light autoradiographic localization of cholinergic muscarinic receptors in rat brain by specific binding of a potent antagonist. *Nature, 253,* 560–561.

Kuhar MJ, Yamamura HI (1976): Localization of cholinergic muscarinic receptors in rat brain by light-microscopic autoradiography. *Brain Res., 110,* 229–243.

Kuhar M, Murrin LC, Malouf AT, Klemm N (1978): Dopamine receptor binding in vivo: The feasibility of autoradiographic studies. *Life Sci., 22,* 203–210.

Laduron PM, Janssen P, Leysen JE (1978): Spiperone: A ligand of choice for neuroleptic receptors. 2. Regional distribution and in vivo displacement of neuroleptic drugs. *Biochem. Pharmacol., 27,* 317–321.

Lentz TL, Chester J (1977): Localization of acetylcholine receptors in central synapses. *J. Cell Biol., 75,* 258–267.

Miebeck RC, Maayani S, Green JP (1980): Characterization and radioautography of ^{3}H-LSD binding by rat brain slices in vitro: The effect of 5-hydroxytryptamine. *Eur. J. Pharmacol., 67,* 371–382.

Mohler H, Battersby MK, Richards JG (1980): Benzodiazepine receptor protein identified and visualized in brain tissue by a photoaffinity label. *Proc. Nat. Acad. Sci. USA, 77,* 1666–1670.

Murrin LC, Kuhar MJ (1979): Dopamine receptors in the rat frontal cortex: An autoradiographic study. *Brain Res., 177,* 279–285.

Niehoff DL, Palacios JM, Kuhar MJ (1979): In vivo receptor binding: Attempts to improve specific/nonspecific ratios. *Life Sci., 25,* 819–826.

Palacios JM, Kuhar MJ (1980): Beta-adrenergic receptor localization by light-microscopic autoradiography. *Science, 208,* 1378–1380.

Palacios JM, Young III WS, Kuhar MJ (1980): Autoradiographic localization of GABA receptors in rat cerebellum. *Proc. Nat. Acad. Sci. USA, 77,* 670–674.

Palacios JM, Niehoff DL, Kuhar MJ (1981a): ^{3}H-Spiperone binding sites in brain: Autoradiographic localization of multiple receptors. *Brain Res., 213,* 277–289.

Palacios JM, Niehoff DL, Kuhar MJ (1981b): Receptor autoradiography with tritium-sensitive film: Potential for computerized densitometry. *Neurosci. Lett., 24,* 111–116.

Palacios JM, Wamsley JK, Kuhar MJ (1981a): The distribution of histamine (H1) receptors in the rat brain: An autoradiographic study. *Neuroscience, 6,* 15–38.

Palacios JM, Wamsley JK, Kuhar MJ (1981b): High affinity GABA receptor autoradiographic localization. *Brain Res., 222,* 285–308.

Pearson J, Brandeis L, Simon E, Hiller J (1980): Radioautography of binding tritiated diprenorphine to opiate receptors in the rat. *Life Sci., 26,* 1047–1052.

Pert CB, Kuhar MJ, Snyder SH (1975): Autoradiographic localization of the opiate receptor in rat brain. *Life Sci., 16,* 1849–1854.

Rogers AW (1973): *Techniques of Autoradiography.* Elsevier Scientific Publishing Co., Amsterdam.

Roth LJ, Stumpf WE (1969): *Autoradiography of Diffusible Substances.* Academic Press, New York.

Roth LJ, Diab IM, Watanabe M, Dinerstein RJ (1974): *Mol. Pharmacol., 10,* 986–998.

Rotter A, Birdsall NJM, Burgen ASV, Field PM, Hulme EC, Raisman G (1979a): Muscarinic receptors in the central nervous system of the rat. I. Technique for autoradiographic localization of the binding of [^{3}H]- propylbenzilylcholine mustard and its distribution in the forebrain. *Brain Res.Rev., 1,* 141–166.

Rotter A, Birdsall NJM, Field PM, Raisman G (1979b): Muscarinic receptor in the CNS of the rat. II. Distribution of binding of [^{3}H]-propylbenzilylcholine mustard in the midbrain and hindbrain. *Brain Res. Rev., 1,* 167–184.

Salpeter MM, Bachman L, Salpeter EE (1969): Resolution in electron-microscope autoradiography. *J. Cell Biol., 41,* 1–12.

Segal M, Dudai Y, Amsterdam A (1978): Distribution of an alpha-bungarotoxin binding cholinergic nicotinic receptor in rat brain. *Brain Res., 148,* 105–119.

Snyder SH, Bennett Jr JP (1976): Neurotransmitter receptors in the brain: Biochemical identification. *Ann. Rev. Physiol., 38,* 153–175.

Stumpf WE, and Roth LG (1966): High resolution autoradiography with dry-mounted, freeze-dried frozen sections. Comparative study of six methods using two diffusible compounds ^{3}H-estradiol and ^{3}H-mesobilirubinogen. *J. Histochem. Cytochem., 14,* 274–287.

Unnerstall JR, Kuhar MJ, Niehoff DL, Palacios JM (1981): Benzodiazepine receptors are coupled to a sub-population of GABA receptors: Evidence from a quantitative autoradiographic study. *J. Pharmacol. Exp. Ther., 218,* 797–804.

Unnerstall JR, Niehoff DL, Kuhar MJ, Palacios JM (1982): Quantitative receptor autoradiography using ^{3}H-Ultrofilm: Application to multiple benzodiazepine receptors. *J. Neurosci. Meth., 6,* 59–73.

Wamsley JK, Lewis MS, Young III WS, Kuhar MJ (1981): Autoradiographic localization of muscarinic cholinergic receptors in rat brainstem. *J. Neurosci., 1,* 176–191.

Yamamura HI, Kuhar MJ, Snyder SH (1974): In vivo identification of muscarinic cholinergic receptor binding in rat brain. *Brain Res., 80,* 170–176.

Yamamura HI, Enna SJ, Kuhar MJ (1978): *Neurotransmitter Receptor Binding.* Raven Press, New York.

Young III WS, Kuhar MJ (1978): Opiate receptor autoradiography: In vitro labelling of tissue slices. In: Van Ree JM, Terenis L, (Eds). *Characteristics and Function of Opioids,* pp. 451–452. Elsevier/North Holland Biomedical Press.

Young III WS, Kuhar MJ (1979a): A new method for receptor autoradiography ^{3}H-opioid receptor labeling in mounted tissue sections. *Brain Res., 179,* 255–270.

Young III WS, Kuhar MJ (1980a): Noradrenergic alpha-1 and alpha-2 receptors.: Light-microscopic autoradiographic localization. *Proc. Nat. Acad. Sci. USA, 77,* 1696–1700.

Young III WS, Kuhar MJ (1980b): Radiohistochemical localization of benzodiazepine receptors in rat brain. *J. Pharmacol. Exp. Ther., 212,* 337–346.

Young III WS, Kuhar MJ (1980c): Serotonin receptor localization in rat brain by light-microscopic autoradiography. *Eur. J. Pharmacol., 62,* 237–239.

Young III WS, Kuhar MJ (1981a): The light microscopic radiohistochemistry of drug and neurotransmitter receptors using diffusible ligands. In: Johnson JE (Ed), *Current Trends in Morphological Techniques, CRC Handbook, Vol. III.,* pp. 119–136. CRC Press.

Young III WS, Kuhar MJ (1981b): Neurotensin receptor localization by light-microscopic autoradiography in rat brain. *Brain Res., 206,* 273–285.

Young III WS, Wamsley JK, Zarbin MA, Kuhar MJ (1980): Opioid receptors undergo axonal flow. *Science, 210,* 76–78.

Zarbin MA, Wamsley JK, Kuhar MJ (1981): Glycine receptor: Light-microscopic autoradiographic localization with ^{3}H-strychnine. *J. Neurosci., 1,* 532–547.

CHAPTER X

Metabolic mapping of functional activity in the central nervous system by measurement of local glucose utilization with radioactive deoxyglucose

LOUIS SOKOLOFF, CHARLES KENNEDY and CAROLYN B. SMITH

1. INTRODUCTION

The brain is a complex, heterogeneous organ composed of many anatomical and functional components with markedly different levels of functional activity that vary independently with time and function. Other tissues are generally far more homogeneous with most of their cells functioning similarly and synchronously in response to a common stimulus or regulatory influence. The central nervous system, however, consists of innumerable subunits, each integrated into its own set of functional pathways and networks and subserving only one or a few of the many activities in which the nervous system participates. Understanding how the nervous system functions requires knowledge not only of the mechanisms of excitation and inhibition but even more so of their precise localization in the nervous system and the relationships of neural subunits to specific functions.

Tissues that do physical and/or chemical work, such as heart, kidney, and skeletal muscle, exhibit a close relationship between energy metabolism and functional activity. From measurement of energy metabolism it is then possible to estimate the level of functional activity. This relationship has been utilized to develop a method that maps functional activity simultaneously in all components of the central nervous system in the normal conscious state and during physiological, pharmacological, or pathological alterations of functional activity (Sokoloff et al. 1977). The method employs radioactive deoxyglucose (DG), an analogue of glucose, to trace glucose metabolism in the brain. The procedure is so designed that the concentration of radioactivity in the tissue is more or less proportional to the rate of glucose utilization. The concentrations of radioactivity in the local cerebral tissues are measured by a quantitative autoradiographic technique. The method not only allows quantification of the actual rates of glucose utilization in the individual cerebral tissues, but the autoradiographs obtained with it provide pictorial representations of the relative rates of glucose utilization in all the cerebral structures seen in autoradiographs of 20 μm serial sections of the entire brain. It is, therefore, now possible to obtain not an anatomical map but a functional map of the entire central nervous system in normal and experimental states.

2. THEORETICAL BASIS OF RADIOACTIVE DEOXYGLUCOSE METHOD

The radioactive deoxyglucose method was developed to measure the local rates of energy metabolism simultaneously in all components of the brain in conscious laboratory animals. It was designed specifically to take advantage of the extraordinary spatial resolution made possible by quantitative autoradiography (Sokoloff et al.

Handbook of Chemical Neuroanatomy. Vol. 1: Methods in Chemical Neuroanatomy.
A. Björklund and T. Hökfelt, editors.
© Elsevier Science Publishers B.V., 1983.

1977). The dependence on autoradiography prescribed the use of radioactive substrates for energy metabolism, the labeled products of which could be assayed in the tissues by the autoradiographic technique. Although oxygen consumption is the most direct measure of energy metabolism, the volatility of oxygen and its metabolic products and the short physical half-life of its radioactive isotopes precluded measurement of oxidative metabolism by the autoradiographic technique. In most circumstances glucose is almost the sole substrate for cerebral oxidative metabolism, and its utilization is stoichiometrically related to oxygen consumption. Radioactive glucose is, however, not fully satisfactory because its labeled products are lost too rapidly from the cerebral tissues. The labeled analogue of glucose, 2-deoxy-D-[^{14}C]glucose, was, therefore, selected because its biochemical properties make it particularly appropriate to trace glucose metabolism and to measure local cerebral glucose utilization by the autoradiographic technique.

The method was derived by analysis of a model based on the biochemical properties of 2-deoxyglucose in brain (Fig. 1A) (Sokoloff et al. 1977). 2-Deoxyglucose is transported bi-directionally between blood and brain by the same carrier that transports glucose across the blood-brain barrier. In the cerebral tissues it is phosphorylated by hexokinase to 2-deoxyglucose-6-phosphate (DG-6-P). Deoxyglucose and glucose are, therefore, competitive substrates for both blood-brain transport and hexokinase-catalyzed phosphorylation. Unlike glucose-6-phosphate, however, which is metabolized further eventually to CO_2 and water, DG-6-P cannot be converted to fructose-6-phosphate, and it is also not a substrate for glucose-6-phosphate dehydrogenase. There is relatively little glucose-6-phosphatase activity in brain and even less deoxyglucose-6-phosphatase activity. Deoxyglucose-6-phosphate, once formed, remains, therefore, essentially trapped in the cerebral tissues, at least for the duration of the experimental period.

If the interval of time is kept short enough, for example, less than one hour, to allow the assumption of negligible loss of [^{14}C]DG-6-P from the tissues, then the quantity of [^{14}C]DG-6-P accumulated in any cerebral tissue at any given time following the introduction of [^{14}C]DG into the circulation is equal to the integral of the rate of [^{14}C]DG phosphorylation by hexokinase in that tissue during that interval of time. This integral is in turn related to the amount of glucose that has been phosphorylated over the same interval, depending on the time courses of the relative concentrations of [^{14}C]DG and glucose in the precursor pools and the Michaelis-Menten kinetic constants for hexokinase with respect to both [^{14}C]DG and glucose. With cerebral glucose consumption in a steady state, the amount of glucose phosphorylated during the interval of time equals the steady state flux of glucose through the hexokinase-catalyzed step times the duration of the interval, and the net rate of flux of glucose through this step equals the rate of glucose utilization.

These relationships can be rigorously combined into a model (Fig. 1A) which can be mathematically analyzed to derive an operational equation (Fig. 1B), provided that the following assumptions are made: (1) steady state for glucose (i.e. constant plasma glucose concentration and constant rate of glucose consumption) throughout the experimental period; (2) homogeneous tissue compartment within which the concentrations of [^{14}C]DG and glucose are uniform and exchange directly with the plasma; and (3) tracer concentrations of [^{14}C]DG (i.e. molecular concentrations of free [^{14}C]DG essentially equal to zero). The operational equation which defines R_i, the rate of glucose utilization per unit mass of tissue, i, in terms of measurable variables is presented in Fig. 1B.

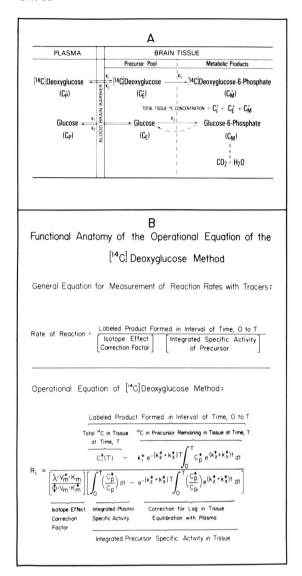

Fig. 1. Theoretical basis of radioactive DG method for measurement of local cerebral glucose utilization (Sokoloff et al. 1977). (A) Diagrammatic representation of the theoretical model. C_i^* represents the total ^{14}C concentration in a single homogeneous tissue of the brain. C_P^* and C_P represent the concentration of [^{14}C]DG and glucose in the arterial plasma, respectively; C_E^* and C_E represent their respective concentrations in the tissue pools that serve as substrates for hexokinase. C_M^* represents the concentrations of [^{14}C]DG-6-P in the tissue. The constants k_1^*, k_2^*, and k_3^* represent the rate constants for carrier-mediated transport of [^{14}C]DG from plasma to tissue, for carrier-mediated transport back from tissue to plasma, and for phosphorylation by hexokinase, respectively; the constants k_1, k_2, and k_3 are the equivalent rate constants for glucose. [^{14}C]DG and glucose share and compete for the carrier that transports both between plasma and tissue and for hexokinase which phosphorylates them to their respective hexose-6-phosphates. The dashed arrow represents the possibility of glucose-6-phosphate hydrolysis by glucose-6-phosphatase activity, if any. (B) Operational equation of the radioactive DG method and its functional anatomy. T represents the time of termination of the experimental period; λ equals the ratio of the distribution space of DG in the tissue to that of glucose; Φ equals the fraction of glucose which once phosphorylated continues down the glycolytic pathway; and K_m^* and V_m^* and K_m and V_m represent the familiar Michaelis-Menten kinetic constants of hexokinase for DG and glucose, respectively. The other symbols are the same as those defined in A.

The rate constants, k_1^*, k_2^*, and k_3^*, are determined in a separate group of animals by a non-linear, iterative process which provides the least squares best-fit of an equation which defines the time course of tissue ^{14}C concentration in terms of the time, the history of the plasma concentration, and the rate constants to the experimentally determined time courses of tissue and plasma concentrations of ^{14}C (Sokoloff et al. 1977). The λ, Φ, and the enzyme kinetic constants are grouped together to constitute a single, lumped constant (see equation). It can be shown mathematically that this lumped constant is equal to the asymptotic value of the product of the ratio of the cerebral extraction ratios of [^{14}C]DG and glucose and the ratio of the arterial blood to plasma specific activities when the arterial plasma [^{14}C]DG concentration is maintained constant. The lumped constant is also determined in a separate group of animals from arterial and cerebral venous blood samples drawn during a programmed intravenous infusion which produces and maintains a constant arterial plasma [^{14}C]DG concentration (Sokoloff et al. 1977).

Despite its complex appearance, the operational equation is really nothing more than a general statement of the standard relationship by which rates of enzyme-catalyzed reactions are determined from measurements made with radioactive tracers (Fig. 1B). The numerator of the equation represents the amount of radioactive product formed in a given interval of time; it is equal to C_i^* the combined concentrations of [^{14}C]DG and [^{14}C]DG-6-P in the tissue at time, T, measured by the quantitative autoradiographic technique, less a term that represents the free unmetabolized [^{14}C]DG still remaining in the tissue. The denominator represents the integrated specific activity of the precursor pool times a factor, the lumped constant, which is equivalent to a correction factor for an isotope effect. The term with the exponential factor in the denominator takes into account the lag in the equilibration of the tissue precursor pool with the plasma.

3. PROCEDURE

The operational equation dictates the variables to be measured to determine the local rates of cerebral glucose utilization. The specific procedure employed is designed to evaluate these variables and to minimize potential errors that might occur in the actual application of the method. If the rate constants, k_1^*, k_2^*, and k_3^*, are precisely known, then the equation is generally applicable with any mode of administration of [^{14}C]DG and for a wide range of time intervals. At the present time the rate constants have been fully determined only in the conscious rat (Sokoloff et al. 1977) (Table 1). Partial determination of the rate constants indicates that they are similar in the monkey (Kennedy et al., 1978). These rate constants can be expected to vary with the condition of the animal, however, and for most accurate results should be re-determined for each condition studied. The structure of the operational equation suggests a more practical alternative. All the terms in the equation that contain the rate constants approach zero with increasing time if the [^{14}C]DG is so administered that the plasma [^{14}C]DG concentration also approaches zero. From the values of the rate constants determined in normal animals and the usual time course of the clearance of [^{14}C]DG from the arterial plasma following a single intravenous pulse at zero time, it has been determined that an interval of 30-45 min after a pulse is adequate for these terms to become sufficiently small so that considerable latitude in inaccuracies of the rate constants is permissible without appreciable error in the estimates of local glucose consumption (Sokoloff et al. 1977). An additional advantage derived from the use of a single pulse of [^{14}C]DG followed by a relatively long interval before killing the animal for measurement of local

TABLE 1. Values of rate constants in the normal conscious albino rat

Structure	Rate constants (min^{-1})			Distribution volume (ml/g) $k_1^*/(k_2^*+k_3^*)$	Half-life of precursor pool (min) $Log_e2/(k_2^*+k_3^*)$
	k_1^*	k_2^*	k_3^*		
Gray matter					
Visual cortex	0.189 ± 0.048	0.279 ± 0.176	0.063 ± 0.040	0.553	2.03
Auditory cortex	0.226 ± 0.068	0.241 ± 0.198	0.067 ± 0.057	0.734	2.25
Parietal cortex	0.194 ± 0.051	0.257 ± 0.175	0.062 ± 0.045	0.608	2.17
Sensory-motor cortex	0.193 ± 0.037	0.208 ± 0.112	0.049 ± 0.035	0.751	2.70
Thalamus	0.188 ± 0.045	0.218 ± 0.144	0.053 ± 0.043	0.694	2.56
Medial geniculate body	0.219 ± 0.055	0.259 ± 0.164	0.055 ± 0.040	0.697	2.21
Lateral geniculate body	0.172 ± 0.038	0.220 ± 0.134	0.055 ± 0.040	0.625	2.52
Hypothalamus	0.158 ± 0.032	0.226 ± 0.119	0.043 ± 0.032	0.587	2.58
Hippocampus	0.169 ± 0.043	0.260 ± 0.166	0.056 ± 0.040	0.535	2.19
Amygdala	0.149 ± 0.028	0.235 ± 0.109	0.032 ± 0.026	0.558	2.60
Caudate-putamen	0.176 ± 0.041	0.200 ± 0.140	0.061 ± 0.050	0.674	2.66
Superior colliculus	0.198 ± 0.054	0.240 ± 0.166	0.046 ± 0.042	0.692	2.42
Pontine gray matter	0.170 ± 0.040	0.246 ± 0.142	0.037 ± 0.033	0.601	2.45
Cerebellar cortex	0.225 ± 0.066	0.392 ± 0.229	0.059 ± 0.031	0.499	1.54
Cerebellar nucleus	0.207 ± 0.042	0.194 ± 0.111	0.038 ± 0.035	0.892	2.99
Mean ± SEM	0.189 ± 0.012	0.245 ± 0.040	0.052 ± 0.010	0.647 ± 0.073	2.39 ± 0.40
White matter					
Corpus callosum	0.085 ± 0.015	0.135 ± 0.075	0.019 ± 0.033	0.552	4.50
Genu of corpus callosum	0.076 ± 0.013	0.131 ± 0.075	0.019 ± 0.034	0.507	4.62
Internal capsule	0.077 ± 0.015	0.134 ± 0.085	0.023 ± 0.039	0.490	4.41
Mean ± SEM	0.079 ± 0.008	0.133 ± 0.046	0.020 ± 0.020	0.516 ± 0.171	4.51 ± 0.90

From Sokoloff et al. 1977.

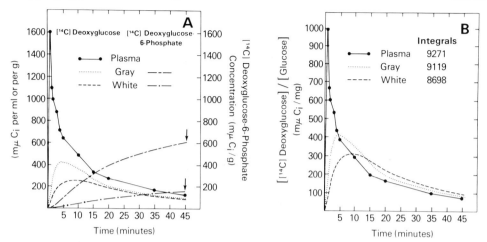

Fig. 2. Graphical representation of the significant variables in the operational equation (Fig. 1B) used to calculate local cerebral glucose utilization. (A). Time courses of [^{14}C]DG concentrations in arterial plasma and in average gray and white matter and [^{14}C]DG-6-P concentrations in average gray and white matter following an intravenous pulse of 50 μCi of [^{14}C]DG. The plasma curve is derived from measurements of plasma [^{14}C]DG concentration. The tissue concentrations were calculated from the plasma curve and the mean values of k_1^*, k_2^*, and k_3^* for gray and white matter in Table 1 according to the second term in the numerator of the operational equation. The [^{14}C]DG-6-P concentration in the tissues was calculated from the integral of the free DG concentration in the tissue and k_3^*; the autoradiographic technique measures the total ^{14}C content at the time of killing, ($C_i^*(T)$), the first term in the numerator of the operational equation. Note that at the time of killing the total ^{14}C content represents mainly [^{14}C]DG-6-P concentration, especially in gray matter. (B). Time courses of ratios of [^{14}C]DG to glucose concentrations (i.e. specific activities) in plasma and average gray and white matter. The curve for plasma was determined by division of the plasma curve in (A) by the plasma glucose concentrations. The curves for the tissues were calculated by the function in brackets in the denominator of the operational equation. The integrals in (B) are the integrals of the specific activities with respect to time and represent the areas under the curves. The integrals under the tissue curves are equivalent to all of the denominator of the operational equation, except for the lumped constant. Note that by the time of killing, the integrals of the tissue curves approach equality with each other and with that of the plasma curve.

tissue ^{14}C concentration is that by then most of the free [^{14}C]DG in the tissues has been either converted to [^{14}C]DG-6-P or transported back to the plasma (Fig. 2); the optical densities in the autoradiographs then represent mainly the concentrations of [^{14}C]DG-6-P and, therefore, reflect directly the relative rates of glucose utilization in the various cerebral tissues.

The following steps are taken in the course of each individual experiment: (1) preparation of the animal; (2) administration of [^{14}C]DG and timed sampling of arterial blood; (3) analysis of arterial plasma for [^{14}C]DG and glucose concentrations; (4) processing of brain tissue; (5) preparation of autoradiographs; (6) densitometric analysis of autoradiographs; (7) calculation of rate of glucose utilization.

3.1. PREPARATION OF ANIMALS

Catheters are inserted into any conveniently located artery and vein. In most of the studies done to date femoral or iliac vessels have been chosen, but tail and axillary sites have also been used. A general anesthesia is employed, fluothane being preferred because of the relatively short recovery period. The catheters must have the usual characteristics for them to remain patent for repeated blood sampling. Those made of polyethylene, in the size designated as PE-50 by the supplier, Clay Adams, are entirely satisfactory, except in animals weighing less than 100 g, which require the use of size PE-10. The catheters, bubble-free, plugged at one end, and filled with dilute herapin solution (100 U/ml) before their insertion, will remain patent for many hours. To minimize the need for extensive flushing of dead space during the sampling period it is desirable that the arterial catheter be as short as possible; 15 cm is suitable for the rat. During recovery from anesthesia the animal is placed in a suitable restraining device. In the case of rats, a loosely fitting, bivalved, plaster cast around the lower trunk is applied with the hind legs taped to a lead brick. For cats, a zippered jacket is satisfactory; for monkeys, a restraining chair. When the experimental condition requires a freely moving animal, a blood sampling system can be devised with a little ingenuity, at least in the case of the rat. Our finding showing no significant difference in values for local cerebral glucose utilization between freely movings rats and rats restrained as described above, however, has deterred our regular use of the more complex preparation. If attention is paid to keeping the concentration of fluothane to a minimum, and the time for the surgical procedure to 15-20 min, recovery is prompt, and the experiment can be initiated within 2-3 h. Immediately before starting the experiment it is useful to measure hematocrit, arterial pH and blood gases, and mean arterial blood pressure to establish the presence of a normal physiologic state.

3.2. ADMINISTRATION OF [¹⁴C]DEOXYGLUCOSE AND THE SAMPLING OF ARTERIAL BLOOD

To ensure that tracer conditions are maintained, the dose of [¹⁴C]DG should be such that the animal receives no more than 2.5 μmoles of DG/kg of body weight. If the specific activity is relatively high (50-60 mCi/mmole) 100-125 μCi/kg can be given. This amount of radioactivity is sufficient to attain a desirable optical density of the autoradiographs in a reasonable period of time, namely 4-6 days of exposure. Economic factors may demand the use of a lower dose, in which case, of course, the exposure must be longer. When smaller doses are employed, it is necessary to ensure that the plastic standards used in making the autoradiographs are sufficiently low in their radioactivity so that their calibrated values cover the range of the concentration of ¹⁴C in the brain sections. If the [¹⁴C]DG is supplied in an ethanol solution, it must be evaporated to dryness and the DG then redissolved in physiological saline. A suitable concentration for its intravenous infusion is 100 μCi/ml. The experimental period is initiated by the infusion of [¹⁴C]DG through the venous catheter as a pulse or as a rapid infusion over a period not exceeding 30 sec. With zero time marking the start of the infusion, sampling is begun from the arterial catheter to monitor the entire time course of the [¹⁴C]DG concentration in the plasma. A suitable sampling schedule is as follows: 15″, 30″, 45″, 1′, 2′, 3′, 5′, 7.5′, 10′, 15′, 25′, 35′ and 45′. Care must be taken to clear the dead space of the catheter prior to each sample. The timed blood samples, 100-200 μl in volume, are collected in herapin-treated, 250 μl plastic tubes. They are immediately centrifuged in a small, high-speed centrifuge such as the Beckman Microfuge, and then are kept on ice until pipetted for the analyses. The use of heparinized tubes may be unnecessary if the animal is heparinized just prior to the experiment. Unless attention is paid to limiting the amount of blood removed in the course of sampling and clearing the dead space, hemorrhagic shock can readily be induced in small animals. Most rats weighing 300-400 g will tolerate the removal of 2 ml over the 45-min experimental period without there being a significant fall in blood pressure. Blood drawn for the purpose of clearing the dead space (3 times the volume of the catheter) may, of course, be returned to the animal. Because of the occasional rat which fails to tolerate even small blood losses, it is necessary to monitor mean arterial blood pressure at intervals during the sampling period. A fall below 90 mm Hg is reason enough to eliminate the animal from an experimental series.

Immediately after the last sample has been taken, the animal is killed. This may be by decapitation in the case of small animals, or alternatively, by an intravenous infusion of thiopental, followed immediately by a saturated solution of KCl to stop the heart.

3.3. ANALYSIS OF ARTERIAL PLASMA FOR [^{14}C]DEOXYGLUCOSE AND GLUCOSE CONCENTRATIONS

The concentration of DG in each plasma sample is measured by means of counting its ^{14}C content. 20 μl of plasma are pipetted into 1 ml of water contained in a counting vial. 10 ml of a suitable phosphor solution are added (e.g. Aquasol, New England Nuclear, Boston, MA). With the aid of internal or external standardization the d.p.m. are determined and the concentration then expressed in μCi/ml. The plasma glucose concentration is most conveniently assayed in a glucose analyzer, such as that made by Beckman Instrument Co. (Fullerton, CA). This is quick and requires only 10 μl of plasma per determination. Also suitable for this purpose is the coupled, glucose-dependent, hexokinase-glucose-6-phosphate dehydrogenase-catalyzed reduction of NADP$^+$which is available in kit form from Calbiochem (La Jolla, CA). Should it be necessary to conserve blood, it is not necessary to measure the glucose concentration in every sample. Analyses in four samples, spaced over the total experimental period, are sufficient to establish the existence of the required steady state for glucose.

3.4. PROCESSING OF BRAIN TISSUE

Some investigators have chosen to perfuse the brain with a fixative immediately after the animal is killed. This serves to improve the quality of histologic sections, which is often desirable to establish the anatomic identity of regions of interest in the autoradiographs. Perfusion fixation is also thought by some to reduce artifacts in the sectioning of the frozen brains, especially those of large animals. For this purpose a 3.5% solution of formaldehyde made in a 0.05 M phosphate buffer adjusted to a pH of 7.4 may be employed. The animal is heparinized immediately before killing. With a cannula placed in the left ventricle and the reservoir of the perfusate 50 cm above the heart level, the perfusion is carried out for 10 min. The brain is then removed and frozen as described below. In order to determine whether this procedure alters the distribution of ^{14}C in the brain, we removed small sections from one hemisphere of a monkey which had undergone the DG procedure just before carrying out the formaldehyde perfusion. The nonperfused and perfused tissues were frozen and mounted side by side when the block was sectioned. In Figure 3 is the autoradiograph prepared from the prefrontal region of this animal. On the left side (nonperfused) the definition of the fine cortical markings, indicative of normal functional columns perpendicular to the surface, is much clearer than it is on the perfused side. Also the optical density is slightly lower on the perfused side. Calculation of the concentration average of ^{14}C in the two sides indicates that the perfusion process washed out 15% of the label.

Until a perfusion procedure which is shown to prevent loss or movement of the label is devised, we recommend that it be omitted and that the brain be frozen immediately after removal. This is done by immersion in isopentane or Freon XII, chilled to $-45°$C

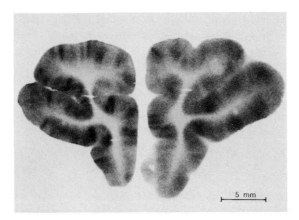

Fig. 3. Autoradiograph of a coronal section of prefrontal cortex of monkey brain following administration of [¹⁴C]DG. The section on the left is from tissue removed and frozen as described in the text immediately after killing. The section on the right was removed and frozen after the brain had been perfused with a formaldehyde fixative solution. Note the poorer resolution of cortical marking on the perfused side. A measurement of average ¹⁴C content on the two sides indicates that the perfusion resulted in a 15% loss of label.

with liquid nitrogen. Many prefer the isopentane because the brain sinks and becomes completely covered. Brain in Freon XII floats and thus tends to freeze unevenly. This results in artifacts from the protrusion of expanding tissue at an unfrozen site on the surface. With constant agitation of the brain in the Freon this, however, can be avoided. There is a tendency for large brains to become grossly distorted in the immersion process. If the brain is placed in a plastic ladle, previously coated with a film of mineral oil, a uniform external configuration of the tissue can be maintained.

After freezing, small brains are mounted on microtome tissue holders with an embedding matrix supplied by Lipshaw Mfg. Co. Brains of larger animals must be cut into two or three smaller blocks in order to accommodate them in the microtome. Cutting the frozen brain into blocks is best done with a small bandsaw, the blade of which is precooled immediately before the cut is made. It is crucial to maintain the brain below −30°C at all times during handling to prevent movement of the label by diffusion. Storage for any prolonged period prior to sectioning should be in a freezer maintained at −70°C. Sectioning of the brain is carried out in a refrigerated microtome at a thickness of 20 μm and at a temperature cycle which does not go above −22°C. Even at this temperature there is some movement of the label in a matter of hours, dictating the need to complete the cutting of one block (or entire small brain as the case may be) at one sitting. Instruments which have proved satisfactory for sectioning are the 'Cryocut' made by the American Optical Co. (Buffalo, NY) and the more refined and elaborate instrument made by the Bright Manufacturing Co. (Huntingdon, England). Errors due to inconsistent thickness of sections and a number of artifacts can be introduced at this stage unless attention is paid to a number of operational details of the microtome such as secure mounting, knife sharpness, anti-roll plate adjustment, and the use of smooth, regularly timed strokes of the knife. The 20 μm sections are picked from the knife surface on glass coverslips to which they adhere by thawing. They are immediately transferred to a hot plate maintained at 60°C on which the momentarily thawed section becomes dry within 5-8 sec. If slides, rather than coverslips are used for this purpose, drying is prolonged and diffusion of isotope occurs, resulting in a reduction in resolution of small structures. The coverslips are then placed on an adhesive-coated paper board, cut to fit in a $10'' \times 12''$ X-ray cassette with a center gap left for a strip holding 6-10 previously calibrated [14C]methylmethacrylate standards. The backing of the standard strip must be carefully made to equal the combined thickness of paperboard and coverslip in order to assure that when the cassette, incorporating a photographic film, is closed there will be uniform contact of all surfaces containing radioactivity with the emulsion.

An alternate system of sectioning brain is that which employs an LKB 2250 PMV cryomicrotome (Stockholm, Sweden), which has a number of advantages, especially in processing brains of large animals. Because of its capability of cutting bone the need for removal of the brain from the calvarium is eliminated. The entire head is sectioned and thus the brain's normal relationship to other tissues is preserved. This is of particular value in studies involving the entire visual pathway as it includes the retina and optic nerves. It has the additional advantage of eliminating various cutting artifacts, in particular those resulting from wrinkling or fragmentation. Sections are remarkably uniform in thickness. Other artifacts, however, may be introduced, the most troublesome of which is that caused by slight shrinkage of the tissue on drying which results in fine lines giving the appearance of parched mud. In one laboratory, in which this system has been extensively employed, there was considerable loss of resolution of fine detail of autoradiographs. The reason for this is uncertain, but it is possible that it results from transient warming of the brain at the time the head is mounted in the embedding medium. Further experience with the system will determine whether or not this serious drawback can be overcome.

3.5. PREPARATION OF AUTORADIOGRAPHS

A number of different photographic films are suitable for contact autoradiography with 14C. The single-coated blue sensitive X-ray film made by Eastman Kodak and designated SB-5 is generally satisfactory when developed acccording to the manufacturer's instructions. If the dose and specific activity of [14C]DG are employed as suggested above, satisfactory images having an optical density range between 0.1 and 1.0 are generated in 4-6 days. Films with finer grain, but requiring a longer period of exposure, are Eastman Kodak's MR-1 and Plus-X.

Quantitative autoradiography requires the simultaneous exposure of standards with brain sections on each film (Fig. 4). [14C]Methylmethacrylate standards are available commercially from Amersham Corporation (Arlington Heights, IL). It is important to note that their 14C content, which may be expressed in μCi/g of plastic material by the manufacturer, is not that which is to be used in the calculations. Each standard must be assigned a value which is equivalent to the 14C concentration in brain, a 20 μm thick, dried section of which will produce the same optical density as the plastic when they are exposed together on the same film. While the supplier may provide the brain-equivalent values for a set of standards which have been calibrated in another laboratory, it may be desirable to establish the values independently. This would be essential, of course, if an investigator chose to cut sections at a thickness other than 20 μm, which at present is that most widely used. If so, then the standards would have to be calibrated for their equivalence to brain sections of the selected thickness. For the calibration procedure any 14C-containing substance may be employed which at equilibrium becomes uniformly distributed in brain after its intravenous administration. For this purpose we have used both [14C]antipyrine and [14C]methylglucose. Either substance given to a normal rat equilibrates adequately in the tissues in approx-

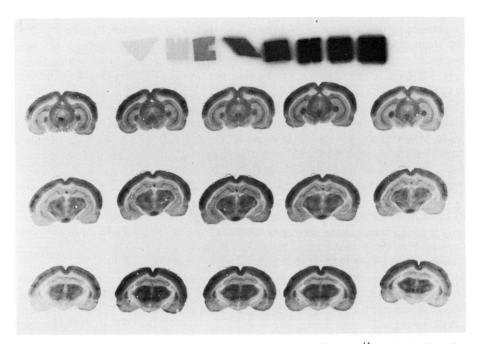

Fig. 4. Autoradiographs of sections of conscious rat brain and calibrated [14C]methylmethacrylate standards used to quantify 14C-concentration in tissues. It is difficult to avoid slight variation in section thickness which is evident in a corresponding slight variation in optical density. Where this is present measurements of optical density must be made in several sections for any given structure.

imately 1 h. Eight to ten rats are each given graded doses of 14C covering a wide range. At the end of the equilibration period each animal is killed, the brain is removed, and the forebrain divided in half. One hemisphere is immediately weighed, then homogenized in a 1:30 dilution of Triton X-100 and made up to a specified volume. The suspension of brain tissue is then assayed for its 14C concentration in a liquid scintillation counter. With a correction for the dilution, the 14C concentration expressed in μCi/unit weight is obtained. The other hemisphere is frozen, sectioned at 20 μm and prepared for autoradiography as described above. The brain sections and standards are then exposed on film in the same cassette. After development of the film, densitometric measurements are made on standards and brain sections (see below). From a plot of the 14C concentration of brains, which had been independently assayed, and their optical densities, a calibration curve can be constructed. This permits assigning a brain-equivalent concentration of 14C to each plastic standard by virtue of its optical density. It is essential, of course, that the graded doses of 14C given to the rats result in a range of optical densities of the brain images which bracket those of the standards. The calibrated values obtained by this procedure are considered valid not just for rat brain but for any species on the assumption of there being no difference in the self-absorption characteristics of dried brain tissue from species to species.

3.6. DENSITOMETRIC ANALYSIS OF AUTORADIOGRAPHS

The autoradiographs provide a pictorial representation of the relative rates of glucose utilization in various structures of the brain, the darker the region the higher the rate of glucose utilization. Most of the major subdivisions in gray matter are clearly delineated because of their differences in optical density from that of an adjacent anatomic area (Fig. 5). Verification of the anatomic identity of a region can be made by staining and histologic study of the section from which the autoradiograph is made. With attention paid to details cited above, the technique can clearly delineate such relatively small structures of the rat brain as the suprachiasmatic nucleus, which measures about 300 μm in coronal section (Fig. 5A). In the normal rat, Layer IV of the cortex, which measures 100-200 μm thick, is also clearly seen as a dark linear band. In

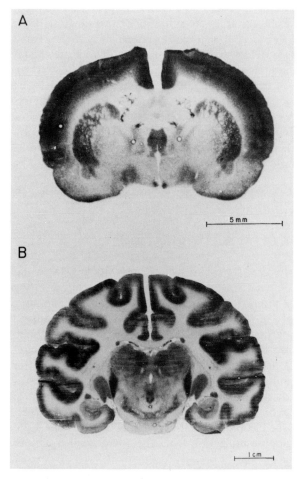

Fig. 5. Autoradiographs of coronal sections of conscious rat (A) and monkey (B) brain made with [^{14}C]DG prepared as described in the text. The pattern produced by differences in optical density permits recognition of most of the component structures. The two small dark spots in the center at the base of the brain in A correspond to the suprachiasmatic nuclei. Layers in the cerebral cortex of the rat can also be distinguished as well as radial markings perpendicular to the cortical surface. In both autoradiographs the right side of the brain is on the right side. Note the right-left symmetry in optical density in all structures except for certain cortical regions in the monkey (B). The monkey from which this brain section was made was engaged in a repetitive task involving the left arm and hand throughout the experiment. This accounts for the increase in markings and locally higher optical density in some cortical regions on the right compared to the homologous cortex on the left.

an analysis of the limit of resolution of autoradiographs when the brain is processed as described, we have shown that at a junction of brain tissue containing [¹⁴C]DG with tissue which is tracer-free the half-distance of the optical density from the junction is less than 50 μm (Goochee et al. 1980). If quantitative resolution is defined as the distance which must separate two sources of equal strength such that the grain density between them falls to half that seen over each source, then the resolution for quantification is no better than 200 μm although structures of smaller dimensions can be visually distinguished.

The determination of the rate of glucose utilization for any given region of the autoradiograph requires an estimate of the concentration of the ¹⁴C concentration in that region. This is done by a measurement of its optical density. Transmission densitometers of the type widely used in photography are suitable for this purpose if the aperture is 0.2—0.5 mm in diameter. For satisfactory readings to be made in very small structures a microdensitometer which provides apertures 100 μm or smaller may be required. One such instrument is that made by Gamma Scientific Corp. (San Diego, CA). Even more useful for the evaluation of very small regions is a system of computerized image analysis described briefly below. Whatever system is employed for densitometry, it is necessary to make optical density readings for a given structure in several sections. The mean value obtained serves both to reduce errors due to variations in section thickness and to give a value which is reasonably representative of the structure in its three dimensions. For larger structures, 12 or more optical density readings should be made. The concentration of ¹⁴C in the structure is determined from the plot of optical density versus the concentration of ¹⁴C of the standards. Each film, of course, has its own standard curve.

3.7. CALCULATION OF RATE OF GLUCOSE UTILIZATION

The operational equation is given in Figure 1B. The measured variables are (1) the entire history of the arterial plasma [¹⁴C]DG concentration, C_P^*, from zero time to the time of killing, T; (2) the steady state arterial plasma glucose level, C_P, over the same interval; and (3) the concentration of ¹⁴C in the tissue, $C_i^*(T)$, which was determined densitometrically from the autoradiographs. The rate constants, k_1^*, k_2^*, and k_3^*, and the lumped constant are not measured in each experiment; the values for these constants are those which have already been determined in our laboratory for the rat (Table 1). Similarly the lumped constant that is used is that determined for a variety of species (Table 2). A full discussion of these constants and their possible variation in special situations is given in the section on theoretical and practical considerations (Section 4). A programmable calculator, such as the Hewlett-Packard Model 9830 or 9845, is employed to calculate values for glucose utilization from the operational equation.

3.8. NORMAL RATES OF LOCAL CEREBRAL GLUCOSE UTILIZATION IN CONSCIOUS ANIMALS

The rates of local cerebral glucose utilization have been measured in the normal conscious and anesthetized albino rat (Sokoloff et al. 1977) and in the conscious Rhesus monkey (Kennedy et al. 1978). The rates in the conscious rat vary widely throughout the brain with the values in white matter distributed in a narrow low range and the values in gray structures broadly distributed around an average about 3 times greater than that of white matter (Table 3). The highest values are in structures of the auditory

TABLE 2. *Values of the lumped constant in the albino rat, Rhesus monkey, cat and dog*

Animal	No. of animals	Mean ± SD	SEM
Albino rat:			
Conscious	15	0.464 ± 0.099[*]	± 0.026
Anesthetized	9	0.512 ± 0.118[*]	± 0.039
Conscious (5% CO_2)	2	0.463 ± 0.122[*]	± 0.086
Combined	26	0.481 ± 0.119	± 0.023
Rhesus monkey:			
Conscious	7	0.344 ± 0.095	± 0.036
Cat:			
Anesthetized	6	0.411 ± 0.013	± 0.005
Dog (Beagle puppy):			
Conscious	7	0.558 ± 0.082	± 0.031

[*] No statistically significant difference between normal conscious and anesthetized rats ($0.3 < P < 0.4$) and conscious rats breathing 5% CO_2 ($P > 0.9$).

Note: The values were obtained as follows: rat (Sokoloff et al. 1977); monkey (Kennedy et al. 1978); cat (M. Miyaoka, J. Magnes, C. Kennedy, M. Shinohara, and L. Sokoloff, unpublished data); dog (Duffy et al. 1979)

TABLE 3. *Representative values for local cerebral glucose utilization in the normal conscious albino rat and monkey (μmoles/100 g/min)*

Structure	Albino rat[*] (10)	Monkey** (7)
Gray matter		
Visual cortex	107 ± 6	59 ± 2
Auditory cortex	162 ± 5	79 ± 4
Parietal cortex	112 ± 5	47 ± 4
Sensory-motor cortex	120 ± 5	44 ± 3
Thalamus: lateral nucleus	116 ± 5	54 ± 2
Thalamus: ventral nucleus	109 ± 5	43 ± 2
Medial geniculate body	131 ± 5	65 ± 3
Lateral geniculate body	96 ± 5	39 ± 1
Hypothalamus	54 ± 2	25 ± 1
Mamillary body	121 ± 5	57 ± 3
Hippocampus	79 ± 3	39 ± 2
Amygdala	52 ± 2	25 ± 2
Caudate-putamen	110 ± 4	52 ± 3
Nucleus accumbens	82 ± 3	36 ± 2
Globus-pallidus	58 ± 2	26 ± 2
Substantia nigra	58 ± 3	29 ± 2
Vestibular nucleus	128 ± 5	66 ± 3
Cochlear nucleus	113 ± 7	51 ± 3
Superior olivary nucleus	133 ± 7	63 ± 4
Inferior colliculus	197 ± 10	103 ± 6
Superior colliculus	95 ± 5	55 ± 4
Pontine gray matter	62 ± 3	28 ± 1
Cerebellar cortex	57 ± 2	31 ± 2
Cerebellar nuclei	100 ± 4	45 ± 2
White matter		
Corpus callosum	40 ± 2	11 ± 1
Internal capsule	33 ± 2	13 ± 1
Cerebellar white matter	37 ± 2	12 ± 1

Note: The values are the means ± standard errors from measurements made in the number of animals indicated in parentheses.

[*] From Sokoloff et al. 1977; **From Kennedy et al. 1978.

system with the inferior colliculus clearly the most metabolically active structure in the brain (Table 3). The value for any selected structure is virtually identical to that of the homologous region on the opposite side. The failure to find this symmetry in values in normal conscious animals strongly points to the presence of disease or defective development such as may be found in the relay nuclei of the auditory pathway in rats with unilateral otitis media, a common disorder in many rat colonies.

The rates of local cerebral glucose utilization in the conscious monkey exhibit similar heterogeneity to those found in the rat, but they are generally one-third to one-half the values in corresponding structures (Table 3). The differences in rates in the rat and monkey brain are consistent with the different cellular packing densities in the brains of these two species.

4. THEORETICAL AND PRACTICAL CONSIDERATIONS

The design of the deoxyglucose method was based on an operational equation, derived by the mathematical analysis of a model of the biochemical behavior of [^{14}C]DG and glucose in brain (Fig. 1). Although the model and its mathematical analysis were as rigorous and comprehensive as reasonably possible, it must be recognized that models almost always represent idealized situations and cannot possibly take into account every single known, let alone unknown, property of a complex biological system. There remained, therefore, the possibility that continued experience with the [^{14}C]DG method might uncover weakness, limitations, or flaws serious enough to limit its usefulness or even to invalidate it. Several years have how passed since its introduction, and numerous applications of it have been made. The results of this experience generally establish the validity and worth of the method. There still remain, however, some potential problems in specialized situations, and several theoretical and practical issues need further clarification.

The main potential sources of error are the rate constants and the lumped constant. The problem with them is that they are not determined in the same animals and at the same time when local cerebral glucose utilization is being measured. The are measured in separate groups of comparable animals and then used subsequently in other animals in which glucose utilization is being measured. The part played by these constants in the method is defined by their role in the operational equation of the method (Fig. 1B).

4.1. RATE CONSTANTS

The rate constants, k_1^*, k_2^*, and k_3^*, have thus far been fully determined for various cerebral tissues only in the normal conscious albino rat (Sokoloff et al. 1977) (Table 1). Partial determination of the rate constants in the normal conscious Rhesus monkey indicates that they are quite similar to those in the rat. All the rat constants vary from tissue to tissue, but the variation among gray structures and among white structures is considerably less than the differences between the two types of tissues (Table 1). The rate constants, k_2^* and k_3^*, appear in the equation only as their sum, and $(k_2^* + k_3^*)$ is equal to the rate constant for the turnover of the free [^{14}C]DG pool in the tissue. The half-life of the free [^{14}C]DG pool can then be calculated by dividing $(k_2^* + k_3^*)$ into the natural logarithm of 2 and has been found to average 2.4 min in gray matter and 4.5 min in white matter in the normal conscious rat (Table 1).

The rate constants vary not only from structure to structure but can be expected to vary with the condition. For example, k_1^* and k_2^* are influenced by both blood flow and transport of [^{14}C]DG across the blood-brain barrier, and because of the competition for the transport carrier, the glucose concentrations in the plasma and tissue affect the transport of [^{14}C]DG and, therefore, also k_1^* and k_2^*. The constant, k_3^*, is related to phosphorylation of [^{14}C]DG and will certainly change when glucose utilization is altered. To minimize potential errors due to inaccuracies in the values of the rate constants used, it was decided to sacrifice time resolution for accuracy. If the [^{14}C]DG is given as an intravenous pulse and sufficient time is allowed for the plasma to be cleared of the tracer, then the influence of the rate constants, and the functions that they represent, on the final result diminishes with increasing time until ultimately it becomes zero. This relationship is implicit in the structure of the operational equation (Fig. 1B); as C_P^* approaches zero, then the terms containing the rate constants also approach zero with increasing time. The significance of this relationship is graphically illustrated in Figure 6. From typical arterial plasma [^{14}C]DG and glucose concentration curves obtained in a normal conscious rat, the portion of the denominator of the operational

INFLUENCE OF RATE CONSTANTS ON INTEGRATED POOL SPECIFIC ACTIVITY

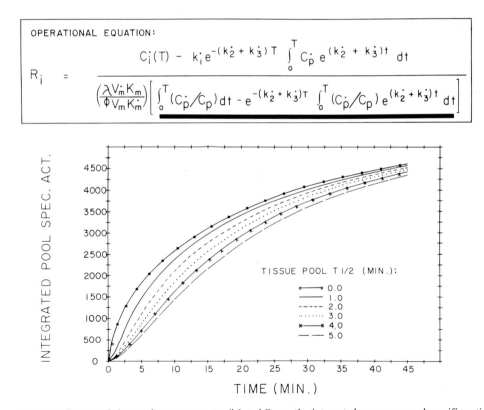

Fig. 6. Influence of time and rate constants, $(k_2^* + k_3^*)$, on the integrated precursor pool specific activity following a pulse of [^{14}C]DG at 0 time. The portion of the equation that is underlined corresponds to the integrated pool specific activity; it was computed as a function of time with different values of $(k_2^* + k_3^*)$, as indicated by their equivalent half-lives, calculated according to T 1/2 = $0.693/(k_2^* + k_3^*)$. (See text.)

equation underlined by the heavy bar was computed with a wide range of values for $(k_2^* + k_3^*)$ as a function of time. The values for $(k_2^* + k_3^*)$ are presented as their equivalent half-lives calculated as described above. The values of $(k_2^* + k_3^*)$ vary from infinite (i.e. T $1/2 = 0$ min) to 0.14/min (i.e. T $1/2 = 5$ min) and more than cover the range of values to be expected under physiological conditions. The portion of the equation underlined and computed represents the integral of the precursor pool specific activity in the tissue. The curves represent the time course of this function, one each for every value of $(k_2^* + k_3^*)$ examined. It can be seen that these curves are widely different at early times but converge with increasing time until at 45 min the differences over the entire range of $(k_2^* + k_3^*)$ equal only a small fraction of the value of the integral. These curves demonstrate that at short times enormous errors can occur if the values of the rate constants are not precisely known, but only negligible errors occur at 45 min, even over a wide range of rate constants of several-fold. In fact, it was precisely for this reason that [^{14}C]DG rather than [^{14}C]glucose was selected as the tracer for glucose metabolism. The relationships are similar for glucose. Because the products of [^{14}C]glucose metabolism are so rapidly lost from the tissues, it is necessary to limit the experimental period to short times when enormous errors can occur if the rate constants are not precisely known. [^{14}C]DG permits the prolongation of the experimental period to times when inaccuracies in rate constants have little effect on the final result.

It should be noted, however, that in pathological conditions, such as severe ischemia or hyperglycemia, the rate constants may fall far beyond the range examined in Figure 6. We have evidence, for example, that this occurs with arterial plasma glucose concentrations above 330 mg%. In such abnormal conditions it may be necessary to redetermine the rate constants for the particular condition under study.

4.2. LUMPED CONSTANT

The lumped constant is composed of 6 separate constants. One of these, Φ, is a measure of the steady-state hydrolysis of glucose-6-phosphate to free glucose and phosphate. Because in normal brain tissue there is little such phosphohydrolase activity (Hers 1957), Φ is normally approximately equal to unity. The other components are arranged in three ratios: λ, which is the ratio of distribution spaces in the tissue for deoxyglucose and glucose; V_m^*/V_m; and K_m/K_m^*. Although each individual constant may vary from structure to structure and condition to condition, it is likely that the ratios tend to remain the same under normal conditions. For reasons described in detail previously (Sokoloff et al. 1977), it is reasonable to believe that the lumped constant is the same throughout the brain and is characteristic of the species of animal, but only in normal tissue. Although reasonable, it is not certain, and there are theoretical possibilities that it may not be so. Empirical experience thus far indicates that it is. The greatest experience has been accumulated in the albino rat. In this species the lumped constant for the brain as a whole has been determined under a variety of conditions (Sokoloff et al. 1977). In the normal conscious rat local cerebral glucose utilization, determined by the [^{14}C]DG method with the single value of the lumped constant for the brain as a whole, correlates almost perfectly ($r = 0.96$) with local cerebral blood flow, measured by the [^{14}C]iodoantipyrine method, an entirely independent method (Sokoloff 1978). It is generally recognized that local blood flow is adjusted to local metabolic rate, but if the single value of the lumped constant did not apply to the individual structures studied, then errors in local glucose utilization would occur that might be expected to obscure the correlation. Also, the lumped constant has been directly determined in the albino rat in the normal conscious state, under barbiturate anesthesia, and during the inhalation of 5% CO_2; no significant differences were observed (Table 2). The lumped constant does vary with the species of animal. It has now also been determined in the Rhesus monkey (Kennedy et al. 1978), cat (M. Miyaoka, J. Magnes, C. Kennedy, M. Shinohara, and L. Sokoloff, unpublished data), and Beagle puppy (Duffy et al. 1979), and each species has a different value (Table 2). The values for local rates of glucose utilization determined with these lumped constants in these species are very close to what might be expected from measurement of energy metabolism in the brain as a whole by other methods (Table 3).

The only conditions thus far found to alter the value of the lumped constant in any species are severe hypoglycemia and hyperglycemia. In rats when the arterial plasma glucose concentration falls to 40 mg% or below the value for the lumped constant rises steeply (Suda et al. 1981). In hyperglycemia with arterial plasma glucose concentrations above 250-300 mg%, there is a slow, moderately progressive fall in the value of the lumped constant with increasing plasma glucose concentration (Schuier et al 1981). There is reason to suspect that the lumped constant might change in pathological conditions. Tissue damage may disrupt the normal cellular compartmentation. There is no assurance that λ, the ratio of the distribution spaces for [^{14}C]DG and glucose, is the same in damaged tissue as in normal tissue. Also in pathological states there may be release of lysosomal acid hydrolases that may hydrolyze glucose-6-phosphate and thus alter the value of Φ.

4.3. ROLE OF GLUCOSE-6-PHOSPHATASE

Confusion has arisen in certain quarters as to the role of glucose-6-phosphatase and the possibility that its presence may lead to an underestimation of calculated values. The model of the method and the operational equation derived from it assume that [^{14}C]deoxyglucose-6-phosphate ([^{14}C]DG-6-P), once formed, remains trapped for the duration of the experiment. This assumption appeared reasonable because of evidence in the literature of very low glucose-6-phosphatase activity in brain (Hers 1957), and low deoxyglucose-6-phosphatase activity in brain was confirmed by direct chemical assay of the hydrolysis of [^{14}C]DG-6-P by whole brain homogenates (Sokoloff et al. 1977). Although low, glucose-6-phosphatase activity is not zero, and [^{14}C]DG-6-P in brain is not retained indefinitely. Its effects become noticeable at 60 min and substantial at 90 min. It is recommended that the experimental period be limited to 45 min. Otherwise, a modified version of the operational equation that takes the effects of phosphatase into account must be employed. Such an equation has been derived (Sokoloff 1982). In damaged tissue phosphohydrolase activity may be increased because of breakdown of cellular compartmentation and release of lysosomal acid hydrolases.

4.4. INFLUENCE OF VARYING PLASMA GLUCOSE CONCENTRATION

Because the operational equation of the method (Fig. 1B) was derived on the basis of the assumption that C_P, the arterial plasma glucose concentration, remains constant during the experimental period, the method was applicable only to experiments in which this assumption was satisfied. This restraint has proved to be cumbersome. A new operational equation has, therefore, been derived which does not require this assumption. The equation is as follows:

$$R = \frac{C_i^*(\tau) - k_1^* e^{-(k_2^* + k_3^*)\tau} \int_0^\tau C_P^* e^{(k_2^* + k_3^*)t} \, dt}{\left[\dfrac{\lambda V_m^* K_m}{\varPhi V_m K_m^*}\right] \int_0^\tau \left[\dfrac{(k_2^* + k_3^*)e^{-(k_2^* + k_3^*)T} \int_0^T C_P^* e^{(k_2^* + k_3^*)t} \, dt}{C_P(0)e^{-(k_2 + k_3)T} + (k_2 + k_3) \, e^{-(k_2 + k_3)T} \int_0^T C_P e^{(k_2 + k_3)t} \, dt}\right] dT}$$

where $(k_2 + k_3)$ equals the turnover rate constant (i.e. $0.693/T \, 1/2$) of the free glucose pool in the brain; $C_P(0)$ equals the arterial plasma glucose concentration at zero time; τ equals the time of killing; and all other symbols are the same as in the equation in Figure 1B.

This new equation requires an estimate of the half-life of the free glucose pool in the tissue. A method has been developed to measure the half-life of the free glucose pool in brain tissue which was found to equal 1.2 and 1.8 min in normal conscious and anesthetized rats, respectively, and to vary with the plasma glucose concentration (Savaki et al. 1978). The equation is relatively insensitive to the value of the half-life of the glucose pool in the range in which it usually falls, and, therefore, only an approximation of this value is sufficient without any serious impairment of the accuracy of the final result. The [14C]DG method can now, therefore, be used in the presence of changing arterial plasma glucose concentrations.

4.5. ANIMAL BEHAVIOR DURING THE EXPERIMENTAL PERIOD

It is desirable that the animal be in a controlled environment with respect to sound and light and that there be a behavioral steady state during the experimental period. While this is not strictly possible in the case of awake, behaving animals, it is well to remember that the measured rates for glucose utilization in brain reflect a kind of integral of the activity in all neural pathways over the 45-min period when the [14C]DG is circulating in the plasma. The results are weighted to reflect predominantly activity of the period between about 5 and 15 min when the [14C]DG is at a relatively high concentration in the precursor pool in the tissue. In studies of seizure activity these considerations may be of particular importance. The results in animals which have a brief generalized seizure followed by a prolonged postical period may be difficult to interpret. Are they indicative of the cerebral metabolism during the seizure, or during the postical depression? Studies should be designed so that the seizure activity or any other behavioral state being investigated, is sustained for at least 10-15 min.

5. THE USE OF [14C]DEOXYGLUCOSE IN METABOLIC MAPPING AND OTHER NONQUANTITATIVE STUDIES

The use of [14C]DG in mapping functional pathways of brain has been previously described (Kennedy et al. 1975; 1976). One may forego the sampling of blood following the administration of [14C]DG and prepare autoradiographs as described. These provide a picture of the relative rates of glucose utilization which is especially useful when studies are designed so that a pathway on one side of the brain is stimulated or deprived and the other side is the control (Buchner et al. 1979; Collins et al. 1976; Kennedy et al. 1975, 1976; McCulloch et al. 1980). In view of the side-to-side symmetry in metabolic rates of the brain under normal circumstances, the finding of even small right-to-left differences in the autoradiographs is significant. While lacking the microscopic resolution of anatomical mapping methods which are dependent upon axoplasmic and trans-synaptic transport, the deoxyglucose procedure results in labeling of the entire functional pathway, unattenuated by synaptic junctions. This is illustrated in the demonstration of the ocular dominance columns in the monkey by studies of monocular stimulation. The reduced function of the pathway subserving the nonstimulated eye is clearly evident beyond the terminals of the geniculostriate pathway in Layer IV of the striate cortex and extends to involve all cortical layers (Kennedy et al. 1976) (Fig. 7).

Another nonquantitative use of [^{14}C]DG is in physiologic alterations and drug-induced behavioral states which result in a redistribution of the rates of glucose utilization in various parts of the brain. Autoradiographs in such induced states show regional differences in optical density resulting in a pattern characteristic for a given state (Hubel et al. 1978; Kliot and Poletti 1979; Meibach et al. 1979; Pulsinelli and Duffy 1979; Schwartz et al. 1979). A difference in this pattern from that in normal resting animals is apparent by inspection. Contrary to a common misconception, it is not possible to make a meaningful comparison of optical density or direct assay of ^{14}C content in any one region of brain of one animal with that for the same region of another animal without monitoring the concentrations of glucose and [^{14}C]DG in the plasma. This is because the ^{14}C concentration for a given brain region is determined not only by its rate of glucose utilization but also by the time course of the relative concentrations of [^{14}C]DG and glucose in the tissue during the experimental period. It cannot be assumed that this is the same in different animals simply because each receives the same dose of [^{14}C]DG/unit weight. Not only are there normal random physiologic variations from animal to animal which affect this time course, (e.g. plasma glucose concentration, cardiac output, the rate of glucose utilization in muscle and other tissues), but there may be systematic alterations which are the result of a given experimental condition. In an effort to circumvent the need for monitoring the plasma content of glucose and [^{14}C]DG and yet to permit comparisons of local metabolic rate to be made between animals, some investigators have employed an index which they considered to be a measure of the relative ratio of glucose utilization. The index is a ratio of the structure's optical density or its ^{14}C content to that in white matter (Schwartz and Gainer 1977; Allen et al. 1981). The validity of such an index, however, rests on the assumption that white matter is unchanged in its metabolic rate when experimental conditions are altered. Because white matter may indeed be altered in its rate of glucose utilization under certain conditions it is not a structure which can be assumed to have a fixed metabolic rate. Had an index of this kind been employed in a recent study of local cerebral glucose utilization in non-rapid-eye-movement sleep, no difference would have been found for most structures between sleep and the waking state. In fact, non-rapid-eye-movement sleep was shown to be accompanied by a 25-30% reduction in glucose utilization in virtually all structures including white matter when the quantitative method as originally described was applied (Kennedy et al. 1982). Unfortunately for those involved in behavioral studies there appears to be no way to eliminate the monitoring of plasma glucose and [^{14}C]DG during the experiment to obtain reliable results.

When qualitative studies of either type described above are done, the preferred route of administration of [^{14}C]DG is as an intravenous pulse. This serves to load the tissue with the labeled substrate early in the experimental period, and yet allows for clearing the tissue of most of the unmetabolized [^{14}C]DG before the end of the experiment.

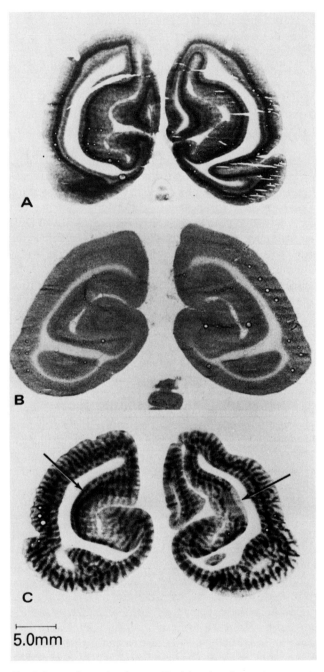

Fig. 7. Autoradiographs of coronal brain sections from Rhesus monkeys at the level of the striate cortex. (A) Animal with normal binocular vision. Note the laminar distribution of the density; the dark band corresponds to Layer IV. (B) Animal with bilateral visual deprivation. Note the almost uniform and reduced relative density, especially the virtual disappearance of the dark band corresponding to Layer IV. (C) Animal with right eye occluded. The half-brain on the left side of the photograph represents the left hemisphere contralateral to the occluded eye. Note the alternate dark and light striations, each approximately 0.3-0.4 mm in width that represent the ocular dominance columns. The columns are most apparent in the dark band corresponding to Layer IV but extend through the entire thickness of the cortex. The arrows point to regions

Thus the signal-to-noise ratio is enhanced. When other routes of administration are used, subcutaneous or intraperitoneal, tissue-specific activity rises only slowly and the free pool likewise is cleared slowly. Much of the optical density in the autoradiographs is due to the unmetabolized deoxyglucose and therefore differences due to variations in metabolism tend to be obscured.

6. RECENT TECHNOLOGICAL ADVANCES

Several recent technological developments, both completed and still in progress, extend the resolution of the [^{14}C]DG method in animals and adapt it for use in man.

6.1. COMPUTERIZED IMAGE-PROCESSING

The regional localization obtained with the [^{14}C]DG method is achieved by the use of quantitative autoradiography. The autoradiographs contain an immense amount of information that cannot be practically recovered by manual densitometry or adequately represented by tabular presentation of the data. A computerized image-processing system has, therefore, been developed to analyze and transform the autoradiographs into color-coded pictorial maps of the rates of local glucose utilization throughout the CNS (Goochee et al. 1980). The autoradiographs are scanned automatically by a computer-controlled scanning microdensitometer. The optical density of each spot on the autoradiograph, from 25-100 μm as selected, is stored in a computer, converted to ^{14}C concentration on the basis of the optical densities of the calibrated ^{14}C-plastic standards, and then converted to local rate of glucose utilization by solution of the operational equation. Colors are assigned to narrow ranges of the rates of glucose utilization, and the autoradiographs are then displayed in a color monitor in color along with a calibrated color scale for identifying the rate of glucose in each spot of the autoradiograph from its color. The display is similar to that used by Lassen et al. (1978) for regional cortical blood flow, but it represents the rates of glucose utilization in all parts of the brain.

6.2. MICROSCOPIC RESOLUTION

The resolution of the present [^{14}C]DG method is at best 200 μm. The use of [^{3}H]DG and LKB Ultrafilm with the standard autoradiographic procedure does not greatly improve the resolution, the limiting factor being the diffusion and migration of the water-soluble labeled compound during the preparation of the tissue sections.

Several investigators have proposed methods for preparing DG-labeled tissue for autoradiography in order to minimize diffusion and migration of the label and at the same time preserve normal cell histology. Conventional fixation with glutaraldehyde and osmium tetroxide has been used both in vivo, i.e. by perfusion (Des Rosiers and Descarries 1978), and in vitro (Basinger et al. 1979). It has been demonstrated (Pilgrim

---

of bilateral asymmetry where the ocular dominance columns are absent. These are presumably areas with normally only monocular input. The one on the left, contralateral to the occluded eye, has a continuous dark lamina corresponding to Layer IV which is completely absent on the side ipsilateral to the occluded eye. These regions are believed to be the loci of the cortical representations of the blind spots. (From Kennedy et al. 1976.)

and Wagner 1981; Ornberg et al. 1979), however, that a significant amount of label is lost during these procedures. Loss of any of the labeled DG-6-P precludes quantification, and unless it can be shown that the label is lost proportionately from all compartments, even qualitative assessment of relative rates of glucose utilization are meaningless. Since it has been shown that most of the labeled DG that remains in the tissue after conventional fixation (Kai Kai and Pentreath 1981; Pentreath et al. 1982) is in the form of deoxyglycogen, selectivity of loss is fairly certain.

There are several other methods available for preparing tissue for autoradiography which may meet the requirements of localizing a water-soluble molecule, such as DG-6-P. The critical requirements are: (1) the tissue must be frozen rapidly at temperatures below −120°C in order to minimize ice crystal formation; (2) the tissue must be kept frozen at very low temperatures in order to prevent diffusion; (3) if moisture is removed, the tissue can be warmed to room temperature, but it must remain totally anhydrous as the introduction of moisture even from the humidity in room air can cause diffusion.

One of the simplest approaches to this problem is the Appleton (1974) technique in which frozen sections are cut under safelight illumination and picked-up onto nuclear track emulsion-coated slides at −12 to −70°C. The slides are exposed in light-tight, dessicated boxes in a freezer. The results of DG studies obtained with this method of preparing autoradiographs (Sharp 1976; Wagner et al. 1979; Pilgrim and Wagner 1981) contrast with the results of the originally described [14C]DG studies by Sokoloff et al. (1977) in that the autoradiographs do not exhibit the heterogeneous levels of glucose utilization normally seen. However, if used with a great deal of care, particularly with regard to the maintenance of frozen tissue sections, high resolution autoradiographs could, theoretically, be achieved with the Appleton technique.

For several reasons freeze-dried or freeze-substituted and plastic-embedded sections may be preferred over frozen sections. The histology is better, the section thickness is more reproducible, the geometry of section and emulsion is more predictable with plastic embedding, and there is the possibility of extending studies to the electron-microscope level. Both of these approaches have been used for the preparation of DG-labeled tissue specimens. Freeze-substitution in acetone at −85°C (Ornberg et al. 1979; Sejnowski et al. 1980; Lancet et al. 1982) or freeze-drying at −70°C (Buchner et al. 1979) followed by embedding in a plastic resin have both been applied with what appear to be good results. Sectioning of the plastic-embedded tissues should be done dry (Baughman and Bader 1977) as it has been shown that some, perhaps as much as 20%, of the label is displaced during flotation of semithin sections on water (Buchner and Buchner 1982). Losses and/or displacement of label may also occur while dipping the sections in emulsion (Stirling and Kinter 1967). It is suggested, therefore, that either the sections be coated with a thin film of carbon (Baker and Appleton 1976) prior to dipping or that they be either coated with a loop of dried emulsion (Caro and Van Tubergen 1962) or sandwiched with a dried emulsion-coated slide. With either approach, freeze-drying or freeze-substitution, the procedure is tedious and requires great care particularly at the stage where the tissue is dry and contact with moisture must be avoided. Results of careful studies such as those of the Drosophila visual system (Fig. 8) (Buchner and Buchner 1980) show that high resolution autoradiographs can be attained.

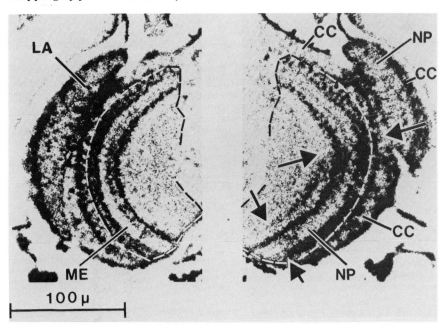

Fig. 8. High resolution [³H]DG autoradiograph of right and left optic lobes (Lamina LA and Medulla ME) of a Drosophila melanogaster. The Drosophila was presented with a flickering visual stimulus to a circular field of the left eye while a moving pattern stimulated the corresponding field of the right eye. The concentric rings of label and their periodic structure reflect the anatomical arrangement of concentric layers and periodic columns of the medulla, respectively. The heavily labeled sector marked by the *4 arrows* in the right medulla corresponds to the visual field that was stimulated by movement. While the cellular cortex (CC) of the lamina is easily identified by its enhanced labeling, the boundary between the cellular cortex and neuropil (NP) of the medulla has been marked by a dashed line. (From Buchner and Buchner 1980.)

6.3. [¹⁸F]FLUORODEOXYGLUCOSE TECHNIQUE

Because the DG method requires the measurement of local concentrations of radioactivity in the individual components of the brain, it cannot be applied as originally designed with quantitative autoradiography to man. Recent developments in computerized emission tomography, however, have made it possible to measure local concentrations of labeled compounds in vivo in man. Emission tomography requires the use of γ-radiation, preferably annihilation γ-rays derived from positron emission. A positron-emitting derivative of DG, 2-[¹⁸F]fluoro-2-deoxy-D-glucose has been synthesized and found to retain the necessary biochemical properties of DG (Reivich et al. 1979). The method has, therefore, been adapted for use in man with [¹⁸F]fluorodeoxyglucose and positron-emission tomography (Phelps et al. 1979; Reivich et al. 1979). The resolution of the method is still relatively limited, approximately 1 cm, but it is already proving to be useful in studies of the human visual system (Phelps et al. 1981) and of clinical conditions, such as focal epilepsy (Kuhl et al. 1979, 1980). This technique is of immense potential usefulness for studies of human local cerebral energy metabolism in normal states and in neurological and psychiatric disorders.

7. REFERENCES

Allen TO, Adler NT, Greenberg JH, Reivich M (1981): Vaginocervical stimulation selectively increases metabolic activity in the rat brain. *Science, 211,* 1070–1072.

Appleton TC (1974): A cryostat approach to ultrathin 'dry' frozen sections for electron-microscopy: A morphological and X-ray analytical study. *J. Microsc. (Oxford), 100/1,* 49–74.

Baker JRJ, Appleton TC (1976): A technique for electron-microscope autoradiography (and X-ray microanalysis) of diffusible substances using freeze-dried fresh frozen sections. *J. Microsc. (Oxford), 108,* 307–315.

Basinger SF, Gordon WC, Lam DMK (1979): Differential labelling of retinal neurons by ^{3}H-2-deoxyglucose. *Nature, 280,* 682–684.

Baughman RW, Bader CR (1977): Biochemical characterization and cellular localization of the cholinergic system in the chicken retina. *Brain Res., 138,* 469–485.

Buchner E, Buchner S (1980): Mapping stimulus-induced nervous activity in small brains by [^{3}H]2-deoxy-D-glucose. *Cell Tissue Res., 211,* 51–64.

Buchner E, Buchner S, Hengstenberg R (1979): 2-Deoxy-D-glucose maps movement-specific nervous activity in the second visual ganglion of Drosophila. *Science, 205,* 687–688.

Buchner S, Buchner E (1982): Functional neuroanatomical mapping in the insects by [^{3}H]2-deoxy-D-glucose at electron-microscopical resolution. *Neurosci. Lett., 28,* 235–240.

Caro LG, Van Tubergen RP (1962): High-resolution autoradiography. I. Methods. *J. Cell Biol., 15,* 173–188.

Collins RC, Kennedy C, Sokoloff L, Plum F (1976): Metabolic anatomy of focal motor seizures. *Arch. Neurol. (Chicago), 33,* 536–542.

Des Rosiers MH, Descarries L (1978): Adaptation de la méthode au désoxyglucose à l'échelle cellulaire: préparation histologique du système nerveux central en vue de la radio-autographie à haute résolution. *CR Acad. Sci. (Paris), 287, Ser. D,* 153–156.

Duffy TE, Cavazzuti M, Gregoire NM, Cruz NF, Kennedy C, Sokoloff L (1979): Regional cerebral glucose metabolism in newborn beagle dogs. *Trans. Amer. Soc. Neurochem., 10,* 171.

Goochee C, Rasband W, Sokoloff L (1980): Computerized densitometry and color coding of [^{14}C]deoxyglucose autoradiographs. *Ann. Neurol., 7,* 359–370.

Hers HG (1957): *Le Métabolisme du Fructose.* Éditions Arscia, Bruxelles, p. 102.

Hubel DH, Wiesel TN, Stryker MP (1978): Anatomical demonstration of orientation columns in macaque monkey. *J. Comp. Neurol., 177,* 361–380.

Kai Kai MA, Pentreath VW (1981): High resolution analysis of [^{3}H]2-deoxyglucose incorporation into neurons and glial cells in invertebrate ganglia: Histological processing of nervous tissue for selective marking of glycogen. *J. Neurocytol., 10,* 693–708.

Kennedy C, Des Rosiers MH, Reivich M, Sharp F, Jehle JW, Sokoloff L (1975): Mapping of functional neural pathways by autoradiographic survey of local metabolic rate with [^{14}C]deoxyglucose. *Science, 187,* 850–853.

Kennedy C, Des Rosiers MH, Sakurada O, Shinohara M, Reivich M, Jehle JW, Sokoloff L (1976): Metabolic mapping of the primary visual system of the monkey by means of the autoradiographic [^{14}C]deoxyglucose technique. *Proc. Nat. Acad. Sci. USA, 73,* 4230–4234.

Kennedy C, Sakurada O, Shinohara M, Jehle J, Sokoloff L (1978): Local cerebral glucose utilization in the normal conscious macaque monkey. *Ann. Neurol., 4,* 293–301.

Kennedy C, Gillin JC, Mendelson W, Suda S, Miyaoka M, Ito M, Nakamura RK, Storch FI, Pettigrew K, Mishkin M, Sokoloff L (1982): Local cerebral glucose utilization in non-rapid eye movement sleep. *Nature, 297,* 325–327.

Kliot M, Poletti CE (1979): Hippocampal afterdischarges: Differential spread of acitivity shown by the [^{14}C]deoxyglucose technique. *Science, 204,* 641–643.

Kuhl D, Engel J, Phelps M, Selin C (1979): Pattern of local cerebral metabolism and perfusion in partial epilepsy by emission computed tomography of ^{18}F-fluorodeoxyglucose and ^{13}N-ammonia. *Acta Neurol. Scand., 60,* 538–539.

Kuhl DE, Engel Jr J, Phelps ME, Selin C (1980): Epileptic patterns of local cerebral metabolism and perfusion in humans determined by emission computed tomography of ^{18}FDG and ^{13}NH$_3$. *Ann. Neurol., 8,* 348–360.

Lancet D, Greer CA, Kauer JS, Shepherd GM (1982): Mapping of odor-related neuronal activity in the olfactory bulb by high-resolution 2-deoxyglucose autoradiography. *Proc. Nat. Acad. Sci. USA, 79,* 670–674.

Lassen NA, Ingvar DH, Skinhøj E (1978): Brain function and blood flow. *Sci. Amer., 239,* 62–71.

440

McCulloch J, Savaki HE, McCulloch MC, Sokoloff L (1980): Retina-dependent activation by apomorphine of metabolic activity in the superficial layer of the superior colliculus. *Science, 207,* 313–315.

Meibach RC, Glick SD, Cox R, Maayani S (1979): Localisation of phencyclidine-induced changes in brain energy metabolism. *Nature, 282,* 625–626.

Ornberg RL, Neale EA, Smith CB, Yarowsky P, Bowers LM (1979): Radioautographic localization of glucose utilization by neurons in culture. *J. Cell Biol. Abstr., 83,* CN142A.

Pentreath VW, Seal LH, Kai Kai MA (1982): Incorporation of [^{3}H]2-deoxyglucose into glycogen in nervous tissues. *Neuroscience, 7,* 759–767.

Phelps ME, Huang SC, Hoffman EJ, Selin C, Sokoloff L, Kuhl DE (1979): Tomography measurement of local cerebral glucose metabolic rate in humans with (F-18)2-fluoro-2-deoxy-d-glucose: Validation of method. *Ann. Neurol., 6,* 371–388.

Phelps ME, Mazziotta JC, Kuhl DE (1981): Metabolic mapping of the brain's response to visual stimulation: Studies in man. *Science, 211,* 1445–1448.

Pilgrim Ch, Wagner H-J (1981): Improving the resolution of the 2-deoxy-D-glucose method. *J. Histochem. Cytochem., 29,* 190–194.

Pulsinelli WA, Duffy TE (1979): Local cerebral glucose metabolism during controlled hypoxemia in rats. *Science, 204,* 626–629.

Rcivich M, Kuhl D, Wolf A, Greenberg J, Phelps M, Ido T, Casella V, Fowler J, Hoffman E, Alavi A, Som P, Sokoloff L (1979): The [^{18}F]fluoro-deoxyglucose method for the measurement of local cerebral glucose utilization in man. *Circ. Res., 44,* 127–137.

Savaki H, Davidsen L, Smith C, Sokoloff L (1978): Turnover of the free glucose pool in brain. *Neurosci. Abstr., 4,* 323.

Schuier F, Orzi F, Suda S, Kennedy C, Sokoloff L (1981): The lumped constant for the [^{14}C]deoxyglucose method in hyperglycemic rats. *J. Cereb. Blood Flow Metab. 1, Suppl. 1,* S63.

Schwartz WJ, Gainer H (1977): Suprachiasmatic nucleus: Use of ^{14}C-labeled deoxyglucose uptake as a functional marker. *Science, 197,* 1089–1091.

Schwartz WJ, Smith CB, Davidsen L, Savaki H, Sokoloff L, Mata M, Fink DJ, Gainer H (1979): Metabolic mapping of functional activity in the hypothalamo-neurohypophysial system of the rat. *Science, 205,* 723–725.

Sejnowski TJ, Reingold SC, Kelley DB, Gelperin A (1980): Localization of [^{3}H]-2-deoxyglucose in single molluscan neurones. *Nature, 287,* 449–451.

Sharp FR (1976): Relative cerebral glucose consumption of neuronal perikarya and neuropil determined with 2-deoxyglucose in resting and swimming rat. *Brain Res., 110,* 127–139.

Sokoloff L (1978): Local cerebral energy metabolism: Its relationships to local functional activity and blood flow. In: Purves MJ, Elliott K (Eds), *Cerebral Vascular Smooth Muscle and Its Control. Ciba Foundation Symposium 56,* pp. 171–197. Elsevier/Excerpta Medica/North-Holland, Amsterdam.

Sokoloff L (1982): The radioactive deoxyglucose method: Theory, procedure, and applications for the measurement of local glucose utilization in the central nervous system. In: Agranoff BW, Aprison MH (Eds), *Advances in Neurochemistry, Vol. 4,* pp. 1–82. Plenum Press, New York.

Sokoloff L, Reivich M, Kennedy C, Des Rosiers MH, Patlak CS, Pettigrew KD, Sakurada O, Shinohara M (1977): The [^{14}C]deoxyglucose method for the measurement of local cerebral glucose utilization: Theory, procedure, and normal values in the conscious and anesthetized albino rat. *J. Neurochem., 28,* 897–916.

Stirling CE, Kinter WB (1967): High-resolution autoradiography of galactose-^{3}H accumulation in rings of hamster intestine. *J. Cell Biol., 35,* 585–604.

Suda S, Shinohara M, Miyaoka M, Kennedy C, Sokoloff L (1981): Local cerebral glucose utilization in hypoglycemia. *J. Cereb. Blood Flow Metab. 1, Suppl. 1,* S62.

Wagner H-J, Pilgrim C, Zwerger H (1979): A system of cells in the unstimulated rat brain characterized by preferential accumulation of [^{3}H]deoxyglucose. *Neurosci. Lett., 15,* 181–186.

CHAPTER XI

Localization of steroid hormone target neurons by autoradiography*

(Anatomical relationships to aminergic and peptidergic systems by combined autoradiography and immunohistochemistry)

MADHABANANDA SAR and WALTER E. STUMPF

1. INTRODUCTION

Steroid hormones influence brain functions by acting directly on specific brain structures or nuclear groups. Some of these effects include the regulation of neuroendocrine functions (Fuxe et al. 1981; Kalra 1981; McCann et al. 1980), activation of sexual behavior in the adult (Dörner 1980; Larsson and Beyer 1981; Gorski and Yanase 1980), and organizational actions in developing brain (Toran-Allerand 1978), as well as modulation of sensory perception (Bereiter and Barker, 1975) memory, and autonomic responses. Precise identification of steroid hormone target sites in the brain is important for the understanding of hormonal action. Both biochemical and histochemical techniques have been employed to localize receptor sites for steroid hormones in brain, pituitary and other tissues. Biochemical approaches (Baulieu et al. 1975; Eisenfeld and Axelrod 1965; Gorski and Gannon 1975; Jensen and Desombre 1972; Kato 1975; Kato and Onouchi 1977; O'Malley and Means 1974) have been used mainly for the study of steroid hormone receptor protein interaction and do not distinguish between individual parts of the organs that contain heterogeneous types of tissues and cells. In contrast, histochemical techniques, such as autoradiography (Stumpf 1970a, 1971, 1976; Stumpf and Sar 1975a) can detect cellular and subcellular target sites by visualizing selective concentration and retention (Stumpf and Sar 1976).

Steroid hormones are small molecules and non-covalently bound to tissue constituents. They may be translocated or lost during tissue preparation. Therefore, the autoradiographic technique used should prevent diffusion and leaching of the labeled compound. Autoradiography is a slow process because of long exposure times. This can be minimized by the use of radiochemically pure compound with high specific activity which will accelerate the latent image formation in emulsion during exposure. Localization of steroid hormones was not possible prior to the development of dry-mount and thaw-mount autoradiography by Stumpf and Roth (1964, 1966) for the localization of diffusible compounds at the cellular and subcellular levels. This technique is sensitive and provides high light-microscopic resolution. It utilizes unfixed and unembedded frozen tissues and, thus, prevents or minimizes translocation and diffusion artifacts. With these techniques the cellular and subcellular localization of steroid

*This work was supported by PHS Grant NSO9914 and NS17479.

Handbook of Chemical Neuroanatomy. Vol. 1: Methods in Chemical Neuroanatomy.
A. Björklund and T. Hökfelt, editors.
© Elsevier Science Publishers B.V., 1983.

442

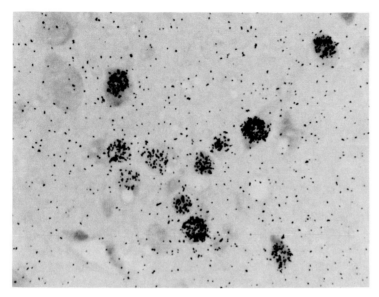

Fig. 1. Thaw-mount autoradiogram of guinea pig brain prepared 1 h after injection of [³H]estradiol showing nuclear concentration of radioactivity in neurons of the arcuate nucleus. Exposure time 96 days, ×670, stained with methylgreen-pyronin. (Reproduced from Sar and Stumpf 1975b.)

hormones have been demonstrated in brain (Sar and Stumpf 1972, 1973b, 1977a,b; Stumpf 1968a, 1970b; Stumpf and Sar 1971, 1975b, 1978, 1979, 1981; Stumpf et al. 1975a,b), pituitary (Sar and Stumpf 1972, 1973a, 1977b, 1979; Stumpf 1968b), and other organs (Sar et al. 1970; Sar and Stumpf 1974, 1976; Sar et al. 1975; Stumpf 1968c, 1969; Stumpf and Sar 1976).

Autoradiographic techniques and their applications for the study of localization of steroid hormones and diffusible compounds have been reviewed (Stumpf 1970a, 1971, 1976; Stumpf and Sar 1975a). In the dry-mount autoradiography, frozen sections are freeze-dried and then mounted on dried emulsion coated slides. In the thaw-mount autoradiography, frozen sections are melted onto dried emulsion coated slides. Thaw-mount autoradiography is now commonly applied for the localization of steroid hormones. This technique excludes the freeze-drying step and is, therefore, more convenient to use. But, wet interaction between tissue section and photographic emulsion, albeit brief, may cause chemographic artifacts. Therefore, the dry-mount technique serves as a control.

Autoradiography has been combined with histofluorescence or immunohistochemistry for the simultaneous demonstration of two different substances in the same tissue preparation. The combined technique of autoradiography and formaldehyde-induced fluorescence permits the visualization of labeled steroid uptake sites and catecholamine cells (Grant and Stumpf 1975; Heritage et al. 1977, 1980). The combined technique of autoradiography and immunohistochemistry is applied for the simultaneous visualization of radioactively labeled cells and peptide or catecholamine producing cells (Sar and Stumpf 1978a, 1979, 1980, 1981a,b).

This chapter reviews these histochemical techniques and their application in brain localization of steroid hormones, peptides and catecholamines.

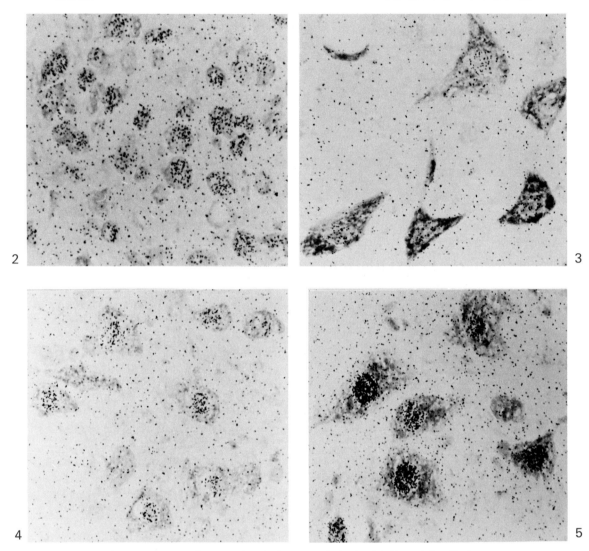

Figs. 2–5. Thaw-mount autoradiograms of rat brain prepared 1 h after injection of [³H]dihydrotestosterone showing nuclear concentration of radioactivity in neurons of the n. preopticus medialis (Fig. 2), n. motorius nervi facialis (Fig. 3), n. ambiguus (Fig. 4) and in the motor neurons of Lamina IX of the thoracic spinal cord (Fig. 5). Exposure time 360 days, ×520, stained with methylgreen-pyronin. (Fig. 2 reproduced from Sar and Stumpf 1977b, and Figs 3 and 5 from Sar and Stumpf 1977a.)

2. AUTORADIOGRAPHY

In both dry-mount and thaw-mount autoradiography, some of the steps for the preparation of autoradiograms are identical. These include freezing, storage and sectioning of frozen tissue, as well as photographic development and staining.

2.1. THAW-MOUNT AUTORADIOGRAPHY

This technique consists of the following steps: (a) freezing of tissue blocks, (b) cryostat sectioning of 4 μm thick sections at $-35°$C to $-40°$C, (c) transferring the frozen sections onto dried emulsion-coated slides, and (d) photographic processing and staining of the slides.

(a) Freezing of tissue blocks

The radioactively (preferably tritium) labeled steroid hormone with high specific activity is injected intravenously, intraperitoneally or subcutaneously into an animal at a physiological or near physiological dose. The radioactively labeled compounds are evaporated to dryness in a stream of dry nitrogen gas and resuspended in 10% ethanol-isotonic saline for injection. The animals are killed by decapitation at different time intervals, depending on the experimental protocol. The brain is removed, placed on a Petri dish kept on ice, and cut into 2 or 3 blocks for mounting on brass mounts. A layer of minced liver on the mount serves as an adhesive for the tissue block. The mount with the tissue is frozen in liquid propane cooled by liquid nitrogen. Prior to the experiment, propane gas is liquefied by cooling it in a 250 ml round-bottom flask immersed in liquid nitrogen in a Dewar with liquid nitrogen. Liquefied propane is then transferred to a beaker cooled with liquid nitrogen. Depending on the size of tissue blocks, slow or fast freezing is applied. For large blocks of tissue, freezing is slower than that for small ones, in order to prevent cracking of the tissue. The temperature of the liquefied propane may be recorded in order to ensure proper freezing of tissue. Freezing in propane at temperatures above $-100°$C may introduce ice crystal formation in the tissues. Freon or isopentane cooled with liquid nitrogen, can also be used as a coolant. Liquid nitrogen is not suitable for freezing of tissues, since it exists at its boiling point and forms vapor around the tissue, thereby preventing rapid freezing and thus causing ice crystal formation. The frozen-mounted tissue is stored indefinitely in a plastic test tube in a liquid nitrogen container.

(b) Cryostat sectioning of 4 μm thick sections at -35 to $-40°$C

Frozen cryostat sectioning of 4 μm thick sections is performed in a cryostat which is maintained at about $-35°$C knife-temperature. The test tube containing the tissue mount is transferred in a liquid nitrogen Dewar from the liquid nitrogen storage container to the cryostat. A long, precooled pair of forceps is used for transferring the tissue within the cryostat to the microtome. For sectioning, a dissecting microscope, equipped with fiber-optics light, is mounted to one side of the cryostat, so that it can be swung over the knife. With the aid of a dissecting microscope, the frozen sections can be judged for quality, and the orientation of the cutting surface of the tissue block and serial sectioning are facilitated. Usually, 4 μm thick sections are cut in the darkroom, with the fiber-optics light on.

(c) Transferring frozen sections onto dried emulsion-coated slides

After 2 or 3 frozen sections have been cut in series, the light is turned off and the safelight (15 watt bulb, Kodak OC filter) is turned on. Sections are transferred from the knife onto a slide coated with a dried emulsion (Kodak NTB 3 or 2) (see below),

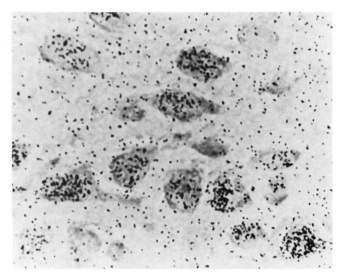

Fig. 6. Thaw-mount autoradiogram of rat brain prepared 15 min after injection of [³H]R5020 showing nuclear concentration of radioactivity in neurons of the arcuate nucleus. Exposure time 72 days, ×880, stained with methylgreen-pyronin.

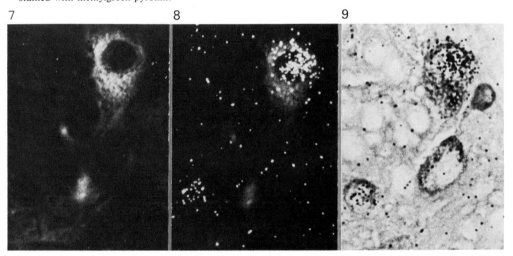

Figs 7–9. Combined formaldehyde-induced fluorescence and dry-mount autoradiography showing localization of [³H]estradiol and catecholamine in neuron of the nucleus reticularis lateralis of the rat brain stem. Visualized under UV light only (Fig. 7), UV light and tungsten light simultaneously (Fig. 8) and after staining with methylgreen-pyronin under tungsten light (Fig. 9). 6 μm, ×470. (Reproduced from Heritage et al. 1977.)

which is then placed in a black box kept at room temperature. After completion of the frozen sectioning, the desiccator box is sealed and stored in a freezer at −15°C for exposure.

(d) Photographic processing and staining of the slides

The optimal time for exposure is determined by developing the slides at different time

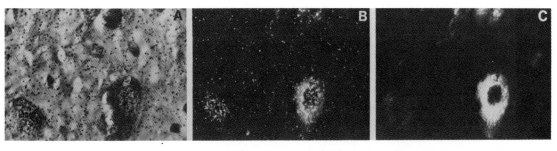

Fig. 10. Combined formaldehyde-induced fluorescence and dry-mount autoradiography showing nuclear concentration of [³H]dihydrotestosterone in catecholamine neurons located adjacent to the nucleus olivaris superior of the rat brain stem. Visualized under tungsten light (Fig. 10A), UV and tungsten light (Fig. 10B) and UV light (Fig. 10C). 6 μm, ×470. (Reproduced from Heritage et al. 1980.)

intervals. Exposure times are variable and dependent upon numerous factors, such as, dose, specific activity, and specific concentration of the labeled compound, route of administration and thickness of the section. Therefore, the exact exposure time for a particular experiment cannot be calculated.

At the end of exposure the slide box is removed from the freezer and allowed to warm to room temperature before removal of the slides. Photographic processing, such as, development, fixation and rinsing is done under constant temperature conditions at 15°C for all fluids. Slides are developed in Kodak D19 developer for 1 min, briefly rinsed in tap water, fixed in Kodak fixer for 5 min and rinsed in tap water for 5 min.

After the photographic procedure, the slides may be stained with methylgreen-pyronin for 30 sec to 1 min, briefly rinsed in tap water, and air-dried before mounting with Permount and a coverslip. Methylene blue-basic fuchsin, which does not obscure silver grains, may be used as an alternate single step stain. Emulsion may be wiped off the back of the slides at the end of staining, before air-drying.

In thaw-mount autoradiography it is necessary to ensure proper control for chemographic artifacts. Chemical interaction between section and photographic emulsion can take place during melting and may create either positive or negative chemography over select tissue constituents. In addition, mechanical pressure may create positive chemography. Control autoradiograms should be prepared from identical specimens without injection of radioactive compound. In negative chemography loss of latent image over the section can occur by direct chemical action. This kind of artifact can be recognized by placing a control section in contact with the emulsion slide that has been fogged by light.

Preparation of emulsion coated slides

Emulsion coating is carried out in a darkroom in the presence of a safelight with filter Wratten series No. 2. Undiluted or diluted (1:1 with distilled water) Kodak NTB3 or NTB2 is used. A water bath is maintained at 42–45°C. The 4 oz emulsion bottle is transferred to a light-proof stainless steel container, which contains some water in order to improve heat transfer. The metal container with the emulsion bottle is placed in the water bath for 1–2 h for the emulsion to melt. Since the commercially provided emulsion bottle is inconvenient for dipping of slides, the melted emulsion is poured slowly, under safelight, into a beaker, which is placed in a container and kept in the water bath for another 30 min to 1 h before dipping of the slides. The extent of time

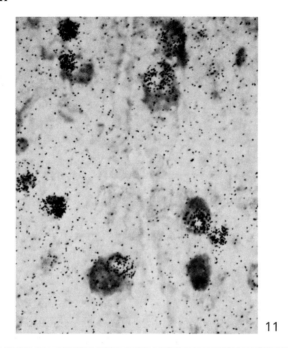

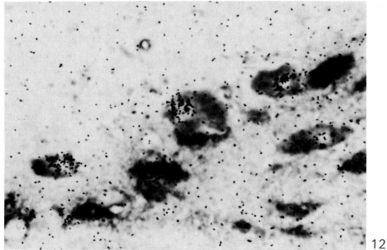

Figs 11–12. Thaw-mount autoradiograms of guinea pig preoptic periventricular nucleus (Fig. 11) and supraoptic nucleus (Fig. 12) prepared 1 h after [³H]estradiol and stained by the immunoperoxidase method with neurophysin I antiserum (1:2000). Note the nuclear concentration of radioactivity in neurophysin-producing cells. Exposure time 90 days, × 760. (Reproduced from Sar and Stumpf 1981b.)

in the water bath permits disappearance of air bubbles, which may have been formed when the emulsion was poured. Microscopic slides with one end and one side frosted, are thoroughly cleaned with absolute alcohol. The clean slides are transferred to plastic slide grips SG-5 (Lipshaw Manufacturing Co., Detroit, MI) which hold 5 slides each. The slides are warmed to 42°C in an incubator before dipping; this facilitates uniform emulsion coating. Dipping may be done by hand, slowly and steadily to assure even coating. The slides held by a slide grip are dipped and withdrawn vertically and transferred to a slide rack for drying at room temperature; this may take 1–2 h and can also be done overnight. The dried emulsion-coated slides are stored in modified Clay-Adam's black boxes with a drying agent (Drierite) compartment. One emulsion-coated slide is immediately developed photographically and the silver grains are counted in order to assess the background before use. Counting of background silver grains is done with an $100\times$ objective and in fields of 1000 μ^2. Generally, there are less than 2 silver grains/1000 μ^2, and emulsion with more than 4 silver grains/1000 μ^2 should not be used.

2.2. DRY-MOUNT AUTORADIOGRAPHY

(a) Frozen sectioning

Freezing of tissue and cutting of frozen sections are identical in both the dry-mount and thaw-mount techniques. In dry-mount autoradiography the frozen sections are freeze-dried and then dry-mounted onto desiccated emulsion slides. Frozen sections (2–4 μm thick) are transferred with the bristles of a fine brush from the knife to Polyvials. Polyvials are placed in a carrier close to the knife. The carrier may contain 5 or more Polyvials, depending on their size. The vials are covered with a fine wire mesh punched out in the center which helps dislodge the sections from the brush and prevents loss of sections during freeze-drying and breaking of the vacuum. Several sections (10–20) may be dropped into one vial. The carrier with the vials containing the frozen sections is then transferred with long precooled forceps to the sample chamber of the Cryosorption Pump (Thermovac Industries Corp., Copiaque, Long Island, NY) within the cryostat for subsequent freeze-drying.

(b) Freeze-drying

Sample chamber and cryopump are assembled within the cryostat with the help of a vacuum created with a forepump, facilitating selfseating of the 0-ring joints and activating the molecular sieve of the cryopump. After a 10- to 15-min evacuation, the mechanical forepump is disconnected and the cryosorption chamber of the assembled cryopump is inserted into a Dewar filled with liquid nitrogen. The liquid nitrogen Dewar with the cryopump is kept inside the cryostat. The cryostat provides the cooling temperature for the specimen chamber of the cryopump. Other methods for freeze-drying may be used; however, it must be ensured that freeze-drying takes place at a low temperature (below $-35°C$) which must not be raised before the end of the procedure.

    Freeze-drying of the sections with the Cryosorption Pump may also be done outside of the cryostat. In this case two Dewars are prepared, one filled with liquid nitrogen and the other with dry ice-alcohol slush as a coolant for the specimens. A vacuum of between 10^{-4} to 10^{-5} Torr is generally maintained. After 24 h the cryosorption pump is removed from the cryostat. The specimen chamber is kept at room temperature until equilibration, while the molecular sieve compartment of the pump remains immersed in liquid nitrogen. The vacuum is broken with dry nitrogen gas and the vials containing the freeze-dried sections are stored in a desiccator at room temperature. The cryopump is removed from the liquid nitrogen and the molecular sieve is reactivated at room temperature or in an oven.

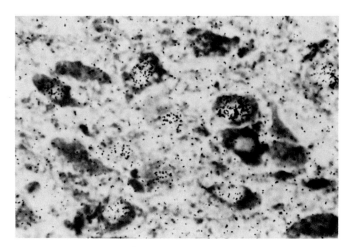

Fig. 13. Thaw-mount autoradiogram of rat lower brain stem prepared 1 h after injection of [³H]estradiol and stained by immunoperoxidase method with DBH antiserum (1:500). Note the nuclear concentration of radioactivity in DBH-stained neurons of the locus ceruleus. ×900. (Reproduced from Sar and Stumpf 1981c.)

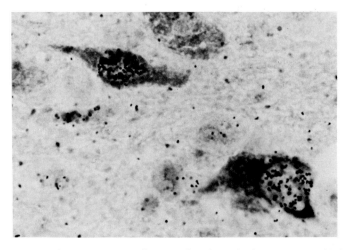

Fig. 14. Thaw-mount autoradiogram of rat lower brain stem prepared 1 h after injection of [³H]estradiol and stained by immunoperoxidase method with DBH antiserum showing nuclear concentration of [³H]estradiol in DBH-positive cells of nucleus tractus solitarii. ×1100. (Reproduced from Sar and Stumpf 1981c.)

(c) Mounting of freeze-dried sections

Freeze-dried sections are placed on a smooth and clean piece of teflon 2 × 1 × 0.16 cm (Crane Packing Co., Morton Grove, IL) with a fine pair of forceps and may be positioned under a dissecting microscope. Checking under a dissecting microscope is useful in order to minimize or remove folds, since folds may introduce pressure artifacts when the slide and teflon are pressed together. Under safelight an emulsion-coated slide is placed over the teflon, and the teflon and the slide are pressed together

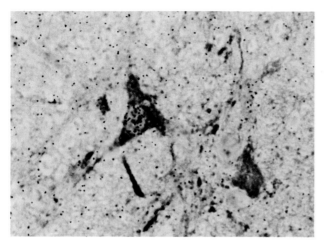

Fig. 15. Thaw-mount autoradiogram of rat lower brain stem prepared 1 h after [³H]estradiol and stained by the immunoperoxidase method with DBH antiserum showing nuclear concentration of [³H]estradiol in DBH-positive neuron of nucleus reticularis lateralis. ×670. (Reproduced from Sar and Stumpf 1981a.)

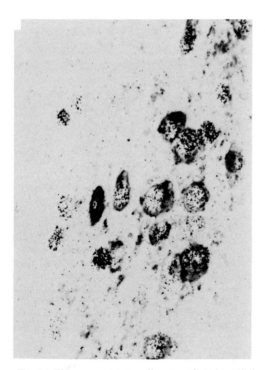

Fig. 16. Thaw-mount autoradiogram of rat hypothalamus prepared 1 h after [³H]estradiol and stained by immunoperoxidase method with tyrosine hydroxylase antibodies. Note the nuclear concentration of [³H]estradiol in tuberoinfundibular dopaminergic neurons. ×950. (Sar, unpublished.)

between the forefingers and thumb. After releasing pressure, the teflon falls off and the tissue adheres to the dried emulsion. The section-mounted slides are then stored in a light-proof desiccator box and exposed at −15°C. After exposure the desiccator box

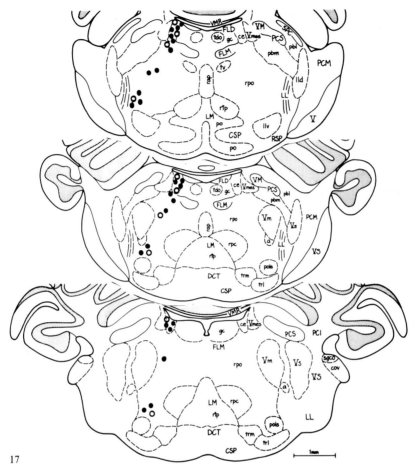

17

Fig. 17 and 18. Schematic drawings (frontal plane) showing immunoreactive dopamine-β-hydroxylase neurons which concentrate [³H]estradiol (●) in pons (Fig. 17) and medulla oblongata (Fig. 18). Some immunoreactive DBH neurons (○) do not show nuclear concentration of radioactivity. (Reproduced from Sar and Stumpf 1981c.) Abbreviations: a = nucleus (n.) alpha; ab = n. ambiguus; ap = area postrema; ce = locus ceruleus; com = n. commissuralis; cov = n. cochlearis ventralis; cum = n. cuneatus medialis; DCT = decussatio corporis trapezoidei; DPY = decussatio pyramidum; FC = fasciculus cuneatus; FLD = fasciculus longitudinalis dorsalis; FLM = fasciculus longitudinalis medialis; gc = griseum centrale; gr = n. gracilis; IAF = fibrae arcuatae internae; LL = lemniscus lateralis; lld = n. lemnisci lateralis dorsalis; llv = n. lemnisci lateralis ventralis; LM = lemniscus medialis; lm = n. reticularis magnocellularis; lp = n. reticularis lateralis parvocellularis; old = n. olivarios accessorius dorsalis; oli = n. olivaris; olm = n. olivaris accessorius medialis; pbl = n. parabrachialis lateralis; pbm = n. parabrachialis medialis; PCI = pedunculus cerebellaris inferior; PCM = pedunculus cerebellaris medius;

with the slides is allowed to equilibrate to room temperature before opening. A slide is removed and the area with the section is breathed on once or twice to moisten the section prior to the photographic development. This assures adherence of the section to the emulsion and prevents loss during photographic development and staining. During the mounting of freeze-dried sections at room temperature, the relative humidity should be between 20 and 40%. If the relative humidity is too high diffusion artifacts and autolysis of tissue may occur, and if it is too low artifacts from electrostatic discharge may result.

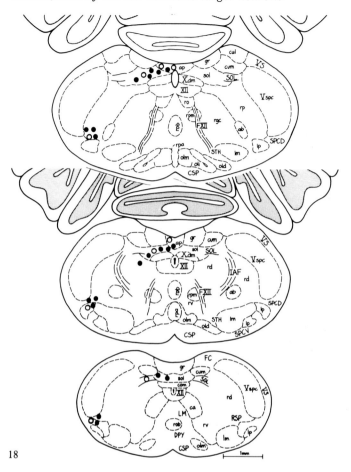

18

PCS = pedunculus cerebellaris superior; po = n. pontis; pols = n. paraolivaris superior; rap = n. raphes pontis; rd = n. reticularis dorsalis medullae oblongata; rgc = n. reticularis gigantocellularis; ro = n. Roller; rob = n. raphe obscusus; rp = n. reticularis parvocellularis; r = n. raphe pallidus; rpc = n. reticularis pontis caudalis; rpm = raphe paramedianus; rpo = n. reticularis pontis oralis; RSP = tractus rubrospinalis; rtp = n. reticularis tegmenti pontis; sgco = substantia gliosa cochlearis; SOL = tractus solitarius; sol = n. tractus solitarii; SPC = tractus spinocerebellaris; SPCD = tractus spinocerebellaris dorsalis; SPCV = tractus spinocerebellaris ventralis; STH = tractus spinothalamicus; tdo = n. tegmentalis dorsalis; trl = n. trapezoides lateralis; trm = trapezoides medialis; tv = n. ventralis thalami; V = nervus trigeminus; VM = tractus mesencephalicus nervi trigemini; Vm = n. motorius nervi trigemini; Vmes = n. tractus mesencephali nervi trigemini; VMR = velum medullare rostrale; VS = tractus spinalis nervi trigemini; Vs = n. sensibilis nervi trigemini; Vspc = n. caudalis tractus spinalis nervi trigemini; Xdm = n. dorsalis motorius nervi vagi; XII = n. nervi hypoglossi.

3. COMBINED AUTORADIOGRAPHY AND FORMALDEHYDE-INDUCED FLUORESCENCE

For simultaneous localization of radioisotopically-labeled substances and catecholamines, autoradiography can be combined with histofluorescence. After injection of radioactively labeled compound, the animals are decapitated at specific times depending on the experimental protocol. The brain is dissected, frozen, and 4–6 μm serial frozen sections are cut and freeze-dried as described in the previous section. After freeze-drying, the sections contained in a Polyvial are exposed for 1–2 h to formaldehyde vapor at 80°C. Formaldehyde vapor is generated by heating paraformaldehyde powder, previously stored for 7–10 days under 50% relative humidity (for details, see Chapter II). The vapor-exposed sections are stored in a desiccator in the dark until dry-mounting. Dry-mounting of sections is done as described in the previous section. After photographic exposure, the slides are developed, fixed and air-dried. The unstained sections are mounted with Entellan and a coverslip and stored in the dark.

The slides are examined with a photo-microscope with fluorescence attachment (Zeiss Mercury lamp HBO w/4-BG-12 excitation and Zeiss '50' emission filters). They are first scanned under ultraviolet light alone to observe and photograph catecholamine cell bodies, fibers and terminals. Once the fluorescing catecholamines are located, a combination of ultraviolet and tungsten light is employed in order to observe the developed silver grains and fluorescing catecholamines simultaneously. Nuclear concentration of radioactivity, representing labeled steroid hormone, is observed as orange-yellow dots over the nuclei of the neurons. The cytoplasm exhibits yellow-green fluorescence which indicates catecholamines.

After fluorescence-microscopy the coverslips may be removed by immersion of the slides in xylene for subsequent staining with methylgreen-pyronin and studied as conventional autoradiograms. In order to avoid artifacts due to possible induction of catecholamine-like fluorescence by the photographic procedure, control freeze-dried sections heated at 80°C but not exposed to formaldehyde gas are dry-mounted on emulsion coated slides and carried through the autoradiographic procedures. The technique has been described in detail (Grant and Stumpf 1981).

4. COMBINED AUTORADIOGRAPHY AND IMMUNOHISTOCHEMISTRY

Both thaw-mount and dry-mount autoradiograms may be used for immunostaining. The immunostaining of autoradiograms consist of the following steps: (a) fixation of exposed slides before autoradiographic development, (b) autoradiographic development, and (c) immunoperoxidase staining. This technique has been described previously (Sar and Stumpf 1979, 1980, 1981b; Stumpf and Sar 1981a).

(a) Fixation of exposed slides before autoradiographic development

After autoradiographic exposure the light-proof slide boxes are removed from the freezer and allowed to assume room temperature. Slides are removed under safelight and fixed for 30-60 sec in 2.5-4% paraformaldehyde solution in 0.01 M phosphate buffer-isotonic saline (PBS), pH 7.5 followed by a brief PBS rinse. Other fixatives, such as 4% buffered formalin or Bouin's fluid may be used. The fixative and PBS are kept at ice temperature. The fixation procedure is the same when dry-mount autoradiograms are used except that the slides are breathed on prior to fixation in order to improve adherence to the emulsion and prevent loss or movement of sections.

(b) Autoradiographic development

After histological fixation the slides are rinsed in PBS and then developed in Kodak D19 developer, diluted 1:1 with PBS, at room temperature for 40-60 sec, rinsed in PBS, and fixed in Kodak fixer for 5 min. After fixation the slides are washed in 2 changes of PBS 5 min each, and subsequently processed for immunostaining.

(c) Immunoperoxidase staining

A modification of the unlabeled antibody technique (Mason et al. 1969; see also, Chapter IV) is applied using the peroxidase-antiperoxidase (PAP) complex (Sternberger 1974). In order to reduce nonspecific staining of autoradiograms by immunoperoxidase staining, the slides are treated either with hydrogen peroxide-egg albumin (Zehr 1978) or phenylhydrazine in PBS pH 7.1 (Straus 1979) followed by egg-albumin. The autoradiograms are incubated with freshly prepared 0.05% phenylhydrazine solution in 0.01 M PBS (pH 7.6), adjusted to pH 7.1 for 1 h at 37°C and washed with 3 changes of PBS 5 min each, followed by a 5-min treatment with egg albumin. After the rinse with PBS, the autoradiograms are incubated with the primary antiserum.

The excess of PBS around the tissue section is wiped off. The primary antibodies raised in rabbit are then applied at optimal dilution over the section. Incubation is carried out at 4°C for 24 or 48 h in a humidified atmosphere. After incubation with the primary antiserum, the slides are washed with PBS and 1% normal sheep serum in PBS for 3 min each followed by incubation for 10 min with second antibodies of sheep anti-rabbit γ-globulin diluted 1:100 (Antibodies Inc., Davis, CA). Following a 3-min wash in PBS the autoradiograms are incubated with rabbit PAP complex (1:50 in PBS) for 20–25 min and washed with PBS for 3 min. The autoradiograms are then incubated for 10 min under constant stirring in the freshly prepared substrate consisting of 200 ml 0.075% diaminobenzidine (DAB) solution in 0.05 M Tris buffer pH 7.6 (Nakane and Pierce 1966) containing 15 μl of 30% hydrogen peroxide. After incubation with the substrate, the slides are washed in Tris buffer and PBS for 3 min each followed by counterstaining with 0.75% methylgreen in PBS. The slides are then dehydrated through ascending grades of alcohol, cleared in 2 changes of xylene and mounted with Permount and a coverslip. Dilution of antisera is made in 0.01 M PBS (pH 7.6) containing 0.1% sodium azide and 1% normal serum of the species in which the second antibodies (anti-γ-globulin) are generated. PAP is diluted in 0.01 M PBS containing 1% normal serum without 0.1% sodium azide, since it inhibits peroxidase activity.

In certain cases the penetration of antibodies into tissue sections may be a limiting factor for immunostaining. For this reason we treat brain sections with 0.3% Triton X-100 in PBS for 5 min, or the antiserum is diluted in PBS containing 0.3% Triton X-100 when autoradiograms are stained for transmitter synthesizing enzymes such as dopamine-β-hydroxylase (DBH) or tyrosine hydroxylase (TH). Treatment with Triton X-100 enhances the immunostaining in certain cases. The specificity of immunostaining of autoradiograms is established by incubating the autoradiograms with preimmune normal serum or with antiserum which has been preabsorbed with the appropriate antigen.

5. APPLICATIONS OF AUTORADIOGRAPHY

Topographical maps on the distribution of target cells for sex and adrenal steroid hormones have been published. Brain autoradiograms were prepared 1 or 2 h after subcutaneous or intravenous injection of tritium labeled hormone with specific activity between 40–120 c/mM at a dose of 0.5–1.0 μg/100 g body weight. The animals were gonadectomized or adrenalectomized at least 48 h prior to the injection of the labeled steroid, in order to diminish endogenous sources of unlabeled hormone. Specificity of hormone localization is generally established by competition studies with injection of unlabeled hormone or its congeners in 100- to 1000-fold excess, prior to the injection of the labeled hormone.

5.1. ESTRADIOL

The distribution of estradiol target cells has been studied in a number of species from different vertebrate classes, including mammals, avians, reptiles, and fishes (for reviews see, Kim et al. 1978; Stumpf and Sar 1976, 1978, 1979, 1981b; Stumpf et al. 1975b, 1976, 1980). There appears to be general agreement regarding the principal sites of accumulation of estradiol concentrating neurons. The intensity of nuclear labeling of hormone varies considerably among cells within a nuclear group, as well as among the different nuclear groups. Glial cells appear unlabeled. Accumulation of estradiol target cells exists in forebrain, midbrain, hindbrain, and spinal cord. The nuclear groups in the forebrain include the n. olfactorius, n. tractus diagonalis, ventral portion of the n. septi lateralis, n. periventricularis, n. paraventricularis, n. supraopticus, zona incerta, n. arcuatus hypothalami, n. ventromedialis hypothalami, n. medialis and corticalis amygdalae, n. centralis amygdalae, hippocampus, certain nuclear groups in the thalamus and n. habenulae lateralis. In the midbrain, hindbrain, and spinal cord, the labeled structures include the central gray, locus ceruleus, n. parabrachialis medialis and lateralis, n. raphae, formatio reticularis, n. tractus solitarii, n. motoris nervi vagi, n. reticularis lateralis and substantia gelatinosa. Ventricular recess organs such as the organun vasculosum laminae terminalis, the subfornicular organ, pineal and area postrema also contain estradiol target cells. The brain distribution of estradiol target cells has been published (Sar and Stumpf 1975b; Stumpf 1968a, 1970b; Stumpf and Sar 1975b; Stumpf et al. 1975a,b).

5.2. ANDROGEN

Results on brain localization of [³H]testosterone and [³H]dihydrotestosterone have been published in the literature (Sar and Stumpf 1972, 1975a, 1977a,b). The topographical distribution of androgen target cells obtained with [³H]dihydro-testosterone in general agrees well with those of [³H]testosterone. However, localization of radioactivity in cells of cerebral cortex has not been observed after [³H]dihydro-testosterone. With 1β–3β[³H]testosterone, Sheridan (1979) observed consistent nuclear concentration of radioactivity in neurons of the nucleus interstitialis striae terminalis and the medial nucleus of the amygdala, suggesting that these are the only sites of androgen-specific action. With [³H]dihydrotestosterone, nuclear concentration of radioactivity is found extensively in neurons at specific hypothalamic and extra-hypothalamic sites. In the forebrain, androgen labeled cells are found in certain nuclei of the lateral septum, preoptic region, anterior and central hypothalamus, epithalamus, amygdala and hippocampus. In the midbrain and hindbrain, a wide distribution of androgen target cells is also reported, with specific localization in motor neurons of cranial nerve nuclei and spinal cord. Target cells are seen in central gray, n. pontis, locus ceruleus, n. raphae, n. dorsalis olivaris accessorius, n. ambiguus, area postrema, n. tractus solitarii and Purkinje cells of the cerebellum. In the spinal cord, target neurons are found in the ventral horn, especially in Lamina IX, as well as in the dorsal horn.

There are several brain sites where a difference in the topographic distribution between androgen and estrogen target cells exists. These include the n. septi lateralis, the hippocampus, the amygdala, the n. ventromedialis hypothalami, the n. pontis, and motor neurons of the cranial nerves and the spinal cord.

5.3. PROGESTIN

Progestin target neurons have been demonstrated in guinea pig hypothalamus after [³H]progesterone (Sar and Stumpf 1973b, 1975b), and in rat hypothalamus after [³H]R5020, a synthetic progestin (Sar and Stumpf 1978b). Estradiol priming has been shown to increase the nuclear uptake of [³H]progesterone or its metabolites. The areas of accumulation of progestin target neurons include n. preopticus medialis, organun vasculosum lamina terminalis, ventrolateral part of the n. ventromedialis hypothalami, n. arcuatus hypothalami, n. interstitialis striae terminalis and n. medialis amygdalae. Recently, progestin target cells in the region of central gray have been reported (Munn et al. 1983).

5.4. CORTICOSTERONE AND ALDOSTERONE

Steroid hormone target cells for gluco- and mineralo-corticosteroids are found in preferentially extrahypothalamic sites (Stumpf and Sar 1978, 1979), while sex steroid hormone target cells are accumulated in both hypothalamic and extrahypothalamic sites (Sar and Stumpf 1972, 1975a,b, 1977a,b; Stumpf 1968a, 1970b). Thaw-mount autoradiograms of the male rat brain, after injection of [³H]corticosterone or [³H]aldosterone, show a nuclear concentration of radioactivity in many neurons and glial cells. An extensive accumulation of target neurons exists in the hippocampus, cortex, amygdala, and in the thalamus, while there is little or no concentration of radioactivity in the preoptic and central hypothalamic neurons. In the midbrain, hindbrain and spinal cord, numerous nuclear groups concentrate hormone in the nuclei of certain neurons. Neurons of reticular formation, and motor neurons of the cranial nerves and spinal cord show heavy concentration of radioactivity. Binding sites for glucocorticoids and mineralocorticoid appear similar, but the binding affinity of these two steroids differs. Also there appears some overlap between the anatomical sites of adrenal steroid hormone target cells and androgen target cells in the brain, such as, hippocampus, amygdala, hindbrain, and spinal cord.

Figures 1-6 show examples of thaw-mount autoradiograms of rat brain prepared after [³H]estradiol (Fig. 1), [³H]dihydrotestosterone (Figs 2-5), and [³H]R5020 (Fig. 6).

6. APPLICATIONS OF COMBINATION TECHNIQUES

6.1. COMBINED AUTORADIOGRAPHY AND FORMALDEHYDE-INDUCED FLUORESCENCE

Effects of sex steroids on gonadal function and behavior have been shown to be mediated in part through interactions with catecholamine producing neurons in the brain (for reviews see, Fuxe et al. 1981; Kalra et al. 1981; McCann et al. 1980). This suggests anatomical relationships between steroid hormone target cells and catecholamine systems in the central nervous system. Through the application of the formaldehyde-induced fluorescence-autoradiography technique, anatomical relationships between steroid hormone target neurons and catecholaminergic systems have been demonstrated (Grant and Stumpf 1975; Heritage et al. 1977, 1981). Nuclear concentration of radioactivity after [³H]estradiol has been shown to exist in dopaminergic neurons in the periventricular-arcuate nucleus of the hypothalamus and in catecholamine neurons of the lower brain stem, such as, n. reticularis lateralis, n. tractus solitarii, ventral tegmental area, and locus ceruleus. In addition, estrogen target neurons appear to be innervated by catecholamine terminals, for instance, in the paraventricular, periventricular, and arcuate nuclei of the hypothalamus, n. tractus solitarii, n. tractus spinalis nervi trigemini and central gray. After [³H]dihydrotestosterone injection, nuclear concentration of radioactivity is observed in catecholamine neurons in the nucleus arcuatus and periventricularis hypothalami, as well as several hindbrain regions, including the n. olivaris inferior, the area dorsomedialis to the n. parabrachialis lateralis, and the locus ceruleus and subceruleus. In addition, in several brain regions [³H]dihydrotestosterone neurons appear to be innervated by catecholamine terminals.

Figures 7-10 show examples of catecholaminergic estrogen neurons (Figs 7-9) and catecholaminergic androgen neurons (Fig. 10).

6.2. COMBINED AUTORADIOGRAPHY AND IMMUNOHISTOCHEMISTRY

Using the combined techniques of autoradiography and immunohistochemistry (Sar and Stumpf 1981b) we have demonstrated morphological relationships between steroid hormone target cells and peptidergic neurons or catecholaminergic neurons (Sar and Stumpf 1980, 1981a,c). Autoradiograms of mouse hypothalamus, prepared after [³H]estradiol and stained by the immunoperoxidase method with neurophysin I antiserum, revealed positive staining in some estradiol target neurons of supraoptic and paraventricular nuclei (Sar and Stumpf 1980). Antiserum to vasopressin also showed immunostaining of estradiol target cells in these two nuclei (Sar and Stumpf 1980). Similarly, in the guinea pig, estradiol target neurons of the preoptic-periventricular nucleus and supraoptic nucleus revealed immunostaining with neurophysin I antiserum.

Certain peptidergic neurons are difficult to detect by immunostaining under normal conditions. Colchicine treatment has been shown to enhance perikaryal staining of enkephalin neurons (Sar et al. 1978). Simultaneous localization of labeled steroid hormone and antibodies to certain neuropeptides can, therefore, be demonstrated by treating the animals with colchicine prior to the administration of tritium labeled steroid hormone. Colchicine treatment does not appear to block the nuclear uptake of radioactivity in neurons after [³H]estradiol. Recently, a pilot experiment was conducted in order to find out if somatostatin producing cells are target for estradiol. Preliminary results in colchicine treated rats demonstrate that certain neurons of the n. periventricularis hypothalami that contained radioactivity in their nuclei after [³H]estradiol, show immunostaining of perikarya with somatostatin antibodies in a few of these neurons (Sar and Stumpf 1983).

Furthermore, with the combination technique of autoradiography and immunohistochemistry, we have demonstrated DBH-positive cells that concentrate [³H]estradiol in the locus ceruleus, lateral tegmental area, nucleus tractus solitarii and nucleus reticularis lateralis (Sar and Stumpf 1981a,c). Similarly, tuberoinfundibular dopaminergic neurons have been shown to concentrate [³H]estradiol in their nuclei. This was also observed when [³H]estradiol autoradiograms of rat hypothalamus were immunostained with tyrosine hydroxylase antibodies (Sar, unpublished observation). These results suggest a genomic action of estradiol in noradrenergic and in dopaminergic neurons. The applications of combination techniques will provide important information on the interaction of steroid hormone(s) with peptidergic and aminergic systems in the central nervous system. Association of steroid hormone with its receptor protein can be demonstrated utilizing [³H]estradiol and estradiol receptor antibodies.

Examples are presented of simultaneous localization of [³H]estradiol and peptidergic neurons (Figs 11–12), noradrenergic neurons (Figs 13–15), and dopaminergic neurons (Fig. 16) in the same section of rat brain. Figures 17 and 18 show topographic distribution of DBH-positive cells that concentrate [³H]estradiol in rat lower brain stem.

7. REFERENCES

Baulieu EE, Atger M, Best-Belpomme M, Corvol P, Courvalin JC, Mester J, Milgrom E, Robel P, Rochefort H, DeCatalogne D (1975): Steroid hormone receptors. *Vitam. Horm. (NY), 33,* 649–731.

Bereiter DA, Barker DJ (1975): Facial receptive fields of trigeminal neurons: Increased size following estrogen treatment in female rats. *Neuroendocrinology, 18,* 115–124.

Dörner G (1980): Sex hormone dependent brain differentiation and sexual behavior. In: Wuttke W, Horowski R (Eds), *Gonadal Steroids and Brain Function, Exp. Brain Res., Suppl. 3,* pp. 208–221. Springer-Verlag, New York.

Eisenfeld AJ, Axelrod J (1965): Selectivity of estrogen distribution in tissues. *J. Pharmacol. Exp. Ther., 150,* 469–475.

Fuxe K, Anderson K, Blake CA, Eneroth P, Gustafsson JA, Agnati LF (1981): Effects of estrogen and combined treatment with estrogen and progesterone on central dopamine, noradrenaline and adrenaline nerve terminal systems of the ovariectomized rat. Relationship of changes in LH and prolactin secretion and in sexual behavior. In: Fuxe K, Gustafsson J-A, Wetterberg L (Eds), *Steroid Hormone Regulation of the Brain,* pp. 73–92. Pergamon Press, New York.

Gorski J, Gannon F (1976): Current models of steroid hormone action: Critique. *Annu. Rev. Physiol., 32,* 422–450.

Gorski RA, Yanase M (1980): Estrogen facilitation of lordosis behavior in the female rat. In: Wuttke W, Horowski R (Eds), *Gonadal Steroids and Brain Function, Exp. Brain Res., Suppl. 3,* pp. 222–237. Springer-Verlag, New York.

Grant LD, Stumpf WE (1975): Hormone uptake sites in relation to CNS biogenic amine systems. In: Stumpf WE, Grant LD (Eds), *Anatomical Neuroendocrinology,* pp. 445–464. S. Karger, Basel.

Grant LD, Stumpf WE (1981): Combined autoradiography and formaldehyde-induced fluorescence methods for localization of radioactively labeled substances in relation to monoamine neurons. *J. Histochem. Cytochem., 29/1A,* 175–180.

Heritage AS, Grant LD, Stumpf WE (1977): (³H)-estradiol in catecholamine neurons of rat brain stem: Combined localization by autoradiography and formaldehyde-induced fluorescence. *J. Comp. Neurol., 176,* 607–630.

Heritage AS, Stumpf WE, Sar M, Grant LD (1980): Brain stem catecholamine neurons are target sites for sex steroid hormones. *Science, 207,* 1377–1379.

Heritage AS, Stumpf WE, Sar M, Grant LD (1981): (³H)-dihydrotestosterone in catecholamine neurons of rat brain stem: Combined localization by autoradiography and formaldehyde-induced fluorescence. *J. Comp. Neurol., 200,* 289–307.

Jensen EV, Desombre ER (1972): Mechanism of action of the female sex hormones. *Ann. Rev. Biochem., 41,* 203–230.

Kalra SP, Kalra PS, Simpkins JW (1981): Regulation of LHRH secretion by gonadal steroids and catecholamines. In: McKerns KW (Ed), *Reproductive Processes and Contraception,* pp. 27–46. Plenum Press, New York.

Kato J (1975): The role of hypothalamic and hypophyseal 5α-dihydrotestosterone, estradiol and progesterone receptors in the mechanism of feedback action. *J. Steroid Biochem., 6,* 979–988.

Kato J, Onouchi T (1977): Specific progesterone receptors in the hypothalamus and anterior hypophysis of the rat. *Endocrinology, 101,* 920–928.

Kim YS, Stumpf WE, Sar M, Martinez-Vargas MC (1978): Estrogen and androgen target cells in the brain of fishes, reptiles and birds: Phylogeny and ontogeny. *Am. Zool., 18,* 425–433.

Larsson K, Beyer C (1981): Sex steroid hormones and sexual behavior. In: Fuxe K, Gustafsson J-A, Wetterberg L (Eds), *Steroid Hormone Regulation of the Brain,* pp. 279–291. Pergamon Press, New York.

Mason TE, Phifer RF, Spicer SS, Swallow RA, Dreskin RB (1969): An immunoglobulin-enzyme bridge method for localizing tissue antigens. *J. Histochem. Cytochem., 7,* 563–569.

McCann SM, Negro-Villar A, Ojeda SR, Advis JP, Lumpkin M, Sammson WK, Vizayan E (1980): Steroid effects on hypothalamic-gonadotropin interactions. In: Wuttke PW, Horowski R (Eds), *Gonadal Steroids and Brain Function, Exp. Brain Res., Suppl. 3,* pp. 142–150. Springer-Verlag, New York.

Munn AR, Sar M, Stumpf WE (1983): Topographic distribution of progestin target cells in hamster brain and pituitary after injection of [³H]R5020. *Brain Res;* in press.

Nakane PK, Pierce Jr GB (1966): Enzyme-labeled antibodies: Preparation and application in the localization of antigens. *J. Histochem. Cytochem., 14,* 929–931.

O'Malley BW, Means AR (1974): Female steroid hormones and target cell nuclei. *Science, 183,* 610–620.

Sar M, Liao S, Stumpf WE (1970): Nuclear concentration of androgens in rat seminal vesicles and prostate by autoradiography. *Endocrinology, 86,* 1008–1011.

Sar M, Stumpf WE (1972): Cellular localization of androgen in the brain and pituitary after the injection of tritiated testosterone. *Experientia, 28,* 1364–1136.

Sar M, Stumpf WE (1973a): Pituitary gonadotropins: Nuclear concentration of radioactivity after injection of ³H-testosterone. *Science, 179,* 389–391.

Sar M, Stumpf WE (1973b): Neurons of the hypothalamus concentrate ³H-progesterone or metabolites of it. *Science, 182,* 1266–1268.

Sar M, Stumpf WE (1974): Cellular and subcellular localization of ³H-progesterone or its metabolites in the oviduct, uterus, vagina and liver of the guinea pig. *Endocrinology, 94,* 1116–1125.

Sar M, Stumpf WE (1975a): Distribution of androgen-concentrating neurons in rat brain. In: Stumpf WE and Grant HLD (Eds), *Anatomical Neuroendocrinology,* pp. 120–133. S. Karger, Basel.

Sar M, Stumpf WE (1975b): Cellular localization of progestin and estrogen in guinea pig hypothalamus by autoradiography. In: Stumpf WE, Grant LD (Eds), *Anatomical Neuroendocrinology,* pp. 142–152. S. Karger, Basel.

Sar M, Stumpf WE (1976): Autoradiography of mammary glands and uteri of mice and rats after injection of ³H-estradiol. *J. Steroid Biochem., 7,* 391–394.

Sar M, Stumpf WE (1977a): Androgen concentration in motor neurons of cranial nerves and spinal cord. *Science, 197,* 77–79.

Sar M, Stumpf WE (1977b): Distribution of androgen target cells in rat forebrain and pituitary after ³H-dihydrotestosterone administration. *J. Steroid Biochem., 8,* 1131–1135.

Sar M, Stumpf WE (1978a): Simultaneous localization of neurophysin I and ³H-estradiol in hypothalamic neurons using a combined autoradiographic and immunohistochemical technique. *J. Histochem. Cytochem., 26,* 277.

Sar M, Stumpf WE (1978b): Progestin-target cells in rat brain and pituitary. *J. Steroid Biochem., 9,* 877.

Sar M, Stumpf WE (1979): Simultaneous localization of steroid and peptide hormones in rat pituitary by combined thaw-mount autoradiography and immunohistochemistry: Localization of dihydrotestosterone in gonadotropes, thyrotropes and pituicytes. *Cell Tissue Res., 203,* 1–7.

Sar M, Stumpf WE (1980): Simultaneous localization of ³H-estradiol and neurophysin I or arginine vasopressin in hypothalamic neurons demonstrated by a combined technique of dry-mount autoradiography and immunohistochemistry. *Neurosci. Lett., 17,* 179–184.

Sar M, Stumpf WE (1981a): Central noradrenergic neurons concentrate ³H-estradiol. *Nature, 289,* 500–502.

Sar M, Stumpf WE (1981b): Combined autoradiography and immunohistochemistry for simultaneous localization of radioactively labeled steroid hormones and antibodies in the brain. *J. Histochem. Cytochem., 29/1A,* 161–166.

Sar M, Stumpf WE (1981c): Estradiol concentration in dopamine-β-hydroxylase containing neurons of lower brain stem demonstrated by combined autoradiography and immunohistochemistry. In: Wuttke W, Horowski R (Eds), *Gonadal Steroids and Brain Function, Exp. Brain Res., Suppl., 3,* pp. 29–36. Springer-Verlag, Berlin.

Sar M, Stumpf WE (1983): Simultaneous localization of steroid hormones and neuropeptides in the brain by combined autoradiography and immunocytochemistry. In: Conn PM (Ed), *Methods in Enzymology, Hormone Action: Neuropeptides.* Academic Press, New York. In press.

Sar M, Stumpf WE, McLean WS, Smith AA, Hanssonn V, Nayfeh SN, French FS (1975): Localization of androgen target cells in the rat testis: Autoradiographic studies. In: French FS, Hansson V, Ritzen EM, Nayfeh SN (Eds), *Hormonal Regulation of Spermatogenesis,* pp. 311–319. Plenum Press, New York.

Sar M, Stumpf WE, Miller RJ, Chang K-J, Guatrecasas P (1978): Immunohistochemical localization of enkephalin in rat brain and spinal cord. *J. Comp. Neurol., 182,* 17–37.

Sheridan PJ (1979): The nucleus interstitialis striae terminalis and the nucleus amygdaloideus medialis: Prime targets for androgen in the forebrain. *Endocrinology, 104,* 130–136.

Sternberger LA (1974): *Immunocytochemistry.* Prentice Hall, Englewood Cliffs, NJ.

Straus W (1979): Peroxidase procedures: Technical problems encountered during their application. *J. Histochem. Cytochem., 27,* 1349–1351.

Stumpf WE (1968a): Estradiol concentrating neurons: Topography in the hypothalamus by dry-mount autoradiography. *Science, 162,* 1001–1003.

Stumpf WE (1968b): Cellular and subcellular ^{3}H-estradiol localization in the pituitary by autoradiography. *Z. Zellforsch. Mikrosk. Anat., 92,* 23–33.

Stumpf WE (1968c): Subcellular distribution of ^{3}H-estradiol in rat uterus by quantitative autoradiography. A comparison between ^{3}H-estradiol and ^{3}H-norethynodrel. *Endocrinology, 83,* 777–782.

Stumpf WE (1969): Nuclear concentration of ^{3}H-estradiol in target tissues. Dry-mount autoradiography of vagina, oviduct, ovary, testis, mammary tumor, liver and adrenal. *Endocrinology, 85,* 31–37.

Stumpf WE (1970a): Localization of hormones by autoradiography and other histochemical techniques: A critical review. *J. Histochem. Cytochem., 18,* 21–29.

Stumpf WE (1970b): Estrogen-neurons and estrogen-neuron systems in the periventricular brain. *Am. J. Anat., 129,* 207–218.

Stumpf WE (1971): Autoradiographic techniques for the localization of hormones and drugs at the cellular and subcellular level. In: Diczfalusy E (Ed), *Proceedings, Third Karolinska Symposium on In Vitro Methods in Reproductive Cell Biology, Acta Endocrinol. (Copenhagen), Suppl. 153,* 205–222.

Stumpf WE (1976): Techniques for the autoradiography of diffusible compounds. In: Prescott DM (Ed), *Methods in Cell Biology, Vol. 13,* pp. 171–193. Academic Press, New York.

Stumpf WE, Roth LJ (1964): Vacuum freeze-drying of frozen sections for dry-mounting, high-resolution autoradiography. *Stain Technol, 39,* 219–233.

Stumpf WE, Roth LJ (1966): High resolution autoradiography with drymounted, freeze-dried, frozen sections. Comparative study of six methods using two diffusible compounds, ^{3}H-estradiol and ^{3}H-mesobilirubinogen. *J. Histochem. Cytochem., 14,* 274–287.

Stumpf WE, Sar M (1971): Estradiol concentrating neurons in the amygdala. *Proc. Soc. Exp. Biol. Med., 136,* 102–106.

Stumpf WE, Sar M (1975a): Autoradiographic techniques for localizing steroid hormones. In: O'Malley BW, Hardman JG (Eds), *Method in Enzymology, Vol. 36, Hormone Action, Part A: Steroid Hormones,* pp. 135–156. Academic Press, New York.

Stumpf WE, Sar M (1975b): Hormone architecture of mouse brain with ^{3}H-estradiol. In: Stumpf WE, Grant LD (Eds), *Anatomical Neuroendocrinology,* pp. 254–261. S. Karger, Basel.

Stumpf WE, Sar M (1976): Autoradiographic localization of estrogen, androgen, progestin and glucocorticosteroid in 'target tissues' and 'non-target tissues'. In: Pasqualini J (Ed), *Receptors and Mechanism of Action of Steroid Hormones, Modern Pharmacology-Toxicology, Vol. 8,* pp. 41–84. Marcel Dekker, New York.

Stumpf WE, Sar M (1978): Anatomical distribution of estrogen, androgen, progestin, corticosteroid and thyroid hormone target sites in the brain of mammals: Phylogeny and Ontogeny. *Am. Zool., 18,* 435–445.

Stumpf WE, Sar M (1979): Glucocorticosteroid and mineral corticosteroid hormone target sites in the brain: Autoradiographic studies with corticosterone, aldosterone and dexamethasone. In: Jones MT, Dallman MF, Gillham B, Chattopadhyay S (Eds), *Interactions Within the Brain-Pituitary Adrenocortical System,* pp. 137–147. Academic Press, New York.

Stumpf WE, Sar M (1981a): Brain localization of hormones and drugs by thaw-mount autoradiography, combined autoradiography-formaldehyde induced fluorescence and combined autoradiography-immunohistochemistry. In: Heym Ch, Forssmann WG (Eds), pp. 245–254. Springer-Verlag, Heidelberg.

Stumpf WE, Sar M (1981b): Steroid hormone sites of action in the brain. In: Fuxe K, Gustafsson J-A, Wetterberg L (Eds), pp. 41–50. Pergamon Press, New York.

Stumpf WE, Sar M, Keefer DA (1975a): Atlas of estrogen target cells in rat brain. In: Stumpf WE, Grant LD (Eds), *Anatomical Neuroendocrinology,* pp. 104–119. S. Karger, Basel.

Stumpf WE, Sar M, Keefer DA (1975b): Anatomical distribution of estrogen in the central nervous system of mouse, rat, tree shrew and squirrel monkey. In: Raspe N (Ed), *Advances in Biosciences, Vol. 15,* pp. 77–88. Pergamon Press, New York.

Stumpf WE, Sar M, Keefer DA, Martinez-Vargas MC (1976): The anatomical substrate of neuroendocrine regulation as defined by autoradiography with ^{3}H-estradiol, ^{3}H-testosterone, ^{3}H-dihydrotestosterone and ^{3}H-progesterone. In: Anand-Kumar TC (Ed), *Neuroendocrine Regulation of Fertility,* pp. 46–56. S. Karger, Basel.

Stumpf WE, Sar M, Kim YS, Keefer DA, Martinez-Vargas MC (1980): Evolutionary aspects of estrogen-sensitive structures in the forebrain. In: Pang PKT, Epple A (Eds), *Evolution of Vertebrate Endocrine Systems,* pp. 85–93. Texas Tech University Press, Lubbock, Texas.

Toran-Allerand CD (1978): Gonadal hormones and brain development: Cellular aspects of sexual differentiation. *Am. Zool., 18,* 553–565.

Zehr DR (1978): Use of hydrogen peroxide-egg albumin to eliminate nonspecific staining in immunoperoxidase techniques. *J. Histochem. Cytochem., 26,* 415–416.

CHAPTER XII

Chemical lesioning techniques: Monoamine neurotoxins*

G. JONSSON

1. INTRODUCTION

Various kinds of lesion techniques and procedures have since long been employed to explore the structural organization and function of the nervous system. The use of chemicals to produce neuronal lesions experimentally was also introduced many years ago, at the end of the last century, although it is only in recent years that this approach has come to be of significant importance in neurobiological research. The first chemical neurotoxins used to induce lesions were $CuSO_4$ and $AgCl$. They are generally cytotoxic in high concentrations and when injected locally into the brain can produce neuronal damage. However, this technique tended to give lesions of unpredictable size, shape and histological characteristics; therefore, it never became popular and, in addition, did not offer any advantages compared to other nonselective lesion techniques (surgical, electrolytic, thermal) that have been developed and extensively used over the years (see, Carpenter and Whittier 1952; Routtenberg 1972; Moore 1978). With the general progress in the knowledge of histo- and biochemical properties of the nervous tissue, in particular those concerning transmitter identified neuronal systems, it was realized that the conventional nonselective lesion techniques are crude and possess many limitations, both with respect to specificity (neuronal versus non-neuronal; classes of neurons) and other unwanted side effects. It therefore became clear that in order to obtain information on more precise neuronal structure-function relationships, it was necessary to have lesion techniques with a target-directed neurodegenerative action making it possible to induce lesions of particular classes of neurons, defined with respect to their chemical messenger (transmitter). The breakthrough in this field was the discovery by Tranzer and Thoenen (1967, 1968) that the noradrenaline (NA) analogue 6-hydroxydopamine (6-OH-DA; 2,4,5-trihydroxyphenylethylamine) could induce an acute and selective degeneration of sympathetic adrenergic nerve terminals with a concomitant loss of neuronal function in many sympathetically innervated organs. Soon after the report of Tranzer and Thoenen (1967) it could be demonstrated that this neurotoxin could be used for the selective denervation of catecholamine (NA and dopamine = DA) neuron systems in the CNS (Ungerstedt 1968; Uretsky and Iversen 1969; Bloom et al. 1969). A few years later Baumgarten and co-workers (Baumgarten et al. 1971, 1972, 1973; Baumgarten and Lachenmeyer 1972) succeeded in discovering and introducing the serotonin (5-hydroxytryptamine = 5-HT) neurotoxins

*Parts of the studies reviewed in this chapter have been supported by grants from the Swedish MRC (04X-2295), Bergvalls Stiftelse, Karolinska Institutet, and Expressen's prenatalforskningsnämnd.

Handbook of Chemical Neuroanatomy. Vol. 1: Methods in Chemical Neuroanatomy.
A. Björklund and T. Hökfelt, editors.
© Elsevier Science Publishers B.V., 1983.

5,6- and 5,7-dihydroxytryptamine (5,6-HT; 5,7-HT) for the selective degeneration of central 5-HT neurons. After their introduction these monoamine neurotoxins (6-OH-DA; 5,6-HT; 5,7-HT) have been extensively used for neuroanatomical studies and analysis of various aspects of monoamine neurotransmitter functions (see, Malmfors and Thoenen 1971; Jonsson et al. 1975; Jacoby and Lytle 1978; Chubb and Geffen 1979). They can be considered to have become standards tools for the experimental production of selective lesions of both the central and peripheral monoamine neuronal systems.

The aim of the present chapter is to review the use of monoamine neurotoxins as denervation tools in both adult and developing animals. The excitotoxic amino acids are dealt with by Coyle and Schwarcz (Chapter XIII). The content will focus mainly on the applicability, certain technical and specificity aspects as well as limitations and pitfalls of using the monoamine neurotoxin denervation techniques. Some more recently discovered neurotoxins that act on monoamine neurons will also be dealt with. The chapter will start with a brief description of certain features of the response of neurons to a damage which form the basis for the use of the lesion approach to study neuronal structure and function. Finally, the chapter will end with a more general discussion on procedures for the evaluation of specificity and extent of neurotoxin induced lesions as well as interpretation problems associated with effects seen following the degeneration of a neuronal system.

2. NEURONAL DEGENERATION PROCESSES

The neuron is a highly differentiated cell which has lost the property of dividing and responds to a damage in a specific manner. This fact forms the basis for the lesion approach to study the neuronal structure and function. Depending on the site and type of damage the degenerative reactions can vary considerably both with respect to time-course and end-result in the chronic state. A transection of the axon (axotomy) will always (in vertebrates) result in a degeneration and disappearance of the distal part (see Fig. 1) which is separated from the soma containing the biochemical machinery responsible for the manufacture of structural and functional macromolecules crucial for the viability of the cell-body and its processes. This degeneration process is denoted *anterograde* or *Wallerian degeneration* which will lead to a denervation of target or effector cells that originally were innervated by the axotomized neuron. Since the axotomy-induced disruption of the connection between neuron and effector cell will prevail for some time and, in most cases, be more or less permanent in the CNS, it will allow the investigator to obtain information on neuronal structure-function relationships. The time-course of the anterograde degeneration varies with species, length of the separated axonal stump and type of neuron. Generally speaking, the most rapid degeneration occurs in unmyelinated fibers and the shorter the axonal stump the faster the process (see, Sachs and Jonsson 1973b). In addition to the anterograde degeneration, an axotomy will in most cases be followed by a series of morphological alterations in the soma that are collectively called the *axon reaction* or 'cell-body response' (see, Lieberman 1971; Grafstein and McQuarrie 1978). These changes involve chromatolysis (dissolution of Nissl substance), swelling and rounding of the soma, eccentricity of the nucleus and often enlargement of the nucleolus. Moreover, there may be a retraction of synapses from the soma and dendrites of the axotomized neuron as well as a proliferation of the glial processes around the soma (see, Barron et al. 1981). The intensity

464

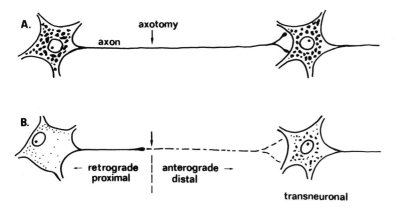

Fig. 1. Schematic illustration of degeneration processes in neurons following axotomy: (A) Normal situation; (B) After *axotomy* at the indicated site (↓). The distal part of the divided axon will always degenerate (*anterograde* or *Wallerian degeneration*) and the speed of this process varies with length of the distal stump and between different categories of neurons. Proximal to the axotomy there is in most neurons a limited *retrograde degeneration* of the distal part of the proximal stump together with an *axon reaction* (chromatolysis, soma swelling and nuclear eccentricity). This reaction is sometimes very severe and will lead to cell death, in particular in developing neurons or after an axotomy close to the soma. In certain neuronal systems *transneuronal degeneration (anterograde* or *retrograde)* may also occur. Anterograde transneuronal degeneration is indicated.

of the axon reaction can vary between different species and classes of neurons (e.g. central, peripheral) and is generally more pronounced the closer the lesion is situated to the cell-body as well as in developing neurons as compared to adult mature neurons (see, Lieberman 1974). The exact signal(s) initiating the axon reaction is unknown, although there are data indicating that the retrograde axoplasmic transport system is involved and that a DNA-dependent RNA-synthesis seems to play a key role (Bisby 1980; Cragg 1970; Grafstein and Forman 1980; Kreutzberg 1981). Whether the retrogradely transported signal is related to the delivery of an agent generated by the axotomy or to a failure to continue the delivery of a normal axonal constituent originating from the target cell is at present unknown. Although the currently held view is that the axon reaction response reflects a switch of command program of the neuron to regeneration and repair processes, it has been observed that the frog spinal cord neurons can start to regenerate without any obvious signs of axon reaction (Carlsen et al. 1982). As to the central monoamine neurons, the data so far available indicate that in contrast to the peripheral sympathetic adrenergic nerves they do not display any classic axon reaction after a lesion, although some changes are observed ultrastructurally (Cheah and Geffen 1973; Reis et al. 1978). It is, however, well established that the monoamine neurons in the CNS exhibit a remarkable sprouting and regrowth capacity (see, Björklund and Stenevi 1979).

There are also alterations in the proximal stump following an axotomy, although these are generally not very pronounced and in many cases only observed as a limited degeneration of the most distal part of the proximal stump. This retrograde degeneration process can, however, sometimes be so extensive that it leads to cell death and complete disappearance of the perikaryon. Such a situation is most frequently seen in developing animals and when the axotomy is very close to the perikaryon. The latter phenomenon is considered to be related to the close axotomy leaving no collateral branches of the axon proximal to the lesion.

Finally, it is now well established that the degenerative alterations following a lesion are not always confined to the damaged neuron, but can also be seen to occur in neurons in direct or indirect synaptic contact with the lesioned neuron. This kind of degeneration is called *transneuronal* or *transsynaptic degeneration* and can be either anterograde or retrograde in nature (see Fig. 1). Transneuronal degeneration has only been reported to occur in certain neuronal systems (see, Smith and Kreutzberg 1976; Pinching and Powell 1971; Ghetti et al. 1975; Hattori and Fibiger 1982), but might be more frequent than generally considered. It is obvious that this degeneration phenomenon represents a potential problem when using the lesion approach as a strategy for establishing structure-function relationships, in particular when using lesions to localize the neuronal origin of various histo- and biochemical markers. Concerning the type of damage that neurotoxic monoamines produce, most of the degenerative processes described above have been observed after a neurotoxin administration, although the time-course and end-result can vary considerably depending on the type of neurotoxin and route of administration determining the site(s) of the neurodegenerative action.

3. CATECHOLAMINE NEUROTOXINS

Following the introduction of 6-OH-DA more than 15 yr ago, a large number of 6-OH-DA related compounds have been synthesized and tested, but none of them has so far been found to be superior to 6-OH-DA as a denervation tool (see, Tranzer and Thoenen 1973; Lundström et al. 1973; Breese 1975). Of these only 6-OH-DOPA and 6-aminodopamine (6-NH$_2$-DA, Fig. 2) have been used to a certain extent. In recent years another class of catecholamine neurotoxins have been introduced, namely the β-halobenzylamines, whose derivatives DSP4 and xylamine (see Fig. 2) have attracted the greatest interest. However, 6-OH-DA is still the best characterized catecholamine neurotoxin and, in addition, appears to have the most general applicability. A great deal of the information available on the use of 6-OH-DA as a denervation tool also has a more general value when employing other chemical neurotoxins for producing lesions in experimental work.

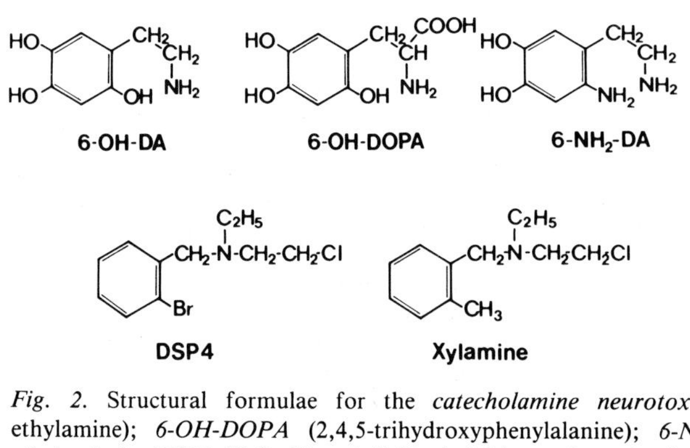

Fig. 2. Structural formulae for the *catecholamine neurotoxins 6-OH-DA* (2,4,5-trihydroxyphenyl-ethylamine); *6-OH-DOPA* (2,4,5-trihydroxyphenylalanine); *6-NH$_2$-DA* (2-amino-4,5-dihydroxyphenyl-ethylamine); *DSP4* (N-(2-chlorethyl)-N-ethyl-2-bromobenzylamine; Xylamine (N-(2-chloroethyl)-N-ethyl-2-methyl-benzylamine.

3.1. 6-HYDROXYDOPAMINE

Mode and mechanism of action

The generally accepted view is that there are two characteristics which are of crucial importance for the selective neurodegenerative action of 6-OH-DA on catecholamine neurons. First, 6-OH-DA is very efficiently taken up and accumulated intraneuronally because of a relatively high affinity to the carrier of the amine uptake mechanism localized at the axonal membrane normally acting to take up and inactivate released catecholamines (Thoenen and Tranzer 1968; Jonsson and Sachs 1971; Ljungdahl et al. 1971). This uptake mechanism is an exclusive constituent of catecholamine neurons and thus accounts for the specificity of 6-OH-DA. Second, 6-OH-DA is very easily auto-oxidized due to a low redox-potential leading to the formation of several potentially cytotoxic molecular species. The selective accumulation of 6-OH-DA is thus responsible for the *specificity*, while the oxidation reactions are related to the *cytotoxic* and *degenerative* actions of the neurotoxin (see, Sachs and Jonsson 1975a; Jonsson 1980). A reflection of this is the observation that 6-OH-NA, in spite of its similar chemical properties to 6-OH-DA, is ineffective as a selective neurodegenerative agent, most likely due to it not being accumulated in adrenergic neurons (Sachs 1973).

Since the uptake mechanism is present in the plasma membrane of the whole neuron, the cytotoxic attack can in principle be on any part of the neuron depending on how the neurotoxin is administered. Experimental data have shown, however, that the axonal nerve terminals are in general the most sensitive structures, while axons are less so and the cell-bodies the least susceptible to neurotoxic action (Malmfors and Sachs 1968; Jonsson and Sachs 1970). Such a differential sensitivity exists for most monoamine neurotoxins (see Fig. 3). The reason for the differential sensitivity between various

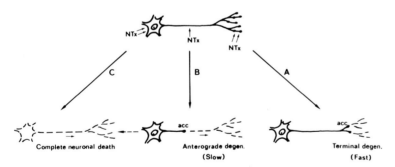

Fig. 3. Schematic illustration of degeneration processes in a monoamine neuron after administration of a monoamine neurotoxin (NTx) acting at different sites. (A) The action of the neurotoxin is mainly at the nerve terminal level leading to a rapid (within hours) degeneration of the terminals with a concomitant accumulation of transmitter and organelles in non-terminal axons (acc.). This type of degenerations is seen, i.e. in sympathetic adrenergic nerves after systemic 6-OH-DA treatment (see also Fig. 4). (B) Following neurotoxin administration over the axon (e.g. after local intracerebral injection) there will be an anterograde degeneration of the distal part of the neuron due to the induced 'chemical axotomy'. This process is relatively slow and will take several days to become completed. Soon after the neurotoxin application there will in addition be a transmitter accumulation in the proximal part of the axon (acc.). If the chemical axotomy is close to the perikaryon a complete degeneration and disappearance of the neuron is likely to occur (←---). (C) Action of the neurotoxin on the perikaryon after local application leads to a complete degeneration of the whole neuron where the axon undergoes anterograde degeneration. It is conceivable that the degeneration of the soma is often caused in this situation by a combination of the effect of a 'close axotomy' and a direct neurotoxic action on the perikaryon. The time-course is in the order of weeks for a complete cell death.

parts of the neuron is not exactly known. In the case of 6-OH-DA it may possibly be explained on the basis of differences in surface-volume relationships, local circulation and diffusion conditions, uptake-accumulation properties and/or certain interneuronal factors interfering with the auto-oxidation reaction of 6-OH-DA (see, Jonsson 1980; Sachs et al. 1975).

Studies on the effects of 6-OH-DA in adrenergic nerve terminals have shown that the neurotoxic actions are initiated when 6-OH-DA reaches a critical concentration intraneuronally (Thoenen and Tranzer 1968; Jonsson and Sachs 1970; Jonsson 1976a). This threshold concentration, which is most likely related to that in the extragranular space, has been calculated to be about 50-100 mM 6-OH-DA (average cytoplasmic concentration; Jonsson 1976a). Consistent with the view of a threshold concentration, it has generally been observed that 6-OH-DA acts mainly in an 'all-or-none' fashion. There is thus a complete disappearance of the biochemical and functional properties in a proportion of adrenergic nerves related to the dose of 6-OH-DA administered, while nerve terminals which have been spared by the neurotoxin display apparently normal properties (Jonsson and Sachs 1972; Jonsson 1976a). Although there is so far little evidence indicating that 6-OH-DA can produce a transient damage of the neuron which is not associated with true degeneration from a structural and biochemical standpoint, such a situation cannot always be excluded and should be watched for.

6-OH-DA can be taken up, stored and released from the amine storage granules, acting like a 'false transmitter'. This action is, however, only seen after low non-degenerative doses (see, Thoenen and Tranzer 1968). The fact that 6-OH-DA has a relatively high affinity for the amine storage granules (Jonsson and Sachs 1971), in conjunction with its ease of oxidation it can be used to identify these structures at the ultrastructural level very early after the 6-OH-DA administration (1 h or less; Bennett et al. 1970; Cobb and Bennett 1971). Granular uptake and storage of 6-OH-DA does not appear to be a prerequisite for the cytotoxic action, although this process might have some minor modulatory effect.

The neurodegenerative effects of 6-OH-DA are initiated very early after its administration, as reflected by a rapid (within 0.5-1 h) and almost complete disappearance of the catecholamine stores, impairment of the uptake properties and a loss of the ability to generate and conduct action potentials (Thoenen and Tranzer 1968; Jonsson and Sachs 1970; Häuesler 1971; Furness et al. 1970). The neurotoxic action of 6-OH-DA is revealed by fluorescence histochemistry (according to Falck-Hillarp for demonstration of NA) as a rapid (within 1-2 h) and long-lasting disappearance of fluorescent NA nerve terminals which is accompanied by pronounced accumulations of transmitter in nonterminal axons (Malmfors and Sachs 1968; Jonsson and Sachs 1970; see also Figs 3 and 4). These accumulations show up in a few hours after the neurotoxin administration and are related to the damage of the nerve terminals leading to a 'pileup' of transmitter in intact axons as a result of the ongoing axoplasmic transport of NA-containing storage granules formed in the soma. The transmitter accumulations seen in monoamine axons after monoamine neurotoxins can be considered as a relatively sensitive index for degenerative effects on the nerve terminals, although not exclusively related to such an action. Transmitter accumulations will also be observed proximal to the site of a neurotoxic action directly on the axons, e.g. after direct application of a neurotoxin on the axons (see, i.e. Ungerstedt 1971; Lidbrink and Jonsson 1974). The degenerative action of 6-OH-DA is moreover reflected by a long-term disappearance of the transmitter enzymes tyrosine hydroxylase and dopamine-β-hydroxylase which are involved in the biosynthesis of catecholamines. Ultrastructural signs of

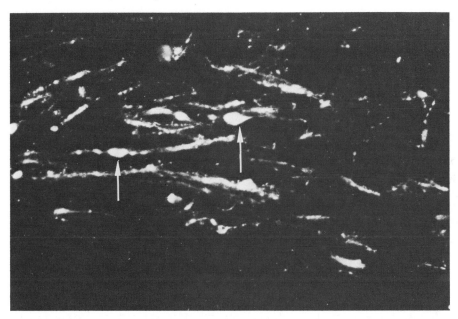

Fig. 4. Fluorescence histochemical demonstration of accumulations (↑) of NA in NA axons (sagittal section) belonging to the dorsal NA bundle after neonatal 6-OH-DA administration (3 × 100 mg/kg s.c., 7 days × 160; from Sachs et al. 1974).

degeneration are seen as early as 1-4 h after 6-OH-DA administration (Furness et al. 1970; Hökfelt et al. 1972; see also, Tranzer and Richards 1971) and these alterations are very similar (dense type of degeneration) to those seen after an axotomy produced by transection or electrocoagulation. If 6-OH-DA is allowed to act directly on the nerve terminals, which is the case after many routes of administration, the degenerative action is much faster than that after an axotomy. This has to be kept in mind when deciding survival time for the sampling of tissue for ultrastructural identification of degeneration. The degenerating structures will in many cases soon be phagocytized and ultimately disappear within a couple of days after which the degeneration process may escape detection.

Concerning the molecular mechanism(s) of the degenerative actions of 6-OH-DA, it is generally agreed that cytotoxicity is linked to the auto-oxidation of 6-OH-DA. This process consists of a series of complex reactions involving the formation of several potentially cytotoxic molecular species, such as quinones (Saner and Thoenen 1971; Tse et al. 1976), 5,6-dihydroxyindole (Blank et al. 1972a) as well as the oxygen oxidation products: hydrogen peroxide (H_2O_2), superoxide (O_2^-) and hydroxyl (.OH) radicals (Heikkila and Cohen 1972, 1973; Cohen and Heikkila 1974). Two theories have been proposed to acount for the degenerative effect of 6-OH-DA at the molecular level. One of them postulates that quinonoid-like oxidation products formed from 6-OH-DA may act as alkylation agents, i.e. form irreversible, covalent bonds with e.g. SH-groups (Saner and Thoenen 1971; Creveling et al. 1975; Jonsson 1976a), while the other theory postulates that the oxygen oxidation products are the cytotoxic agents producing degeneration (Heikkila and Cohen 1975). It is conceivable that both alkylation and actions of oxygen oxidation products can alter structural and functional properties of membrane constituents leading to an initiation of degeneration (see Fig. 5). There is

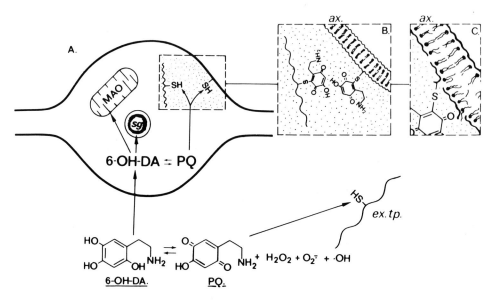

Fig. 5. Schematic representation of possible molecular mechanisms at the adrenergic nerve terminals after 6-OH-DA administration leading to neurodegeneration. 6-OH-DA is efficiently taken up and accumulated intraneuronally by the axonal 'membrane pump' where 6-OH-DA is rapidly oxidized to PQ (*para*-quinone) with simultaneous formation of H_2O_2 and radicals ($O_2^{\cdot-}$.OH). The PQ or some reactive intermediate may then undergo rapid nucleophilic reaction (irreversible covalent binding) with i.e. SH-groups of proteins in the cytoplasm and the axonal membrane (ax.). This latter alkylation process together with actions of H_2O_2 and radicals are likely to initiate the degeneration of the neuron. Part of the 6-OH-DA in the cytoplasm can also be deaminated by monoamine oxidase (MAO) in mitochondria or be taken up and stored by amine storage granules (sg.). PQ and oxygen oxidation products formed from 6-OH-DA in the extraneuronal compartment may react with extraneuronal tissue proteins (ex.tp.) leading to the so-called nonspecific cytotoxic effects of 6-OH-DA. The specificity of 6-OH-DA is completely dependent on its selective, rapid and efficient uptake-accumulation in adrenergic neurons (modified after Jonsson 1976a).

also experimental support for both theories and studies using a variety of poly-hydroxyphenyl derivatives have provided evidence for the view that both processes can act simultaneously (Borchardt et al. 1977; Graham et al. 1978). It has, however, not been possible to assess the relative importance of any one or the other of the proposed mechanisms. At the present stage of knowledge it therefore appears that the cytotoxic action of 6-OH-DA is caused by a series of complex chemical reactions involving both the alkylation mechanisms and the action of oxygen oxidation products. Other contributory mechanisms have also been proposed involving the effects of 6-OH-DA on the energy metabolism of the neuron (Heikkila and Cohen 1972; Liang et al. 1975; Wagner and Trendelenburg 1971).

6-OH-DA as denervation tool

A great deal of information has accumulated over the years as to the use of 6-OH-DA as a denervation tool for various species and catecholamine neuron systems. It is beyond the scope of this chapter to review all this information, and the reader is recommended to consult the following publications for further detailed information on experimental procedures: Kostrezewa and Jacobowitz (1974), Breese (1975), Malmfors and Thoenen (1971), Jonsson et al. (1975), Moore (1978). The intention here is to present some general guidelines and discuss certain aspects of principal importance. It should be pointed out that according to general experience there is a considerable heterogeneity in the response to 6-OH-DA between various central and peripheral catecholamine neuron systems as well as between different species. There is also, as already mentioned, a variable susceptibility between different parts of the single neuron. Different results, mainly with respect to degree of denervation quantitatively, have moreover been reported from different laboratories employing more or less identical lesion parameters. All this emphasizes the necessity of empirically establishing optimal lesion conditions for each given catecholamine system that is intended to be denervated, which implicitly means that the lesion has to be evaluated by adequate techniques.

In practical experimental work it is important to use freshly prepared solutions of 6-OH-DA in saline or artificial cerebrospinal fluid (for intracisternal, intraventricular or intracerebral injections) containing an antioxidant (e.g. 0.2 mg/ml ascorbic acid). The risk of 6-OH-DA oxidation can be further reduced by sparging the solvent with nitrogen or some other inert gas. Although ascorbic acid is an efficient antioxidant and can increase the neurotoxic potency of 6-OH-DA (see, Jonsson 1980), it should be kept in mind that the use of ascorbic acid is a double-edged approach, since a high concentration of ascorbic acid can by itself have general cytotoxic effects (see, Waddington and Crow 1979), which is of particular significance when using intracerebral injections. The potential cytotoxicity of ascorbic acid should be controlled. Moreover, it is recommended that the substance of 6-OH-DA used should be stored under dry, dark and cold conditions to minimize auto-oxidation.

PNS-'chemical sympathectomy'

The most efficient and consistent 6-OH-DA induced degeneration of the sympathetic adrenergic nerves is obtained by using the intravenous (i.v.) route of administration. For ordinary doses a bolus injection can be made, whereas if higher doses of 6-OH-DA (100 mg/kg or more) are administered, the injection must be made slowly in order to avoid lethal effects (see, Malmfors 1971). An i.v. injection of 50 mg/kg 6-OH-DA will in several species (mouse, rat, guinea-pig, rabbit) produce a very efficient denervation (NA reduction of 90% or more) of adrenergic nerves in most organs, e.g. iris, heart, salivary glands. In the mouse an efficient sympathectomy can be obtained even with a dose of 20 mg/kg i.v. For chemical sympathectomy in the cat, see Häusler et al. (1969). An often used procedure is to inject the same dose of 6-OH-DA twice (16-h interval). Such an approach will generally not produce a more efficient sympathectomy, although the NA denervations obtained will be more consistent. The adrenergic nerves innervating the vas deferens are relatively resistant; hence, very high doses (100-500 mg/kg, i.v. injected slowly) are needed in order to obtain a fairly complete denervation. Using doses of 6-OH-DA up to 50 mg/kg will not produce any notable damage of the cell-bodies in the sympathetic ganglia, while after high doses (250-500 mg/kg, i.v.) a moderate decrease of the number of the cell-bodies has been found in the rat (Malmfors 1971). Although 6-OH-DA can be considered to be very selective for the sympathetic adrenergic nerves, signs of nonspecific cytotoxic effects have been observed after high doses (i.e. endothelial damage, hemolysis, damage of tubules of the kidney). Similar to the catecholamines, 6-OH-DA does not easily pass the blood-brain barrier (BBB), and opening of the BBB either by infusion of hyperosmotic solutions or hypertension is needed for a passage of catecholamines into the brain (Hardebo et al.

1979). However, there is both bio- and histochemical evidence for this barrier not being completely impermeable and protective to the neurotoxic actions of 6-OH-DA (Sachs and Jonsson 1973a). A 6-OH-DA dose of 100 mg/kg i.v. will thus produce in the rat a moderate (−25%) but permanent NA depletion in the cerebral cortex. In this context it should be mentioned that neither acute nor chronic 6-OH-DA induced sympathectomy has been found to modify the BBB dysfunction (increased permeability) induced by hypertension (Hardebo et al. 1980; Johansson and Henning 1980). On the other hand it has been observed that 6-OH-DA induced degeneration of central NA neurons (primarily the *locus ceruleus* system) leads to an enhanced protein leakage into the brain after experimentally induced hypertension (Ben-Menachem et al. 1982; Johansson 1979).

With time there will be a regeneration of the adrenergic nerves with a functional recovery after a 6-OH-DA induced sympathectomy. The time-course will depend on the 6-OH-DA dose used, which most likely reflects the level of axonal damage; with a higher dose an axonal damage closer to the cell-bodies will occur resulting in a slower recovery (Jonsson and Sachs 1972a, 1973b). The regeneration will generally take several months, although the process commences within the first week after the neurotoxin administration. It should be pointed out that there are several techniques available to produce a sympathectomy, all of which have their advantages and disadvantages, although the 'chemical sympathectomy' using 6-OH-DA appears to be the most simple one with the most general applicability (see, Thoenen 1972; Jonsson 1982a).

CNS-lesioning of central catecholamine neurons

Since 6-OH-DA does not easily pass the BBB, the neurotoxin has to be injected intraventricularly (IVT), intracisternally (IC) or directly into the brain tissue (intracerebrally) to induce degeneration of central catecholamine neurons. It should be pointed out here that the route of administration and injection technique are factors of crucial importance for the end-result. This makes it very difficult to give any precise general statements as to the sensitivity of the various catecholamine neuron systems in the CNS. There is thus a considerable variation — from very susceptible to almost completely resistant systems. Given the situation that the whole neurons of the various catecholamine systems can be exposed to a comparable concentration of 6-OH-DA, it is the general experience that the nerve terminal projections originating from the nucleus locus ceruleus are the most sensitive structures, while terminals originating from the lateral tegmental NA cell-body groups innervating, e.g. the hypothalamus, are less sensitive. The DA systems also exhibit a differential susceptibility; from being fairly sensitive (the nigrostriatal DA system) to almost completely resistant (the tuberoinfundibular DA system; see, Jonsson et al. 1972). The latter system with its nerve terminals in the median eminence which is 'outside' the BBB might, however, be affected after very high doses of 6-OH-DA given systemically (i.v.). The central adrenaline (A) systems also appear to be very resistant to the action of 6-OH-DA, although the question of 6-OH-DA neurotoxicity on these systems is somewhat unclear at present (vide infra).

Intracisternal or intraventricular 6-OH-DA administration

Following this route of 6-OH-DA administration, there is a dose-dependent, long-lasting reduction of both NA and DA and disappearance of NA and DA nerves as demonstrated by fluorescence histochemistry and bochemistry (Uretsky and Iversen 1969, 1970; Breese and Taylor 1970, 1971; Ungerstedt 1971) as well as histological and ultrastructural signs of selective degeneration (Bloom et al. 1969; Hedreen and Chalmers 1972). Similar to the situation in the PNS, the neurotoxic action is brought about very rapidly and dramatic reductions of the catecholamine levels are seen already a couple of hours after the 6-OH-DA administration (Bell et al. 1970). IC and IVT injections of very large doses of 6-OH-DA (500-1000 µg in 25-50 µl solvent) have been found to produce remarkably specific neurotoxic effects on catecholamine neurons with relatively limited general cytotoxic effects, both from a structural and biochemical point of view (see, Ungerstedt 1971; Jacks et al. 1972), although a certain damage of the ependymal cells has been noted after high doses, and this may lead to hydrocephalus (Decarries and Saucier 1972; Poirier et al. 1972). Hedreen (1975) has observed that there is a clearly less local general cytotoxic damage after an IC compared to an IVT injection. The latter type of 6-OH-DA administration is, however, generally more effective in producing catecholamine denervations. It is likely that the nonspecific effects may be more pronounced in larger animals (e.g. cat, monkey), where higher doses of 6-OH-DA have to be administered IC or IVT to obtain comparable effects (see, Kraemer et al. 1981). In the cat, doses of 2-4 × 2.5 mg of 6-OH-DA have been used for IVT injections resulting generally in moderate catecholamine denervations (Laguzzi et al. 1972; Petitjean et al. 1972; Howard and Breese 1974; see also, Pujol et al. 1975). Attempts to use IVT injections of 6-OH-DA in the Rhesus monkey have been found unsatisfactory (Kraemer et al. 1981).

In the rat, a commonly used 6-OH-DA dose for IVT (lateral ventricle) injection is 200 µg in 20-50 µl solvent, which can be repeated (16-20 h interval). A second or a third 6-OH-DA injection is not likely to markedly increase the extent of the catecholamine denervation, but rather improve the reproducibility. An IVT injection of 6-OH-DA (200 µg) will lead to a rather heterogenous denervation pattern with very marked NA denervations (75% or more) in the locus ceruleus innervated areas (cerebral cortex, hippocampus, cerebellum and spinal cord), while the effects are less pronounced in the hypothalamus and pons-medulla. The action of 6-OH-DA on the DA neurons will be mainly on the nigrostriatal system (60-80% DA reduction) where the areas close to the lateral ventricles will be most markedly affected, thus reflecting a pronounced denervation gradient. Most of the catecholamine cell-bodies will generally survive after an IC or an IVT injection of 6-OH-DA, although this statement does not always hold, especially after high doses. Decarries and Saucier (1972) have reported a complete disappearance of the whole locus ceruleus after a slow IVT (lateral ventricle) infusion (4 min) of 300 µg 6-OH-DA in 50 µl saline. Both an IC and IVT administration of 6-OH-DA will thus lead to a very heterogenous denervation pattern regionally and there can also be a differential time-course of the degeneration process depending on the primary site of action of the neurotoxin; from very rapid when the 6-OH-DA hits directly the nerve terminals (within hours), to fairly slow when the 6-OH-DA acts primarily on axons leading to an anterograde degeneration, which will take several days to become completed (see, Ungerstedt 1971; see also Fig. 3). It can also be advantageous to administer 6-OH-DA bilaterally using the IVT route of administration to avoid asymmetrical effects (see, Gershanik et al. 1979). After high 6-OH-DA doses (IC or IVT) there is generally very limited regrowth of catecholamine nerves. It is likely, however, that the degree of regeneration increases with smaller doses. Although generally speaking both the IC and the IVT routes of 6-OH-DA administration can be considered to produce reasonably specific catecholamine denervations, it is clear that the very heterogenous denervation pattern produced regionally using this approach make them less attractive and limit their use, in particular in functional studies.

Intracerebral 6-OH-DA injection

The local intracerebral 6-OH-DA injection technique was introduced by Ungerstedt (1968, 1971) for the selective denervation of one principal catecholamine system. This denervation technique generally involves stereotoxic placing of an injection cannula (metal or glass) in a brain region where catecholamine cell-bodies or axons are situated. The cannula is connected to an injection device making it possible to infuse microliter quantities of the 6-OH-DA solution. For most types of lesions 1-10 μg 6-OH-DA have been infused in 1-10 μl at a rate of 1-5 μl/min. This approach has been extensively used to denervate various catecholamine neurons systems where the best documented procedures are those for the denervation of the nigro-neostriatal DA system and the dorsal tegmental NA bundle originating from the locus ceruleus innervating many forebrain regions, i.e. the cerebral cortex and the hippocampus (Ungerstedt 1971, 1973; Hökfelt and Ungerstedt 1973; Sotelo et al. 1973; Agid et al. 1973; Javoy et al. 1975; Lidbrink and Jonsson 1974). Infusion of 8 μg 6-OH-DA in 4 μl into the substantia nigra or over the NA axons in the mesencephalon (dorsal NA bundle) will produce rather selective DA and NA denervations, respectively. The neuro- and histochemical sequel following the latter lesion is presented in Figure 6. There is a gradual disappearance with time of

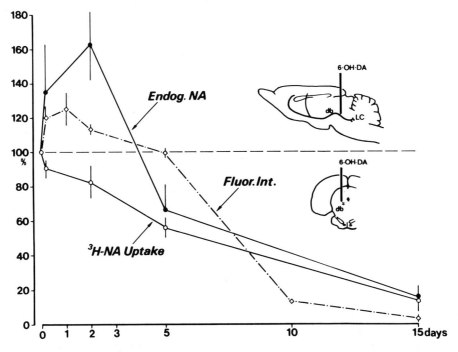

Fig. 6. Time-course of the effects of a 6-OH-DA induced lesion of the dorsal NA bundle (db) on endogenous NA levels, [³H]NA uptake and fluorescence intensity of NA nerve terminals (demonstrated histochemically and estimated semiquantitatively) in rat cerebral cortex. The lesion was performed by infusion of 8 μg 6-OH-DA/4 μl over the NA axons in the posterior mesencephalon as indicated. The values are expressed as % of control. LC = locus ceruleus (from Lidbrink and Jonsson 1974).

both endogenous NA levels and [³H]NA uptake in vitro as well as of the NA nerve terminals as demonstrated by fluorescence histochemistry, reflecting the anterograde degeneration of the NA neurons. There is (up to 2 days) an acute increase of the NA levels, most likely related to a continued, and even increased, NA synthesis, which in the absence of neuronal firing and reduction of NA release leads to an increase of the steady-state levels of NA. This is consistent with the finding that the acute NA increase can be blocked by inhibition of NA biosynthesis by administering a tyrosine hydroxylase inhibitor (Lidbrink and Jonsson 1974). An acute rise in the transmitter concentration following an axotomy has also been observed in the sympathetic adrenergic nerves (Sedvall 1964; Sachs and Jonsson 1973b) and in particular in the striatal DA nerve terminals after both surgical axotomy and 6-OH-DA (Andén et al. 1972; see also, Breese 1975). The acute increase of catecholamines in the terminals after axonal damage thus seems to be a fairly general phenomenon. The time-course of the disappearance of the NA levels and the NA uptake mechanism in the cerebral cortex with maximal reductions of the parameters after about 10-14 days (Fig. 6) is very similar to that reported for the disappearance of the catecholamine biosynthetic enzymes tyrosine hydroxylase and DA-β-hydroxylase after an axotomy (Reis et al. 1977, 1978). After injection of 6-OH-DA into the substantia nigra the disappearance of the biochemical DA parameters as well as of morphological DA neuron markers is much faster and the degeneration is completed within 48 h. This certainly reflects, at least partly, the fact that the DA axons are much shorter than those of the NA neurons innervating the forebrain. While the NA perikarya of the locus ceruleus remain after a 6-OH-DA injection over the dorsal NA bundle, the DA perikarya degenerate and disappear completely. This is most likely due to a direct neurotoxic action of 6-OH-DA on the DA perikarya, and possibly partly also a result of a retrograde degeneration process due to a 6-OH-DA induced 'close axotomy'. Degeneration of the locus ceruleus NA perikarya can be obtained by a direct injection of 6-OH-DA into the locus ceruleus (Koda et al. 1978).

Concerning the specificity of the local intracerebral injection technique, the general experience is that the solution injected should not contain more than 2 μg/μl of 6-OH-DA (infused at a rate of 1-5 μl/min) in order to avoid extensive nonspecific, generally cytotoxic effects (see, Bloom 1975). It should be kept in mind that there are always great risks for obtaining nonspecific cytotoxic effects using the intracerebral injection technique. The reason for this is that 6-OH-DA is a generally cytotoxic agent and its specificity is exclusively dependent on its selective accumulation. Any tissue element can thus be damaged if exposed to high enough concentrations of 6-OH-DA, a situation that can easily occur when 6-OH-DA is infused directly into the nervous tissue at a relatively rapid speed. The mere introduction of the injection cannula will always produce a certain mechanical damage, which in the chronic state will be surrounded by a reactive gliosis. This is a general response of the CNS tissue after a mechanical damage (see, Moore 1978). Further away from the tip of the cannula there will be a zone where more or less all structures will be damaged due to the general cytotoxic effects of 6-OH-DA. The extension of this zone is largely a function of the concentration of 6-OH-DA used, although the infusion speed will certainly also affect it. The zone of nonspecific damage can be kept rather small with infusion parameters referred to above (2 μg/μl; 1 μl/min; totally 8 μg 6-OH-DA), although it has been noted in single animals that quite an extensive nonspecific damage can occur (see, Hökfelt and Ungerstedt 1973). While the exact reason for this is unknown, it may possibly be related to a clogging of the tip of the infusion cannula when introduced into the brain. In such a situation a certain pressure has to be achieved before the clogging is removed leading to an initial rapid outflow of the 6-OH-DA solution that can result in a pronounced nonspecific damage. This potential problem may be overcome by clearing the outlet of the cannula before starting the infusion. Outside the zone of general tissue damage there will be an area where only certain structures are affected and this is the zone of the specific action of 6-OH-DA on catecholamine neurons. The size of this zone is mainly a function of the volume of 6-OH-DA solution infused, although 6-OH-DA concentration and infusion speed are also factors of significance. This rather simplified picture of the degenerative consequences following a local 6-OH-DA infusion can, however, vary considerably from region to region in the CNS as well as according to the injection technique used. Another possible complicating factor is the recent finding that 6-OH-DA may damage BBB (Cooper et al. 1982). The information available at present on the dose, volume, and infusion conditions for the selective denervation of various catecholamine neuron systems should therefore be regarded as guidelines (Agid et al. 1973; Hökfelt and Ungerstedt 1973; Ungerstedt 1971, 1973; Lidbrink 1974; Lidbrink and Jonsson 1974; Fuxe et al. 1975; Heybach et al. 1978; Koda et al. 1978; Hansen et al. 1981). The optimal lesion conditions have to be worked out empirically whereby the specificity and extent of the lesion in each particular case should be evaluated by adequate morphological, biochemical and physiological techniques depending on the purpose of the lesion. For a successful outcome of the 6-OH-DA induced lesion, especially with respect to achieving a rather complete denervation, the neuroanatomical considerations for deciding the infusion point are of course also of utmost importance. If the CNS region containing the catecholamine structures that are intended to be lesioned is fairly large e.g. in large animals (monkey), for specificity reasons it may be advisable to make multiple injections instead of trying to produce the lesion by one infusion of a large volume of 6-OH-DA solution (cf. Kraemer et al. 1981).

Another type of technique for intracerebral infusion of 6-OH-DA has been introduced in recent years where osmotic minipumps (Alzet) are employed to deliver the neurotoxin (Pettigrew and Kasamatsu 1978; Kasamatsu et al. 1979, 1981). This procedure has been used for local denervation of the cerebral cortex of catecholamine nerve terminals in the cat. The 6-OH-DA infusion is performed by placing a cannula about 1/2 mm in the grey matter of the cortex and fixing the cannula to the skull bone with dental cement. The cannula is connected to an osmotic minipump (delivery rate: 1 μl/h) filled with 4 mM 6-OH-DA solution containing ascorbic acid and placed subcutaneously at the neck. This delivery system will produce a 6-OH-DA infusion at a speed of 1 μl/h for 1 week and lead to an almost complete NA denervation locally in an area 6-8 mm around the cannula (Fig. 7; Kasamatsu et al. 1981). Further away from the infusion point there will be a partial denervation which decreases with distance from the tip of the cannula and the cortex is largely unaffected 15 mm away from the infusion point. There will also be a degeneration of the DA nerve terminals, although less pronounced (see Fig. 7). It is of interest that despite the fairly high 6-OH-DA concentrations used, the nonspecific cytotoxic damage is rather limited being confined to the area just around the infusion cannula; this is most probably due to the slow infusion rate (1 μl/h). This local denervation technique can also be used in a similar way to denervate locally the rat cerebral cortex of NA nerve terminals (Kojima and Jonsson, unpublished). In the cat it has been noticed that there is a considerable regrowth in the denervated area with time which is initially fairly rapid, although it will take several months before the restoration is almost complete (Nakai et al. 1983).

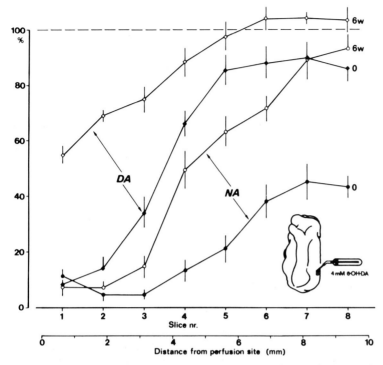

Fig. 7. The spatial distribution of endogenous NA and DA in cat visual cortex locally perfused with 4 mM 6-OH-DA delivered by an osmotic minipump (1 μl/h, 7 days). The analyses were performed either directly or 6 weeks after termination of the 6-OH-DA perfusion. The results are expressed as % of control (data from Nakai et al. 1983).

Specificity

Two main specificity problems have to be considered when using 6-OH-DA as a denervation tool: the general cytotoxic effects, and its actions on different monoamine neurons. As to the latter problem, 6-OH-DA has very potent neurotoxic actions on both NA and DA neurons and if only one of the neuron types is intended to be lesioned, certain measures have to be undertaken to secure specificity. The simplest way to obtain a selective DA denervation is to inject a potent NA uptake inhibitor (e.g. desipramine = DMI, or protriptyline = PTP; 20-25 mg/kg i.p.) 15-30 min before the 6-OH-DA administration. This pretreatment results in a protection of the NA neurons, leaving the DA neurons exposed to degenerative action. A similar strategy should also be possible for a selective NA denervation, although no such satisfactory approach has yet been reported mainly due to the lack of potent and selective DA inhibitors. Benztropine has been tried for this purpose but with limited success; amfonelic acid, which is a potent DA inhibitor, might be a better alternative (see, Shore 1976; Ross and Kelder 1979; Fuller and Hemrick-Luecke 1980).

Whether 6-OH-DA has any neurotoxic action on central adrenaline (A) is somewhat unclear at present although the general finding is that A neurons are relatively resistant, a notion based mainly on data obtained by the analysis of PNMT (phenylethanol-amine-N-methyltransferase = NA-N-methyltransferase) as an A neuron marker (Jonsson et al. 1976; Reid et al. 1976; Fuxe et al. 1975). It has been observed, however, that PNMT activity is reduced in the hypothalamus after intrategmental injections of large doses of 6-OH-DA over the A axons (Fuxe et al. 1976). Moreover, after an IVT injection of 6-OH-DA the endogenous A levels in both the hypothalamus and the brain stem are reduced, while the PNMT activity remains unaltered (see, Fuller 1982). It has been suggested that the discrepancy between the two A-neuron markers is related to a compensatory increase in PNMT activity in the remaining neurons (Burgess et al. 1980), a situation which resembles that reported for NA-neurons in the hippocampus after 6-OH-DA (Acheson et al. 1980). These authors noted that tyrosine hydroxylase activity and NA levels were acutely reduced to a similar extent, while later the enzyme activity recovered more quickly. It would thus appear as if 6-OH-DA can have a certain neurotoxic action on A-neurons, although more conclusive structural studies are needed to substantiate this view.

6-OH-DA is generally considered as a fairly specific catecholamine neurotoxin without affecting 5-HT neurons, at least in mice and rats. The overwhelming majority of investigations have also demonstrated this to be the case; however, a word of precaution might be appropriate here since a few studies have also shown that 6-OH-DA can affect 5-HT neurons to a certain degree, e.g in the hippocampus (De Montigny et al. 1980; see also, Breese 1975). Since it is known that the uptake mechanism of 5-HT neurons is not absolutely specific for 5-HT but also has a certain affinity for catecholamines, it is perhaps not astonishing that 5-HT neurons can be damaged by 6-OH-DA in certain cases. This potential specificity problem is more likely to occur after local intracerebral 6-OH-DA injections. Species differences have also been observed, since it has been demonstrated that 5-HT neurons are affected by 6-OH-DA in the cat (Laguzzi et al. 1971; Pujol et al. 1975). It therefore seems advisable to watch out for potential neurotoxic actions of 6-OH-DA on 5-HT neurons. Such control should preferably be both histo- and biochemical (transmitter levels and uptake), since a small reduction of the 5-HT levels alone cannot be taken as evidence for a neurodegenerative action, especially in the chronic state of a lesion. Moderate alterations of the transmitter levels can also be related to an alteration of the functional state of the neuron. However, if there is a specificity problem for 6-OH-DA with respect to 5-HT neurons — a property that 6-OH-DA shares with the NA neurotoxin DSP4 — it is possible to circumvent it by pretreatment (30 min before 6-OH-DA) with a preferential 5-HT uptake blocker (Ross et al. 1976), such as chlorimipramine (20 mg/kg i.p.) or zimelidine (10 mg/kg i.p.). Finally, it should be pointed out that the use of different uptake blockers to improve selectivity and secure specificity has limitations in the sense that it is not always possible to obtain complete protection against the neurotoxic action of 6-OH-DA. The exact reasons for this are unknown, but may in part be related to the uptake blockade being overcome when the neurons are exposed to high concentrations of 6-OH-DA.

Concerning the nonspecific, generally cytotoxic effects of 6-OH-DA, it has already been mentioned that this is a problem mainly encountered when using the local intracerebral injection technique. Some authors have found this so problematic and therefore conclude that 6-OH-DA is no more specific than any other conventional nonselective lesion technique (Poirier et al. 1972; Butcher et al. 1974; Butcher 1975). Although this view appears to be far too extreme, it is clear that great care has to be taken to minimize the nonspecific cytotoxic effects. The factors of importance here have already been discussed (6-OH-DA concentration, amount of 6-OH-DA infused, and rate of infusion). The optimal lesion conditions for a given system have to be tested out empirically. It is possible that the modification of the rate of 6-OH-DA infusion should be exploited more than it has been in the past, in view of the results obtained after local 6-OH-DA infusion using osmotic minipumps for neurotoxin delivery (Kasamatsu et al. 1981). There are also other possibilities to optimize the lesion, e.g. by pretreatment with a MAO inhibitor (e.g. pargyline 100 mg/kg i.p., 15-30 min before 6-OH-DA). Since 6-OH-DA is a substrate for MAO, inhibition of this enzyme will increase the neurotoxic potency of 6-OH-DA; hence, lower doses can be used and will thereby improve specificity. (For various possibilities of modifying the neurotoxic potency of 6-OH-DA see, Jonsson 1980). From a functional standpoint in particular, the use of uptake inhibitors to prevent the neurodegenerative action of 6-OH-DA may also be valuable for securing specificity. An example of this is the finding that pretreatment with PTP abolishes both the NA denervation in the cerebral cortex and the alterations in EEG behavior produced by a local injection of 6-OH-DA in the 'dorsal NA bundle' (Lidbrink and Jonsson 1975). Such information indicates strongly that 6-OH-DA produces a specific NA lesion both from the structural and functional standpoints.

3.2. β-HALOBENZYLAMINES

This is a fairly recently discovered group of compounds that has been shown to possess neurotoxic effects on, in particular, central NA neurons. The original observation was made by Ross and co-workers when testing a series of tertiary N-haloalkyl-2-bromobenzylamine derivatives (Ross et al. 1973). These authors found that one of the compounds, N-(2-chloroethyl)-N-ethyl-2-bromobenzylamine (DSP4, Fig. 2), is capable of producing a long-lasting inhibition of [^{3}H]NA uptake and a reduction of NA levels and DA-β-hydroxylase, suggesting a neurotoxic action on NA neurons (Ross 1976; Ross and Reyni 1976). More recently, another series of β-halobenzylamines closely related to DSP4 have been described and one of the derivatives, xylamine (N-2-chloroethyl-N-ethyl-2-methylbenzylamine, Fig. 2), appears to have actions very similar to that of DSP4 (Kammerer et al. 1979; Cho et al. 1980; Fischer and Cho 1982; Dudley et al. 1981). An interesting property of DSP4 and xylamine is their lipophilicity which makes them both pass the BBB and blood-placenta barrier (Jaim-Etcheverry and Zieher 1980; Jonsson et al. 1981, 1982; Dudley et al. 1981). It is therefore possible to employ systemic injections to affect NA neurons in the CNS, both in adult animals and fetuses. Although the ultrastructural evidence is still lacking, all histo- and biochemical data are compatible with the view that DSP4 and xylamine can produce a selective neurotoxic damage of NA neurons, most likely associated with neuronal degeneration.

Mode and mechanism of action

The information on the mode of action of DSP4 is still rather limited, but the studies so far have shown that DSP4 acts on the NA neurons in a manner similar to that of 6-OH-DA, as revealed by neuro- and histochemical analyses. DSP4 has its most potent neurotoxic action on the NA nerve terminals, while the cell-bodies have not been noted to be affected. There is rapid depletion of the endogenous NA stores and a loss of the ability of the nerve terminals to take up, accumulate and store exogenously adminstered NA following a systemic DSP4 administration (Jonsson et al. 1981). The effects are dose-dependent and are already maximal after 4-6 h in the mouse, while it takes a somewhat longer time in the rat (see Fig. 8). Also, soon after the DSP4 administration there is a 'pileup' of NA in the axons, reflecting the neurotoxic action at the terminal level. Moreover, the neurotoxin induces a disappearance of the DA-β-

479

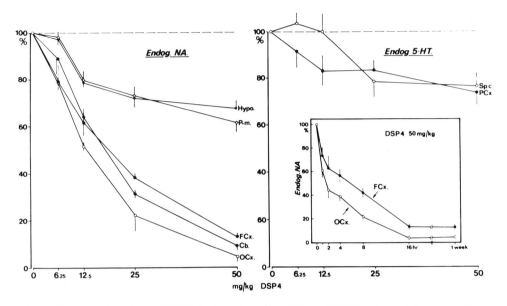

Fig. 8. Effect of various doses of DSP4 (i.p.) on the regional NA and 5-HT levels in adult rat brain 1 week after the neurotoxin administration. The acute time-course of the NA depletion in cortical regions following DSP4 (50 mg/kg i.p.) is inserted in the right diagram. The values are expressed as % of control FCx = frontal; OCx = occipital; PCx = parietal cortex; Cb = cerebellum; Hypo = hypothalamus; P-m = pons-medulla; Sp.c. = spinal cord (from Archer et al. 1983).

hydroxylase (a vesicular enzyme) activity and the neuron is no longer able to synthesize NA from L-DOPA. The DSP4 induced neurotoxic effects can be prevented by pretreatment with a NA uptake inhibitor (DMI; 25 mg/kg, 30 min before DSP4) indicating that DSP4 has to act directly on the NA nerve terminals to elicit its neurotoxic effects. It is, however, not known whether toxicity is mediated via an action on the NA uptake carrier and/or other presynaptic receptors or whether the compound has to be accumulated like 6-OH-DA intraneuronally and act from this site. Experiments with reserpine show that intact granular uptake-storage mechanisms are not a prerequisite for neurotoxicity. There are also data indicating that DSP4 has MAO inhibitory properties, but it is known if this is related to neurotoxicity (Lyles and Callingham 1981).

Regarding the molecular mechanism of the neurotoxic action of DSP4 very little is known, although it is conceivable from chemical considerations that the neurotoxic effects are mediated via an alkylation reaction whereby DSP4 is converted to an aziridinium ion, which is a potent electrophile that readily reacts with tissue nucleophiles to form irreversible covalent bonds. Such an alkylation of neuronal constituents of vital importance for the neuron might account for the neurotoxic effects (see, Jonsson et al. 1981; Dudley et al. 1981).

Effects of DSP4 on peripheral and central NA neurons

Most studies conducted with DSP4 so far have employed the *systemic* route of administration. For both rats and mice 50 mg/kg i.p. is a fairly safe dose and does not cause any lethal effects. DSP4 is, however, a rather labile compound which rapidly cyclizes (t1/2 ~ 10 min) at neutral pH to its quarternary aziridinium derivative (Ross et al. 1973). Although this latter compound is likely to be the neurotoxic molecular species, it does not pass the BBB (Zieher and Jaim-Etcheverry 1980). Therefore, DSP4 has to be injected immediately after being dissolved in order to obtain maximal effects in the CNS.

PNS

Systemic administration of a large dose of DSP4 produces acutely a rapid and marked NA depletion and disappearance of [^{3}H]NA uptake and DA-β-hydroxylase activity in sympathetically innervated organs (e.g. heart, salivary glands, iris; Ross 1976, Jaim-Etcheverry and Zieher 1980; Jonsson et al. 1981). A pronounced reduction of the adrenergic nerve density as well as a 'pileup' of NA transmitter in non-terminal axons (sign of neurotoxicity) is observed by fluorescence histochemistry. No detectable effects on the NA perikarya in ganglia are seen. However, there is a fairly rapid recovery and within a couple of weeks an almost complete restoration of the adrenergic nerves is seen. This is quite different from the situation found after 6-OH-DA where the recovery takes several months. It might therefore be argued that DSP4 does not produce any true degenerative effects on the sympathetic adrenergic nerves, but rather a transient damage only. Although this is an unclear point at present, the rapid recovery observed could be due to the neurotoxic action of DSP4 being limited to the most distal parts of the adrenergic nerve terminals. Such a situation could very well be compatible with the rapid recovery observed, since it is known that the outgrowth of sympathetic adrenergic nerves is a very rapid process (Olson and Malmfors 1970). The reason for the relatively slow recovery process after 6-OH-DA may be related to this neurotoxin having a greater neurotoxic potency than DSP4 leading to a damage of the axons closer to the perikarya, which for obvious reasons requires a longer time for regeneration. In view of the clearly less marked effects of DSP4 than 6-OH-DA, it appears that 6-OH-DA is the neurotoxin of choice for producing sympathectomy in experimental work (see, Jonsson 1982). On the other hand, the fact that DSP4 produces only short-lasting effects in the periphery can be considered as an advantage for using the neurotoxin in CNS studies.

CNS

Systemically administered DSP4 produces a rapid and dose-dependent reduction of NA which is maximal within 6-16 h (Fig. 8). The NA reduction is accompanied by a reduction of the in vitro uptake of [^{3}H]NA in the NA nerves as well as a reduction of DA-β-hydroxylase activity and disappearance of NA nerve terminals demonstrated by fluorescence histochemistry. The NA perikarya are not notably affected. Regional analysis has shown that those regions innervated by NA nerve terminals originating from the nucleus locus ceruleus are preferentially affected, e.g. the neocortex, olfactory bulb, hippocampus, cerebellum and spinal cord (Fig. 9). According to data from biochemical analysis a dose of 50 mg/kg will produce an almost complete NA denervation in the locus ceruleus innervated regions in both rats and mice (Jonsson et al. 1981; Archer et al. 1983), whereas regions mainly innervated by other NA systems (e.g. hypothalamus and pons-medulla) are clearly less affected. It is unlikely that this difference is due to an absolute specificity for the locus ceruleus system, but rather related to this system being the most susceptible one. The preferential action on the locus ceruleus system is also supported by the finding that most of the NA accumulations seen in NA axons after DSP4 are mainly confined to the dorsal NA bundle (Jonsson et

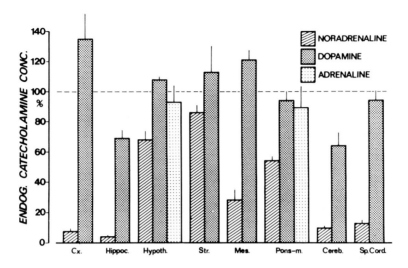

Fig. 9. Effect of DSP4 (50 mg/kg i.p., 10 days) on the regional catecholamine levels in adult rat brain. The results are expressed as % of control (data from Jonsson et al. 1981).

al. 1981). DSP4 produces a long-lasting disappearance of the biochemical markers for NA nerves, but there will with time (after several months) be a certain recovery, e.g. in the frontal cortex (Jonsson, unpublished).

As to the specificity of DSP4, it has been observed that this compound is very selective for central NA neurons in the mouse without affecting the DA, A and 5-HT neurons (Jonsson et al. 1981). DSP4 is also very selective in the rat for the NA neurons among the various catecholamine systems, although in this species DSP4 has been observed to have a minor, long-lasting neurotoxic action on the 5-HT neurons (see also Fig. 8). This is perhaps not unexpected in view of the fact that DSP4 has a certain affinity for the 5-HT uptake system (Ross 1976). The nonselective action of DSP4 on 5-HT neurons can be prevented by pretreatment with the preferential 5-HT blocker zimelidine (10 mg/kg i.p., 30 min before DSP4). All the neurotoxic actions of DSP4 on NA neurons recorded can be abolished by DMI pretreatment (25 mg/kg i.p.) and this pharmacological approach can therefore serve as a very useful control when using DSP4 in experimental work.

From the data available it appears that DSP4 and xylamine have very similar effects on both central and peripheral NA neurons (see, Cho et al. 1980; Fischer and Cho 1982; Dudley et al. 1981). In a recent comparative study it was observed that xylamine and DSP4 had almost the same quantitative effects on the regional NA depletion (both acutely and chronically) in the CNS of mice after a dose of 50 mg/kg i.p. (Jonsson, unpublished).

Very little information is available at present on the effects of DSP4 using routes of administration other than the systemic one. It has been reported that an IVT injection of 300 μg DSP4 resulted in an 80% depletion of NA in the hippocampus (measured 18 days after the injection) without affecting the 5-HT levels and choline-O-acetyltransferase activity in this region (Ladinsky et al. 1980). Whether this route of DSP4 administration has any advantage over the systemic one is at present unknown. Local intracerebral injections of DSP4 have also been tried, although with ambiguous results (Ross, personal communication).

3.3. OTHER CATECHOLAMINE NEUROTOXINS

Although 6-OH-DA and DSP4 can at present be considered to be the most useful catecholamine neurotoxin in experimental work where 6-OH-DA has the most general applicability, there are also other neurotoxins of interest. Of the 6-OH-DA related compounds 6-OH-DOPA and 6-NH$_2$-DA (Fig. 2) have been used to a certain extent. Other compounds that have received attention with respect to neurotoxic actions on catecholamine neurons are guanethidine and (+)-amphetamine.

6-OH-DOPA

The amino acid 6-OH-DOPA can produce a selective degeneration of both central and peripheral NA neurons and its neurotoxicity is mediated by decarboxylation of 6-OH-DOPA to 6-OH-DA (Corrodi et al. 1971; Jacobowitz and Kostrzewa 1971; Sachs and Jonsson 1972a,b; Kostrzewa and Jacobowitz 1972, 1973; Sachs et al.1973; Clarke et al. 1972). While 6-OH-DA cannot pass the BBB, 6-OH-DOPA can readily enter the brain after a systemic injection. The effect of 6-OH-DOPA in the CNS is selective for NA neurons leaving 5-HT and DA neurons apparently unaffected, although the denervation pattern is rather heterogenous with respect to various NA neuron systems; the terminal fields originating from the locus ceruleus appear to be the most susceptible ones. The main problem associated with the use of 6-OH-DOPA is its relatively high degree of general toxicity and high doses are needed to produce substantial NA denervations. The highest dose of 6-OH-DOPA tolerated by rats and mice is 100 mg/kg i.p., although its effect can be potentiated by pretreatment with a MAO inhibitor (e.g. nialamide or pargyline; 100 mg/kg i.p., 15-30 min before 6-OH-DOPA). In spite of this, the degree of NA denervation is generally not more than 50-60%.

6-NH$_2$-DA

This compound has a neurotoxic potency and action on catecholamine neurons very similar to that of 6-OH-DA (Jonsson and Sachs 1973a; Heikkila et al 1973; Blank et al. 1972b; Borchardt 1975; Siggins et al. 1975). However, 6-NH$_2$-DA has proved to be more generally cytotoxic than 6-OH-DA and has therefore not been used as a denervation tool to any greater extent.

Guanethidine

This is an adrenergic neuron blocking agent which has been used to treat hypertension for many years. Guanethidine has been demonstrated to cause a degeneration of sympathetic adrenergic neurons after chronic treatment (Jensen-Holm and Juul 1971; Burnstock et al. 1971; Eränkö and Eränkö 1971; Heath et al. 1972). Guanethidine does not pass the BBB and that is why its action is restricted to the PNS. Moreover, it has been observed that chronic intracerebral injection of guanethidine is ineffective in causing degeneration of the central catecholamine neurons (Evans et al. 1975). A single injection of this compound is known to produce a NA depletion and an inhibition of the action-potential evoked release of NA from adrenergic nerves (see, Furness 1979). Treatment with large doses (10-20 mg/kg i.p., daily for 1-2 weeks or more) of guanethidine chronically leads to a marked and selective degeneration of sympathetic adrenergic neurons. There is a differential sensitivity between various sympathetically innervated organs, and the most sensitive neurons appear to be the short adrenergic neurons innervating the vas deferens and other genital organs (Gannon et al. 1971; Evans et al. 1972; Bittiger et al. 1977; Evans 1979). An interesting feature of the action of guanethidine is that it induces degeneration of the whole adrenergic neuron and thus produces a permanent sympathectomy, unlike 6-OH-DA which acts mainly on the nerve terminals resulting in a later structural and functional recovery. The selectivity of the neurodegenerative action of guanethidine is certainly related to its selective and efficient accumulation in adrenergic nerves, while the cytotoxicity has been proposed to be associated with an inhibitory action of the compound on oxidative phosphorylation (see, Bittiger et al. 1977). Although basically an interesting neurotoxin with respect to both its mode and mechanism of action, guanethidine has received only limited interest as a denervation tool, mainly because of its restricted applicability and the time-consuming and tedious administration procedure needed to induce degeneration. Guanethidine may, however, have some advantages for the production of a sympathectomy in developing animals (Johnson et al. 1975).

(+)-Amphetamine

An increasing body of evidence has accumulated in recent years demonstrating that the administration of large doses of (+)-amphetamine can have neurotoxic actions on central DA neurons of the rat (Ellison et al. 1978; Fuller and Hemrick-Luecke 1980), mouse (Steranka and Sanders-Bush 1980; Nwanze and Jonsson 1981; Jonsson and Nwanze 1982), and cat (Trulson and Jacobs 1979). Similar observations have been made after repeated injections of metamphetamine (Hotchkiss et al. 1979; Wagner et al. 1980; Hotchkiss and Gibb 1980; Lorez 1981). The action of (+)-amphetamine is stereoselective and mainly on a vulnerable population of DA nerve terminals in the striatum without notably affecting the DA perikarya in the mesencephalon. Metamphetamine has also been observed to affect DA terminals in the nucleus accumbens (Ricuarte et al. 1982). The DA denervation in the striatum has been found to be at best about 50% as monitored by measuring endogenous DA levels. Pharmacological analysis has shown that the action of (+)-amphetamine is most likely directly on the DA nerve terminals (Fuller and Hemrick-Luecke 1982; Steranka 1982), but the exact mode of the neurotoxic action is known. Although (+)-amphetamine at present does not offer any advantageous alternative for the selective denervation of DA neurons in the CNS, the observations made are of interest for the development of new specific denervation procedures.

4. SEROTONIN NEUROTOXINS

There are at present two types of compounds available for the selective destruction of 5-HT neurons, namely the dihydroxytryptamines and the halogenated amphetamines. A large number of dihydroxytryptamine derivatives have been synthesized and tested, but all the data so far indicate that the first compounds (5,6- and 5,7-dihydroxytryptamine; 5,6-HT and 5,7-HT, see Fig. 10) discovered are the best suited as denervation tools (Baumgarten et al. 1975a, 1977, 1981; Baumgarten and Björklund 1976). Of the halogenated amphetamines, *p*-chloroamphetamine (pCAM, Fig. 10) is the most potent and frequently used one (see, Fuller 1978).

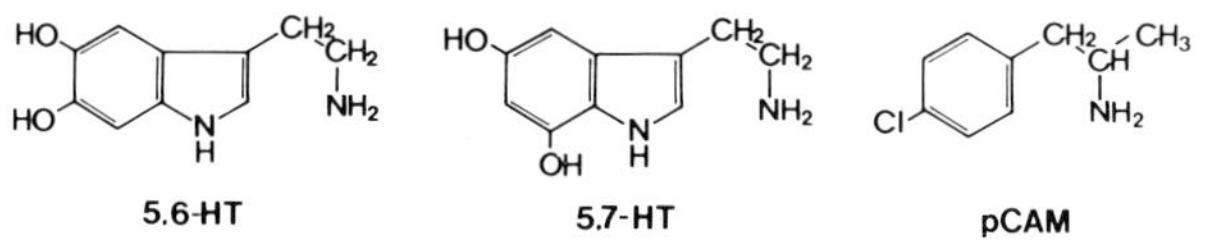

Fig. 10. Structural formulae for the *serotonin* neurotoxins *5,6-HT* (5,6-dihydroxytryptamine); *5,7-HT* (5,7-dihydroxytryptamine) and *pCAM* (*p*-chloroamphetamine).

4.1. 5,6- AND 5,7-DIHYDROXYTRYPTAMINE

Mode and mechanism of action

These compounds appear to act on the 5-HT neurons very much like the 6-OH-DA does on the catecholamine neurons. The specificity of 5,6-HT and 5,7-HT is thus related to the selective accumulation of the neurotoxin in 5-HT neurons, while the degenerative action is most likely brought about by cytotoxic compounds formed by auto-oxidation and/or by enzymatic conversion of the dihydroxytryptamines accumulated intraneuronally. An unresolved question here is also the relative importance of alkylation reactions versus actions of oxygen oxidation products in the initiation of the degeneration. Although the similarities in the action of the dihydroxytryptamines and 6-OH-DA are obvious, it is also evident from many studies that there are distinct differences at the molecular level as well as clear differences between the two dihydroxytryptamines themselves (see Baumgarten et al. 1975a, 1981; Jonsson 1980).

5,6- and 5,7-dihydroxytryptamines as denervation tools

Since neither 5,6-HT nor 5,7-HT passes the BBB, these neurotoxins have to be introduced directly into the brain, either intracisternally, intraventricularly or intracerebrally, in order to elicit the damage to 5-HT neurons. Both compounds are rather unstable in solution and hence the same precautions as those with 6-OH-DA have to be undertaken to minimize breakdown. The solutions should be prepared just before injection (see, Baumgarten et al. 1977).

After an IVT injection, both 5,6-HT and 5,7-HT cause a dose-dependent destruction of 5-HT-neurons (Baumgarten et al. 1971, 1972b, 1973, 1977; Breese et al. 1974; Breese and Cooper 1975). The action is mainly on the nerve terminals, although marked cell-body losses have also been observed (Nygren and Olson 1977). The general experience is that the highest dose of 5,6-HT that rats can tolerate without lethal effects is 75 μg (in 20-25 μl solvent), while 5,7-HT is clearly less toxic and doses up to 200 μg (or more) can be injected without serious consequences. Both neurotoxins can in the highest dose-ranges produce very substantial 5-HT denervations after IVT and IC administration, although the time-course of degeneration can vary somewhat and the degree of denervation varies considerably in various CNS regions. The IC route of administration produces somewhat less extensive 5-HT denervations, than after an IVT injection, but the specificity problems appear to be less pronounced (see Baumgarten et al. 1977). When monitoring the 5-HT denervation after IVT administration by recording the 5-HT levels, it is seen that there is initially a rapid drop of the 5-HT levels within a few hours and thereafter a more gradual 5-HT depletion which occurs over several days (see, Baumgarten et al. 1977). The initial, rapid 5-HT reduction conceivably reflects the action of the neurotoxin directly on the nerve terminals, while the protracted 5-HT disappearance is likely to reflect an axonal damage by the neurotoxin leading to an anterograde degeneration which takes several days to be completed depending on the site of damage. As to the regional heterogeneity of the degree of denervation, high doses of 5,6- or 5,7-HT will both produce very marked 5-HT denervations in the spinal cord (90% or more), while the extent of denervation is variable in other regions, mainly depending on their relation to the ventricular system. The extent of 5-HT denervation after 5,7-HT (200 μg IVT) is clearly more pronounced than that after 5,6-HT (75 μg IVT), except in the spinal cord. The denervation in the striatum and remaining forebrain (mainly cerebral cortex) has thus been found to be about 50% after 5,6-HT, while it is very marked (80-90%) in the same regions after 5,7-HT. Unilateral IVT injections of most neurotoxins tend to produce asymmetrical effects (see, Garshanik et al. 1979), although it has been proposed that in the case of 5,7-HT this can be overcome by administering the neurotoxin as a pulse injection (Jenner and Baumgarten 1980; Baumgarten et al. 1981). It should also be mentioned that these authors observed a more pronounced 5-HT degenerative effect of 5,7-HT if the injection was performed under ether anesthesia as compared to nembutal anesthesia. (For further details on suitable anesthesia procedures, see Baumgarten et al. 1977.) A varying degree of regeneration of 5-HT neurons has been observed after 5,6- and 5,7-HT induced lesions of 5-HT neurons, although the most extensive regenerative phenomena have been observed after 50-75 μg (IVT) of 5,7-HT (Björklund et al. 1973a,b; Nygren et al. 1974; Wiklund et al. 1978; Björklund and Stenevi 1979).

The neurotoxic dihydroxytryptamines can also be used to produce a denervation of principal 5-HT neuron systems by local intracerebral injection, similar to that described for 6-OH-DA. Results from procedures for denervation of ascending 5-HT systems in the rat have been reported (Björklund et al. 1973b; Daly et al. 1973, 1974; Fuxe and Jonsson 1974; Hole et al. 1976; Lorens et al. 1976; Fuxe et al. 1978; Lorden et al. 1979; see also, Baumgarten et al. 1977) as well as for descending 5-HT systems (Saner et al. 1974). A commonly used concentration of 5,6- or 5,7-HT for such lesions is 1 μg/μl and a total amount of 4 μg is infused. Optimal lesion parameters have to be worked out empirically, however, based preferably on both morphological and biochemical evaluation of the lesion and the methodological problems are in many respects similar to those seen for 6-OH-DA. (For further information, see Baumgarten et al.1977.) The general experience is that a more efficient denervation is achieved when the injection is aimed more directly over the 5-HT axon bundles as compared to injections directly into 5-HT cell-body groups.

Specificity

Both 5,6-HT and 5,7-HT can be regarded to have potent neurotoxic actions on 5-HT neurons and properly used they can produce reasonably selective and almost complete 5-HT denervations. There are, however, a number of specificity problems associated with the use of these compounds which have to be considered in experimental work. Generally speaking, 5,6-HT appears to possess a greater specificity than 5,7-HT in affecting more selectively 5-HT neurons only while 5,7-HT also has, in addition to effects on 5-HT neurons, neurotoxic actions on NA and DA neurons. Thus, an intraventricular injection of 5,6-HT will almost exclusively affect the 5-HT neurons among the monoamine neurons, while 5,7-HT will also have a substantial degenerative effect on NA neurons, as well as on DA neurons, although generally to a lesser degree (Baumgarten et al. 1979; Liston et al. 1982). The nonselective effect of 5,7-HT on NA neurons can be circumvented by pretreatment with the preferential NA uptake blocker DMI (25 mg/kg i.p., 30 min before 5,7-HT), a procedure which will prevent the effects of 5,7-HT on NA neurons without affecting its action on 5-HT neurons (Björklund et al. 1975; Gershon and Baldessarini 1975; Sachs and Jonsson 1975d). In a recent study by Baumgarten et al. (1979), pretreatment with nomifensine (25 mg/kg i.p.) was shown to give good protection to the nonselective actions of 5,7-HT, administered IVT, on both NA and DA neurons. 5,6-HT can be considered to be rather specific for 5-HT neurons among the various monoamine neurons, but the main problem with this neurotoxin is its property of being rather generally cytotoxic. It has thus been observed that on injection of a high dose of 5,6-HT IVT leads to a nonselective damage of non-myelinated fiber systems as well as to a deposition of brownish pigments on the walls of the ventricles (Baumgarten et al. 1973). The general cytotoxic effects are not so pronounced for 5,7-HT.

With the use of local intracerebral injections of 5,6- or 5,7-HT, the specificity problems are in many respects similar to those for 6-OH-DA (see, Baumgarten et al. 1977). It is always difficult to completely avoid the nonspecific general cytotoxic effects, which are particularly pronounced after 5,6-HT. Such effects are readily apparent if 8-10 μg of 5,6-HT is injected. Therefore, 5,7-HT appears to be the neurotoxin of choice for denervation of 5-HT neurons using intracerebral injections, in spite of its more general effects on the various monoamine neurons (see, Daly et al. 1974). In order to increase the specificity of 5,7-HT the pharmacological approach employing uptake inhibitors described above can be used, although it is not always possible to obtain a complete counteracting effect by the inhibitors. It is advisable to check specificity by monitoring all relevant monoamine neurons, irrespective of whether 5,6-HT or 5,7- HT is used as denervation tool. For the sake of completeness it should be mentioned that both 5,6- and 5,7-HT can induce degeneration of the sympathetic adrenergic nerves after systemic administration.

4.2. *p*-CHLOROAMPHETAMINE

This compound (Fig. 10) belongs to a class of substances commonly denoted halogenated amphetamines, some of which have been shown to possess a selective neurotoxic action on central 5-HT neurons. The first discovered and apparently most potent of these neurotoxic substances is *p*- or 4-chloroamphetamine (pCAM; Sanders-Bush et al. 1972, 1975). It was originally observed that pCAM causes a profound and long-lasting reduction of 5-HT levels and tryptophan hydroxylase activity in rat brain. pCAM readily passes the BBB and can therefore be administered systemically, although the neurotoxic effects can also be elicited after intraventricular administration (Sherman et al. 1975). Maximal neurotoxic effects of pCAM can be produced in rats after administration of 10-20 mg/kg i.p., while higher doses are needed in mice (50 mg/kg i.p.). Initially pCAM produces a rapid 5-HT depletion, which becomes totally irreversible within 32-48 h (Fuller et al. 1975b). Thus it appears that the neurodegenerative action of the neurotoxic dihydroxytryptamines is more rapidly elicited than that of pCAM. The neurotoxic effect of pCAM and related neurotoxic compounds can be abolished by pretreatment with 5-HT uptake blockers such as clorimipramine and zimelidine (Meek et al. 1971; Fuller et al. 1975a; Ross 1976), demonstrating that the neurotoxic action of pCAM is brought about by a direct action on the 5-HT neurons, although it is not clear whether or not pCAM has to be accumulated intraneuronally to produce the neurodegeneration. The exact molecular mechanism(s) of action of pCAM leading to degeneration of 5-HT neurons is unknown. Reactive metabolites formed from pCAM have been suggested but this is very speculative at the present state of knowledge (Ames and Frank 1982). The neurotoxic action of pCAM is very selective for 5-HT neurons, without any notable effects on other monoamine neurons.

From the data available it is clear that pCAM and related neurotoxic compounds are not generally neurotoxic for all 5-HT neuron systems. There is thus a marked regional variability in the effects on 5-HT neurons. Although there is some controversy in the literature as to the precise 5-HT neuron systems that are preferentially affected by the neurotoxic halogenated amphetamines, biochemical and histochemical data have shown that pCAM mainly affects the ascending 5-HT systems while the descending ones are left more or less intact (see, Köhler et al. 1978; Fuller 1978). There are thus almost complete 5-HT denervations in certain forebrain regions, e.g. cerebral cortex, while practically no effects are found in the spinal cord. pCAM also appears to have minor effects in the mesencephalon and the hypothalamus. It should also be mentioned that pCAM has been shown to have no detectable effects on the central 5-HT neurons when administered in the neonatal stage (Clemens et al. 1978). The reason for the variable sensitivity noted between different 5-HT systems as well as between immature and adult neurons is totally unknown and only stresses the fact that pCAM is, in contrast to 5,6- and 5,7-HT, not a generally applicable denervation tool for 5-HT neurons. Although this limits the use of pCAM, it is clear that this compound represents an interesting neurotoxin for studies of brain regions where it is possible to obtain almost complete 5-HT denervations (e.g. cerebral cortex), since pCAM can be easily administered (i.p.-injection) and possesses apparently less specificity problems than 5,6- and 5,7-HT. This latter statement may be of particular relevance in functional studies (see, Fuller 1978; Ögren et al. 1981; Ögren 1982).

5. MONOAMINE NEUROTOXINS AND DEVELOPMENT

Several of the monoamine neurotoxins described have been found suitable for experimental work in developing animals. While both 6-OH-DA and 6-OH-DOPA as well as DSP4 are useful for studies on immature catecholamine neurons, the general experience is that 5,7-HT is the only one of the 5-HT neurotoxins that can be employed in ontogenetic studies. 5,6-HT is not very well tolerated by developing rats (Breese et al. 1974; Sachs and Jonsson 1975d; Jonsson et al. 1978) and pCAM appears to be ineffective on 5-HT neurons, at least during the neonatal stage (Clemens et al. 1978). It should also be mentioned that guanethidine can be used to obtain a chemical sympathectomy in developing rats (Johnson et al. 1975).

5.1. 6-HYDROXYDOPAMINE AND 6-OH-DOPA

Both rats and mice have been found to tolerate the administration of 6-OH-DA or 6-OH-DOPA in the neonatal stage. For systemic treatments, doses up to 100 mg/kg (s.c. or i.p.) can be administered to newborn animals without any serious consequences. This dose can be repeated several times on consecutive days. The systemic route of 6-OH-DA administration for CNS studies can only be used during the first postnatal week in rat due to the development of a BBB for 6-OH-DA around 7-10 days after birth (Sachs 1973; Fig. 11). Other alternatives are to administer 6-OH-DA IC or IVT and us-

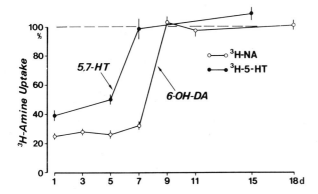

Fig. 11. Effect of 6-OH-DA (3 × 100 mg/kg s.c., 24 h interval) or 5,7-HT (2 × 100 mg/kg s.c., 24 h interval) administered to rats of various ages on the in vitro uptake of [^{3}H]NA and [^{3}H]5-HT, respectively in the cerebral cortex of adult rats. The first dose of neurotoxin was administered on postnatal Day 1, 3, 5 .. etc. The results are expressed as % of control (data from Sachs 1973; Sachs and Jonsson 1975d).

ing these modes of administration doses up to 100 μg of 6-OH-DA (in 2-10 μl) can be administered from the day of birth. Systemically administered 6-OH-DA has been found to have very minute effects on body weight gain and the general development of rats (Sachs et al. 1974), whereas a 6-OH-DA injection IC that leads to a DA denervation causes growth deficits (Breese et al. 1973a,b; Smith et al. 1973). It is also possible to employ an intracerebral injection of 6-OH-DA, although this approach has so far been used only to a limited extent. 6-OH-DA does not pass the blood-placenta barrier and the neurotoxin has therefore to be applied directly into the fetus. For prenatal studies 6-OH-DOPA and DSP4 can be of value since they pass this barrier readily.

Studies in rats have shown that the developing catecholamine neurons respond differently to 6-OH-DA, both in the PNS and CNS, as compared to mature neurons. It has thus been reported that systemic administration of 6-OH-DA in the neonatal stage can produce a selective and permanent destruction of the NA perikarya in sympathetic ganglia leading to a permanent sympathectomy (Angeletti and Levi-Montalchini 1970; Angeletti 1971; Jaim-Etcheverry and Zieher 1971). This is in contrast to the situation in the adult stage when the effects on NA perikarya are rather limited and only seen after very high doses of 6-OH-DA (Malmfors 1971). The reason for the difference is considered to be related to the 6-OH-DA induced disruption of the connection between the neuron and its target cell which supplies the perikaryon with NGF (nerve growth factor) via retrograde axoplasmic tranport. Since the sympathetic adrenergic neurons are dependent on the supply of NGF for their survival and development, the consequence will be a cell-body death after 6-OH-DA administration neonatally (Aloe et al. 1975). A cell-body death is seen after all procedures where a disruption of the connection between the sympathetic neurons and their effector cells is produced in the neonatal stage (see, Johnson 1978).

Systemic administration of 6-OH-DA (1-3 × 100 mg/kg s.c.) during the first postnatal week causes selective and permanent changes in the postnatal development of NA neurons in the CNS (Clark et al. 1972; Sachs and Jonsson 1972a; Singh and De Champlain 1972; Jonsson et al. 1973, 1974; Konkol et al. 1978; Bendeich et al. 1978; Schmidt and Bhatnager 1979). This treatment appears to alter the development of the locus ceruleus NA neuron system preferentially, although lateral tegmental NA cell-groups also appear to be partially involved (Jonsson and Sachs 1976; Sachs and

Jonsson 1975b,c; Versteeg et al. 1977; Levitt and Moore 1980). The effects of 6-OH-DA are very selective on the NA system leaving the other monoamine neurons apparently unaffected. The consequences following a systemic 6-OH-DA administration in the neonatal stage are characterized by pronounced and permanent denervations of distant NA nerve terminal projections (e.g. in the cerebral cortex, hippocampus and spinal cord) as well as a hyperinnervation in regions close to the NA cell-bodies (e.g. in the pons-medulla and the cerebellum, see Fig. 12). No significant changes in the number and fluorescence morphology of the NA cell-bodies are seen after neonatal 6-OH-DA treatment (Jonsson et al. 1979; Sachs and Jonsson 1975b). Administration of various doses of 6-OH-DA (10-100 mg/kg s.c.) have disclosed a clear dose-response relationship in the sense that there is, with increasing 6-OH-DA dose, a more pronounced NA denervation in the cerebral cortex which is accompanied by an increasing degree of hyperinnervation in the pons-medulla (Sachs and Jonsson 1975b). These and other data indicate a close relationship between the NA denervation and hyperinnervation (see, Jonsson and Hallman 1982a,b; Jonsson and Sachs 1982). It has therefore been proposed that the altered development of the NA neurons induced by 6-OH-DA is mainly due to a 'pruning effect' (see, Schneider 1973, 1981), i.e. the permanent denervation of certain axonal branches (to cerebral cortex and spinal cord) leads to a proliferative outgrowth of the terminals in intact axon collateral systems resulting in a hyperinnervation (in the pons-medulla and cerebellum) reflecting a strict developmental program of the NA neurons with respect to their expression of the size of their nerve terminal arborizations (see, Jonsson and Hallman 1982b; Jonsson and Sachs 1982). It has also been suggested that the hyperinnervation growth response after neonatal 6-OH-DA is a result of a specific interaction between the locus ceruleus neurons and their target areas, presumably by release of target-specific factors acting on ingrowing axons and their cell-bodies (Iacovitti et al. 1981; Reis et al. 1981; Schmidt et al. 1980, 1981; see also, Sievers and Klemm 1982).

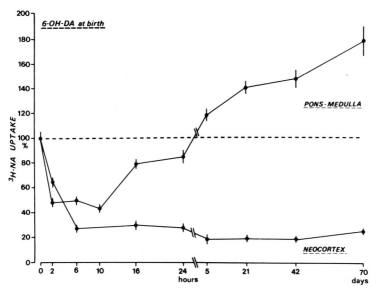

Fig. 12. Effect of neonatal 6-OH-DA treatment (100 mg/kg s.c.) on the in vitro uptake of [³H]NA in cerebral cortex and pons-medulla during the postnatal development. The results are expressed as % of control (from Sachs and Jonsson 1975b; Sachs et al. 1974).

Similar alterations in the development of the central NA neurons as those seen after systemic 6-OH-DA treatment have also been observed after systemic 6-OH-DOPA treatment 50-100 mg/kg s.c. (Zieher and Jaim-Etcheverry 1973, 1975; Jaim-Etcheverry and Zieher 1975, 1977; Kostrzewa and Harper 1974; Kostrzewa 1975; Kostrzewa and Garey 1977; Kostrzewa et al. 1978), although certain differences have been noted (Zieher and Jaim-Etcheverry 1979).

The IC mode of 6-OH-DA administration in developing rats is a procedure that has been extensively used (Breese and Traylor 1971, 1972; Lytle et al 1972; Schmidt et al. 1980; see also, Breese 1975). Injection of small doses of 6-OH-DA (10-30 μg) will mainly affect the NA neurons with alterations similar to those observed after systemic 6-OH-DA injection (see, Sachs and Jonsson 1975c). Larger doses (100 μg) will produce permanent NA denervations, although regionally quite variable, from almost complete denervations (in the cerebral cortex, cerebellum and spinal cord), to more moderate effects in the pons-medulla. It has been shown that this treatment produces NA cell-body losses (Sievers et al. 1981a) and there will in addition be a marked and permanent DA denervation in the striatum. Treatment schedules have been devised for the preferential denervation of NA and DA neurons, respectively (see, Breese 1975). It has also been observed that high doses of 6-OH-DA (100 μg IC) will lead to rather marked and apparently nonspecific alterations in the morphological development of the cerebellum, which has been proposed to be related to a 6-OH-DA induced damage of cerebellar pial fibroblasts (Sievers et al. 1981a,b; Allen et al. 1981). Minor nonspecific changes in cerebellar development were also noted after systemic 6-OH-DA (100 mg/kg s.c.) administration (Sievers et al. 1981a).

For the use of 6-OH-DA to induce catecholamine denervations in developing rats employing the IVT injection technique, see Pappas et al. (1976, 1980) and Peters et al. (1977), while for intracerebral injections of 6-OH-DA, see Lanfumey et al. (1981), Jonsson and Sachs (1982) and Pappas et al. (1982).

For prenatal studies, 6-OH-DA has to be injected directly into the fetus. Although this is a relatively difficult approach with great risks for high mortality among the fetuses, there are a few studies which have reported a successful outcome using this procedure (Tassin et al. 1975; Thierry et al. 1975; Lidov and Molliver 1982). These authors administered 100-400 μg/g in a volume of 10 μl saline into the abdomen of each fetus and could thereby obtain a marked, permanent and selective NA denervation (-85%) in the cerebral cortex. Other alternatives for the production of prenatal lesions of central NA neurons are to administer 6-OH-DOPA (50-100 mg/kg i.v.), or DSP4 (25-50 mg/kg i.v.) to pregnant rats (see, Jaim-Etcheverry and Zieher 1975, 1980; Jonsson et al. 1981).

5.2. DSP4

Developing rats tolerate this neurotoxin fairly well after doses up to 50 mg/kg s.c. and neonatal administration of such a dose produces an alteration of the postnatal development of central NA neurons very similar to that seen after neonatal 6-OH-DA treatment (Jonsson et al. 1982). In contrast to 6-OH-DA, injections of even large doses DSP4 in the neonatal stage will have only minor effects on the peripheral sympathetic adrenergic neurons, indicating that the neurotoxic potency of DSP4 on the NA neurons is clearly less pronounced than that of 6-OH-DA. The DSP4 induced changes in the CNS are dose-dependent and after 50 mg/kg (s.c.) marked and permanent NA depletions are found in the cerebral cortex and the spinal cord, whereas NA increases occur

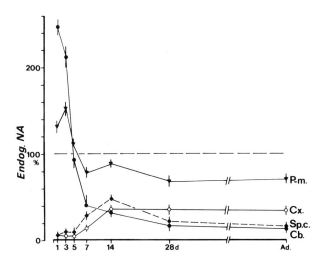

Fig. 13. Effects of DSP4 (50 mg/kg) administered at various developmental stages (1, 3, 5, 14 and 28 days-old and adults = Ad) on the endogenous NA levels in various brain regions 2 months after the DSP4 treatment. The values are expressed as % of age-matched controls (data from Jonsson et al. 1982).

in the pons-medulla and in particular in the cerebellum (see Fig. 13). The central effects of DSP4 are preferential in the locus ceruleus NA system without any detectable actions on DA- and A-systems, although a moderate neurotoxic effect on 5-HT neurons is noted. This latter effect is somewhat more pronounced than that seen after DSP4 to adult rats (cf., Jonsson et al. 1981), but can be almost completely prevented by pretreatment with the 5-HT uptake blocker zimelidine (10 mg/kg s.c.). Since DSP4 easily passes the BBB, this neurotoxin can be used to compare the effects at various developmental stages. Administration of DSP4 to rats of different ages thus produces marked and permanent NA depletions of the distant NA nerve terminal projections (cerebral cortex, spinal cord) after treatment at all ages, while increases of NA levels in the pons-medulla and cerebellum are seen only in animals treated with DSP4 up to the age of 3-5 days. DSP4 treatment in older rats produces substantial and permanent NA reductions in both these regions (Fig. 13). For prenatal studies, DSP4 can be administered to pregnant rats in doses of 25-50 mg/kg (i.v.).

5.3. 5,7-DIHYDROXYTRYPTAMINE

As already mentioned, 5,7-HT appears to be the 5-HT neurotoxin of choice for developmental studies, since 5,6-HT is very toxic (Breese et al. 1974; Krieger 1975; Sachs and Jonsson 1975d) and pCAM appears to be ineffective (Clemens et al. 1978). So far only data on the effects of 5,7-HT on the postnatal development of 5-HT neurons have been reported. For IC injections doses up to 50-100 μg of 5,7-HT (in 10 μl) are reasonably well tolerated by newborn rats (Lytle et al. 1975; Breese and Cooper 1975), although such high doses may be too high to be completely devoid of general cytotoxic actions (see, Baumgarten et al. 1977). Even doses in the range of 40-50 μg have been shown to produce marked neurodegenerative effects on 5-HT neurons (Baumgarten et al. 1975b; Breese et al. 1978), although as always with this route of administration, there will be a marked regional heterogeneity in the denervation pattern.

Systemic administration of 5,7-HT for studies on central 5-HT neurons can only be used in the neonatal stage, since the BBB for 5,7-HT matures before the end of the first postnatal week (Fig. 11; Jonsson et al. 1978). Doses up to 200 mg/kg (s.c.) can be injected without lethal effects and 50-200 mg/kg of 5,7-HT (s.c.) given to newborn rats produces an alteration of the postnatal development of central 5-HT neurons in an analogous manner as that seen for NA neurons after neonatal 6-OH-DA, 6-OH-DOPA or DSP4 treatment systemically (Sachs and Jonsson 1975d; Jonsson 1976b; Jonsson et al. 1978; Ponzio and Jonsson 1978; see also, Jonsson and Hallman 1982b). There is thus a permanent denervation of distant 5-HT nerve terminal projections in the cerebral cortex and spinal cord, whereas a marked 5-HT hyperinnervation is present in regions close to the 5-HT cell-bodies, which do not appear to be notably affected by the 5,7-HT treatment. The nonselective neurodegenerative effects of 5,7-HT on NA neurons produced by both systemic or IC injection of 5,7-HT can be largely prevented by pretreatment with a NA uptake blocker, e.g. DMI (Sachs and Jonsson 1975d; Breese et al. 1978).

6. GENERAL COMMENTS

The introduction of target-directed chemical neurotoxins for the selective destruction of monoamine neurons no doubt represents a great methodological progress for the analysis of the basic aspects of monoaminergic neurotransmission, both from structural and functional viewpoints. Although these monoamine neurotoxins are capable of producing reasonably specific lesions when properly used, it is clear from the experience obtained over the years that there are a number of complications and factors that have to be considered when using them as denervation tools. As already emphasized, the most important consideration is a *careful evaluation of the specificity and the extent of the neurotoxin induced lesion,* preferably in quantitative terms. None of these neurotoxins possesses a specificity that allows their use on a 'blind basis', but each particular lesion has to be evaluated employing adequate morphological, biochemical, pharmacological and/or physiological indices, depending on the purpose of the lesion.

For most of the monoamine neurotoxins the question of structural specificity can be regarded to consist of at least 3 sub-problems: (1) presence of general cytotoxic effects; (2) degenerative actions on more than one type of monoamine transmitter neurons; (3) denervation of more than one principal monoamine neuronal system, neuroanatomically and functionally defined. The most relevant specificity problems for each neurotoxin and possibilities to test and circumvent them have already been dealt with. The intention here is to comment on the methodology that can be used to evaluate the lesion. All the three specificity aspects can be approached by the use of morphological and neurochemical techniques, although the last point (3) is to a large extent a question of neuroanatomical considerations. As to the general cytotoxic effects, this can usually be analyzed fairly well using conventional neurohistological and ultrastructural techniques, although it should be kept in mind that it is always difficult to exclude minor, general nonspecific damage induced by the lesion in spite of no obvious structural evidence for that. The second problem — related to the specificity for one transmitter type only among the various monoamine neurons — has to be investigated by specific ultrastructural, histo- and neurochemical techniques. Such an analysis will provide adequate qualitative information, but it will, in addition, be of great importance to get information on the extent or degree of denervation of the particular neuron system that the lesion has produced. The most precise information on this point can generally be obtained by using quantitative morphological techniques for neuron specific markers (transmitters or transmitter synthesizing enzymes). These techniques are generally, however, very time-consuming and therefore not always feasible as evaluation instruments. Another limitation of the quantitative morphological procedures is that they are often poorly defined with respect to the limit of detectability in precise quantitative terms. The situation is in that case generally more favorable for the neurochemical techniques, where endogenous transmitter level, enzyme activity and content as well as transmitter uptake can be monitored easily. The main question that this approach raises is how the neurochemical parameters recorded are related to neuronal structure in quantitative terms. It should be pointed out that the neurochemical techniques are best suited for analysis at the nerve terminal level, while morphological techniques are definitely superior for the evaluation of alterations in the perikarya and main axons. The neurochemical analysis should moreover be performed in relevant tissue regions, since rather marked changes locally may escape detection if too much tissue is sampled. The most attractive neurochemical technique for the evaluation of a lesion is the measurement of transmitter uptake (initial rate) in vitro, which can be considered to be a measure of axonal surface area and hence a measure of nerve terminal density. If the kinetic parameters (K_m and V_{max}) are controlled, transmitter uptake gives a fairly reliable index of nerve terminal density; a weak point, however, is the difficulty in giving a precise definition of 'blank value' or 'extraneuronal uptake' (see, Jonsson et al. 1974; Sachs and Jonsson 1975b; Jonsson and Sachs 1973b) and this may lead to problems in obtaining accurate measurements when extensive denervations are at hand, i.e. in the range of about 0-20% of control. Concerning the use of endogenous transmitter levels to monitor changes in the nerve terminal field, it is known that substantial alterations in the steady-state levels may occur in both directions without changes in nerve density; e.g. acutely after an axotomy (see Fig. 6). Such changes are, however, most likely to occur in the acute stage of an experimental manipulation, while the general experience is that a lesion induced change in the transmitter levels agrees very well with uptake data, indicating that endogenous transmitter levels in most cases reflect nerve density, at least in the subchronic and chronic stage (see Fig. 6). An exception is the developing and regenerating neurons which appear to contain less transmitter than normal, and that is why measurements of transmitter levels tend to give an underestimation of the real nerve density in such situations (see, Jonsson and Sachs 1972, 1973b). It is also known that small changes in endogenous transmitter levels chronically may reflect alterations in the functional state of the neuron rather than a change in nerve density. The main advantage with measurement of transmitter levels is that the techniques available are specific, rapid and simple, although it may be advisable to record both transmitter uptake and levels in order to be on the safe side.

The situation is somewhat more complex when recording the content and activity of transmitter specific enzymes, since these parameters are not always constant in the single neuron under various experimental conditions. Of particular relevance in this context is that there appears to be a switch in the priorities of the synthesizing capacity of the soma after an axonal damage, in favor of structural proteins for repair processes, during which transmitter enzyme formation may be reduced. Measurement of transmitter enzymes can, however, be considered as a very sensitive and specific way of monitoring the consequences following a lesion, especially when evaluating extensive lesions.

When using morphological and neurochemical evaluation techniques in combination with pretreatment with an appropriate uptake inhibitor (e.g. DMI) to prevent a neurotoxin induced lesion, valuable information on the functional specificity of a lesion can also be obtained (see, Lidbrink and Jonsson 1975). It should be kept in mind, however, that the use of uptake inhibitors in order to secure specificity and/or to improve selectivity does not always produce the intended complete protection towards the neurotoxin induced damage. This should be watched for. It is furthermore advisable to test the specificity for all monoamine neurotoxins by analyzing their potential degenerative action on each relevant monoamine neuron, due to the fact that each monoamine neuron type does not have an uptake mechanism with absolute specificity. In view of the discussion above it is clear that no single analysis technique will provide reasonably safe information on the specificity and extent of a monoamine neurotoxin induced lesion; hence, such evaluation should be based on both morphological and neurochemical techniques where independent markers or parameters should be analyzed.

Another aspect which might be pertinent to comment upon here is that the lesion strategy is commonly used with a relatively static view as to changes of the structural organization of the nervous tissue following a lesion. It is, however, now well established that the post-lesion state is by no means a static situation. On the contrary, the period following the acute degenerative phase is characterized by active and dynamic processes, which can lead to a substantial structural reorganization which may have important functional consequences. Reparative processes involving both neurons and glia cells thus start very soon after inducing the lesion and continue over months, which appears to be of particular relevance with respect to central monoamine neurons, since they have been shown to have a marked regrowth capacity after neurotoxin induced lesions (see, Björklund and Stenevi 1979). The degree of regenerative response and reorganization depends very much on the site(s) of neurodegenerative damage. The most extensive regrowth has been observed when the damage is restricted to the distal parts of the axonal arborizations. For furhter information on various growth responses of central monoamine neurons seen after monoamine neurotoxin lesions in adult and developing animals, see Björklund and Stenevi (1979) and Jonsson and Hallman (1982b). The information available underlines the importance of evaluating the lesion both in the acute and chronic stages when using the lesion approach to establish structure-function relationships (see also, Jonsson 1982b).

Finally, it should be mentioned that the degenerative changes following a lesion are not always exclusively restricted to the damaged neurons, but there may also be transneuronal or transsynaptic degeneration processes (see Fig. 1). This phenomenon has recently been observed in the striatum, after lesion of both the glutaminergic corticostriatal (induced by cortical aspiration) and dopaminergic nigrostriatal (6-OH-DA induced) projections (Hattori and Fibiger 1982). These authors found that degenerating dendritic spines postsynaptic to the degenerating striatal boutons were detectable already 2-3 days after either type of lesion. It is clear that this degeneration phenomenon constitutes a potential problem when employing lesions to localize the neuronal location of various histo- and biochemical markers (transmitters, enzymes, receptors). Although this is not always an easily analyzed degeneration process, it is evident that transneuronal effects might be of significant importance and should therefore be considered.

ACKNOWLEDGEMENTS

The author is very grateful to Mrs Christina Seiger for typing the manuscript.

7. REFERENCES

Acheson AL, Zigmond MJ, Stricker EM (1980): Compensatory increase in tyrosine hydroxylase activity in rat brain after intraventricular injections of 6-hydroxydopamine. *Science, 207,* 537–540.

Agid Y, Javoy F, Glowinski J, Bouvet D, Sotelo C (1973): Injection of 6-hydroxydopamine into the substantia nigra of the rat. II. Diffusion and specificity. *Brain Res., 58,* 291–301.

Allen C, Sievers J, Berry M, Jenner S (1981): Experimental studies on cerebellar foliation. II. A morphometric analysis of cerebellar fissuration defects and growth retardation after neonatal treatment with 6-OH-DA in the rat. *J. Comp. Neurol., 203,* 771–783.

Aloe L, Mugnaini E, Levi-Montalcini R (1975): Light- and electron-microscopic studies of the excessive growth of sympathetic ganglia in rats injected daily from birth with 6-OH-DA and NGF. *Arch. Ital. Biol., 113,* 236–253.

Ames MM, Frank SK (1982): Stereochemical aspects of *para*-chloroamphetamine metabolism. *Biochem. Pharmacol., 31,* 5–9.

Andén N-E, Bédard P, Fuxe K, Ungerstedt U (1972): Early and selective increase in brain dopamine levels after axotomy. *Experientia, 28,* 300–301.

Angeletti PU (1971): Chemical sympathectomy in newborn animals. *Neuropharmacology, 10,* 55–59.

Angeletti PU, Levi-Montalcini R (1970): Sympathetic nerve cell destruction in newborn mammals by 6-hydroxydopamine. *Proc. Nat. Acad. Sci. USA, 65,* 114–121.

Archer T, Jonsson G, Johansson G, Ross SB (1983): A parametric study of the effects of the noradrenaline neurotoxin DSP4 on avoidance acquisition and noradrenaline neurons in the CNS of the rat. *Br. J. Pharmac.,* in press.

Barron KD, Dentinger MP, Rodichok LD (1981): The axon reaction of central and peripheral mammalian neurons: A comparison. In: Gorio A, Millesi H, Mingrino S (Eds), *Posttraumatic Peripheral Nerve Regeneration,* pp. 17–26. Raven Press, New York.

Baumgarten HG, Björklund A (1976): Neurotoxic indolamines and monoamine neurons. *Ann. Rev. Pharmacol. Toxicol., 16,* 101–111.

Baumgarten HG, Lachenmayer L (1972): 5,7-Dihydroxytryptamine: Improvement in chemical lesioning of indolamine neurons in mammalian brain. *Z. Zellforsch., 135,* 399–414.

Baumgarten HG, Björklund A, Lachenmayer L, Nobin A, Stenevi U (1971): Long-lasting selective depletion of brain serotonin by 5,6-dihydroxytryptamine. *Acta Physiol. Scand., Suppl.,* 373.

Baumgarten HG, Evetts KD, Holman RB, Iversen LL, Vogt M, Wilson G (1972a): Effects of 5,6-dihydroxytryptamine on monoaminergic neurons in the central nervous system of the rat. *J. Neurochem., 19,* 1587–1597.

Baumgarten HG, Lachenmayer L, Schlossberger H-G (1972b): Evidence for a degeneration of indolamine containing nerve terminals in rat brain, induced by 5,6-dihydroxytryptamine. *Z. Zellforsch., 125,* 553–569.

Baumgarten HG, Björklund A, Lachenmayer L, Nobin A (1973): Evaluation of the effects of 5,7-dihydroxytryptamine on serotonin and catecholamine neurons in the rat CNS. *Acta Physiol. Scand., Suppl.,* 391.

Baumgarten HG, Björklund A, Lachenmayer L, Rensch A, Rosengren E (1974): De- and regeneration of the bulbospinal serotonin neurons in the rat following 5,6- or 5,7-dihydroxytryptamine treatment. *Cell Tissue Res., 152,* 271–281.

Baumgarten HG, Björklund A, Nobin A, Rosengren E, Schlossberger HG (1975a): Neurotoxicity of hydroxylated tryptamines: Structure-activity relationships. *Acta Physiol. Scand., Suppl.,* 429.

Baumgarten HG, Victor SJ, Lovenberg W (1975b): A developmental study of the effects of 5,7-dihydroxytryptamine on regional tryptophan hydroxylase in rat brain. *Psychopharmacol. Comm., 1,* 75–88.

Baumgarten HG, Lachenmayer L, Björklund A (1977): Chemical lesioning of indolamine pathways. In: Myers RD (Ed), *Methods in Psychobiology, Vol. 3,* pp. 47–98. Academic Press, New York.

Baumgarten HG, Jenner S, Schlossberger H-G (1979): Serotonin neurotoxins: Effects of drugs on the destruction of brain serotonergic, noradrenergic and dopaminergic axons in adult rat by intraventricularly, intracisternally or intracerebrally administered 5,7-dihydroxytryptamine and related compounds. In: Chubb IW, Geffen LB (Eds). *Neurotoxins, Fundamental and Clinical Advances,* pp. 221–226. Adelaide University Union Press, Adelaide.

Baumgarten HG, Jenner S, Klemm HP (1981): Serotonin neurotoxins: Recent advances in the mode of administration and molecular mechanism of action. *J. Physiol. (Paris), 77,* 309–314.

Bell JL, Iversen LL, Uretsky NJ (1970): Time course of the effects of 6-hydroxydopamine on catecholamine-containing neurones in rat hypothalamus and striatum. *Br. J. Pharmacol., 40,* 790–799.

Ben-Menachem E, Johansson BB, Svensson T-H (1982): Increased vulnerability of the blood-brain barrier to acute hypertension following depletion of brain noradrenaline. *J. Neural Transm., 53,* 159–167.

Bendeich EG, Konkol RJ, Krigman MR, Breese GR (1978): Morphological evidence for 6-hydroxydopamine induced sprouting of noradrenergic neurons in the cerebellum. *J. Neurol. Sci., 38,* 47–57.

Bennett T, Burnstock G, Cobb JLS, Malmfors T (1970): An ultrastructural and histochemical study of the short-term effects of 6-hydroxydopamine on adrenergic nerves in the domestic fowl. *Br. J. Pharmacol., 38,* 802–809.

Bisby MA (1980): Retrograde axonal transport. *Adv. Cell. Neurobiol., 1,* 69–117.

Bittiger H, Maître L, Krinke G, Schnider K, Hess R (1977): A study of long-term effects of guanethidine on peripheral noradrenergic neurones of the rat. *Toxicology, 8,* 63–78.

Björklund A, Steveni U (1979): Regeneration of monoaminergic and cholinergic neurons in the mammalian central nervous system. *Physiol. Rev., 59,* 62–100.

Björklund A, Nobin A, Steveni U (1973a): Regeneration of central serotonin neurons after axonal degeneration induced by 5,6-dihydroxytryptamine. *Brain Res., 50,* 214–220.

Björklund A, Nobin A, Steveni U (1973b): The use of neurotoxic dihydroxytryptamines as tools for morphological studies and localized lesioning of central indolamine neurons. *Z. Zellforsch., 145,* 479–501.

Björklund A, Baumgarten HG, Rensch A (1975): 5,7-Dihydroxytryptamine: Improvement of its selectivity for serotonin neurons in the CNS by pretreatment with desipramine. *J. Neurochem., 24,* 833–835.

Blank CL, Kissinger PT, Adams RN (1972a): 5,6-Dihydroxyindole formation from oxidized 6-hydroxy-dopamine. *Eur. J. Pharmacol., 19,* 391–394.

Blank CL, Murrill E, Adams RN (1972b): Central nervous system effects of 6-aminodopamine and 6-hydroxydopamine. *Brain Res., 45,* 635–637.

Bloom FE (1975): Monoaminergic neurotoxins: Are they selective? *J. Neural Transm., 37,* 183–187.

Bloom FE, Algeri S, Groppetti A, Revuelta A, Costa E (1969): Lesions of central norepinephrine terminals with 6-OH-dopamine: Biochemistry and fine structure. *Science, 166,* 1284–1286.

Borchardt RT (1975): Catechol-O-methyltransferase: A model to study the mechanism of 6-hydroxy-dopamine interaction with proteins. In: Jonsson G, Malmfors T, Sachs Ch (Eds), *Chemical Tools in Catecholamine Research, Vol. 1,* pp. 33–40. North-Holland Publ. Co., Amsterdam.

Borchardt RT, Burgess SK, Reid JR, Liang YO, Adams RN (1977): Effects of 2- and/or 5-methylated analogues of 6-hydroxydopamine on norepinephrine and dopamine-containing neurons. *Mol. Pharmacol., 13,* 805–818.

Breese GR (1975): Chemical and immunochemical lesions by specific neurotoxic substances and antisera. In: Iversen LL, Iversen SD, Snyder SH (Eds), *Handbook of Psychopharmacology, Vol. 1,* pp. 137–189. Plenum Press, New York.

Breese GR, Cooper BR (1975): Behavioral and biochemical interactions of 5,7-dihydroxytryptamine with various drugs when administered intracisternally to adult and developing rats. *Brain Res., 98,* 517–527.

Breese GR, Traylor TD (1970): Effect of 6-hydroxydopamine on brain norepinephrine and dopamine: Evidence for selective degeneration of catecholamine neurons. *J. Pharmacol. Exp. Ther., 174,* 413–427.

Breese GR, Traylor TD (1971): Depletion of brain noradrenaline and dopamine by 6-hydroxydopamine. *Br. J. Pharmacol., 42,* 88–99.

Breese GR, Traylor TD (1972): Developmental characteristics of brain catecholamines and tyrosine hydroxylase in rat: Effects of 6-hydroxydopamine. *Br. J. Pharmacol., 44,* 210–222.

Breese GR, Cooper BR, Smith RD (1973a): Biochemical and behavioral alterations following 6-hydroxy-dopamine administration into brain. In: Usdin E, Snyder SH (Eds). *Frontiers in Catecholamine Research,* pp. 701–706. Pergamon Press, New York.

Breese GR, Smith RD, Cooper BR, Grant LD (1973b): Alterations in consummatory behaviour following intracisternal injection of 6-hydroxydopamine. *Pharmacol. Biochem. Behav., 1,* 319–328.

Breese GR, Cooper BR, Grant LD, Smith RD (1974): Biochemical and behavioural alterations following 5,6-dihydroxytryptamine administration into brain. *Neuropharmacology, 13,* 177–187.

Breese GR, Vogel RA, Mueller RA (1978): Biochemical and behavioural alterations in developing rats treated with 5,7-dihydroxytryptamine. *J. Pharmacol., 201,* 587–595.

Burgess SK, Eiden LE, Tessel RE (1980): 6-Hydroxydopamine differentially affects PNMT activity and epinephrine content in rat hypothalamus: Evidence for compensatory enhancement in neuronal function. *Soc. Neurosci. Abstr., 6,* 441.

Burnstock G, Evans B, Gannon BT, Heath JW, James V (1971): A new method of destroying adrenergic nerves in adult animals using guanethidine. *Br. J. Pharmacol., 43,* 295–301.

Butcher LL (1975): Degenerative processes after punctuate intracerebral administration of 6-hydroxy-dopamine. *J. Neural Transm., 37,* 189–208.

Butcher LL, Eastgate SM, Hodge GK (1974): Evidence that punctuate intracerebral administration of 6-hydroxydopamine fails to produce selective neuronal degeneration: Comparison with copper sulphate and factors governing the deportment of fluids injected into brain. *Naunyn-Schmiedebergs Arch. Pharmakol., 285,* 31–70.

Carlsen RC, Kiff J, Ryugo K (1982): Suppression of the cell body response in axotomized frog spinal neurons does not prevent initiation of nerve regeneration. *Brain Res., 234,* 11–25.

Carpenter MB, Whittier JR (1952): Study of methods for producing experimental lesions in the central nervous system with special reference to stereotaxic technique. *J. Comp. Neurol., 97,* 73–132.

Cheah TB, Geffen LB (1973): Effects of axonal injury on norepinephrine, tyrosine hydroxylase and monoamine oxidase levels in sympathetic ganglia. *J. Neurobiol., 4,* 443–452.

Cho AK, Ransom RW, Fischer JB, Kammerer RC (1980): The effects of xylamine, a nitrogen mustard on [^{3}H]norepinephrine accumulation in rabbit aorta. *J. Pharmacol. Exp. Ther., 214,* 324–327.

Chubb IW, Geffen LB (1979): *Neurotoxins: Fundamental and Clinical Advances.* Adelaide University Press, Adelaide.

Clark DW, Laverty R, Phelan EL (1972): Long-lasting peripheral and central effects of 6-hydroxydopamine in rats. *Brit. J. Pharmacol., 44,* 233–243.

Clarke DE, Smookler HH, Hadinata J, Chi C, Barry III H (1972): Acute effects of 6-hydroxydopa and its interaction with dopa on brain amine levels. *Life Sci., 11,* 97–102.

Clemens JA, Fuller RW, Perry KW, Sawyer BD (1978): Effects of *p*-chloramphetamine on brain serotonin in immature rats. *Commun. Psychopharmacol., 2,* 11–16.

Cobb JLS, Bennett T (1971): An electron-microscopic examination of the short-term effects of 6-hydroxy-dopamine on the peripheral adrenergic nervous system. In: Malmfors T, Thoenen H (Eds), *6-Hydroxydopamine and Catecholamine Neurons,* pp. 33–45. North-Holland Publ. Co., Amsterdam.

Cohen G, Heikkila RE (1974): The generation of hydrogen peroxide, superoxide radical and hydroxyl radical by 6-hydroxydopamine, dialuric acid and related cytotoxic agents. *J. Biol. Chem., 249,* 2447–2452.

Cooper PH, Novin D, Butcher LL (1982): Intracerebral 6-hydroxydopamine produces extensive damage to the blood-brain barrier in rats. *Neurosci. Lett., 30,* 13–18.

Corrodi H, Clark WG, Masouka DI (1971): The synthesis and effects of DL-6-hydroxydopa. In: Malmfors T, Thoenen H (Eds), *6-Hydroxydopamine and Catecholamine Neurons,* pp. 187–192. North-Holland Publ. Co., Amsterdam.

Cragg BG (1970): What is the signal for chromatolysis. *Brain Res., 23,* 1–21.

Creveling CR, Rotman A, Daly JW (1975): Interactions of 6-hydroxydopamine and related compounds with proteins: A model for the mechanism of cytotoxicity. In: Jonsson G, Malmfors T, Sachs Ch (Eds), *Chemical Tools in Catecholamine Research,* pp. 23–32. North-Holland Publ. Co., Amsterdam.

Daly J, Fuxe K, Jonsson G (1973): Effects of intracerebral injections of 5,6-dihydroxytryptamine on central monoamine neurons: Evidence for selective degeneration of central 5-hydroxytryptamine neurons. *Brain Res., 49,* 476–482.

Daly J, Fuxe K, Jonsson G (1974): 5,7-Dihydroxytryptamine as a tool for the morphological and functional analysis of central 5-hydroxytryptamine neurons. *Res. Commun. Chem. Pathol. Pharmacol., 1,* 175–187.

De Montigny C, Wang RY, Reader TA, Aghajanian GK (1980): Monoaminergic denervation of the rat hippocampus: Microiontophoretic studies on pre- and postsynaptic supersensitivity to norepinephrine and serotonin. *Brain Res., 200,* 363–376.

Descarries L, Saucier G (1972): Disappearance of the locus ceruleus in the rat after intraventricular 6-hydroxydopamine. *Brain Res., 37,* 310–316.

Dudley MW, Butcher LL, Kammerer RG, Cho AK (1981): The actions of xylamine on central adrenergic neurons. *J. Pharmacol. Exp. Ther., 217,* 834–840.

Ellison G, Eison MS, Huberman HS, Daniel F (1978): Long-term changes in dopaminergic innervation of caudate nucleus after continuous amphetamine administration. *Science, 201,* 276–278.

Eränkö L, Eränkö O (1971): Effect of guanethidine on nerve cells and small intensely fluorescent cells in sympathetic ganglia of newborn and adult rats. *Acta Pharmacol. Toxicol., 30,* 403–416.

Evans BK (1979): Influence of neuronal activity levels on the cytotoxic effects of guanethidine. *J. Pharmacol. Exp. Ther., 209,* 205–214.

Evans B, Gannon BJ, Heath JW, Burnstock G (1972): Long-lasting damage to the internal male genital organs and their adrenergic innervation following chronic treatment with the antihypertensive drug guanethidine. *Fertil. Steril., 23,* 657–667.

Evans BK, Singer G, Armstrong S, Saunders PE, Burnstock G (1975): Effects of chronic intracranial injection of low and high concentrations of guanethidine in the rat. *Pharmacol. Biochem. Behav., 3,* 219–228.

Fischer JB, Cho AK (1982): Inhibition of [³H]norepinephrine uptake in organ cultured rat superior cervical ganglia by xylamine. *J. Pharmacol. Exp. Ther., 220,* 115–119.

Fuller RW (1978): Neurochemical effects of serotonin neurotoxins. *Ann. NY Acad. Sci., 305,* 178–181.

Fuller RW (1982): Pharmacology of brain epinephrine neurons. *Ann. Rev. Pharmacol. Toxicol., 22,* 31–55.

Fuller RW, Hemrick-Luecke S (1980): Long-lasting depletion of striatal dopamine by a single injection of amphetamine in iprindole-treated rats. *Science, 209,* 305–307.

Fuller RW, Hemrick-Luecke SK (1982): Further studies on the long-term depletion of striatal dopamine in iprindole-treated rats by amphetamine. *Neuropharmacology, 21,* 433–438.

Fuller RW, Baker J-C, Perry KW, Molloy BB (1975a): Comparison of 4-chloro-, 4-bromo- and 4-fluoroamphetamine in rats: Drug levels in brain and effects on brain serotonin metabolism. *Neuropharmacology, 14,* 739–746.

Fuller RW, Perry KW, Molloy (1975b): Reversible and irreversible phases of serotonin depletion by 4-chloroamphetamine. *Eur. J. Pharmacol., 33,* 119–124.

Furness J (1979): Toxic effects of drugs on catecholamine receptors. In: Chubb IW, Geffen LB (Eds), *Neurotoxins: Fundamental and Clinical Advances,* pp. 213–220. Adelaide University Union Press, Adelaide.

Furness JB, Cambell GR, Gillard SM, Malmfors T, Chobb JLS, Burnstock G (1970): Cellular studies of sympathetic denervation produced by 6-hydroxydopamine in the vas deferens. *J. Pharmacol. Exp. Ther., 174,* 111–122.

Fuxe K, Jonsson G (1974): Further mapping of central 5-hydroxytryptamine neurons: Studies with neurotoxic dihydroxytryptamines. In: Costa E, Gessa GL, Sandler M (Eds), *Serotonin - New Vistas, Adv. Biochem. Psychopharmacol., Vol. 10,* pp. 1–12. Raven Press, New York.

Fuxe K, Eneroth P, Gustavsson JÅ, Hökfelt T, Jonsson G, Löfström A, Skett P (1975): Effects of 6-OH-DA induced lesions of the ascending noradrenaline and adrenaline pathways to the tel- and diencephalon on FSH, LH and prolactin secretion in the ovariectomized female rat. In: Jonsson G, Malmfors T, Sachs Ch (Eds), *Chemical Tools in Catecholamine Research, Vol. I,* pp. 273–283. North-Holland Publ. Co., Amsterdam.

Fuxe K, Ögren S-O, Agnati LF, Jonsson G, Gustafsson JÅ (1978): 5,7-Dihydroxytryptamine as a tool to study the functional role of central 5-hydroxytryptamine neurons. *Ann. NY Acad. Sci., 305,* 346–369.

Gannon BJ, Iwayama T, Burnstock G, Gerkens J, Mashford M (1971): Prolonged effects of chronic guanethidine treatment on the sympathetic innervation of the genitalia of male rats. *Med. J. Aust., 2,* 207–208.

Gershanik OS, Heikkila RE, Duvoisin RC (1979): Asymmetric action of intraventricular monoamine neurotoxins. *Brain Res., 174,* 345–350.

Gershon S, Baldessarini RJ (1975): Selective destruction of serotonin terminals in rat forebrain by high doses of 5,7-dihydroxytryptamine. *Brain Res., 85,* 140–145.

Ghetti B, Horoupian DS, Wisniewsky HM (1975): Acute and long-term transneuronal response of dendrites of lateral geniculate neurons following transection of the primary visual afferent pathway. In: Kreutzberg W (Ed), *Advances in Neurology, Vol. 12,* pp. 401–424. Raven Press, New York.

Grafstein B, Forman DS (1980): Intracellular transport in neurons. *Physiol. Rev., 60,* 1167–1283.

Grafstein B, McQuarrie IG (1978): Role of the nerve cell body in axonal regeneration. In: Cotman CW (Ed), *Neuronal Plasticity,* pp. 155–195. Raven Press, New York.

Graham DG, Tiffany SM, Bell Jr WR, Gutknecht WF (1978): Autoxidation versus covalent binding of quinones as the mechanism of toxicity of dopamine, 6-hydroxydopamine and related compounds toward C1300 neuroblastoma cells in vitro. *Mol. Pharmacol., 14,* 644–653.

Häusler G (1971): Early pre- and postjunctional effects of 6-hydroxydopamine *J. Pharmacol. Exp. Ther., 178,* 49–62.

Häusler G, Haefely W, Thoenen H (1979): Chemical sympathectomy of the rat with 6-hydroxydopamine. *J. Pharmacol. Exp. Ther., 170,* 50–61.

Hansen S, Stanfield EJ, Everitt BJ (1981): The effects of lesions of lateral tegmental noradrenergic neurons on components of sexual behaviour and pseudopregnancy in female rats. *Neuroscience, 6,* 1105–1117.

Hardebo JE, Edvinsson L, Owman Ch, Rosengren E (1977): Quantitative evaluation of the blood-brain barrier capacity to form dopamine from circulating L-DOPA. *Acta Physiol. Scand., 99,* 377–384.

Hardebo J-E, Edvinsson L, MacKenzie ET, Owman Ch (1979): Histofluorescence study on monoamine entry into the brain before and after opening of the blood-brain barrier by various mechanisms. *Acta Neuropathol., 47,* 145–150.

Hardebo JE, Edvinsson L, Johansson BB (1980): Cerebrovascular sympathetic denervation and blood-brain barrier function in conscious rats. *Acta Physiol. Scand., 110,* 375–379.

Hattori T, Fibiger HC (1982): On the use of lesions of afferents to localize neurotransmitter receptor sites in the striatum. *Brain Res., 238,* 245–250.

Heath JW, Evans BK, Gannon BJ, Burnstock G, James VB (1972): Degeneration of adrenergic neurones following guanethidine treatment: An ultrastructural study. *Virchows Arch. B., 11,* 182–197.

Hedreen J (1975): Increased nonspecific damage after lateral ventricle injection of 6-OHDA compared with fourth ventricle injection in rat brain. In: Jonsson G, Malmfors T, Sachs Ch (Eds), *Chemical Tools in Catecholamine Research, Vol. I,* pp. 91–100. North-Holland Publ. Co., Amsterdam.

Hedreen JC, Chalmers JP (1972): Neuronal degeneration in rat brain induced by 6-hydroxydopamine: A histochemical and biochemical study. *Brain Res., 47,* 1–36.

Heikkila R, Cohen G (1972): Further studies on the generation of hydrogenperoxide by 6-hydroxydopamine. *Mol. Pharmacol., 8,* 241–248.

Heikkila RE, Cohen G (1973): 6-Hydroxydopamine: Evidence for superoxide radical as an oxidative intermediate. *Science, 181,* 456–457.

Heikkila RE, Cohen G (1975): Prevention of 6-OH-DA induced neurotoxicity. In: Jonsson G, Malmfors T, Sachs Ch (Eds), *Chemical Tools in Catecholamine Research, Vol. I,* pp. 7–14. North-Holland Publ. Co., Amsterdam.

Heikkila RE, Mytilineou C, Côlé LJ, Cohen G (1973): The biochemical and pharmacological properties of 6-aminodopamine: Similarity with 6-hydroxydopamine. *J. Neurochem., 21,* 111–116.

Heybach JP, Coover GD, Leints CE (1978): Behavioral effects of neurotoxic lesions of the ascending monoamine pathways in the rat brain. *J. Comp. Physiol. Psychol., 92,* 58–70.

Hole K, Fuxe K, Jonsson G (1976): Behavioral effects of 5,7-dihydroxytryptamine lesions of ascending 5-hydroxytryptamine pathways. *Brain Res., 107,* 385–399.

Hökfelt T, Ungerstedt U (1973): Specificity of 6-hydroxydopamine induced degeneration of central monoamine neurons: An electron- and fluorescence-microscopic study with special reference to intracerebral injection on the nigrostriatal dopamine system. *Brain Res., 60,* 269–297.

Hökfelt T, Jonsson G, Sachs Ch (1972): Fine structure and fluorescence morphology of adrenergic nerves after 6-hydroxydopamine in vivo and in vitro, *Z. Zellforsch., 131,* 529–543.

Hotchkiss AJ, Gibb JW (1980): Long-term effects of multiple doses of methamphetamine on tryptophan hydroxylase and tyrosine hydroxylase activity in rat brain. *J. Pharmacol. Exp. Ther., 214,* 257–262.

Hotchkiss AJ, Morgan ME, Gibbs JW (1979): The long-term effects of multiple doses of methamphetamine on neostriatal tryptophan hydroxylase, tyrosine hydroxylase, choline acetyltransferase and glutamate decarboxylase activities. *Life Sci., 25,* 1373–1378.

Howard JL, Breese GR (1974): Physiological and behavioural effects of centrally administered 6-hydroxydopamine in cats. *Pharmacol. Biochem. Behav., 2,* 537–543.

Iacovitti L, Reis DJ, Joh TH (1981): Reactive proliferation of brain stem noradrenergic nerves following neonatal cerebellectomy in rats: Role of target maturation on neuronal response to injury during development. *Develop. Brain Res., 1,* 3–24.

Jacoby JH, Lytle LD (1978): Serotonin neurotoxins. *Ann. NY Acad. Sci., Vol. 305.*

Jaim-Etcheverry G, Zieher LM (1971): Permanent depletion of peripheral norepinephrine in rats treated at birth with 6-hydroxydopamine. *Eur. J. Pharmacol., 13,* 272–276.

Jaim-Etcheverry G, Zieher LM (1975): Alterations of the development of central adrenergic neurons produced by 6-hydroxydopa. In: Jonsson G, Malmfors HT, Sachs Ch (Eds), *Chemical Tools in Catecholamine Research, Vol. I,* pp. 173–180. North-Holland Publ. Co., Amsterdam.

Jaim-Etcheverry G, Zieher LM (1977): Differential effects of various 6-hydroxydopa treatment on the development and peripheral noradrenergic neurons. *Eur. J. Pharmacol., 45,* 105–112.

Jaim-Etcheverry G, Zieher LM (1980): DSP4: A novel compound with neurotoxic effects on noradrenergic neurons of adult and developing rats. *Brain Res., 188,* 513–523.

Jacks BR, DeChamplain J, Cordeau J-P (1972): Effects of 6-hydroxydopamine on putative transmitter substances in the central nervous system. *Eur. J. Pharmacol., 18,* 353–360.

Jacobowitz D, Kostrzewa R (1971): Selective action of 6-hydroxydopa on noradrenergic terminals: Mapping of preterminal axons of the brain. *Life Sci., 10,* 1329–1342.

Javoy F, Agid Y, Sotelo C (1975): Specific and nonspecific catecholaminergic neuronal destruction by intracerebral injection of 6-OH-DA in the rat. In: Jonsson G, Malmfors T, Sachs Ch (Eds), *Chemical Tools in Catecholamine Research,* pp. 75–82. North-Holland Publ. Co., Amsterdam.

Jenner S, Baumgarten HG (1980): Regional depletion of monoamines and distribution of radioactivity in the rat brain following slow or fast injection of 5,7-dihydroxytryptamine or [^{14}C]5,7-DHT into the left lateral ventricle and the effects of anaesthesia on these parameters. *Neurosci. Lett., Suppl. 5,* S449.

Jensen-Holm J, Juul P (1971): Ultrastructural changes in the rat superior ganglion following prolonged guanethidine administration. *Acta Pharmacol. Toxicol., 30,* 308–320.

Johansson BB (1979): Neonatal 6-hydroxydopamine treatment increases the vulnerability of the blood-brain barrier to acute hypertension in conscious rats. *Acta Neurol. Scand., 60,* 198–203.

Johansson BB, Henning M (1980): 6-Hydroxydopamine and the blood-brain barrier in adult conscious rats. *Acta Physiol. Scand., 110,* 1–4.

Johnson EM (1978): Destruction of the sympathetic nervous system in neonatal rats and hamsters by vinblastine: Prevention by concomitant administration of nerve growth factor. *Brain Res., 141,* 105–118.

Johnson EM, Cantor E, Douglas JR (1975): Biochemical and functional evaluation of the sympathectomy produced by the administration of guanethidine to newborn rats. *J. Pharmacol. Exp. Ther., 193,* 503–512.

Jonsson G (1976a): Studies on the mechanisms of 6-hydroxydopamine cytotoxicity. *Med. Biol., 54,* 406–420.

Jonsson G (1976b): Developmental characteristics of central monoamine neurons and their reciprocal relations. *Exp. Neurol., 53,* 801–814.

Jonsson G (1980): Chemical neurotoxins as denervation tools in neurobiology. *Ann. Rev. Neurosci., 3,* 169–187.

Jonsson G (1982a): Sympathectomy: Past, present and future. In: Kalsner S (Ed), *Trends in Autonomic Pharmacology,* pp. 133–145. Urban & Schwarzenberg Inc., Baltimore.

Jonsson G (1982b): Lesion methods in neurobiology. In: Heym Ch, Forssmann WG (Eds), *Techniques in Neuroanatomical Research,* pp. 71–99. Springer-Verlag, Berlin.

Jonsson G, Hallman H (1982a): Modulation of 6-hydroxydopamine induced alteration of the postnatal development of central noradrenaline neurons. *Brain. Res. Bull., 9,* 635–640.

Jonsson G, Hallman H (1982b): Response of central monoamine neurons following an early neurotoxic lesion. *Bibl. Anat., No. 23,* 76–92.

Jonsson G, Nwanze E (1982): Selective (+)-amphetamine neurotoxicity on striatal dopamine nerve terminals in the mouse. *Br. J. Pharmacol., 77,* 335–345.

Jonsson G, Sachs Ch (1970): Effects of 6-hydroxydopamine on the uptake and storage of noradrenaline in sympathetic adrenergic neurons. *Eur. J. Pharmacol., 9,* 141–155.

Jonsson G, Sachs Ch (1971): Uptake and accumulation of [^{3}H]6-hydroxydopamine in adrenergic nerves. *Eur. J. Pharmacol., 16,* 55–62.

Jonsson G, Sachs Ch (1972a): Neurochemical properties of adrenergic nerves regenerated after 6-hydroxydopamine. *J. Neurochem., 19,* 2577–2585.

Jonsson G, Sachs Ch (1972b): Degenerative and nondegenerative effects of 6-hydroxydopamine on adrenergic nerves. *J. Pharmacol. Exp. Ther., 180,* 625–635.

Jonsson G, Sachs Ch (1973a): 6-Aminodopamine induced degeneration of catecholamine neurons. *J. Neurochem., 21,* 117–124.

Jonsson G, Sachs Ch (1973b): Histochemical and neurochemical studies on adrenergic nerves regenerated after chemical sympathectomy produced by 6-hydroxydopamine. In: Fujiwara M (Ed), *Fluorescence Histochemistry of Biogenic Amines.,* pp. 67–81. Igaku-Shoin Ltd., Tokyo.

Jonsson G, Sachs Ch (1976): Regional changes in [^{3}H]noradrenaline uptake, catecholamines and catecholamine synthetic and catabolic enzymes in rat brain following neonatal 6-hydroxydopamine treatment. *Med. Biol., 54,* 286–297.

Jonsson G, Sachs Ch (1982): Changes in the development of central noradrenaline neurons after axonal lesions neonatally. *Brain Res. Bull., 9,* 641–650.

Jonsson G, Fuxe K, Hökfelt T (1972): On the catecholamine innervation of the hypothalamus, with special reference to the median eminence. *Brain Res., 40,* 271–281.

Jonsson G, Pycock Ch, Sachs Ch (1973): Plastic changes of central noradrenaline neurons after 6-hydroxydopamine. In: Usdin E, Snyder S (Eds), *Frontiers in Catecholamine Research,* pp. 459–461. Pergamon Press, New York.

Jonsson G, Pycock Ch, Fuxe K, Sachs Ch (1974): Changes in the development of central noradrenaline neurons following neonatal administration of 6-hydroxydopamine. *J. Neurochem., 22,* 621–626.

Jonsson G, Malmfors T, Sachs Ch (1975): *Chemical Tools in Catecholamine Research I. 6-Hydroxydopamine as a Denervation Tool in Catecholamine Research.* North-Holland Publ. Co., Amsterdam.

Jonsson G, Fuxe K, Hökfelt T, Goldstein M (1976): Resistance of central phenylethanolamine-N-methyl transferase containing neurons to 6-hydroxydopamine. *Med. Biol., 54,* 421–426.

Jonsson G, Pollare T, Hallman H, Sachs Ch (1978): Developmental plasticity of central serotonin neurons after 5,7-dihydroxytryptamine treatment. *Ann. NY Acad. Sci., 305,* 328–345.

Jonsson G, Wiesel FA, Hallman H (1979): Developmental plasticity of central noradrenaline neurons — Changes in transmitter functions. *J. Neurobiol., 10,* 337–353.

Jonsson G, Hallman H, Ponzio F, Ross S (1981): DSP4-(N-2-chloroethyl-N-ethyl-2-bromobenzylamine) — A useful denervation tool for central and peripheral noradrenaline neurons. *Eur. J. Pharmacol., 72,* 173–188.

Jonsson G, Hallmann H, Sundström E (1982): Effects of the noradrenaline neurotoxin DSP4 on the postnatal development of central noradrenaline neurons in the rat. *Neuroscience, 7,* 2895–2907.

Kammerer RC, Amivi B, Cho AK (1979): Inhibition of uptake of catecholamines by benzylamine derivatives. *J. Med. Chem., 22,* 352–355.

Kasamatsu T, Pettigrew JD, Ary M (1979): Restoration of visual cortical plasticity by local microperfusion of norepinephrine. *J. Comp. Neurol., 185,* 163–182.

Kasamatsu T, Itakura T, Jonsson G (1981): Intracortical spread of exogenous catecholamines: Effective concentration for modifying cortical plasticity. *J. Pharmacol. Exp. Ther., 217,* 841–850.

Koda LY, Schulman JA, Bloom FE (1978): Ultrastructural identification of noradrenergic terminals in rat hippocampus: Unilateral destruction of the locus ceruleus with 6-hydroxydopamine. *Brain Res., 145,* 190–195.

Köhler C, Ross SB, Szrebo B, Ögren SO (1978): Long-term biochemical effects of *p*-chloroamphetamine in the rat. *Ann. NY Acad. Sci., 305,* 645–663.

Konkol RJ, Bendeich EG, Breese GR (1978): A biochemical and morphological study of the altered growth pattern of central catecholamine neurons following 6-hydroxydopamine. *Brain Res., 140,* 125–135.

Kostrzewa R (1975): Effects of neonatal 6-hydroxydopa treatment on monoamine content of rat brain and peripheral tissues. *Res. Commun. Chem. Pathol. Pharmacol., 11,* 567–579.

Kostrzewa RM, Garey RE (1977): Sprouting of noradrenergic terminals in rat cerebellum following neonatal treatment with 6-hydroxydopa. *Brain Res., 124,* 385–391.

Kostrzewa RM, Harper JW (1974): Effect of 6-hydroxydopa on catecholamine containing neurons in brain of newborn rats. *Brain Res., 69,* 174–181.

Kostrzewa R, Jacobowitz D (1972): The effect of 6-hydroxydopa on peripheral adrenergic neurons. *J Pharmacol. Exp. Ther., 183,* 284–297.

Kostrzewa R, Jacobowitz D (1973): Acute effects of 6-hydroxydopa on central monoaminergic neurons. *Eur. J. Pharmacol., 21,* 70–80.

Kostrzewa RM, Jacobowitz DM (1974): Pharmacological actions of 6-hydroxydopamine. *Pharmacol. Rev., 26,* 199–288.

Kostrzewa RM, Klara JW, Robertson J, Walker LC (1978): Studies on the mechanism of sprouting of noradrenergic terminals in rat and mouse cerebellum after neonatal 6-hydroxydopa. *Brain Res. Bull., 3,* 525–531.

Kraemer GW, Breese GR, Prange AJ, Morgan EC, Lewis JK, Keumitz JW, Bushnell PJ, Howard JL, McKinney WT (1981): Use of 6-hydroxydopamine to deplete brain catecholamines in the Rhesus monkey: Effects on urinary catecholamine metabolites and behavior. *Psychopharmacology, 73,* 1–11.

Kreutzberg GW (1981): The regeneration program of the neuron: An introduction. In: Gorio A, Millesi H, Mingrino S (Eds), *Posttraumatic Peripheral Nerve Regeneration,* pp. 3–6. Raven Press, New York.

Krieger DF (1975): Effects of intraventricular neonatal 6-OH-dopamine or 5,6-dihydroxytryptamine administration on the circadian periodicity of plasma corticoid levels in the rat. *Neuroendocrinology, 17,* 62–74.

Ladinsky H, Consolo S, Tirelli AS, Ferloni GL (1980): Evidence for noradrenergic mediation of the oxotremorine-induced increase in acetylcholine content in rat hippocampus. *Brain Res., 187,* 494–498.

Laguzzi L, Petitjean F, Pujol JF, Jouvet M (1971): Effects de l'injection intraventriculaire de 6-hydroxydopamine sur les états de sommeil et les monoamines cérébrales du chat. *CR Soc. Biol. (Paris), 165,* 1649–1653.

Laguzzi R, Petitjean F, Pujol JF, Jouvet M (1972): Effects de l'injection intraventriculaire de 6-hydroxydopamine. II. Sur le cycle veille-sommeils du chat. *Brain Res., 48,* 295–310.

Lanfumey L, Arluison M, Adrien J (1981): Destruction of noradrenergic cell-bodies by intracerebral 6-hydroxydopamine in the newborn rat. *Brain Res., 214,* 445–450.

Levitt P, Moore RY (1980): Organization of brain stem noradrenaline hyperinnervation following neonatal 6-hydroxydopamine treatment in rat. *Anat. Embryol., 158,* 133–150.

Liang Y-O, Wightman RM, Plotsky P, Adams RN (1975): Oxidative interaction of 6-hydroxydopamine with CNS constituents. In: Jonsson G, Malmfors T, Sachs Ch (Eds), *Chemical Tools in Catecholamine Research,* pp. 15–22. North-Holland Publ. Co., Amsterdam.

Lidbrink P (1974): The effect of lesions of ascending noradrenaline pathways on sleep and waking in the rat. *Brain Res., 74,* 19–40.

Lidbrink P, Jonsson G (1974): Noradrenaline nerve terminals in the cerebral cortex — Effects on noradrenaline uptake and storage following axonal lesion with 6-hydroxydopamine. *J. Neurochem., 22,* 617–626.

Lidbrink P, Jonsson G (1975): On the specificity of 6-hydroxydopamine induced degeneration of central noradrenaline neurons after intracerebral injection. *Neurosci. Lett., 1,* 35–39.

Lidov HG, Molliver ME (1982): The structure of cerebral cortex in the rat following prenatal administration of 6-hydroxydopamine. *Dev. Brain Res., 3,* 81–108.

Lieberman AR (1971): The axon reaction: A review of the principal features of perikaryal responses to axon injury. *Int. Rev. Neurobiol., 14,* 49–124.

Lieberman AR (1974): Some factors affecting retrograde neuronal responses to axonal lesions. In: Bellairs R, Gray EG (Eds), *Essays on the Nervous System,* pp. 71–105. Clarendon Press, Oxford.

Liston DR, Franz DN, Gibb JW (1982): Biochemical evidence for alteration of neostriatal dopaminergic function by 5,7-dihydroxytryptamine. *J. Neurochem., 38,* 1329–1335.

Ljungdahl Å, Hökfelt T, Jonsson G, Sachs Ch (1971): Autoradiographic demonstration of uptake and accumulation of [^{3}H]6-hydroxydopamine in adrenergic nerves. *Experientia, 27,* 297–299.

Lorden JF, Oltmans GA, Dawson R, Callahan M (1979): Evaluation of the nonspecific effects of catecholamine and serotonin neurotoxins by injection into the medial forebrain bundle of the rat. *Pharmacol. Biochem. Behav., 10,* 79–80.

Lorens SA, Guldberg HC, Hole K, Köhler C, Szrebro B (1976): Activity, avoidance learning and regional 5-hydroxytryptamine following intrabrain stem 5,7-dihydroxytryptamine and electrolytic midbrain raphe lesions in the rat. *Brain Res., 108,* 97–113.

Lorez H (1981): Fluorescence histochemistry indicates damage of striatal dopamine nerve terminals in rats after multiple doses of methamphetamine. *Life Sci., 28,* 911–916.

Lundström J, Ong H, Daly J, Creveling CR (1973): Isomers of 2,4,5-trihydroxyphanethylamine (6-hydroxydopamine): Long-term effects on the accumulation of [^{3}H]norepinephrine in mouse heart in vivo. *Mol. Pharmacol., 9,* 505–513.

Lyles GA, Callingham BA (1981): The effect of DSP-4 (N-(2-chloroethyl)-N-ethyl-2-bromobenzylamine) on monoamine oxidase activities in tissues of the rat. *J. Pharm. Pharmacol., 33,* 632–638.

Lytle L, Shoemaker W, Cottman K, Wurtman R (1972): Long-term effects of postnatal 6-hydroxydopamine treatment on tissue catecholamine levels. *J. Pharmacol. Exp. Ther., 183,* 56–64.

Lytle LO, Jacoby JH, Nelson MF, Baumgarten HG (1974): Long-term effects of 5,7-dihydroxytryptamine administered at birth on the development of brain monoamines. *Life Sci., 15,* 1203–1217.

Malmfors T (1971): The effects of 6-hydroxydopamine on the adrenergic nerves as revealed by the fluorescence histochemical method. In: Malmfors T, Thoenen H (Eds), *6-Hydroxydopamine and Catecholamine Neurons.* pp. 47–58. North-Holland Publ. Co., Amsterdam.

Malmfors T, Sachs Ch (1968): Degeneration of adrenergic nerves produced by 6-hydroxydopamine. *Eur. J. Pharmacol., 3,* 89–92.

Malmfors T, Thoenen H (1971): *6-Hydroxydopamine and Catecholamine Neurons.* North-Holland Publ. Co., Amsterdam.

Meek JL, Fuxe F, Carlsson A (1971): Blockade of *p*-chloromethamphetamine induced 5-hydroxytryptamine depletion by chlorimipramine, chlorpheniramine and meperidine. *Biochem. Pharmacol., 20,* 707–709.

Moore RY (1978): Surgical and chemical lesion techniques. In: Iversen LL, Iversen SD, Snyder SH (Eds), *Handbook of Psychopharmacology, Vol. 9,* pp. 1–39. Plenum Press, New York.

Nakai K, Jonsson G, Kasamatsu T (1983): Regrowth of central norepinephrine fibers in cat visual cortex following localized lesions with 6-hydroxydopamine. *J. Comp. Neurol.,* in press.

Nwanze E, Jonsson G (1981): Amphetamine neurotoxicity on dopamine nerve terminals in the caudate nucleus of mice. *Neurosci. Lett., 26,* 163–168.

Nygren L-G, Fuxe K, Jonsson G, Olsen L (1974): Functional regeneration of 5-hydroxytryptamine nerve terminals in the rat spinal cord following 5,6-dihydroxytryptamine induced degeneration. *Brain Res., 78,* 377–394.

Nygren L-G, Olson L (1977): Intracisternal neurotoxins and monoamine neurons innervating the spinal cord: Acute and chronic effects on cell and axon counts and nerve terminal densities. *Histochemistry, 52,* 281–306.

Ögren SO (1982): Central serotonin neurones and learning in the rat. In: Osborne NN (Ed), *Biology of Serotonergic Transmission,* pp. 317–334. John Wiley & Sons, Baltimore.

Ögren SO, Fuxe K, Archer T, Hall H, Holm A-C, Köhler C (1981): Studies on the role of central 5-HT neurons in avoidance learning: A behavioural and biochemical analysis. In: Haber B, Gabay S, Issidorides MR, Alivisatos SGA (Eds), *Serotonin: Current Aspects of Neurochemistry and Function,* pp. 681–705. Plenum Press, New York.

Olson L, Malmfors T (1970): Growth characteristics of adrenergic nerves in the adult rat. *Acta Physiol. Scand., Suppl.,* 348.

Pappas BA, Saari M, Peters DAV (1976): Regional brain catecholamine levels after intraventricular 6-hydroxydopamine in the neonatal rats. *Res. Commun. Chem. Pathol. Pharmacol., 14,* 751–754.

Pappas BA, Gallivan JV, Dugas T, Saari M, Ings R (1980): Intraventricular 6-hydroxydopamine in the newborn rat and locomotor responses to drugs in infancy: No support for the dopamine depletion model of minimal brain dysfunction. *Psychopharmacology, 70,* 41–46.

Pappas B, Ings R, Roberts D (1982): Neonatal intraspinal 6-hydroxydopamine, 5,7-dihydroxytryptamine or their combination-effects on nociception and morphine analgesia. *Eur. J. Pharmacol., 86,* 157–166.

Peters DAV, Pappas BA, Taub H, Saari M (1977): Effect of intraventricular injections of 6-hydroxy-dopamine in neonatal rats on the catecholamine levels and tyrosine hydroxylase activity in brain regions at maturity. *Biochem. Pharmacol., 26,* 2211–2215.

Petitjean F, Laguzzi R, Sordet F, Jouvet M, Pujol F (1972): Effets de l'injection intraventriculaire de 6-hydroxydopamine. I. Sur les monoamines cérébrales du chat. *Brain Res., 48,* 281–294.

Pettigrew JD, Kasamatsu T (1978): Local perfusion of noradrenaline maintains visual cortical plasticity. *Nature (London), 271,* 761–763.

Pinching AJ, Powell TPS (1971): Ultrastructure features of transneuronal cell degeneration in the olfactory system. *J. Cell Sci., 8,* 253–268.

Poirier LJ, Langelier P, Roberge A, Boucher R, Kitsikis A (1971): Nonspecific histopathological changes induced by the intracerebral injection of 6-hydroxydopamine (6-OH-DA). *J. Neurol. Sci., 16,* 401–416.

Ponzio F, Jonsson G (1978): Effects of neonatal 5,7-dihydroxytryptamine treatment of the development of serotonin neurons and their transmitter metabolism. *Dev. Neurosci., 1,* 80–89.

Pujol JF, Kan JP, Buda M, Petitjean F, Mouset J, Jouvet M (1975): Is 6-hydroxydopamine a specific tool for the study of functional roles of catecholaminergic neurons in the sleep-waking cycle? In: Jonsson G, Malmfors T, Sachs Ch (Eds), *Chemical Tools in Catecholamine Research, Vol. I,* pp. 259–271. North-Holland Publ. Co., Amsterdam.

Reid JL, Zivin JA, Kopin IJ (1976): The effects of spinal cord transection and intracisternal 6-hydroxy-dopamine on phenylethanolamine-N-methyltransferase (PNMT) activity in rat brain stem and spinal cord. *J. Neurochem., 26,* 629–631.

Reis DJ, Gilad GM, Pickel VM, Ross RA, Joh TH (1977): Dynamic changes in the activities and amounts of neurotransmitter-synthesizing enzymes in mesolimbic and other central catecholamine neurons in response to axonal injury and during collateral sprouting. In: Costa E, Gessa GL (Eds), *Non-striatal Dopaminergic Neurons,* pp. 331–341. Raven Press, New York.

Reis DJ, Ross RA, Gilad G, Joh TH (1978): Reaction of central catecholaminergic neurons to injury: Model systems for studying the neurobiology of central regeneration and sprouting. In: Cotman CW (Ed), *Neuronal Plasticity,* pp. 197–226. Raven Press, New York.

Reis DJ, Ross RA, Iacovitti L, Gilad G, Joh TH (1981): Changes in neurotransmitter synthesizing enzymes during regenerative, compensatory and collateral sprouting of central catecholamine neurons in adult and developing rats. In: Flohr H and Precht W (Eds), *Lesion-induced Neuronal Plasticity in Sensorimotor Systems,* pp. 87–102. Springer-Verlag, Berlin.

Ricuarte GA, Guillery RW, Seiden LS, Schuster CR, Moore RY (1982): Dopamine nerve terminal degeneration produced by high doses of methylamphetamine in the rat brain. *Brain Res., 236,* 93–103.

Ross SB (1976): Long-term effects of N-2-chloroethyl-N-ethyl-2-bromobenzylamine hydrochloride on noradrenergic neurons in the rat brain and heart. *Br. J. Pharmacol., 58,* 521–527.

Ross SB, Kelder D (1979): Inhibition of [^{3}H]dopamine accumulation in reserpinized and normal rat striatum. *Acta Pharmacol. Toxicol., 44,* 329–335.

Ross SB, Renyi AL (1976): On the long-lasting inhibitory effect of N-(2-chlorethyl)-N-ethyl-2-bromoben-zylamine (DSP4) on the active uptake of noradrenaline. *J. Pharm. Pharmacol., 28,* 458–459.

Ross SB, Johansson JG, Lindborg B, Dahlbom R (1973): Cyclizing compounds. I. Tertiary N-(2-bromoben-zyl)-N-haloalkylamine with adrenergic blocking action. *Acta Pharm. Suec., 10,* 29–42.

Ross SB, Ögren SO, Renyi L (1976a): (Z)-Dimethylamino-1-(4-bromophenyl)-1-(3-pyridyl) propene (H102/09): A new selective inhibitor of the neuronal 5-hydroxytryptamine uptake. *Acta Pharmacol. Toxicol., 39,* 152–166.

Ross SB, Ögren SO, Renyi AL (1976b): Antagonism of the acute and long-term biochemical effects of 4-chloramphetamine on the 5-HT neurons in the rat brain by inhibitors of the 5-hydroxytryptamine uptake. *Acta Pharmacol. Toxicol., 39,* 456–476.

Routtenberg A (1972): Intracranial injection and behaviour: A critical review. *Behav. Biol., 7,* 601–641.

Sachs Ch (1972): Failure of 6-hydroxynoradrenaline to produce degeneration of catecholamine neurons. *Eur. J. Pharmacol., 20,* 149–155.

Sachs Ch (1973): Development of the blood-brain barrier for 6-hydroxydopamine. *J. Neurochem., 20,* 1753–1760.

Sachs Ch, Jonsson G (1972a): Degeneration of central noradrenaline neurons after 6-hydroxydopamine in newborn animals. *Res. Commun. Chem. Pathol. Pharmacol., 4,* 203–220.

Sachs Ch, Jonsson G (1972b): Degeneration of central and peripheral noradrenaline neurons produced by 6-hydroxy-DOPA. *J. Neurochem., 19,* 1561–1575.

Sachs Ch, Jonsson G (1972c): Selective 6-hydroxy-DOPA induced degeneration of central and peripheral noradrenaline neurons. *Brain Res., 40,* 563–568.

Sachs Ch, Jonsson G (1973a): Changes in central noradrenaline neurons after systemic 6-hydroxydopamine administration. *J. Neurochem., 21,* 1517–1524.

Sachs Ch, Jonsson G (1973b): Quantitative microfluorimetric and neurochemical studies on adrenergic nerves after axotomy. *J. Histochem. Cytochem., 21,* 902–911.

Sachs Ch, Jonsson G (1975a): Mechanisms of action of 6-hydroxydopamine. *Biochem. Pharmacol., 24,* 1–8.

Sachs Ch, Jonsson G (1975b): Effects of 6-hydroxydopamine on central noradrenaline neurons during ontogeny. *Brain Res., 99,* 277–291.

Sachs Ch, Jonsson G (1975c): Changes in the development of central noradrenaline neurons following neonatal 6-OH-DA administration. In: Jonsson G, Malmfors T, Sachs Ch (Eds), *Chemical Tools in Catecholamine Research, Vol. I,* pp. 163–171. North-Holland Publ. Co., Amsterdam.

Sachs Ch, Jonsson G (1975d): 5,7-Dihydroxytryptamine induced changes in the postnatal development of central 5-hydroxytryptamine neurons. *Med. Biol., 53,* 156–164.

Sachs Ch, Jonsson G, Fuxe K (1973): Mapping of central noradrenaline pathways with 6-hydroxy-DOPA. *Brain Res., 63,* 249–261.

Sachs Ch, Pycock Ch, Jonsson G (1974): Altered development of central noradrenaline neurons during ontogeny by 6-hydroxydopamine. *Med. Biol., 52,* 55–65.

Sachs Ch, Jonsson G, Heikkila R, Cohen G (1975): Control of the neurotoxicity of 6-hydroxydopamine by intraneuronal noradrenaline in rat iris. *Acta Physiol. Scand., 93,* 345–351.

Sanders-Bush E, Bushing JA, Sulser F (1972): Long-term effects of *p*-chloroamphetamine on tryptophan hydroxylase activity and on the levels of 5-hydroxytryptamine and 5-hydroxyindoleacetic acid in brain. *Eur. J. Pharmacol., 20,* 385–388.

Sanders-Bush E, Bushing JA, Sulser FJ (1975): Long-term effects of *p*-chloroamphetamine and related drugs on central serotonergic mechanisms. *J. Pharmacol. Exp. Ther., 192,* 33–41.

Saner A, Thoenen H (1971): Model experiments on the molecular mechanism of action of 6-hydroxydopamine. *Mol. Pharmacol., 7,* 147–154.

Saner A, Pieri L, Moran J, Da Prada M, Pletscher A (1974): Decrease of dopamine and 5-hydroxytryptamine after intracerebral application of 5,6-dihydroxytryptamine. *Brain Res., 76,* 109–117.

Schmidt RH, Bhatnagar RK (1979): Regional development of norepinephrine, dopamine-β-hydroxylase and tyrosine hydroxylase in the rat brain subsequent to neonatal treatment with subcutaneous 6-hydroxydopamine. *Brain Res., 166,* 293–308.

Schmidt RH, Kasik SA, Bhatnagar RK (1980): Regenerative critical periods for locus ceruleus in postnatal pups following intracisternal 6-hydroxydopamine: A model for noradrenergic development. *Brain Res., 191,* 173–190.

Schmidt RH, Björklund A, Loren I (1981): Neuron-target interactions in the development of central catecholamine systems. In: Garrod and Feldman (Eds), *Development in the Nervous System,* pp. 85–106. Cambridge University Press, London.

Schneider GE (1973): Early lesions of superior colliculus: Factors affecting the formation of abnormal retinal projections. *Brain Behav. Evol., 8,* 73–109.

Schneider GE (1981): Early lesions and abnormal neuronal connections. *TINS, 4,* 187–192.

Sedvall G (1964): Noradrenaline storage in skeletal muscle. *Acta Physiol. Scand., 60,* 39–50.

Sherman A, Gál EM, Fuller RW, Molloy BB (1975): Effects of intraventricular p-chloroamphetamine and its analogues on cerebral 5-HT. *Neuropharmacology, 14,* 733–737.

Shore PA (1976): Actions of amfonelic acid and other nonamphetamine stimulants on the dopamine neurons. *J. Pharm. Pharmacol., 28,* 855–857.

Sievers J, Klemm HP (1982): Locus ceruleus — Cerebellum: Interaction during development. *Bibl. Anat., No. 23,* 56–75.

Sievers J, Berry M, Baumgarten H (1981a): The role of noradrenergic fibers in the control of postnatal cerebellar development. *Brain Res., 207,* 200–208.

Sievers J, Mangold U, Berry M, Allen C, Schlossberger H-G (1981b): Experimental studies on cerebellar foliation. I. A qualitative morphological analysis of cerebellar fissuration defects after neonatal treatment with 6-OH-DA in the rat. *J. Comp. Neurol., 203,* 751–769.

Siggins GR, Forman DS, Bloom FE, Sims KL (1975): Degenerative effects of 6-aminodopamine on peripheral and central adrenergic nerves. In: Jonsson G, Malmfors T, Sachs Ch (Eds), *Chemical Tools in Catecholamine Research, Vol. I,* pp. 59–66. North-Holland Publ. Co., Amsterdam.

Singh B, De Champlain J (1972): Altered ontogenesis of central noradrenergic neurons following neonatal treatment with 6-hydroxydopamine. *Brain Res., 48,* 432–437.

Smith BH, Kreutzberg GW (1976): Neuron-target cell interactions. *Neurosci. Res. Program Bull., 14,* 3.

Smith RD, Cooper BR, Breese GR (1973): Growth and behavioral changes in developing rats treated intracisternally with 6-hydroxydopamine: Evidence for involvement of brain dopamine. *J. Pharmacol. Exp. Ther., 185,* 609–619.

Sotelo C, Javoy F, Agid Y, Glowinski J (1973): Injection of 6-hydroxydopamine in the substantia nigra of the rat. I. Morphological study. *Brain Res., 58,* 269–290.

Steranka LR (1982): Long-term decreases in striatal dopamine, 3,4-dihydroxyphenylacetic acid and homovanillic acid after a single injection of amphetamine in iprindole-treated rats: Time-course and time-dependent interactions with amfonelic acid. *Brain Res., 234,* 123–136.

Steranka LR, Sanders-Bush E (1980): Long-term effects of continuous exposure to amphetamine on brain dopamine concentration and synaptosomal uptake in mice. *Eur. J. Pharmacol., 65,* 439–443.

Tassin JP, Velley L, Stinus L, Blanc G, Glowinski J, Thierry AM (1975): Development of cortical and nigroneostriatal dopaminergic systems after destruction of central noradrenergic neurons in foetal or neonatal rats. *Brain Res., 83,* 93–106.

Thierry A-M, Velley L, Stinus L, Tassin JP, Blanc G, Blowinski J (1975): Development of the mesocortical and nigrostriatal dopaminergic systems following various 6-hydroxydopamine treatments. In: Jonsson G, Malmfors T, Sachs Ch (Eds), *Chemical Tools in Catecholamine Research, Vol. I,* pp. 205–210. North-Holland Publ. Co., Amsterdam.

Thoenen H (1972): Surgical, immunological and chemical sympathectomy. Their application in the investigation of the physiology and pharmacology of the sympathetic nervous system. In: Blaschko H, Muscholl E (Eds), *Catecholamines,* pp. 813–844. Springer-Verlag, Berlin.

Thoenen H, Tranzer JP (1968): Chemical sympathectomy by selective destruction of adrenergic nerve endings with 6-hydroxydopamine. *Naunyn-Schmiedebergs Arch. Pharmakol. Exp. Path., 261,* 271–288.

Tranzer JP, Richards JG (1971): Fine structural aspects of the effect of 6-hydroxydopamine on peripheral adrenergic neurons. In: Malmfors T, Thoenen H (Eds), *6-Hydroxydopamine and Catecholamine Neurons,* pp. 15–31. North-Holland Publ. Co., Amsterdam.

Tranzer JP, Thoenen H (1967): Ultramorphologische Veränderungen der sympathischen Nervenendigungen der Katze nach Vorbehandlung mit 5- und 6-Hydroxy-Dopamine. *Naunyn-Schmiedebergs Arch. Pharmakol. Exp. Path., 257,* 343.

Tranzer JP, Thoenen H (1968): An electron-microscopic study of selective, acute degeneration of sympathetic nerve terminals after administration of 6-hydroxydopamine. *Experientia, 24,* 155–156.

Tranzer JP, Thoenen H (1973): Selective destruction of adrenergic nerve terminals by chemical analogues of 6-hydroxydopamine. *Experientia, 29,* 314–315.

Trulson ME, Jacobs BB (1979): Chronic amphetamine administration to cats: Behavioural and neurochemical evidence for decreased central serotonergic function. *J. Pharmacol. Exp. Ther., 211,* 375–384.

Tse DCS, McCreery RL, Adams RN (1976): Potential oxidative pathways of brain catecholamines. *J. Med. Chem., 19,* 37–40.

Uretsky NJ, Iversen LL (1969): Effects of 6-hydroxydopamine on noradrenaline-containing neurones in the rat brain. *Nature (London), 221,* 557–559.

Uretsky NJ, Iversen LL (1970): Effects of 6-hydroxydopamine on catecholamine containing neurones in rat brain. *J. Neurochem., 17,* 269–278.

Ungerstedt U (1968): 6-Hydroxydopamine induced degeneration of central monoamine neurons. *Eur. J. Pharmacol., 5,* 107–110.

Ungerstedt U (1971): Use of intracerebral injections of 6-hydroxydopamine as a tool for morphological and functional studies on central catecholamine neurons. In: Malmfors T, Thoenen H (Eds), *6-Hydroxydopamine and Catecholamine Neurons,* pp. 315–332. North-Holland Publ. Co., Amsterdam.

Ungerstedt U (1973): Selective lesions of central catecholamine pathways: Application in functional studies. In: Ehrenpreis S, Kopin IJ (Eds), *Chemical Approaches to Brain Function,* pp. 73–96. Academic Press, New York.

Versteeg DHG, Wijnen HJLM, De Kloet ER, De Jong W (1977): Differential effects of neonatal 6-hydroxydopamine treatment on the catecholamine content of hypothalamic nuclei and brain stem regions. *Neurosci. Lett., 7,* 341–346.

Waddington JL, Crow TJ (1979): Drug-induced rotational behaviour following unilateral intracerebral injection of saline-ascorbate solution: Neurotoxicity of ascorbic acid and monoamine-independent circling. *Brain Res., 161,* 371–376.

Wagner GD, Ricaurte GA, Seiden LS, Schuster CR, Miller RJ, Westley J (1980): Long-lasting depletions of striatal dopamine and loss of dopamine uptake sites following repeated administration of methamphetamine. *Brain Res., 181,* 151–160.

Wagner K, Trendelenburg U (1971): Effect of 6-hydroxydopamine on oxidative phosphorylation and on monoamine oxidase activities. *N-S. Arch. Pharmakol., 269,* 112–116.

Wiklund L, Björklund A, Nobin A (1978): Regeneration of serotonin neurons in the rat brain after 5,6-dihydroxytryptamine induced axotomy. *Ann. NY Acad. Sci., 305,* 370–384.

Zieher LM, Jaim-Etcheverry G (1973): Regional differences in the long-term effect of neonatal 6-hydroxy-dopa treatment on rat brain noradrenaline. *Brain Res., 60,* 199–207.

Zieher LM, Jaim-Etcheverry G (1975): 6-Hydroxydopa during development of central noradrenergic neurons produces different long-term changes in rat brain noradrenaline. *Brain Res., 86,* 271–281.

Zieher LM, Jaim-Etcheverry G (1979): 6-Hydroxydopamine during development: Relation between opposite regional changes in brain noradrenaline. *Eur. J. Pharmacol., 58,* 217–223.

Zieher L, Jaim-Etcheverry G (1980): Neurotoxicity of N-(2-chloroethyl)-N-ethylbromobenzylamine hydrochloride (DSP4) on noradrenergic neurons is mimicked by its cyclic aziridinium derivative. *Eur. J. Pharmacol., 65,* 249–256.

CHAPTER XIII

The use of excitatory amino acids as selective neurotoxins

JOSEPH T. COYLE and ROBERT SCHWARCZ

1. INTRODUCTION

Recent years have witnessed an increasing emphasis in neuroscientific research on the precise characterization of defined pathways within the CNS. Thus, the neurochemist must determine the properties associated with specific neuronal populations; and behavioralists and neurophysiologists are increasingly confronted with the task of determining the functional role played by identified neuronal groups in the brain. Selective lesion of the neurons of interest is often the first strategy for resolving these questions. Traditionally, this has been accomplished by thermocoagulation or surgical extirpation. These methods, however, present well recognized problems that limit interpretation. Most importantly, the observed alterations may reflect damage not to the neurons of interest but rather to axons passing through the lesioned area resulting in anterograde or retrograde degeneration. In addition, ablative techniques cannot be used to characterize local circuit neurons since they destroy all neuronal and non-neuronal elements with their circumference of effect. Although highly selective neurotoxins such as 6-hydroxydopamine and 5,7-dihydroxytryptamine have been developed, their specificity restricts their use to a very few defined neuronal systems such as the catecholaminergic and serotonergic neurons. However, a technique has recently emerged for producing perikaryal specific lesions through administration of glutamate or the so-called excitotoxins, i.e. compounds which are structurally and neurophysiologically related to this excitatory acidic amino acid. In this chapter, we shall review the practical aspects of the excitotoxin lesion technique.

2. HISTORICAL BACKGROUND

The excitotoxin lesion technique grew out of observations made two decades ago by Lucas and Newhouse (1957) on the cytotoxic effects of systemically administered glutamic acid on the retina of neonatal mice. These investigators were exploring the possible therapeutic effects of glutamic acid, an amino acid found in particularly high concentration in the nervous system, on a form of hereditary retinal degeneration. Contrary to their expectations, they observed that administration of glutamic acid to normal neonatal mice caused an acute degeneration of the neurons in the inner layers of the retina. Subsequent studies revealed that not only neurons in the inner layers of the retina but also neurons with cell bodies in the arcuate nucleus and in the circumventricular organs, which lie outside the blood-brain barrier, were vulnerable to the

Handbook of Chemical Neuroanatomy. Vol. 1: Methods in Chemical Neuroanatomy.
A. Björklund and T. Hökfelt, editors.
© Elsevier Science Publishers B.V., 1983.

cytotoxic effects of systemically administered glutamate in the neonatal rodent (Olney 1969a). Although the mechanism responsible for this selective neuronal damage was obscure, neurophysiologic studies had previously provided evidence that acidic amino acids like glutamate have excitatory effects on central neurons (Curtis and Watkins 1960). In fact, virtually all neurons in the brain could be depolarized by iontophoretic application of glutamic acid (Curtis and Johnston 1974).

The disparate information on the neurotoxic and excitatory effects of the acidic amino acids was first integrated by Olney. His electron-microscopic studies demonstrated that the initial signs of toxicity appeared within minutes of systemic treatment with glutamate and were typified by profound swelling of affected neuronal dendrites which rapidly spread to involve the neuronal perikarya (Olney 1971). A critical feature of the acute lesion was the absence of cytopathological changes in neuronal terminals or axons traversing the lesioned area. Finally, Olney demonstrated a close correlation between the neuroexcitatory potency and the neurotoxic effects of a variety of acidic amino acids. He concluded that the neurotoxic effects of these agents resulted from their depolarizing action, which caused influx of sodium and water into the dendrites bearing their receptors; as axons and non-neuronal elements do not possess these excitatory receptors, they were not vulnerable. Thus, he coined the term 'excitotoxins' for these substances that appeared to kill neurons on the basis of their excitatory effects (Olney 1974).

Neurophysiologists have identified a number of conformationally restricted or synthetic analogues structurally related to glutamate whose excitatory effects were much more potent than glutamate. These substances include kainic acid, isolated from the seaweed *Diginea simplex* (Shinozaki and Konishi 1970), ibotenic acid, isolated from the mushroom *Amanita muscara* (Johnston et al. 1968), quisqualic acid, isolated from the *quisqualus* nut (Shinozaki and Shibuya 1974) and the synthetic compound N-methyl-D-aspartic acid. While it was initially thought that the heterocyclic analogues of glutamate were merely potent agonists at a 'glutamate receptor', recent studies have indicated a variety of receptors which respond rather selectively to kainic acid, quisqualic acid and N-methyl-D-aspartic acid (McLennan 1981; Watkins and Evans 1981). For some of these potent analogues, Olney has shown that systemic administration causes neurotoxic effects similar to those seen with glutamic acid (Olney et al. 1971, 1974).

Systemic administration of excitotoxins suffers from the obvious limitation that the lesions occur only in those few areas of the CNS with a deficient blood-brain barrier; and neuronal vulnerability is rather limited to the perinatal period. To make a precisely localized perikaryal-specific lesion, Coyle and Schwarcz (1976) first described the neurotoxic effects of direct infusion of the potent glutamic acid analogue, kainic acid, in the striatum of the rat. Neurochemical and histologic studies established that the injection of kainic acid caused a selective degeneration of neurons with cell bodies intrinsic to the striatum but spared, acutely, extrinsic axons passing through or terminating in the region. In subsequent studies, it was shown that several other potent excitatory analogues of glutamic acid also exhibited selective neuronal toxicity after direct intracranial injection (Schwarcz et al. 1978). However, in keeping with current understanding of a multiplicity of excitatory amino acid receptors, it has become increasingly apparent that these analogues including kainic acid, ibotenic acid and N-methyl-D-aspartic acid exhibit different patterns of neurotoxicity (Zaczek et al. 1981). Currently, the two most commonly used excitotoxins for intracerebral lesions are kainic acid and ibotenic acid whose properties will be reviewed in detail together with those of glutamic acid, the 'original' excitotoxin (Fig. 1).

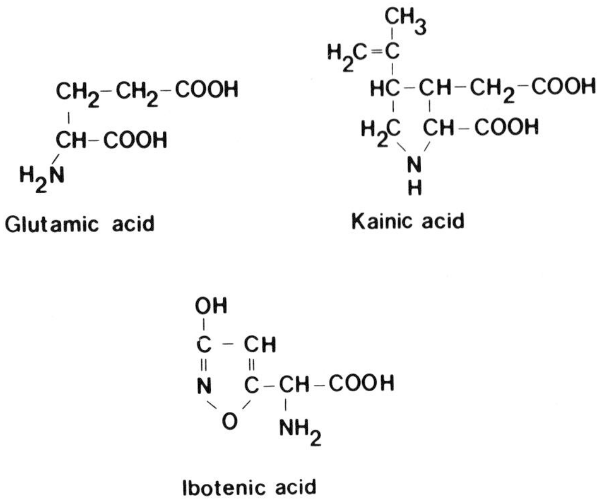

Fig. 1. Molecular structures of glutamic acid, kainic acid and ibotenic acid.

3. GLUTAMIC ACID

The current status of glutamate as a neurotoxin, summarized in an excellent recent review by Nemeroff (1981), is still obscured by the variations of experimental designs used in different laboratories. By far, the most extensive use of glutamate is that as an ablative or provocative tool in neuroendocrinology. There is little dispute that neuronal cell bodies of the arcuate nucleus of the hypothalamus of infant rodents degenerate after systemic administration of monosodium glutamate (MSG). The lowest effective doses were found to be 0.5 g/kg (oral) and 0.35 g/kg (subcutaneous) in 10-day-old mice. Optimal parenteral doses (2-5 g/kg, repeated every 48 h until Day 10 after birth) result in the destruction of 80-90% of all local neuronal somata. Both light- and electron-microscopic examinations indicate a severe reduction of arcuate neurons within hours after MSG-treatment. The subfornical organ and the area postrema are also very susceptible to MSG, showing identical 'axon-sparing' lesions in response to the toxin (Olney 1979). While other hypothalamic areas exhibit some degree of vulnerability vis-a-vis MSG, extrahypothalamic brain regions, with the exception of the cingulate cortex (Rascher 1981), appear to be unaffected even by repeated administration of very high doses of MSG. Importantly, parenteral MSG also results in hypothalamic damage in adult rodents.

The arcuate nucleus has long been known to constitute an essential relay station in the modulation of neuroendocrine function (Weindl 1973). It was therefore not unexpected that destruction of arcuate cells would produce severe deficits in various hormonal systems. Adult animals treated with MSG during infancy indeed show reduced content of growth hormone and luteinizing hormones in the anterior pituitary (Redding et al. 1971; Nagasawa et al. 1974), greatly reduced serum growth hormone levels and elevated serum prolactin levels (Nemeroff et al. 1977a,b). The latter, however, can be demonstrated in males only. Reproductive dysfunction, together with decrease in gonad size, indicates marked disturbances in sex hormonal status in both male and female rodents (Holzwarth-McBride et al. 1976; Pizzi et al. 1977). Moreover, the weight of the anterior pituitary appears to be reduced in MSG-treated rats when compared to age- and sex-matched controls (Bakke et al. 1978). While the effect on adrenal weight in animals exposed to MSG is controversial, plasma corticosterone levels in mice and female rats are dramatically increased (Olney 1979). Finally, there exist pronounced histological changes in the thyroid glands of MSG-treated mice that are indicative of hypothyroidism and these findings are corroborated by a significant reduction of both serum tri-iodothyronine and the free thyroxine index (Nemeroff et al. 1977b; Dhindsa et al. 1981).

This brief summary of the reported alterations in endocrine organs and their function after neonatal MSG-treatment is merely intended to demonstrate the possibilities for the design and conduct of studies of any of the hormonal systems listed. Clearly, ablation of arcuate neurons with MSG causes multiple and complex endocrine changes. Carefully controlled experiments, which include dose-response studies and which address critical parameters such as species and strain differences, routes of administration and age of initiation and duration of MSG-treatment, are needed in the future.

MSG-induced selective degeneration of arcuate neurons has also been employed to examine neuronal pathways that originate in the nucleus. With the aid of MSG-lesions, it could be demonstrated that substantial portions of brain α-melanocyte-stimulating hormone (Eskay et al. 1979), adrenocorticotropic hormone, β-lipotropin and β-endorphin (Krieger et al. 1979; Bodnar et al. 1980) have their primary source in the neuronal perikarya of the arcuate nucleus. The same lesions, however, do not result in a concomitant decrease of these peptide hormones in the pituitary, thus differentiating at least two different cellular subpopulations. In other words, in the hypothalamic region, glutamate can be used as an excitotoxic tool like kainate or ibotenate (see below) for the study of pathways for neuroactive substances and neurochemical changes distant from their site of origin. The best established neurotransmitters contained in arcuate perikarya appear to be dopamine and acetylcholine since MSG-treatment results in a significant reduction in local dopamine levels as assessed both histofluorimetrically and biochemically, and in an equally pronounced decrease in choline acetyltransferase activity (Nemeroff 1981). Thus, MSG can be employed as a tool to unravel hypothalamic microcircuitry and the involvement of specific neurotransmitter systems in endocrine function.

The interaction of neurotransmitters and hormones in the arcuate region can also be assessed by acute treatment with subtoxic doses of MSG or related excitatory amino acids in adult rats. In accordance with the excitotoxic hypothesis, such subtoxic doses should depolarize (excite) all those neurons which degenerate after exposure to larger amounts of the same amino acid. Thus, in the provocative paradigm, doses, which are 25% or less of those causing toxicity, are administered and changes in the serum levels of hormones are measured within minutes. This attractive approach may mimic physiological conditions much more closely than the ablative method described above. However, comparatively few studies utilizing the provocative approach have been published to date (Olney et al. 1976; Terry et al. 1977). Elevations in serum luteinizing hormone, testosterone and prolactin and decrease in serum growth hormone have been observed; but mechanisms responsible for these alterations must be considered tentative (see Nemeroff 1981 for discussion). Data on the modulation of these acute MSG-effects by inhibitory amino acids like GABA and taurine are even more fragmentary but may offer a valuable new method for the examination of the hypothalamo-pituitary-gonadal axis (Olney 1979).

The retina constitutes the only other region of the central nervous system where MSG has been successfully employed as a lesion tool. In fact, it was the selective neurotoxic effects of MSG on the inner layers of the mouse retina that had originally initiated research on MSG-neurotoxicity (see above). In subsequent years, both light- and electron-microscopic analyses have confirmed the resistance to MSG of photoreceptor and Müller cells while ganglion and amacrine cells proved quite vulnerable (Olney 1969b; Olney et al. 1971). Both systemic administration of MSG (2-5 g/kg) early in development and intraocular injections of large quantities (500 μg) of the amino acid have been used for the examination of neurotransmitter localization and of the distribution, between retinal cell types, of enzymes related to synaptic transmission (Lund-Karlsen and Fonnum 1976; Schwarcz et al. 1978).

Intracerebral injections of very high amounts (and concentrations) of GLU in adult rodents cause only minimal neuronal damage in the immediate vicinity of the injection site (Olney and De Gubareff 1978). Even chronic infusions of large quantities (600 μg/24 h for 14 days) do not result in nerve cell loss (Mangano and Schwarcz submitted for publication). This lack of neurotoxicity may be related to such factors as the rapid metabolism of or its efficient reuptake into presynaptic nerve endings or glia. On the practical side, the absence of neurodegenerative qualities renders glutamate useless as an axon-sparing lesioning tool in extrahypothalamic brain regions.

4. KAINIC ACID

4.1. CHARACTERISTICS

Kainic acid is a dicarboxyl-containing pyrrolidine (Fig. 1) that has been isolated from the seaweed *Diginea simplex* which grows off the coast of Japan. Kainic acid has within its structure the sequence of glutamic acid (Fig. 1). Neurophysiologic studies indicate that it is 30- to 100-fold more potent than glutamic acid as a neuronal excitant (Biscoe et al. 1976). Structure-activity studies of the stereoisomers, derivatives and analogues of α-kainic acid have revealed a remarkable degree of specificity for its effects (Biscoe et al. 1976). The isopropylene side-chain, in particular, plays a critical role in its activity since reduction of the double bond, as in dihydrokainic acid, or reversal of its spacial orientation, as in α-allo-kainic acid, markedly attenuate the neuroexcitatory effects. In contrast, domoic acid, which has a more extended side-chain, is 2- to 3-fold more potent than kainate as a neuroexcitant. Blockade of the ring nitrogen by alkylation or esterification of the carboxyl groups also markedly attenuate the activity of the compound. α-Keto-kainate, which has a ketone group substituted for the methylene group, retains approximately 10% of the activity of the parent compound. Ligand binding studies with [^{3}H]kainic acid have identified a receptor recognition site in neuronal membranes in mammalian CNS whose characteristics closely correlate with those identified by neurophysiologic studies (London and Coyle 1979; Coyle et al. 1981). Since the excitatory effects of kainic acid are not antagonized by drugs which block the excitatory effect of glutamic acid, quisqualic or N-methyl-D-aspartic acid, it appears that kainic acid acts at a different receptor than these other agonists (Watkins and Evans 1981).

The neurotoxic effects of kainic acid appear to be mediated by the same receptors responsible for its excitatory effects on mammalian neurons. Thus, structure-activity studies of neurotoxic action indicate a close correlation between the neurophysiologic potency and their neurotoxic effects when injected into the rat striatum (Schwarcz et al. 1978; Zaczek et al. 1982). Kainate lesions result in a marked reduction in the

[^{3}H]kainate binding sites, consistent with their localization on vulnerable neurons (Biziere and Coyle 1979; London and Coyle 1979). Furthermore, the development of neuronal vulnerability to locally injected kainic acid in the immature striatum coincides with the ontogenetic increase in the specific binding sites for [^{3}H]kainic acid (Campochiaro and Coyle 1978); and recent autoradiographic findings suggest that the density of kainate receptor sites correlates with neuronal sensitivity to its toxic effects (Foster et al. 1981).

4.2. MECHANISM OF NEUROTOXICITY

While the potent neuroexcitatory effects of kainic acid are consistent with the excitotoxin hypothesis, a number of features of its action indicate that this concept is an oversimplification. Although there is an excellent correlation between neuroexcitatory potency and neurotoxic effects of kainate and its structural analogues, kainic acid is disproportionally more potent as a neurotoxin than congeners thought to act at different receptors such as quisqualic acid and N-methyl-D-aspartic acid (Zaczek and Coyle 1982). A peculiar feature of the neurotoxic effects of kainic acid, noted early on in its use, was the marked variation in neuronal vulnerability. Thus, certain neurons in close proximity to the injection site are spared whereas other neurons, in some cases quite distant from the lesion, degenerate (Schwarcz and Coyle 1977a; Weurthele et al. 1978). Striking examples are the CA_{3-4} pyramidal cells in the hippocampal formation (Fig. 2), which degenerate in the rat after striatal lesion with kainic acid, and the mesencephalic nucleus of the fifth nerve, which is impervious to direct injection (Colonnier et al. 1979). This uneven vulnerability seems inconsistent with the virtually universal sensitivity of neurons to the excitatory effects of glutamate (Curtis and Johnston 1974).

Several studies have shown that the prior ablation of major excitatory afferents eliminates or markedly attenuates the neurotoxic effects of kainic acid in several brain regions including the striatum (Biziere and Coyle 1978; McGeer et al. 1978), hippocampus (Nadler and Cuthbertson 1980; Köhler et al. 1979a) and optic tectum (Street et al. 1980). However, this has not been a universal finding (Bird and Gulley 1979). In the rat striatum, for example, destruction of the main excitatory input from the cerebral cortex, which presumably uses glutamate as its neurotransmitter, protects against the neurotoxic effects of intrastrially injected kainate (Biziere and Coyle 1978a; McGeer et al. 1978). In this region, the cortical lesion does not significantly reduce the density of [^{3}H]kainate binding sites in the striatum (Biziere and Coyle 1979) nor alter striatal neuronal sensitivity to the excitatory effects of kainic acid (McLennan 1980). Thus, there appears be a dissociation between neuronal excitation and vulnerability to kainic acid, which indicates that excitation per se is unlikely to be responsible for the neuronal degeneration.

A striking feature of kainic acid is its convulsant properties. Systemic (Olney et al. 1974), intraventricular (Nadler et al. 1978) or intracerebral injection (Schwarcz et al. 1978; Ben-Ari et al. 1980) of kainic acid can precipitate a prolonged episode of seizures. And the marked sensitivity of the rat to kainic acid-induced limbic seizures is associated with an unusual proclivity of the agent to cause degeneration of certain limbic neurons including the hippocampal pyramids, the amygdaloid nuclei and pyriform cortex. Prior treatment with anticonvulsants that interfere with seizure spread markedly attenuates the neurotoxic action of kainic acid within the limbic system (Zaczek et al. 1978, 1980). These observations have led to the suggestion that the toxic effects of kainic acid within

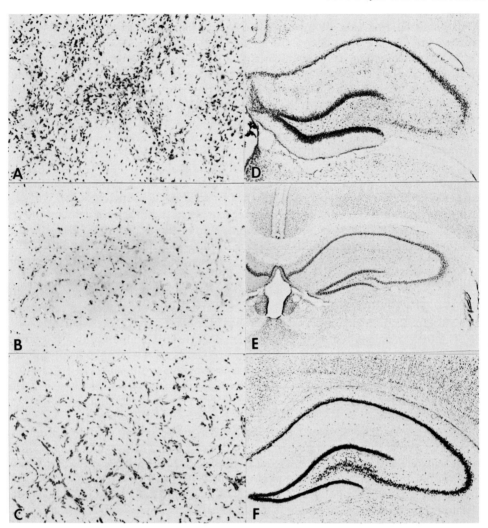

Fig. 2. Histopathology of excitotoxin lesion in Nissl-stained sections. (A) Rat striatum 5 days after intrastriatal injection of 4.6 nmoles of kainic acid. Note the loss of the striatal neuronal perikarya and the astrocytic response that spares the myelinated bundles in internal capsule fibers; × 27. (B) Mouse striatum 2 days after intrastriatal injection of 1.6 nmoles of kainic acid. Note the hypocellular appearance of the striatum and the absence of neuronal perikarya; × 27. (C) Rat striatum 10 days after intrastriatal injection of 64 nmoles of ibotenic acid. Note the absence of neuronal perikarya; × 27. (D) Dental gyrus of the rat 5 days after intrastriatal injection of 4.6 nmoles of kainic acid. Note the selective loss of the CA_{3-4} pyramidal cells in the hilus; × 10. (E) Dentate gyrus of the mouse 2 days after intrastriatal injection of 1.6 nmoles of kainic acid. Note the integrity of the CA_{3-4} pyramidal cells in the hilus; × 5. (F) Dentate gyrus of the rat 10 days after intrastriatal injection of 64 nmoles of ibotenic acid. Note the integrity of the CA_{3-4} pyramidal cells in the hilus; ×5.

the limbic regions result directly from the convulsions. However, other analogues such as N-methyl-D-aspartic acid and quisqualic acid can produce severe seizures without the attendant damage associated with kainic acid (Zaczek et al. 1981b; Zaczek and Coyle 1982). Moreover, it is noteworthy that the hippocampal pyramidal neurons most sensitive to kainic acid possess a remarkably high density of kainate receptors (Foster et al. 1981). Finally, there is a certain degree of species specificity with regard to this effect since mice (Retz and Coyle 1982) do not exhibit the propensity for limbic damage with intrastriatal injection of kainic acid (Fig. 2).

Taken together, these studies indicate that the mechanism of neurotoxicity of kainic acid is complex and probably indirect. Several studies point to a requirement for receptor sites responsive to kainic acid on sensitive neurons. The activity of excitatory afferents appears to modulate neuronal sensitivity in many areas. Kainic acid is relatively metabolically inert and, therefore, capable of considerable diffusion within the brain (Zaczek et al. 1980). It is likely that kainate's enhancement of excitatory neurotransmission leading to seizures increases neuronal vulnerability in distant areas to which it diffuses; consequently, it is difficult to separate the 'convulsant' effects of kainic acid from its direct action upon vulnerable neurons. Metabolic studies have provided evidence that neuronal degeneration is associated with an increase in glucose utilization and consumption of high energy phosphates (Biziere and Coyle 1978; Wooten and Collins 1980; Retz and Coyle 1982). But the precise mechanism or proximate cause responsible for neuronal degeneration precipitated by kainic acid remains to be defined.

4.3. PRACTICAL CONSIDERATIONS FOR IN SITU KAINATE LESIONS

Because of its potent neurotoxic effects, kainic acid has much to recommend as a method for producing perikaryal specific lesions in the vertebrate central nervous system. There is a wealth of evidence that, when used appropriately, in situ injection of kainic acid results in an axon-sparing type of lesion that minimally damages even the finest unmyelinated axons in the central nervous system. In a worst case example, Mason and Fibiger (1979) found only a 25% decrease in the norepinephrine content of the ipsilateral cerebral cortex after direct injection into the dorsal noradrenergic bundle, a dose of kainic acid which resulted in extensive degeneration of the surrounding neurons. Indeed, the convulsant effects of the agent, which depletes cortical norepinephrine stores, might account for even this modest reduction (Nelson et al. 1980).

Because of its remarkable potency, the injection solution of kainate does not have to be particularly concentrated. Kainic acid, purchased from Sigma Chemical Co. (the available commercial supplier), is generally dissolved in a final concentration of 1-10 mM with gentle heating in 140 mM NaCl solution containing 25 mM sodium phosphate, pH 7.4. Accurate placement of the infusion requires stabilizing of the anesthetized animal in a stereotaxic apparatus (Fig. 3). After drilling a burr hole in the calvarium, a fine Hamilton cannula connected to a Hamilton syringe (1-5 μl) by Tygon tubing (0.4 mm o.d.) is positioned at the appropriate brain coordinates with the stereotaxic arm. It should be emphasized that published coordinates are only approximate and may deviate significantly from the correct coordinates, depending upon the size and strain of the animal. Accordingly, it is often useful to make trial injections with a dye such as India ink or dextran blue in order to establish the precise coordinates for a desired lesion. In a large animal such as the monkey, where this is not possible, the coordinates might be identified by other techniques; for example, we have mapped out the caudate, putamen and globus pallidus in the monkey by neurophysiologic methods in order to accurately place kainate lesions within these strcutures (DeLong and Coyle 1979).

The dose of kainic acid selected clearly depends upon the size of the lesion desired. Current experience indicates that a number of factors affect the extent of the lesion

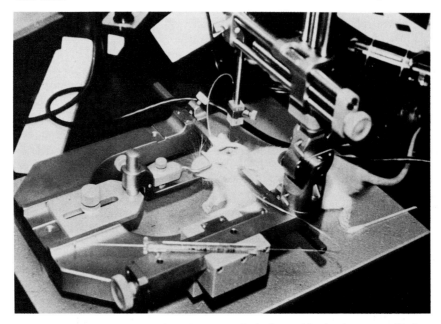

Fig. 3. Stereotaxic injection of excitotoxin. An anesthetized rat, with calvarium exposed is situated in a David Kopf small animal stereotaxic apparatus. Note the cannula attached by Tygon tubing to the Hamilton microliter syringe for ease of manipulation.

with a given dose of kainate. Because of the marked variation in neuronal sensitivity to kainic acid, particularly small doses may be effective in eliminating the neurons in some regions whereas greater doses will be required to produce comparable lesions in other regions. The limited dose-response studies have demonstrated a non-linear relationship between dose and the extent of the lesion with small increments in dose resulting in much more extensive lesions (Schwarcz and Coyle 1977a,b). Species differences, possibly even strain differences (Sanberg et al. 1979) and age (Gaddy et al. 1979) are important, yet poorly defined, variables affecting lesion size. For example, a dose of kainate which, in the rat causes a modest lesion of the striatum, produces a lesion with a 2- to 3-fold greater radius in the monkey striatum (DeLong and Coyle 1979).

Anesthetics and anticonvulsants reduce the neurotoxic action of kainic acid, presumably by interfering with excitatory neurotransmission; the degree of attenuation of neurotoxicity appears to correlate with the duration of anesthesia (Zaczek et al. 1978, 1980, 1981a). Accordingly, we have eschewed the use of the relatively long-acting anesthetics such as the combination of chloral hydrate/pentobarbital in favor of brief anesthesia with ether; this has allowed considerable reduction in the dose of kainate without remarkably affecting the size of lesions but with fewer problems with distant damage (Zaczek et al. 1980). Consequently, over the last 5 yr there has been a tendency to use progressively lower doses to accomplish kainate lesions or to use multiple small injections where extensive lesions are required; thus, the typical dose for intracerebral injection has fallen from an early level of 10 nmoles to 1-2.5 nmoles.

One must be aware that the potent excitatory effects of kainic acid can acutely disrupt neuronal function in structures contiguous to the injection site with attendant complications of morbidity and mortality. In the rat, kainic acid injections into the limbic system or structures near the limbic system precipitate a severe seizure disorder that may result in death from status epilepticus. Some investigators have recommended pretreatment of the animals with diazepam to avoid this complication (Ben-Ari et al. 1980). Midbrain lesions are often associated with a transient phase of adipsia and aphagia that can prove fatal within the first several days after the injection (Stricker et al. 1978). This complication is particularly severe and may even be incompatible with the recovery of spontaneous feeding when bilateral lesions are made. The nucleus solitarius, which regulates peripheral sympathetic tone, is exquisitely sensitive to kainic acid; thus, injections affecting this area may produce a syndrome of malignant hypertension and heart failure (Talman et al. 1979). And it is likely that other centers controlling fundamental homeostatic processes are vulnerable to kainic acid and may be responsible for morbidity and mortality associated with kainate injections into the brain stem.

To restrict the spread of the lesion, several strategies can be considered. First, the smallest dose that results in the desired lesion under optimal anesthesia conditions should be used. Secondly, the dose should be administered in the smallest manageable volume in order to reduce nonspecific pressure damage as well as reflux along the cannula track (McGeer and McGeer 1978). In the same vein, the infusion should be made slowly — at least over 2 min; and, in some cases, infusions over 30 min have been performed. After a delay, the cannula is then removed with mild backpressure to prevent leakage along the cannula track. Recently, some investigators have reported success in restricting the lesion by the iontophoretic expression of kainic acid from cannulas.

The neurotoxic effects of kainic acid appear to be remarkably rapid in onset. Profound alterations in glucose metabolism and high energy phosphate levels have been noted in lesioned areas by 30 min after injection (Retz and Coyle 1982); and electrophysiologic studies indicate that the affected neurons cease firing within 10 min of an injection (DeLong and Coyle 1979; and unpublished). Severe cytologic alterations, particularly of the dendrites, are also apparent quite early (Olney et al. 1979) although the actual degeneration of the neurons takes place more slowly over 48-72 h (Coyle et al. 1978). For these reasons, it is unlikely that the acute behavioral manifestations of the kainate lesion reflect excessive activity of the affected neurons since they are irreversibly damaged within minutes of the injection; more likely, these acute behavioral alterations represent the profound activation of adjacent neuronal systems as subtoxic levels of kainic acid diffuse beyond the lesion site.

5. IBOTENIC ACID

5.1. CHARACTERISTICS

Historically, the isoxazole ibotenic acid, extracted from the mushroom *Amanita muscaria* (Good et al. 1965; Eugster and Takemoto 1967), was the first in a long list of naturally occurring heterocyclic amino acids whose neuroexcitatory properties were recognized (Johnston et al. 1968). Although ibotenic acid contains only one carboxyl group in its molecular structure (Fig. 1), its hydroxyl group apparently renders it sufficiently acidic to act as a potent excitant. Decarboxylation to muscimol, a powerful GABA-agonist, may in part account for reports on the inhibitory qualities of ibotenate (MacDonald and Nistri 1978; Curtis et al. 1979). However, such loss of CO_2 has as yet not been shown to occur enzymatically under physiological conditions (as its occurs, by the action of glutamate decarboxylase, in the analogous pair glutamate-GABA). On the other hand, ibotenate is known to be both thermolabile and photosensitive and decomposition may take place in a non-enzymatic fashion.

In neurophysiological terms, ibotenate has been categorized as an agonist at the 'N-methyl-D-aspartate' receptor (McLennan and Lodge 1979; Watkins and Evans 1981). Classification of these sites has been greatly facilitated by the development of receptor-specific antagonists such as D-α-aminoadipic acid or α-amino-ω-phosphono carboxylic acids (Biscoe et al. 1977; Stone et al. 1981). However, because of the lability of ibotenate and its complicated chemical synthesis, [^{3}H]ibotenic acid has as yet not become available and binding studies with labeled N-methyl-D-aspartate have so far been unsuccessful. Pharmacologically valuable ligand binding experiments may therefore have to await the advent of labelled antagonists of high specific activity. While it can be anticipated that the pronounced differences between receptor sites recognizing kainic and ibotenic acid (Schwarcz and Fuxe 1979; London and Coyle 1979; Coyle et al. 1981) would be confirmed and extended by such studies, they may also be instrumental in further delineating the relationship, at the receptor level, between glutamate and ibotenate (Foster and Roberts 1978).

The neurotoxic properties of ibotenate after intracerebral injection were first identified in the course of structure-activity experiments conducted to analyze the molecular mechanisms surrounding the toxic events which are triggered by the local application of kainate (Schwarcz et al. 1978). Lesions caused by ibotenate are of the axon-sparing type common to all excitotoxins and may therefore be mediated through specific receptors (see above) localized on the dendrosomatic parts of vulnerable neurons (Schwarcz et al. 1979a). Esterification of the single carboxyl group renders the isoxazole nontoxic upon intracerebral application (Schwarcz and Eugster, unpublished). Mechanistic in vivo and in vitro and morphological analyses indicate that ibotenate microinjections are of particular interest from both theoretical and practical viewpoints.

5.2. MECHANISM OF NEUROTOXICITY

While electrophysiological data indicate a good quantitative correlation between the excitatory and toxic properties of ibotenic and thus support the excitotoxic concept, there can be little doubt that there exist fundamental differences at, but possibly not beyond (Retz and Coyle 1982), the receptor level between kainate and ibotenate. The neurotoxic effects of ibotenate appear to be more direct than those of kainate. In contrast to the latter, ibotenate-toxicity does not seem to be attenuated by prior deafferentation of the injected brain region. Thus, in the hippocampal paradigm, transection of either perforant path (Köhler et al. 1979a) or fornix-fimbria (Schwarcz and Köhler 1980) has no influence on the ibotenate-induced degeneration of granule cells in the area dentata. It remains to be seen if ibotenate 'receptors' — in the hippocampus and throughout the brain — are localized exclusively on neuronal perikarya and dendrites and if they are identical with or resemble a subpopulation of glutamate receptors. Unlabeled ibotenate, unlike kainate, potently displaces [^{3}H]glutamate from brain membranes (Foster and Roberts 1978) and a close relationship between the two sites, possibly mediating neurotoxic effects, has been postulated. In other words, ibotenate (but not kainate) may mimic the actions of a postsynaptically acting endogenous excitatory amino acid (maybe glutamate), an overactivity of which might be responsible for axon-sparing neurodegenerative disorders (Schwarcz et al. 1979b).

One of the most prominent differences between ibotenate and kainate regards their epileptogenicity. Ibotenate does not reliably cause electroencephalographic seizures at intracerebral doses < 3 μg, i.e. it is at least 1000 times weaker a convulsant than kainate (Aldinio et al. 1981). Although the threshold doses for neurotoxic and convulsant effects of ibotenate are quite close to each other, it is of theoretical significance that the drug can cause neuronal degeneration without concomitant seizure activity. The reason for such drastic differences in the convulsive properties among excitotoxins is unclear at present but appears to be unrelated to the receptors per se since N-methyl-D-aspartate, apparently acting at the same sites as ibotenate, has been demonstrated to possess powerful epileptogenic qualities (Zaczek et al. 1981b). Thus, convulsions elicited by some excitotoxins constitute an additional complicating feature. The molecular mechanism surrounding such seizures appears to be quite separate from the axon-sparing characteristics of kainate, ibotenate and congeners.

Another interesting peculiarity of ibotenate is its pronounced effect on the developing central nervous system. Unlike kainate, which is devoid of neurodegenerative properties when applied intracerebrally during the early stages in ontogeny (Campochiaro and Coyle 1978), ibotenate causes extensive lesions when injected into rat pup striatum or hippocampus (Köhler and Schwarcz 1981). While the reasons for this discrepancy between the two excitotoxins remain to be scrutinized in more detail and extended to related amino acids, ibotenate lesions during early postnatal period may become of considerable interest for practical purposes.

5.3. PRACTICAL CONSIDERATIONS

When applied stereotaxically into the rodent brain, ibotenate causes specific neuronal lesions which are quite different from those resulting from a kainate injection (Schwarcz et al. 1979a; Garey and Hornung 1980; Guldin and Markowitsch 1981). Neuronal degeneration is spherically circumscribed and can easily be limited in size by reduction of dose and/or injection volume (as a rule of thumb, ibotenate is approximately 5- to 20-fold less potent than kainate upon intracerebral injection). Moreover, neither hemorrhagic necrosis nor neuronal degeneration distant from the site of primary application has been observed; and species differences may be less pronounced than for kainate lesions (Fisher et al. 1982). It is also evident that the pronounced variation in neuronal vulnerability to kainate within and between brain regions is greatly reduced (although present in some instances) for ibotenate. Thus, hippocampal granule cells are the least kainate-susceptible neurons in the limbic system but degenerate readily after exposure to ibotenate (Köhler et al. 1979b). Similarly, cells in the medial septum can be selectively ablated by ibotenate but are resistant even to high doses (1 μg) of kainate. However, there exist neuronal populations in the brain which are not affected by ibotenate, e.g. the unipolar cells of the mesencephalic trigeminal nucleus and the arcuate nucleus of the hypothalamus (Köhler and Schwarcz, submitted). Also, as for kainate, injections of ibotenate into hindbrain nuclei, probably due to leakage of the toxin to respiratory centers of the brain, frequently lead to death of the animal in the acute phase (sometimes within minutes).

The greatest advantage of ibotenate lies in the production of restricted, perikaryal specific lesions. This selectivity is of obvious importance for neuroanatomical and functional studies and has already been successfully applied for investigations of such structures as the substantia nigra, locus ceruleus and globus pallidus (Schwarcz et al. 1979a; Johnston et al. 1981). For practical purposes, it is advisable to keep the injection volume < 0.5 μl if small lesions are desired. The amount of ibotenate used for small lesions may vary from 2-10 μg.

The optimal stereotaxic procedure for ibotenate lesions is identical to that described above for kainate. Ibotenic acid, extracted from the mushrooms *Amanita muscaria* or *Amanita pantherina* or synthesized de novo, can now be purchased from commercial suppliers (Biosearch, CA, or Regis Chemical Co., IL). Although the drug is not inexpensive (10 mg cost approximately $60.00), solutions can be made up at physiological pH and subsequently stored at −20°C without appreciable loss of neurotoxic properties. Repeated freezing and thawing is therefore acceptable if precautions are taken to avoid exposure to light and temperature > 5°C. Ibotenic acid is soluble in physiological buffers (pH 7.4) at concentrations usually required for successful intracerebral application. However, continued mixing for 5-10 min is necessary to dissolve the drug completely. Alternatively, the powder can be rapidly dissolved in microliter amounts of 2 N NaOH, and the desired volume of buffer added subsequently.

While a dependency of the evolution or extent of the lesion on the anesthetic used has as yet not been reported for ibotenate, the typical sleep pattern of injected animals in the acute postinjection phase should be noted. It was this particular narcosis-potentiating property of ibotenate that had originally led to its isolation and identification (see, Eugster 1968). Animals injected with ibotenate may sleep for long periods of time (up to 8 h) even when only low doses (5 μg) of the drug are applied. Ibotenate-induced sedation is characterized by loss of reflexes after the effects of the anesthetic subside. Analgesia, on the other hand, is not very pronounced. This particular state of consciousness may well be due to the presence of ibotenate metabolites, such as muscimol, in brain and will have to be taken into account in acute behavioral experiments using ibotenate. While this property of ibotenic acid thus constitutes an obvious drawback for such research, behavioral assessment of ibotenate-lesioned animals appears to be feasible after the first 24 postoperative hours. Unlike kainate, ibotenate does not appear to cause adipsia and aphagia even when applied in large doses and chronically lesioned animals display a virtually normal array of spontaneous behaviors.

6. CHARACTERIZATION OF THE LESION

When excitotoxins are injected into a previously uncharacterized brain region or in a different species, it is essential to determine the specificity of the lesion. The three principal concerns are that the toxin kills the neuronal cell bodies of interest, that it does not damage critical axons of passage, and that subsequent alterations in behavior or neurochemistry do not result from damage distant to the site of injection. At the very least, Nissl-stained sections through the lesion site, prepared within a week of injection, should be scrupulously examined to identify the location and extent of the lesion. Adjacent structures should be scrutinized to determine whether neurons distant from the primary site of injection are affected. Since it is more difficult to detect the absence of neurons than the presence of abnormal staining characteristics, the use of ammonical silver stains such as the Fink-Heimer technique within 2-5 days after injection may highlight sets of neurons that degenerate distant from the site of the injection (Fig. 4). This technique can also be useful in visualizing the axon terminals of the affected afferents from the lesion site (Zaczek et al. 1980).

The demonstration of the axon-sparing effects of the lesion may be more problematic; however, preservation of myelinated tracts through the lesion site and their lack of involvement in the subsequent gliotic reaction can be considered as suggestive

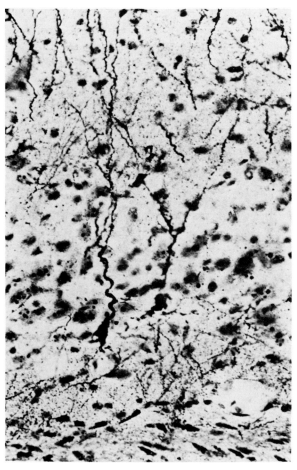

Fig. 4. Fink-Heimer stained kainate-induced degenerating neurons. The section was obtained through the dentate gyrus 24 h after intrastriatal injection of 4.6 nmoles of kainic acid in the rat. Note the 2 impregnated degenerating pyramidal cells from the CA_4 region.

evidence. Additional studies might include retrograde transport labeling techniques (Divac et al. 1978), electron-microscopy and immunocytochemistry or histochemistry (Coyle et al. 1978). Neurochemical analysis of presynaptic markers associated with axons passing through or terminating in the area have also proved useful in determining the specificity of the lesion.

7. EVOLUTION OF THE LESION

In evaluating the effects of the excitotoxin lesion, one must keep in mind the evolving nature of the lesion, which affects interpretations of histologic, neurochemical or behavioral alterations (Fig. 5). As noted above, neuronal cell death at the site of the injection occurs quite rapidly although the subsequent process of dissolution and clearance of neuronal constituents takes place much more gradually. Combined neurochemical and histologic analyses indicate that 2-3 days are required for the acute

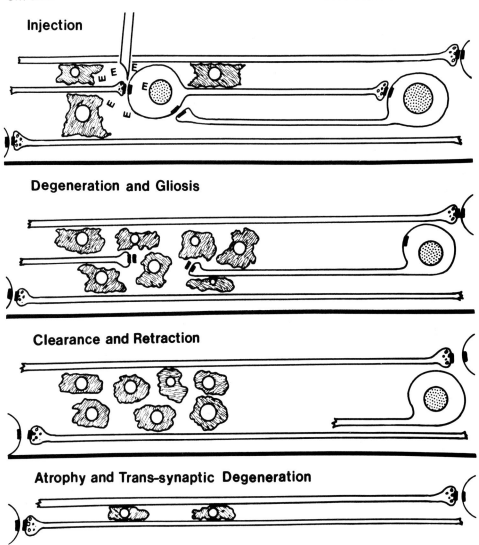

Fig. 5. Schematic representation of the evolution of excitotoxin lesion.

degenerative process associated with the complete disruption of the affected neurons as well as maximal reduction in presynaptic markers associated with them, such as neurotransmitter synthetic enzymes, uptake processes or neurotransmitters themselves (Schwarcz and Coyle 1977; Coyle et al. 1978). Those constituents that require a high level of cellular integrity, such as dopamine-sensitive adenylate cyclase in the striatum, may decrease quite rapidly. Other elements, which seem less dependent on cellular integrity such as neurotransmitter receptor-ligand binding sites may be cleared much more slowly from the lesion site (Herndon et al. 1980).

An important cellular concomitant of the lesion is the proliferation of, or invasion by, reactive astrocytes that phagocytize the degenerated remnants of the neurons. The gliotic reaction appears within a few days of the lesion and becomes particularly prominent over the subsequent weeks, gradually resolving thereafter (Coyle et al. 1978). It should be noted that this gliotic reaction markedly alters the metabolic and neurochemical characteristics of the lesion site as markers associated with these cells increase dramatically (Minneman et al. 1978). Of course, death of neurons with perikarya within the confines of the lesions is associated with degeneration of their axons to projection areas. This response is accompanied not only by a decrease in the presynaptic markers associated with the axonal terminals but also, in some cases, a gliotic reaction along their fiber tracts (Zaczek et al. 1980).

At the very initial stages after the lesion, the weight of the affected area does not change significantly although cellular edema occurs as demonstrated by a reduction in the amount of protein per mg of tissue wet weight. With the loss of neurons and their associated neuropil, the lesion site undergoes progressive atrophy, resulting in alterations in neuroanatomic relationships as the spared axons and the surrounding surviving neurons collapse upon the lesion (Zaczek et al. 1978). Loss of postsynaptic neurons within the lesion results in retraction or, at least, a rearrangement of surviving afferents (Nadler et al. 1980). Krammer (1980) has provided evidence of a more gradual transsynaptic degeneration that occurs in response to loss of efferents from the lesioned area. Thus, in evaluating the effects of an excitotoxic lesion, one must keep in mind the phase in its evolution.

8. SUMMARY

Subcutaneous administration of glutamate to infant rodents has become a useful method for investigating hypothalamic neurons, whether for identifying the arcuate synaptic chemistry or for characterizing regulation of the brain-pituitary-gonadal axis. Both ablation and provocative approaches have been successfully employed for these purposes. Intracerebral microinjection of kainate has been used widely to produce perikaryal specific lesions. Along with the well-described advantages of kainate lesions, certain drawbacks have been uncovered. Of these, variation of neuronal vulnerability between and within brain regions is the most prominent one, leading to uneven lesions and often resulting in neuronal loss distant from the primary site of injection. However, depending upon an investigator's interest, this limitation may be turned to an advantage for specific purposes. Thus, the lower vulnerability of the large neurons in the striatum bears striking parallels to the pathology of Huntington's disease (Coyle and Schwarcz 1976) and the unusual sensitivity of certain limbic neurons (Nadler et al. 1978) to kainate has proved a useful model system for studying temporal lobe epilepsy in the rat. Ibotenate now appears to be the excitotoxin of choice when discrete and circumscribed perikaryal selective lesions at the injection site are required. Ibotenate's particular properties, which may be in part due to a different mechanism of action than kainate, will have to be analyzed further before broad use as a neurotoxin can be recommended.

9. REFERENCES

Aldinio C, French ED, Schwarcz R (1981): Seizures and neuronal degeneration: Relationships investigated by intrahippocampal kainic and ibotenic acid. *Soc. Neurosci. Abstr., 7,* 589.
Bakke JL, Lawrence N, Bennett J, Robinson S, Bowers CY (1978): Late endocrine effects of administering monosodium glutamate to neonatal rats. *Neuroendocrinology, 26,* 220–228.
Ben-Ari Y, Tremblay E, Ottersen OP (1980): Injections of kainic acid into the amygdaloid complex of the

rat: An electrographic, clinical and histologic study in relation to the pathology of epilepsy. *Neuroscience, 5,* 515–528.

Bird S, Gulley RL (1979): Evidence against a presynaptic mechanism for kainate neurotoxicity in the cochlear nucleus. *Neurosci. Lett., 15,* 55–60.

Biscoe TJ, Evans RH, Headley PM, Martin MR, Watkins JC (1976): Structure-activity relations of excitatory amino acids on frog and rat spinal neurons. *Br. J. Pharmacol., 58,* 373–382.

Biscoe TJ, Evans RH, Francis AA, Martin MR, Watkins JC (1977): D-α-Aminoadipate as a selective antagonist of amino acid-induced and synaptic excitation of mammalian spinal neurons. *Nature, 270,* 743–745.

Biziere K, Coyle JT (1978a): Influence of cortico-striatal afferents on striatal kainic acid neurotoxicity. *Neurosci. Lett., 8,* 303–310.

Biziere K, Coyle JT (1978b): Effects of kainic acid on ion distribution and ATP levels of striatal slices incubated in vitro. *J. Neurochem., 31,* 513–520.

Biziere K, Coyle JT (1979): Effects of cortical ablation on the neurotoxicity and receptor binding of kainic acid in striatum. *J. Neurosci. Res., 4,* 383–398.

Bodnar RJ, Abrams GM, Zimmermann EA, Krieger DT, Nicholson G, Kizer JS (1980): Neonatal monosodium glutamate: Effects upon analgesic responsivity and immunocytochemical ACTH/β-lipotropin. *Neuroendocrinology, 30,* 280–284.

Campochiaro P, Coyle JT (1978): Ontogenetic development of kainate neurotoxicity: Correlates with glutamatergic innervation. *Proc. Nat. Acad. Sci. USA, 75,* 2025–2029.

Colonnier M, Geriade M, Landry P (1979): Selective resistance of sensory cells of the mesencephalic trigeminal nucleus to kainic acid-induced lesions. *Brain Res., 172,* 522–556.

Coyle JT, Schwarcz R (1976): Lesion of striatal neurones with kainic acid provides a model for Huntington's chorea. *Nature, 263,* 244–246.

Coyle JT, Molliver ME, Kuhar MJ (1978): Morphologic analysis of kainic acid lesion of the rat striatum. *J. Comp. Neurol., 180,* 301–324.

Coyle JT, Zaczek R, Slevin J, Collins J (1981): Neuronal receptor sites for kainic acid: Correlations with neurotoxicity. In: Di Chiara G, Gessa GL (Eds), *Glutamate as a Neurotransmitter,* pp. 337–346. Raven Press, New York.

Curtis DR, Johnston GAR (1974): Amino acid transmitters in the mammalian central nervous system. *Ergeb. Physiol. Biol. Chem. Exp. Pharmakol., 69,* 97–188.

Curtis DR, Watkins JC (1960): The excitation and depression of spinal neurones by structurally related amino acids. *J. Neurochem., 6,* 117–141.

Curtis DR, Lodge D, McLennan H (1979): The excitation and depression of spinal neurones by ibotenic acid. *J. Physiol., 291,* 19–28.

DeLong M, Coyle JT (1979): Globus pallidus lesions in monkey produced by kainic acid: Histologic and behavioral effects. *Appl. Neurophysiol., 42,* 95–97.

Dhindsa KS, Omran RG, Bhup R (1981): Histological changes in the thyroid gland induced by monosodium glutamate in mice. *Acta Anat., 109,* 97–102.

Divac I, Markowitsch HJ, Pritzel M (1978): Behavioral and anatomical consequences of small intrastriatal injections of kainic acid in the rat. *Brain Res., 151,* 523–532.

Eskay RL, Brownstein MJ, Long RT (1979): α-Melanocyte-stimulating hormone: Reduction in adult rat brain after monosodium glutamate treatment of neonates. *Science, 205,* 827–829.

Eugster CH (1968): Wirkstoffe aus dem Fliegenpilz. *Naturwissenschaften, 55,* 305–313.

Eugster CH, Takemoto T (1967): Zur Nomenklatur der neuen Verbindungen aus Amanita-Arten. *Helv. Chim. Acta, 50,* 126–127.

Fisher SK, Frey KA, Agranoff BW (1982): Loss of muscarinic receptors and of stimulated phospholipid labelling in ibotenate-treated hippocampus. *J. Neurosci.,* in press.

Foster AC, Roberts PJ (1978): High-affinity L-^{3}H-glutamate binding to postsynaptic receptor sites on rat cerebellar synaptic membranes. *J. Neurochem., 31,* 1467–1477.

Foster AC, Mena EE, Monaghan DT, Cotman CW (1981): Synaptic localization of kainic acid binding sites. *Nature, 289,* 73–75.

Gaddy JR, Britt MD, Neill DB, Haugler HJ (1979): Susceptibility of rat neostriatum to damage by kainic acid: Age dependence. *Brain Res., 176,* 192–196.

Garey LJ, Hornung JP (1980): The use of ibotenic acid lesions for light- and electron-microscopic study of anterograde degeneration in the visual pathway of the cat. *Neurosci. Lett., 19,* 117–123.

Good R, Muller GFR, Eugster CH (1965): Isolierung und Charakterisierung von Pramuscimol und Muscazon aus Amanita muscaria. *Helv. Chim. Acta, 48,* 927–930.

Guldin WO, Markowitsch HJ (1981): No detectable remote lesions following massive intrastriatal injections of ibotenic acid. *Brain Res., 225,* 446–451.

Herndon RM, Addicks E, Coyle JT (1980): Ultrastructural analysis of kainic acid lesion to the cerebellar cortex. *Neuroscience, 5,* 1015–1026.

Holzwarth-McBride MA, Hurst EM, Knigge KM (1976): Monosodium glutamate induced lesions of the arcuate nucleus. I. Endocrine deficiency and ultrastructure of the median eminence. *Anat. Rec., 186,* 185–196.

Johnston GAR, Curtis DR, De Groat WC, Duggan AW (1968): Central actions of ibotenic acid and muscimol. *Biochem. Pharmacol., 17,* 2488–2489.

Johnston MV, McKinney M, Coyle JT (1981): Neocortical cholinergic innervation: A description of extrinsic and intrinsic components in the rat. *Exp. Brain Res., 43,* 159–172.

Köhler C, Schwarcz R (1981): Kainic and ibotenic acid neurotoxicity: Methodological and mechanistic considerations In: *Abstracts, 8th Meeting of the International Society of Neurochemistry,* pp. 272.

Köhler C, Schwarcz R, Fuxe K (1979a): Hippocampal lesions indicate differences between the excitotoxic properties of acidic amino acids. *Brain Res., 175,* 366–371.

Köhler C, Schwarcz R, Fuxe K (1979b): Intrahippocampal injections of ibotenic acid provide histological evidence for a neurotoxic mechanism different from kainic acid. *Neurosci. Lett., 15,* 223–228.

Krammer EB (1980): Anterograde and transsynaptic degeneration 'en cascade' in basal ganglia induced by intrastriatal injection of kainic acid: An animal analogue of Huntington's disease. *Brain Res., 196,* 209–221.

Krieger DT, Liotta AC, Nicholson G, Kizer JS (1979): Brain ACTH and endorphin reduced in rats with monosodium glutamate-induced arcuate nucleus lesions. *Nature, 278,* 562–563.

London ED, Coyle JT (1979): Specific binding of [^{3}H]kainic acid to receptor sites in rat brain. *Mol. Pharmacol., 15,* 492–505.

Lucas DR, Newhouse JP (1957): The toxic effect of sodium L-glutamate on the inner layers of the retina. *Arch. Ophthalmol., 58,* 193–204.

Lund-Karlsen R, Fonnum F (1976): The toxic effect of sodium glutamate on rat retina: Changes in putative transmitters and their corresponding enzymes. *J. Neurochem., 27,* 1437–1441.

MacDonald JF, Nistri A (1978): A comparison of the action of glutamate, ibotenate and other related amino acids on feline spinal interneurones. *J. Physiol. (London), 275,* 449–465.

Mason S, Fibiger HC (1979): On the specificity of kainic acid. *Science, 204,* 1339–1341.

McGeer EG, McGeer PL (1978): Some factors influencing the neurotoxicity of intrastriatal injections of kainic acid. *Neurochem. Res., 3,* 501–517.

McGeer EG, McGeer PL, Singh K (1978): Kainate-induced degeneration of neostriatal neurons dependency on corticostriatal tract. *Brain Res., 139,* 381–383.

McLennan H (1980): The effect of decortication on the excitatory amino acid sensitivity of striatal neurons. *Neurosci. Lett., 18,* 313–316.

McLennan H (1981): On the nature of the receptors for various excitatory amino acids in the mammalian central nervous system. In: Di Chiara G, Gessa GL (Eds), *Glutamate as a Neurotransmitter,* pp. 253–262. Raven Press, New York.

McLennan H, Lodge D (1979): The antagonism of amino acid-induced excitation of spinal neurones in the cat. *Brain Res., 169,* 83–90.

Minneman KP, Quick M, Emson P (1978): Receptor-linked cyclic-AMP systems in rat neostriatum: Differential localization revealed by kainic acid injection. *Brain Res., 151,* 507–521.

Nadler JV, Cuthbertson GJ (1980): Kainic acid neurotoxicity toward hippocampal formation: Dependence on specific excitatory pathways. *Brain Res., 195,* 47–56.

Nadler JV, Perry BW, Cotman CW (1978): Intraventricular kainic acid preferentially destroys hippocampal pyramid cells. *Nature, 271,* 676–677.

Nadler JV, Perry BW, Gentry C, Cotman CW (1980): Fate of the hippocampal mossy fiber projection after destruction of its postsynaptic targets with intraventricular kainic acid. *J. Comp. Neurol., 196,* 549–569.

Nagasawa H, Yanai R, Kikuyama S (1974): Irreversible inhibition of pituitary prolactin and growth hormone secretion and of mammary gland development in mice by monosodium glutamate administered neonatally. *Acta Endocrinol., 75,* 249–259.

Nelson M, Zaczek R, Coyle JT (1980): Effects of sustained seizures produced by intrahippocampal injection of kainic acid on noradrenergic neurons: Evidence for local control of norepinephrine release. *J. Pharmacol. Exp. Ther., 214,* 694–702.

Nemeroff CB (1981): Monosodium glutamate-induced neurotoxicity: Review of the literature and call for further research. In: Miller SA (Ed), *Nutrition and Behavior,* pp. 177–211. Franklin Institute Press, Philadelphia.

Nemeroff CB, Grant LD, Bissette G, Ervin GN, Harrell LE, Prange Jr AJ (1977a): Growth, endocrinological and behavioral deficits after monosodium L-glutamate in the neonatal rat: Possible involvement of arcuate dopamine neuron damage. *Psychoneuroendocrinology, 2,* 179–196.

Nemeroff CB, Konkol RJ, Bissette G, Youngblood W, Martin JB, Brazeau P, Rone MS, Prange Jr AJ, Breese GR, Kizer JS (1979b): Analysis of the disruption in hypothalamic-pituitary regulation in rats treated neonatally with monosodium L-glutamate (MSG): Evidence for the involvement of tuberoinfundibular cholinergic and dopaminergic systems in neuroendocrine regulation. *Endocrinology, 101,* 613–622.

Olney JW (1969a): Brain lesions, obesity and other disturbances in mice treated with monosodium glutamate. *Science, 164,* 719–721.

Olney JW (1969b): Glutamate-induced retinal degeneration in neonatal mice. Electron-microscopy of the acutely evolving lesion. *J. Neuropathol. Exp. Neurol., 28,* 455–474.

Olney JW (1971): Glutamate-induced neuronal necrosis in the infant mouse hypothalamus. An electron-microscopic study. *J. Neuropathol. Exp. Neurol., 30,* 75–90.

Olney JW (1974): Toxic effects of glutamate and related amino acids on the developing central nervous system. In: Nyhan WL (Ed), *Heritable Disorders of Amino Acid Metabolism,* pp. 501–512. John Wiley and Sons, New York.

Olney JW (1979): Excitotoxic amino acids: Research applications and safety implications. In: Filer Jr LJ, Garattini S, Kare MR, Reynolds WA, Wurtman RJ (Eds), *Glutamic Acid: Advances in Biochemistry and Physiology,* pp. 287–319. Raven Press, New York.

Olney JW, De Gubareff T (1978): Glutamate neurotoxicity and Huntington's chorea. *Nature, 271,* 557–559.

Olney JW, Ho OL, Rhee V (1971): Cytotoxic effects of acidic and sulphur containing amino acids on the infant mouse central nervous system. *Exp. Brain Res., 14,* 61–76.

Olney JW, Rhee V, Ho OL (1974): Kainic acid: A powerful neurotoxic analogue of glutamate. *Brain Res., 77,* 507–512.

Olney JW, Cicero TJ, Meyer ER, De Gubareff T (1976): Acute glutamate induced elevations in serum testosterone and luteinizing hormone. *Brain Res., 112,* 420–424.

Olney JW, Fuller T, De Garbreff T (1979): Acute dendrotoxic changes in the hippocampus of kainate treated rats. *Brain Res., 176,* 91–100.

Pizzi WJ, Barnhart JE, Fanslow DJ (1977): Monosodium glutamate administration to the newborn reduces reproductive ability in female and male mice. *Science, 196,* 452–454.

Rascher K (1981): Monosodium glutamate-induced lesions in the rat cingulate cortex. *Cell Tissue Res., 220,* 239–250.

Redding TW, Schally AV, Arimura A, Wakabayashi I (1971): Effect of monosodium glutamate on some endocrine functions. *Neuroendocrinology, 8,* 245–255.

Retz KC, Coyle JT (1982): Effects of kainic acid on high-energy metabolites in the mouse. *J. Neurochem., 38,* 196–203.

Sanberg PR, Pisa M, McGeer E (1979): Strain differences and kainic acid neurotoxicity. *Brain Res., 166,* 431–435.

Schwarcz R, Coyle JT (1977a): Striatal lesions with kainic acid: Neurochemical characteristics. *Brain Res., 127,* 235–249.

Schwarcz R, Coyle JT (1977b): Kainic acid: Neurotoxic effects after intraocular injection. *Invest. Ophthalmol., 16,* 141–148.

Schwarcz R, Fuxe K (1979): [³H]Kainic acid binding: Relevance for evaluating the neurotoxicity of kainic acid. *Life Sci., 24,* 1471–1480.

Schwarcz R, Köhler C (1980): Evidence against an exclusive role of glutamate in kainic acid neurotoxicity. *Neurosci. Lett., 19,* 243–249.

Schwarcz R, Scholz D, Coyle JT (1978a): Structure-activity relations for the neurotoxicity of kainic acid derivatives and glutamate analogues. *Neuropharmacology, 17,* 145–151.

Schwarcz R, Zaczek R, Coyle JT (1978b): Microinjection of kainic acid into the rat hippocampus. *Eur. J. Pharmacol., 50,* 209–220.

Schwarcz R, Hökfelt T, Fuxe K, Jonsson G, Goldstein M, Terenius L (1979a): Ibotenic acid-induced neuronal degeneration: A morphological and neurochemical study. *Exp. Brain Res., 37,* 199–216.

Schwarcz R, Köhler C, Fuxe K, Hökfelt T, Goldstein M (1979b): On the mechanism of selective neuronal degeneration in the rat brain: Studies with ibotenic acid. In: Chase TN, Wexler NS, Barbeau A (Eds), *Advances in Neurology, Vol. 23, Huntington's Disease,* pp. 655–668. Raven Press, New York.

Shinozaki H, Konishi S (1970): Actions of several anthelmintics and insecticides on rat cortical neurones. *Brain Res., 24,* 368–371.

Shinozaki H, Shibuya I (1974): A new potent excitant, quisqualic acid: Effects on crayfish neuromuscular junction. *Neuropharmacology, 13,* 665–672.

Stone TW, Perkins MN, Collins JF, Curry K (1981): Activity of the enantiomers of 2-amino-5-phosphonovaleric acid as stereospecific antagonists of excitatory amino acids. *Neuroscience, 6,* 2249–2252.

Street P, Stella M, Cuenod M (1980): Kainate-induced lesion in the optic tectum: Dependency upon optic nerve afferents or glutamate. *Brain Res., 187,* 47–57.

Stricker EM, Seindloff AF, Zigmond MJ (1978): Intrahypothalamic injections of kainic acid produce feeding and drinking deficits in rats. *Brain Res., 158,* 470–473.

Talman W, Perrone MH, Doba N, Reis DJ (1979): Fulminating hypertension produced by local injection of kainic acid into the nucleus tractus solitarii in the rat. *Neurosci. Abstr., 5,* 51.

Terry LC, Epelbaum J, Brazeau P, Marin JB (1977): Monosodium glutamate: Acute and chronic effects on growth hormone (GH), prolactin (Prl) and somatostatin (SRIF) in the rat. *Fed. Proc., 36,* 500.

Watkins JC, Evans RH (1981): Excitatory amino acid transmitter. *Annu. Rev. Pharmacol., 21,* 165–204.

Weindl A (1973): Neuroendocrine aspects of circumventricular organs. In: Martini L, Ganong WF (Eds), *Frontiers in Neuroendocrinology,* pp. 1–32. Oxford University Press, London.

Weurthele SM, Lovell KM, Jones MZ, Moore KE (1978): A histological study of kainic acid-induced lesions in the rat brain. *Brain Res., 147,* 489–497.

Wooten GF, Collins R (1980): Regional brain glucose utilization following intrastriatal injection of kainic acid. *Brain Res., 201,* 173–184.

Zaczek R, Coyle JT (1982): Excitatory amino acid analogues: Neurotoxicity and seizures. *Neuropharmacology, 21,* 15–16.

Zaczek R, Nelson M, Coyle JT (1978a): Effects of anaesthetics and anticonvulsants on the action of kainic acid in the rat hippocampus. *Eur. J. Pharmacol., 52,* 323–327.

Zaczek R, Schwarcz R, Coyle JT (1978b): Long-term sequelae of striatal kainate lesion. *Brain Res., 152,* 626–632.

Zaczek R, Simonton S, Coyle JT (1980): Local and distant neuronal degeneration following intrastriatal injection of kainic acid. *J. Neuropathol. Exp. Neurol., 39,* 245–264.

Zaczek R, Nelson M, Coyle JT (1981a): Kainic acid neurotoxicity and seizures. *Neuropharmacology, 20,* 183–199.

Zaczek R, Collins JF, Coyle JT (1981b): N-methyl-D-aspartic acid: A convulsant with weak neurotoxic properties. *Neurosci. Lett., 24,* 181–186.

Subject index

Prepared by R. Warren, Ph.D., Edinburgh

538

staining 218, 221
second antibody 199
sensitivity 169, 171, 184
staining intensity 200
tracer cross-reactivity 172
vasoactive intestinal polypeptide 164, 165
peroxidase double-staining
184, 185
colors 184
phenylethanolamine-N-methyl-
transferase
adrenaline neuron marker
477, 478
β-phenylethylamine 53
phenylethylamines
see also monoamines
metabolism 51
β-phenylisopropyl hydrazine
309
5′-phosphonucleotides
cytochemistry 132,
134–137
photodecomposition of
fluorophores 64
physostigmine
cholinesterase histochemistry 20–23
Pictet–Spengler cyclization
reaction 53, 55, 59, 60
pineal gland
chromaffin reaction 128,
129
uranaffin reaction 134,
138
pinealocytes 128, 129, 138
melatonin 60
monoamine fluorescence
53, 60
plastics, embedding 161, 197
platelet
amine analog accumulation
139, 140
amine storage and fixative
125–127
cancer and amine content
125–127
origins 134
reserpine effect 130, 140,
142
uranaffin reaction model
134, 135
polyethylene glycol embedding
90, 160

potassium permanganate
fixative solution 124
monoamine reaction 124
primuline
see also fluorescent tracers
characteristics 231, 233
emission and excitation
spectra 231, 233, 235
granular 253, 255
immunocytochemistry, com-
bination with 252, 257
protein binding 236
sources 270
substantia nigra fluores-
cence 253, 254
survival time 237
progestin, target cell distribu-
tion 457
proline
[³H] and acetylcholines-
terase demonstration
37–39
retrograde transport, CNS
368–381, 382
perikaryal labeling 368,
382
transmitter role 381
propidium iodide
see also fluorescent tracers
brain stem excitation and
emission spectra
243–245
characteristics 231, 233
emission and excitation
spectra 231, 233, 235
fluorescence 91
fluorescence intensity 247
immunocytochemistry, com-
bination with 252–257
monoamine cell emission
246
monoamine visualization,
combination with
243–246
problems and remedies
271
sources 270
survival time 237
propiomelanocorticotropin
152
propionylcholine hydrolysis 3
protein
carrier and nonspecific
staining 223, 224

cross-linking and immuno-
genicity 214
hapten carriers 151, 152,
190, 214
protein A
coupling and labeling 147,
148, 168
IgG binding types 191
reactivity 147
size 159
pseudo-cholinesterase 3
Purkinje cells
GABA uptake 330
retrograde GABA labeling
368, 372

quartz optics and slides 100
quisqualic acid 509
seizures 513

R5020
brain cell concentration
446, 457
radioautography
see autoradiography
radioimmunoassay 149
immunocytochemistry dis-
crepancy 149
specificity 169
radioimmunocytochemical
method 169
advantages 170
antibody dilution 201
autoradiography 170
disadvantages 172
gastrin 171
labeling 201
method 201, 202, 219
neurophysin detection 218,
222
pancreatic polypeptide 171
PAP use 171, 218, 219
principle 170
specificity 181
tracer 201
radiolabels
neuronal transport 37–40
sizes 159
raphe magnus
PAP and RICH combined
staining 218, 221
receptors
autoradiography of drug
and neurotransmitter

545

548